MECHANISMS
OF DISEASE

A TEXTBOOK OF
COMPARATIVE GENERAL PATHOLOGY

THIRD EDITION

MECHANISMS OF DISEASE

A TEXTBOOK OF
COMPARATIVE GENERAL PATHOLOGY

DAVID O. SLAUSON, DVM, PhD

Diplomate, American College of Veterinary Pathologists
Distinguished Professor of Comparative Medicine, Emeritus
Department of Pathology
University of Tennessee College of Veterinary Medicine
Knoxville, Tennessee
and
Adjunct Professor of Pathology
Department of Microbiology and Pathology
Washington State University College of Veterinary Medicine
Pullman, Washington

BARRY J. COOPER, BVSc, PhD

Diplomate, American College of Veterinary Pathologists
Professor of Pathology
Department of Biomedical Sciences
Cornell University College of Veterinary Medicine
Ithaca, New York

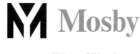

An Affiliate of Elsevier

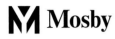

An Affiliate of Elsevier

Editorial Manager: Linda L. Duncan
Senior Developmental Editor: Teri Merchant
Project Manager: Catherine Jackson
Production Editor: Carl Masthay
Designer: Amy Buxton

THIRD EDITION
Copyright © 2002 by Mosby

Previous editions copyrighted 1982, 1990

Permissions may be sought directly from Elsevier's Health Sciences Rights Department in Philadelphia, USA: phone: (+1)215-238-7869, fax: (+1)215-238-2239, email: healthpermissions@elsevier.com. You may also complete your request on-line via the Elsevier Science homepage (http://www.elsevier.com), by selecting 'Customer Support' and then 'Obtaining Permissions'.

Mosby
An Affiliate of Elsevier
11830 Westline Industrial Drive
St. Louis, Missouri 63146

Printed in the United States of America

Library of Congress Cataloging-in-Publication Data

Slauson, David O.
    Mechanisms of disease : a textbook of comparative general pathology/
David O. Slauson, Barry J. Cooper.—3rd ed.
        p. ; cm.
    Includes bibliographical references and index.
    ISBN: 0-323-00228-5 (alk. paper)
        1. Pathology, Comparative. I. Cooper, Barry J. II. Title.
    [DNLM: 1. Pathology. 2. Pathology, Veterinary. QZ 33 S631m
2002]
RB114.S58 2002
636.089'607—dc21   2001020553

Last digit is the print number: 04 05 CL/MV 9 8 7 6 5 4 3

CONTRIBUTORS

Philip N. Bochsler, DVM, PhD
Diplomate, American College of Veterinary
  Pathologists
Associate Professor of Pathology
Department of Pathology
The University of Tennessee College of Veterinary
  Medicine
Knoxville, Tennessee

Talmage T. Brown, Jr., DVM, PhD
Diplomate and Past President, American College of
  Veterinary Pathologists
Professor of Pathology
Department of Microbiology, Pathology, and
  Parasitology
North Carolina State University School of
  Veterinary Medicine
Raleigh, North Carolina

Gary L. Cockerell, DVM, PhD
Diplomate and Past President, American College of
  Veterinary Pathologists
Investigative Toxicology
Pharmacia Corporation
Kalamazoo, Michigan

Barry J. Cooper, BVSc, PhD
Diplomate, American College of Veterinary
  Pathologists
Professor of Pathology
Department of Biomedical Sciences
Cornell University College of Veterinary Medicine
Ithaca, New York

Howard B. Gelberg, DVM, PhD
Diplomate, American College of Veterinary
  Pathologists
Professor of Pathology and Dean, College of
  Veterinary Medicine
Oregon State University
Corvallis, Oregon

David O. Slauson, DVM, PhD
Diplomate, American College of Veterinary
  Pathologists
Distinguished Professor of Comparative Medicine,
  Emeritus
Department of Pathology
University of Tennessee College of Veterinary
  Medicine
Knoxville, Tennessee
Adjunct Professor of Pathology
Department of Microbiology and Pathology
Washington State University College of Veterinary
  Medicine
Pullman, Washington

Maja M. Suter, Dr med Vet, PhD
Diplomate, American College of Veterinary
  Pathologists
Professor of Pathology
Director, Institute of Veterinary Pathology
Faculty of Veterinary Medicine
University of Bern
Bern, Switzerland

PREFACE

Our aim for this book remains to introduce students to disease concepts inherent in clinical medicine through the study of pathogenic mechanisms. It is primarily aimed at beginning students of pathology who will ultimately become clinicians. Previous editions of this book have also been considered a useful sourcebook of basic material for residents and graduate students and a compact review of disease mechanisms for persons preparing for national board examinations. We would hope that such a dual function might continue and are gratified by the enthusiasm with which the book has been received.

Pathology is a changing science, yet its roots remain exceedingly intact. Disease is still often caused by various forms of microbes and toxins, but our continuing fascination with *how* disease occurs has produced greatly increased levels of resolution and an enriched understanding of the complex mechanisms by which mammals become sick. Paralleling this increased comprehension has been an explosion of detailed information that confounds even purposeful efforts to surround and comprehend it. A partial list of newer relevant items in contemporary pathobiology includes chemokines, interleukins, cyclooxygenase, protein C, acumentin, defensins, integrins, selectins, TNF-α, perforins, prions, p53, *myc, ras,* cyclins, NADPH-oxidase, G proteins, antithrombin III, lipomodulin, PAF, *bcl*-2, PCR, RLFP, FISH, leucine zippers, and the TATA box. Is this pathology? Whatever happened to pneumonia and mastitis?

The question begs an answer, and the answer begs an explanation. Pneumonia and mastitis are still with us; our contemporary molecular brilliance has yet to be translated into truly effective therapy for many clinical situations, but the great and recurring optimism of medicine is that understanding will lead to solutions. Clinical medicine is changing because advances in the biological understanding of disease have allowed therapy to be more specific and less empirical. We always knew that pneumonia and mastitis could be caused by bacteria; Koch's postulates told us so. The real story, however, was not the bacteria themselves but their molecular products and the influence of those products on host tissues and defense mechanisms. We have long known that genetics was important in disease pathogenesis, but even so we have likely underestimated its contribution. Now we are beginning to

understand disease at increasingly molecular levels of detail, and we must rethink many of the old explanations regarding pathogenesis; they were not incorrect but simply inadequate.

Disciplinary lines have become blurred. Contemporary pathology is a blend of the disease-oriented aspects of what used to be the intellectual provinces of such diverse disciplines as immunology, cell biology, biochemistry, internal medicine, and physiology. Does this mean that pathology has lost its identity as a discipline? Not at all. Pathologists have both contributed to and profited from the advances in all these various areas of science. This blending of disciplines has produced much progress and a few problems for the authors of textbooks. One relates to organization. Shall we discuss the activation of the complement system under inflammation, in which complement activation is clearly of importance, or as part of the immunopathogenesis of the hypersensitivities? We have had to do some blending and to make some arbitrary decisions in such matters.

A second problem relates to deciding what level of detail is appropriate for contemporary students. We continue to believe that modern students require sophisticated explanations of disease mechanisms to best equip them for the future but simultaneously recognize the curricular limitations of time and the obstacles to learning created by information overload. Teachers must act as guides and provide appropriate road maps. Students have neither the time nor the inclination for resplendent exercises in scientific trivial pursuit, nor do we. The reading lists at the end of each chapter are not comprehensive but should provide motivated veterinary students and candidates for pathology boards with a more comprehensive entry to the considerable literature of contemporary pathobiology.

The role of the teacher of pathology has also changed. We recognize that it is clearly no longer sufficient to merely relate the traditional stories of disease at a simplistic level, but good judgment must prevail in selecting the borders that define an appropriate level of detail. We must be prepared to filter and summarize the abundant literature to present a contemporary picture of disease that avoids the hazards of inadvertent drowning in informational minutiae. We need to be continually aware of the leaps and bounds by which medical science advances and to remind ourselves from time to time that much of what we teach today may be obsolete within the professional lifetime of our students. We must therefore abandon any sentimental attachments to the so-called cult of coverage and continue actively to stress the importance of lifelong learning. To achieve these important goals for the new millennium means we must hope to convey a sense of the excitement of discovery and the pleasure of independent thinking that comes with successful problem solving. We must help our students to understand that the "pathobiology of disease" is exciting largely because the "biology of health" is so complicated and inspiring. The conflict for contemporary pathology lies not in whether the study of lesions is still appropriate but in how best to present lesions in the modern light of what we now know about how those lesions came to be. We must make the lesions come to life.

> "Bitzer," said Thomas Gradgrind, "your definition of a horse."
>
> "Quadruped. Gramnivorous. Forty teeth, namely twenty-four grinders, four eye-teeth, and twelve incisive. Sheds coat in the spring; in marsh countries sheds hoofs too. Hoofs hard, but requiring to be shod with iron. Age known by marks in mouth." Thus (and much more) Bitzer.
>
> "Now. . . ," said Mr. Gradgrind, "you know what a horse is."
>
> CHARLES DICKENS, Hard Times

If we approach the teaching of pathology the way Mr. Gradgrind approached the defining of *Equus caballus*, our students will respond similarly, and all of the fascinating biology of the diseased state will be reduced to a list of lesions that might be used to merely define, say, infectious bovine rhinotracheitis. But Thomas Gradgrind was wrong, and Bitzer's definition of a horse came from a dictionary. It classified a horse, but it did not capture the inherent excitement of the beast. No racing fan ever bet on a "gramnivorous quadruped," no jockey ever rode one, and no artist ever painted one. One of the greatest contemporary challenges for teachers of pathology is to capture for our students the excitement of disease mechanisms as they might occur in the living and breathing patient.

An additional challenge can be illustrated by even a quick trip to the library. The constant and unending flow of published observations germane to the study of disease mechanisms has become cumbersome to the point of being almost unmanageable, and all of us have had to become innovative in facing the dilemma of keeping up with it. We are pleased to recognize in this regard that "none of us is as smart as all of us," and welcome several new contributers to this third edition. All these distinguished pathologists are also experienced and dedicated teachers. We believe that their classroom experience is important.

A major goal for this third edition has been to contemporize the information presented to reflect current knowledge about disease mechanisms without a major expansion in text volume. To accomplish this required a substantial massage of much of the text material. We have occasionally had to be ruthless about what was included and what was left behind; what we have chosen to present reflects our best collective wisdom regarding the needs of contemporary students, and we assume full responsibility for our decisions.

Lastly, we have made a substantial effort here to present a contemporary synopsis of disease pathogenesis in a palatable and readable way and continue to believe that no more exciting blend of science can be found than what is aimed at an understanding of disease.

David O. Slauson
Barry J. Cooper

ACKNOWLEDGMENTS

It is a pleasure to be able to record a measure of genuine thanks to the many individuals who have directly or indirectly contributed to the completion of this book. Our wives have been generous in their support and understanding of the additional work load associated with the completion of this task and have grown accustomed to our carrying home large piles of paper and hovering over the word processor at night. We also are greatly indebted to our very busy colleagues who agreed to serve as chapter authors; we believe the quality of their contributions is consistently high, showing once again that "if you want the job done right, give it to a busy person."

Several other colleagues have again been kind enough to read significant portions of the manuscript and to share important micrographs with us, and we are grateful for their active interest and involvement. One of the senior authors (DOS) wishes to extend special thanks to Drs. Fairfield Bain and Doug Byars of Hagyard-Davidson-McGee, P.S.C., Lexington, Kentucky, for their professional hospitality and personal friendship during a difficult stretch of time. All the authors are indebted to key staff members whose considerable talents once again produced a readable manuscript from often illegible notes.

Harcourt Health Sciences has been tenacious for excellence from the beginning, and our editors, Linda Duncan and Teri Merchant, have been steadily supportive and unfailingly patient with our penchant for altering deadlines. We hope that the final product pleases them.

Last, it would be wrong not to mention the numerous unseen contributions made by our students of pathology over the years. In a very real way, it has been their probing questions, effusive spirit, indefatigable good humor, and consistent enthusiasm for pathology that caused this book to be written in the first place. Students always believe that we are their teachers, but it is we who learn from them.

Teachers
When I was young my teachers were the old.
I gave up fire for form till I was cold.
I suffered like a metal being cast.
I went to school to age to learn the past.
Now I am old my teachers are the young.
What can't be molded must be cracked and
  sprung.
I strain at lessons fit to start a suture.
I go to school to youth to learn the future.
                                    ROBERT FROST

CONTENTS

CHAPTER 1

Pathology—The Study of Disease

David O. Slauson
Barry J. Cooper

OUTLINE

The study of pathology is an important and exciting milestone for students of biomedical science. For them it is an introduction to the study of disease and the mechanisms that underlie it. From the study of pathology should emerge the concepts upon which a satisfying career in medicine can be built. We are firmly committed to the idea that the best medical practice, both diagnostic and therapeutic, is based on a thorough understanding of the mechanisms of disease. Pathology is concerned with these mechanisms.

Students must rationalize and comprehend many apparent conflicts on their route to an understanding of disease. The vital host defenses linked together in the inflammatory response also constitute the major pathways of tissue injury. The same coagulation factors that produce the beautiful and life-saving hemostatic plug are responsible for the ugly and life-threatening thrombus. The injured endothelial cell produces both tissue thromboplastin to start the clot and plasminogen activators to initiate clot removal. Macrophages and neutrophils perform phagocytic heroics on our behalf while simultaneously releasing enzymes that degrade our tissues. To gain an understanding of these things is to acquire an appreciation of how and why diseases are complicated affairs.

Disease is a manifestation of physiology gone wrong and ultimately reflects some structural or functional alteration in the cells of which all living things are made. To understand disease, we must turn our attention toward understanding the changes that occur in living tissues in response to various kinds of stimuli. Students often first encounter pathology with some apprehension feeling that they are poorly prepared to study disease when in fact they are usually well equipped. They are well versed in the normal structure and function of tissues. The typical student, however, generally believes that *finally* all of that basic material has been surmounted so that something applicable to medicine can now be learned. Students usually consider pathology a worthwhile pursuit, but all too often they do not seem to appreciate that understanding normal structure and function is the ultimate basis for understanding disease and that it is in no sense irrelevant to medicine.

Students seem surprised to discover that, in the disease state, there are, with rare exceptions, no new cellular functions and new metabolic pathways at work. Rather, pathways that already exist are accentuated, diminished, or lost. The same is largely true for structural changes. Only rarely are truly new structures involved in disease states; rather there are increases, decreases, or alterations in structures already present in the normal animal. Even the grossest lesion is usually produced by the same rigorous, lawful, molecular and cellular interactions that govern normalcy. Disease is difficult to understand, but our success or failure at doing so more often lies in the realm of logic than in the realm of application. The Statements of the Obvious in Box 1-1 may help place this into perspective.

WHAT IS PATHOLOGY?

Broadly speaking, pathology is the study of disease. According to the dictionary, it is the "study of the essential nature of disease, especially the structural and functional consequences thereof." Pathology, however, is different things to different people. To the student it is an introduction to disease, an introduction to the abnormal processes that manifest themselves as clinical signs in sick animals. The clinician sees pathology as one of the means by which a diagnosis can be made. To the pathologist it is the study of lesions associated with disease and the mechanisms that underlie them. These various views of pathology are not incompatible. They simply reflect the varied interests of individuals. Pathology is the study of disease. It is the study of morphological lesions, that is, structural abnormalities that characterize particular diseases. Most importantly in the context of this book, it is the study of how and why these lesions develop and their functional consequences.

BOX 1-1 **Statements of the Obvious**

The proportions and organization of both the cellular and extracellular constituents of a tissue determine the structural and functional characteristics of the tissue.

The structural and functional characteristics determine the adaptability of each tissue. Tissue adaptability decreases with aging and in many disease states.

Any agent or condition that exceeds a tissue's capacity to adapt results in an injury or disease process.

Understanding the mechanism and site of action of a disease-producing agent or condition should allow one to be able to predict the effects of this perturbance on the host.

Knowing the structural and functional changes occurring in the tissues allows one to predict the clinical presentation.

The clinical presentation, conversely, allows us to draw conclusions about the structural and functional changes that have occurred in the tissue. These conclusions can then be used to decide on a differential list of causes for each disease process.

Courtesy Dr. R.R. Minor, Ithaca, N.Y.

As a subject for study, pathology bridges the gap between the basic sciences and clinical medicine. It has one foot in the sciences of tissue structure and function, anatomy and histology, physiology and biochemistry. The other foot is in the clinics.

At the simplest level, pathology identifies lesions and often can provide a diagnosis for clinicians. The science of pathology, however, did not grow simply from a need to recognize and name lesions and diseases. It arose from the attempts of practicing clinicians to *understand* disease. The first pathologists were clinicians who studied the structural abnormalities of the tissues in an attempt to explain the illnesses of their patients. Gradually pathology evolved into a specialty, but today it still retains its roots in morphology and in understanding the nature of disease. General pathology, the subject of this book, involves the study of the mechanisms by which tissues are injured. It provides the basic principles that allow us to understand specific diseases, whether they involve the lung, the liver, the kidneys or any other organ system.

The study of disease can be approached in many different ways. We can emphasize the expressions of various disease processes because they lead to the recognizable alterations in tissues that we call *lesions*. We can emphasize the study and classification of these lesions into recognizable patterns and forms useful to understanding disease and to making definitive diagnoses. We can emphasize the causative agents, the bacteria, viruses, fungi, toxins, and so on, responsible for causing disease. We can emphasize the functional consequences of various kinds of organic diseases and thus emphasize *pathophysiology*. All of these are important, but these approaches are by their very nature too often aimed at asking "What is it?" rather than "Why is it?" or "How is it?"

Students beginning to learn about disease must emphasize the *how* and the *why* over the *what* if they are to become flexible clinicians able to think their way through disease problems encountered in clinical patients. A fascinating world of disordered structure and function lies before us in any diseased creature if only we can have the eyes to see it. To enumerate a list of clinical signs and then a list of lesions is not enough, for it is the relation of one to the other that counts. Sometimes this is easy, sometimes difficult, and sometimes impossible to determine. Sometimes our ignorance, however we might try to mask it in attractive scientific phraseology, still sounds like ignorance. But if we try to understand disease as to its *hows* and *whys,* we undertake a persistent endeavor that is the ultimate challenge of medicine.

Pathology can never be purely a science; it is made up of too many variables and immeasurables.

The dog with verrucous mitral endocardiosis and the cow with infectious bovine viral rhinotracheitis are not internal combustion engines. We can interpret them, but we cannot memorize their circuitry and replace their spark plugs. Our best effort is to try to understand *why* their systems failed by knowing *how* such systems fail. In other words, knowing *what* disease they have is ultimately less useful than understanding the mechanisms by which that disease came to be. The former approach gives a name to the disease to help us communicate among ourselves, but the latter forces a reconstruction of the moving series of events involved in the disease process itself.

WHAT DO PATHOLOGISTS DO?

Clearly, not all the many people who study disease would call themselves "pathologists." Traditionally pathologists have been regarded as those who study the morphological manifestations of disease. To some extent this is still true. Most pathologists today are trained to study the morphological manifestations of disease but also are vitally interested in the functional changes with which such lesions are associated. Most are interested in *why* such lesions develop. Pathologists are medical specialists who have spent many years in specific training, often leading to *specialty board certification*. In North America, veterinary pathologists are certified by the American College of Veterinary Pathologists, the oldest and largest specialty group recognized by the American Veterinary Medical Association.

Many pathologists have particular interests, and many subspecialties have developed within the field of pathology. *Medical pathology* deals with the diseases of man, and *veterinary pathology* with the diseases of animals other than man. Many veterinary pathologists would regard themselves as *comparative pathologists* because their interests encompass the diseases of all species, including man. The study of the pathogenesis of animal diseases often allows considerable insight into similar disease processes in man, and information gained from the study of human diseases is usually pertinent to veterinary medicine as well. *Diagnostic pathologists* study tissue abnormalities, using either *gross* pathology or *histopathology* (microscopic pathology) or both, to identify the nature of the disease. They may study the whole animal, in the case of the postmortem examination (necropsy), or they may study samples of tissue taken from the living patient as a diagnostic procedure (biopsy). *Surgical pathologists* specialize in the study of biopsy material. *Specialty pathologists* might have a specific interest in particular organ systems and would, for example, be recognized as neuropathologists, pulmonary pathologists, or renal pathologists. Other specialty pathologists might be experts in *environmental pathology, toxicological pathology,* or *zoo and wildlife pathology.*

Such advanced levels of specialization are a natural outcome of the rapid advances in research and the virtual explosion of information available about disease and disease mechanisms. It is a tough chore for even a specialist to keep up with his or her field in today's world, and pathologists who believe they know all the answers probably do not understand all the questions. One beneficial outgrowth of specialization is *consultation.* The renal pathologist asks the neuropathologist to examine the brain lesions in a case awaiting a final diagnosis, and the neuropathologist seeks the opinion of the renal pathologist on a difficult kidney case. Both individuals profit from the knowledge of the other. Most pathologists try to keep up with the entire field of pathology in a broad sense, and most have recognized the necessity for specialization.

Immunopathologists are particularly interested in tissue injury that is associated with or caused by the immune system. *Clinical pathologists* are especially important in the laboratory analysis of disease as it occurs in living patients. They provide a wide variety of investigative tests and help to interpret them to support or deny diagnoses. They utilize hematology, cytology, serum chemistry, clinical endocrinology, and similar procedures to help make specific diagnoses. *Experimental pathologists* manipulate, analyze, and sometimes recreate abnormalities of structure and function so that we may better understand the mechanisms that underlie disease. Of course, there is some overlap in these interests. Diagnostic pathologists may utilize the techniques of immunopathology, for example, and experimental pathologists also may be diagnostic pathologists.

An important and emerging subspecialty or area of emphasis of interest to students might be called *molecular pathology.* Increasing knowledge of the molecular and genetic basis of disease and the huge advances in biotechnology for analyzing nucleic acids and gene products are changing the practice of pathology and medicine. It is difficult to overstate the importance that molecular technology and genetics have brought to modern diagnostics, and the contemporary practice of medicine and pathology increasingly requires a legitimate understanding of the basis and application of exciting new technologies such as polymerase chain reaction (PCR) amplification, *in situ* hybridization, microchip and array technology, probe production and nucleic acid labeling, Southern and Northern blot analysis, sequence analysis, restriction fragment length polymorphism, and methods of mutation screening (Box 1-2). This technology is likely to continue to expand rapidly, and education in molecular medicine and pathology needs to become a central part of our core instruction for students lest we permit them to fall behind the leading edge.

General pathology is a traditional academic subdivision of pathology that remains in use to distinguish it from *special pathology,* or the pathology of specific diseases as they affect specific organs and organ systems. As such, general pathology deals with common denominators of disease and the mechanisms of disease production. The topics of general pathology include cellular injury and death, circulatory disorders common to many tissues, inflammation and repair, immunopathology, growth disturbances and neoplasia, and the nature and causes of disease, including genetics. These are the subjects of general pathology because they have common mechanistic features useful to a general understanding of specific disease states. All tumors have some features in common. Inflammation, whether it affects the heart or the lungs or the kidneys, has a large number of common features. Hence, what is learned in general pathology is applicable to disease problems involving any organ system. As such, it is a mechanism-oriented discipline.

THE TOOLS OF PATHOLOGY

The wide range of interests covered by pathology necessitates the use of a wide variety of tools, or techniques, to study lesions. Although highly sophisticated and expensive equipment is necessary for some special procedures, the best pathological examination usually begins with rather simple tools indeed: the *eyes* and the *hands* of the pathologist. A great deal can be learned from a specimen by the

---

BOX 1-2 **Technology for Modern Pathology**

DNA and RNA isolation and quantitation
Probe production and labeling
Polymerase chain reaction (PCR) and reverse transcription–PCR (RT-PCR)
Southern and Northern blot analysis
Pulsed-field gel electrophoresis
Immunofluorescence and chemiluminescence
ELISA plate and microwell arrays
In situ hybridization
DNA sequence analysis and ribotyping
Oligonucleotide sequencing and analysis
Microsatellite allele assessment
Restriction fragment length polymorphism analysis
Mutation screening and genetic databasing

fundamental processes of careful examination and inspection, and most good pathologists are quite astute observers. Skillful palpation and visual scrutiny are often learned talents, and experience can be an invaluable teacher. Individuals preparing for careers in pathology must spend 3 years in mentored training before they are "eligible" to take the American College of Veterinary Pathologists examination for Board Certification in Veterinary Pathology.

The *light microscope* familiar to all remains the basic tool of the pathologist. It provides magnification of tissue changes up to a maximum of about 1000 times normal and is most commonly used to study sections of tissues taken from animals. The sections used in histopathology are simply very thin slices of tissue prepared from larger pieces of tissue preserved in formaldehyde or other fixative and embedded in a medium such as paraffin wax. The sections are stained with dyes, which allow the various components of the tissue to be visualized. The usual stain for routine sections is *hematoxylin and eosin* (H&E) (Fig. 1-1), but a wide variety of special stains may be used to illustrate special components of the tissue. For example, the periodic acid–Schiff (PAS) reaction is used to demonstrate carbohydrate substances such as glycogen. Toluidine blue stain can be used to illustrate mast cell granules and so

distinguish these cells from others. Numerous different stains can illustrate organisms in tissues. There are many special stains, each of which has special usefulness to the pathologist (Table 1-1).

Histochemical stains are those that react with known specific chemical groups or substances in the tissue. For example, there are available stains that can identify iron in tissues and distinguish it from other substances. Enzyme histochemical stains identify the presence of specific enzymes in the tissue. These are widely used, for example, in the study of muscle lesions to distinguish different types of muscle fibers (Fig. 1-2). For some of these techniques, sections cut from fresh, frozen (rather than fixed) tissue are required.

Other special techniques utilizing the light microscope are *dark-field, phase-contrast,* and *fluorescence* microscopy. The last technique is especially useful in immunopathology where deposits of immunoglobulin, complement proteins, or other substances can be detected. If, for example, we wanted to illustrate deposits of IgG in the glomeruli of a horse with glomerulonephritis, we would apply a specific antiserum against equine IgG that binds to the IgG in the renal tissue (Fig. 1-3). The antiserum is conjugated to a dye such as fluorescein, which is fluorescent under ultraviolet (UV) radiation. The suspect tissue is examined in a microscope fitted with UV illumination, and the IgG deposits, if present, are

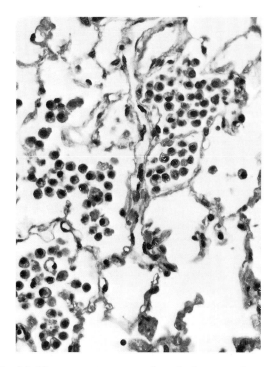

Fig. 1-1 Tissue section stained with hematoxylin and eosin (H&E). In this routine preparation, nuclei are stained blue *(dark)* with the hematoxylin while cytoplasmic and extracellular elements are stained pink *(light)* with the eosin. This section of lung from a dog contains many alveolar macrophages.

TABLE 1-1   Examples of Commonly Used Stains in Pathology

STAIN	USE
Hematoxylin and eosin (H&E)	Routine staining
Phosphotungstic acid–hematoxylin (PTAH)	Cross-striations in muscle, fibrin
Masson trichrome	Connective tissues, collagen
van Gieson's stain	Elastin fibers, collagen
Oil red O (frozen sections)	Fat, lipid
Periodic acid–Schiff reaction (PAS)	Carbohydrate
Best's carmine	Glycogen
Congo red	Amyloid
Crystal violet	Amyloid
Acid-fast	Bacteria
Brown-Brennan (B&B)	Bacteria, gram positive or negative
Levaditi's method	Spirochetes
von Kossa's	Calcium salts
Luxol fast blue (LFB)	Myelin
Gomori's silver	Fungi
Toluidine blue	Mast cell granules

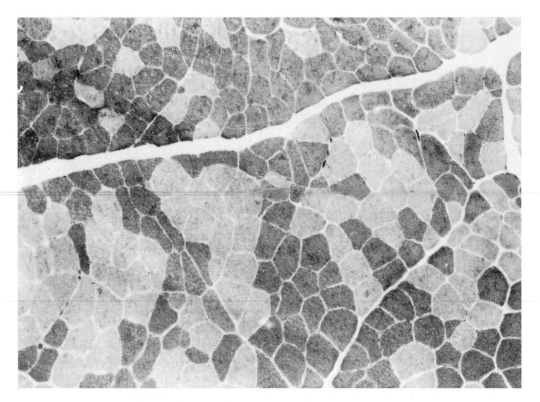

Fig. 1-2 Enzyme histochemistry of muscle. ATPase stain differentiates Type I fibers *(light)* from Type II fibers *(dark).* In this case there is abnormal grouping of fiber types typical of denervation followed by reinnervation. The lesion in this dog could not be appreciated without enzyme histochemistry.

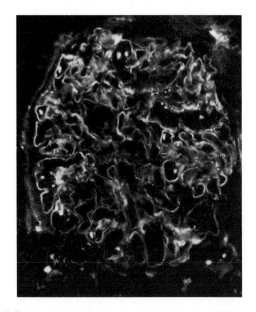

Fig. 1-3 Fluorescence microscopy. This section of kidney has been stained with fluorescein-labeled antibody against equine IgG. It demonstrates linear deposition of host IgG in the glomerulus. *(Micrograph courtesy Dr. R.M. Lewis, Ithaca, N.Y.)*

revealed by fluorescence against a dark background. This technique has been modified by labeling of antisera with the enzyme horseradish peroxidase so that instead of fluorescence, a colored reaction product of a substrate oxidized by the enzyme is detected and can be seen in the ordinary light microscope. Any substance against which an antiserum can be raised can be detected by these techniques, and they are now widely used in pathology.

Electron microscopy is also a leading method for the examination of the morphological changes in diseased tissues. Its major advantage is high resolution, which greatly exceeds that of light microscopy, and magnification of well over 100,000 times normal is possible. Structures far too small to be seen in the light microscope can thus be resolved by the electron microscope (Fig. 1-4). For *transmission* electron microscopy, small pieces of fixed tissue are embedded in special plastics, and extremely thin sections are cut. Stains that are electron dense are used, and the image formed by the beam of electrons is recorded on photographic film. *Scanning* electron microscopy is used to study the three-dimensional structure of tissue (Fig. 1-5). It is particularly useful in demonstrating surface microanatomic changes, which cannot easily be appreciated with the transmission electron micro-

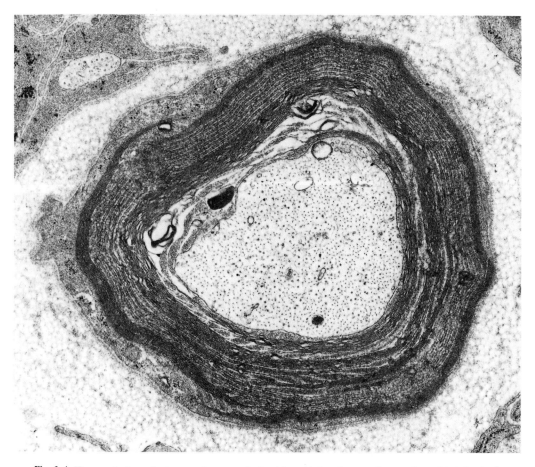

Fig. 1-4 Transmission electron micrograph. In this peripheral nerve from a dog with inherited neuropathy there is abnormal compaction of myelin lamellae. The increased resolution provided by electron microscopy allows such lesions to be visualized.

scope. Finally, special methods of preparation can be used for electron microscopy.

Deposition of substances such as immunoglobulins can be demonstrated by *immunoelectron microscopy* using antisera linked to electron-dense substances or to enzymes using methods that produce an electron-dense product. These techniques are similar to those used at the light microscopic level but provide much higher resolution.

Tissues embedded in plastic also can be used for high-resolution light microscopy. Because one can cut sections from plastic that are much thinner than the 4 to 5 μm usually provided by paraffin-embedding techniques, a much better level of resolution is provided (Fig. 1-6).

Pathologists, especially experimental pathologists, use many other techniques to measure the functional consequences of lesions. These include essentially all the techniques of contemporary investigative biology. As the answers to research questions become more and more complicated, the ap-

proaches used in many types of experiments in modern pathology increasingly involve studies at the cellular and molecular level of resolution. The data generated by such research is very important, for it provides the basis on which we eventually are able to first understand and then predict the clinical consequences of particular morphological lesions.

The rapidly emerging *molecular technology* plays an ever-increasing role in diagnostic and investigative pathology, but it is our view that the occasional suggestion that "H&E" histopathology will be superseded are both unrealistic and premature. Pathologists and their students must remain open to the new technology and what it can help us accomplish while ever mindful that our traditional goal of optimizing the benefit to patients remains central.

THE LANGUAGE OF PATHOLOGY

The study of pathology introduces the student to an extensive new vocabulary. Many of these terms will

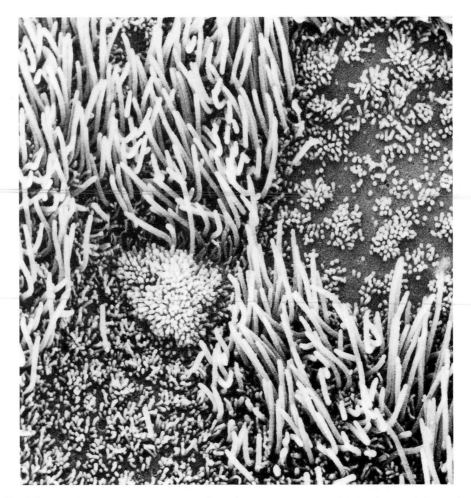

Fig. 1-5 Scanning electron micrograph (SEM). The three-dimensional structure of these ciliated bronchial epithelial cells is revealed here as are the microvilli on adjacent goblet cells. SEM is a useful, high-resolution means of studying cell surfaces. *(Micrograph courtesy Dr. W.L. Castleman, Gainesville, Fla.)*

become evident throughout this book. Here we will limit ourselves to a few particular terms that are of general importance. A *lesion* is an abnormality in a tissue. Generally when we use this term, we are referring to a structural abnormality, but sometimes the word is used in reference to a functional abnormality. We might, for example, use the term "biochemical lesion" to describe a functional abnormality. Such a lesion may or may not have a morphological counterpart. *Pathogenesis* is the term used to describe the way in which a disease or lesion develops. That is, it is the sequence of events and mechanisms that underlie a disease process. The lesion itself is an observation; its pathogenesis is the explanation of how and why it developed.

Disease itself is hard to define. What does it mean to be sick? It is the culmination of those various defects, abnormalities, excesses, deficiencies, and injuries as they occur at the cell and tissue level that ultimately results in clinically apparent dysfunction. Disease may sometimes go undetected at the clinical

level even though the lesions underlying the disease have been present in the tissues for a long time. Most of us can recall from our experience some situation where a person "suddenly" became ill, but the underlying lesions had in fact been present for months. Cancer often presents in this way.

Diseases and indeed lesions are often difficult to categorize, and the terminology can be confusing. Let us take the specific example of leptospirosis in a dog. Leptospirosis names the disease and, as such, is the *definitive diagnosis*. The dog probably has subacute nonsuppurative interstitial nephritis, which names the lesion and gives us a *morphological diagnosis*. Because the cause in our example is *Leptospira canicola*, the *etiological diagnosis* for the renal lesions would be leptospiral nephritis.

Other examples can be given. *Escherichia coli* (the cause) results in colibacillosis (the disease), which is basically an acute to subacute catarrhal enteritis (the morphological diagnosis). *Mycobacterium paratuberculosis* (the cause) produces a

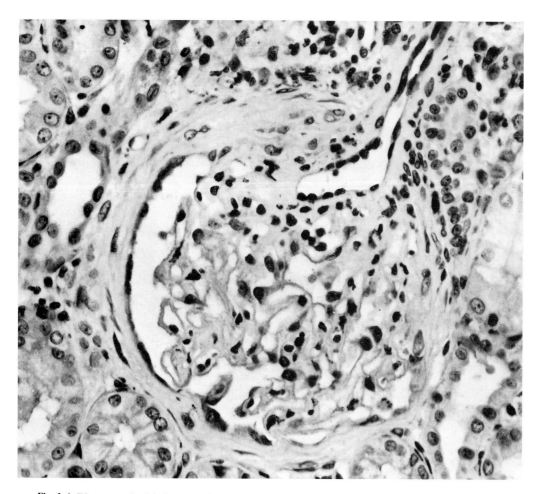

Fig. 1-6 Plastic embedded tissue. In this 2 μm thick section of a glomerulonephritic dog kidney, the thickened capillary walls in the glomerulus and the adhesions to Bowman's capsule are clearly evident. These changes are often hard to evaluate in routine material.

chronic granulomatous enterocolitis (the morphological diagnosis) in cattle that have Johne's disease (the name of the disease and the definitive diagnosis). One of the important jobs of diagnostic pathologists is to find, interpret, and name such changes to reach a diagnosis. In some situations, particularly with surgical biopsies, this information will allow the pathologist to offer a *prognosis* or estimate the future behavior of any lesion or change in tissue with respect to its influence on the whole organism.

AN APPROACH TO THE STUDY OF PATHOLOGY

Pathology and in fact medicine as a whole can be approached in two ways. We can learn to *recognize* disease entities and to treat them by certain set maneuvers. Unfortunately, disease varies in its manifestations, and such an approach is bound to fail frequently. Alternatively we can try to *understand* the disease process and to make logical diagnoses and formulate treatments based on the functional ab-

normalities that we have shown to be present. In practice we utilize both methods, but it is essential that we understand, as well as we can, the biological processes that underlie disease.

If we can understand basic pathobiological mechanisms, we can find our way through new or unfamiliar disease syndromes. If we understand, we can generate rational rather than empirical methods to treat disease. We need only to look at the recent history of medicine to see that our attempts to understand disease have led to much more effective means to control it.

We can appreciate disease at any one of a variety of levels, ranging from the whole animal, or organismal level, to the molecular level. Between these extremes we might understand any particular disease process at the level of the organs, the tissues, the cells, or the subcellular organelles involved. Consider, for example, a dog that shows evidence of the disease diabetes mellitus (Fig. 1-7). At the crudest level of understanding we have a sick or possibly even a dead dog. If we look at the organ level, we find

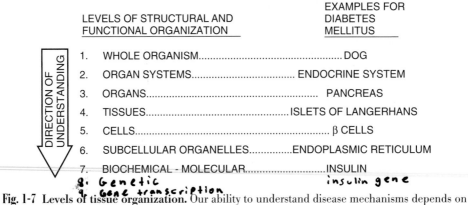

LEVELS OF STRUCTURAL AND FUNCTIONAL ORGANIZATION	EXAMPLES FOR DIABETES MELLITUS
1. WHOLE ORGANISM	DOG
2. ORGAN SYSTEMS	ENDOCRINE SYSTEM
3. ORGANS	PANCREAS
4. TISSUES	ISLETS OF LANGERHANS
5. CELLS	β CELLS
6. SUBCELLULAR ORGANELLES	ENDOPLASMIC RETICULUM
7. BIOCHEMICAL - MOLECULAR	INSULIN
8. Genetic	insulin gene
9. Gene transcription	

DIRECTION OF UNDERSTANDING

Fig. 1-7 Levels of tissue organization. Our ability to understand disease mechanisms depends on the level of resolution where reliable information is available. For diabetes mellitus, the molecular basis is known. This is not true for many diseases.

that the animal has a large, yellow liver, which we recognize as fatty change (lipidosis), or the accumulation of lipid in the liver cells. If we look in more detail we find that the islets of Langerhans in the pancreas are vacuolated. These are observations. They allow us to make a probable diagnosis of diabetes mellitus. However, it is only the appreciation of molecular or functional changes in this case that allows us to really understand the basis of this disease. Diabetes mellitus was recognized for many years as a disease syndrome without a real understanding of its basis. It was not until the discovery of insulin and the role it played in controlling blood glucose levels that we really began to understand diabetes mellitus. With this understanding came the opportunity to treat the disease with exogenous insulin. As a result many people and animals enjoy a relatively normal life despite their having this disease.

It is a basic tenet of pathology that all disease is essentially a manifestation of cellular injury. Such injury leads to changes in the structure and function of tissues and organs. The changes in function are what we recognize as clinical signs. The changes in structure are what we recognize as morphological lesions. To understand disease we must understand the changes in structure and function that occur in response to a variety of stimuli. In reading this book the student may sometimes wonder about the relevance of such detailed discussions of disease mechanisms. We would suggest that at such times the example of diabetes mellitus be reconsidered. It is on the basis of detailed understanding that future advances in medicine, including therapy, will be made.

Injury versus Reaction to Injury

We also should make a distinction here between injury and the reaction to injury. Very often it is the reaction to injury, rather than the injury itself, that produces the clinical manifestations of disease.

Take, for example, a simple, focal bacterial infection in the skin. We perceive such an infection as local swelling, heat, redness, and pain. These changes are for the most part not brought about by the bacteria themselves but by the host reaction that we call "inflammation." The bacteria may or may not be capable of injuring host tissues, but they are recognized by host defense systems, and, through a variety of complex mechanisms, the local blood flow is increased, fluid and plasma proteins leak out of vessels, and phagocytic cells migrate into the lesion. It is the latter changes that we appreciate, not the presence of the bacteria or their direct effects.

Biology versus Pathobiology

In beginning the study of pathology the student is not entering a strange new world. Pathology is a subdiscipline of biology. With rare exceptions there are no new metabolic or biochemical pathways involved in disease, nor are new structures usually involved. Rather, structures and functional pathways that *already exist* are altered, either accentuated, diminished, or lost altogether. It is the departure from the normal day-to-day balance or steady state that produces disease. From this observation the concept of pathophysiology emerges. *Pathophysiology* is the alteration of normal functions that constitutes the disease process.

"It is in her moments of abnormalities that nature reveals its secrets." GOETHE

Consider, for example, the rather common clinical problem of uremia (renal failure). If a dog presented in uremia dies and a necropsy is performed, the pathologist might find numerous lesions. These might include chronic inflammation of the kidneys, mineralization of a variety of tissues, softening of the bones, and enlargement of the parathyroid glands. However, it was not this list of lesions that led to the dog entering the hospital. It was the pathophysiology of the disease that did that. What the owner of the dog observed was abnormal function, that is, *clinical signs*. The complaint of the owner might well have been that the dog had bad breath, difficulty in eating, increased water consumption, and polyuria manifested by nightly urination on the living room carpet.

It is the job of the clinician to understand how the pathophysiology of renal disease can lead to these signs. In this case, the pathophysiology of the disease relates to the function of the kidneys in electrolyte and water homeostasis. Loss of functional kidney tissue leads to loss of body water and to calcium and phosphorus imbalances, and loss of concentrating ability because of kidney lesions leads to polyuria. The animal becomes dehydrated and drinks more (polydipsia), which is often accompanied by frequent urination (polyuria), often at night (nocturia). The calcium-phosphorus imbalance leads to stimulation and hyperplasia of the parathyroid glands. The parathyroid hormone secreted leads to removal of calcium from bones in an attempt to maintain blood calcium homeostasis. As a result, the bones become soft. Loss of renal function also leads to accumulation of nitrogenous wastes. These contribute to the offensive ammoniacal breath odor common to animals in renal failure, and the measurement of nitrogenous wastes in the blood, particularly urea nitrogen, is a common aid to the diagnosis of renal failure. This whole pathophysiological syndrome is called "uremia."

As students of disease, therefore, we should direct our attention toward understanding the phenomena that lead to the disease state (that is, toward its pathogenesis), its morphological expressions, and its functional consequences (or pathophysiology). There is no more exciting form of detective work than starting with a sick animal and working backward through clinical signs and clinicopathological tests of organ function to arrive at an understanding of the disease and its lesions that permits an accurate diagnosis. A thorough understanding of disease mechanisms gained from the study of pathology will be of great value in supporting this satisfying approach to clinical medicine.

It is our sincere hope that this book will help students to be excited by the prospect of understanding disease. The attitudes formed by students now will influence their whole future. Those who appreciate trying to understand disease will enjoy their professional life; those who are willing to settle for dogma will miss out on much of the challenge and pleasure of a medical career. It is a matter of learning how to think and how to interpret. There are fewer absolutes, and more uncertainties. The "art" and the "science" of medicine become united. To see how enjoyable this kind of medical thinking can be, Lewis Thomas's superb little book *Lives of a Cell* is highly recommended.

Causes and Pathogenesis of Disease

Disease can be caused by a great variety of agents. These include infectious agents (viruses, bacteria, fungi, and parasites), chemical agents, and physical agents such as heat, cold, radiation, and direct trauma. There are literally thousands of individual etiological agents that can be the cause of disease. It is important to realize, however, that this long list is not reflected by an equally long list of host reactions, and regardless of how long the list of individual etiological agents becomes, mammalian organisms have really only six basic forms of expression of injury (Box 1-3).

In other words, the pathogenetic mechanisms and morphological and functional expressions of disease are limited, regardless of the cause.

Many agents cause disease through common pathways. For example, the virus that causes feline infectious enteritis, a parvovirus, attacks mitotically active cells in the intestinal glands. These same cells are particularly susceptible to radiation injury. The result of each of these forms of injury therefore is the same. There is necrosis of intestinal gland cells, and the lesions are essentially the same in each case despite having quite different causes. This is not to say that there is not still a bewildering variety of mechanisms that may be involved in disease processes. The variety, however, reflects the complexity of *normal* biological processes, not the number of potential causes of diseases.

The complexity of biological interactions that occur in the whole animal often make the study of disease very difficult. Often we can identify a cause and can observe the effect, that is, the disease. The pathobiological processes connecting the two, however, may present a puzzle that is impossible to understand when working with the whole animal. For this reason most detailed research these days is done on isolated tissues or cells *in vitro*. Much of our understanding of immunological phenomena, for example, is derived from studying lymphocytes and macrophages *in vitro*. In this way we can assemble small parts of the puzzle without the confusion of interactions that occur in the whole animal. Nevertheless, the objective is essentially to understand these processes in the setting of the intact animal. The puzzle is not yet complete and essentially it never will be. There always will be new questions about normal and abnormal biological processes.

BOX 1-3   **Classes and Causes of Tissue Lesions**

CLASSES	CAUSES
DISRUPTIVE DEFECTS	**GENETIC ABNORMALITIES**
Incision (a cut) not a laceration	Autosomal
Abrasion (friction lesion)	Sex-linked
Excoriation (friction lesion)	Dominant
Laceration (stretch lesion)	Recessive
Contusion (stretch lesion deep in tissues)	Polygenic etc.
Fracture (stretch lesion of bone)	
Constriction or dilatation	**PHYSICAL INJURY**
Rupture	Trauma
	Obstruction
DEGENERATIVE DEFECTS	Pressure
Degeneration	Ionizing radiation
Hydropic	Ultrasonic vibration
Fatty	UV radiation etc.
Hyaline	
Fibrinoid	**THERMAL INJURY**
Necrosis	Heat ($>+5°$ C)
Coagulation	Superficial
Liquefaction	Deep
Caseous	Electric current
Fat	Microwaves
Mineralization	Cold ($<-15°$ C) etc.
Metastatic	
Dystrophic	**CHEMICAL INJURY**
	Exogenous
VASCULAR DEFECTS	Toxins
Hyperemia	Poisons
Congestion	Drugs
Edema	Food substances
Thrombosis	Endogenous
Ischemia	Metabolites
Hemorrhage	Cytolytic or inhibitory substances (AgAb + complement)
INFLAMMATION	Free radicals
Acute	Oxidants etc.
Subacute	
Chronic	**INFECTIONS OR INFESTATIONS**
Suppurative	Bacterial
Nonsuppurative	Fungal
Granulomatous	Viral
Focal	Protozoal
Multifocal	Parasitic
Diffuse	Mycoplasmal etc.
DEFECTS OF GROWTH AND DIFFERENTIATION	**METABOLIC ABNORMALITIES**
Atrophy	Hormone imbalance
Hypertrophy	Enzyme defects
Aplasia	Membrane defects
Hypoplasia	Structural protein defects etc.
Hyperplasia	
Metaplasia	**NUTRITIONAL INJURY**
Neoplasia	Undernutrition
	Overnutrition
DEVELOPMENTAL (CONGENITAL DEFECTS)	Nutritional imbalance
All of above	Nutritional deficiencies etc.

Courtesy Dr. R.R. Minor, Ithaca, N.Y.

Presumably the answers will provide the same sort of advances in our ability to modify or treat disease that we have already experienced in the past.

Continuity, Interactions, and Lesions

Emerging from our discussions of the complexity of the disease process is an important concept. It is that *when we look at lesions we are seeing a static representation of a dynamic process.* In other words, the disease process is composed of continually evolving, interacting mechanisms. Lesions may be progressing and becoming more severe, they may be resolving, or their severity may be relatively constant. However, they are rarely static. They rarely remain exactly the same over long periods. This concept is analogous to a motion-picture film (Fig. 1-8). If we look at a single frame, we see a still picture. But we know that this is only a representation of a moment in a continuum. In the same way, when we look at a histological slide, we are seeing one moment in the continuum of the development of the lesion.

How do we interpret this "still" picture? Can we tell in what direction it was evolving? The answer often is, "Yes, we can." Consider again the motion-picture frame. Let us assume it showed a person running. We can tell easily from a single frame whether the person was running forward or backward. Why? Because our *experience* has taught us to recognize these things. We have seen many people running, and we know from experience *how* and *why* a person running forward would look different from one running backward. If we had never seen a person running, we would probably *not* be able to make these assumptions. The interpretation of lesions is the same. We learn from experience to interpret the still picture we see as a lesion, as part of a dynamic disease process. The role of experimental pathology is partly to teach us these things. By looking at multiple samples taken at different points in time, for example, we can learn how lesions evolve. These lessons allow us to interpret the likely progress of naturally occurring lesions and to predict the likely outcome of a disease process. In other words, we can suggest a prognosis.

Returning to our opening question, What is pathology? It is the study of biological functions that, for some reason, are not proceeding normally.

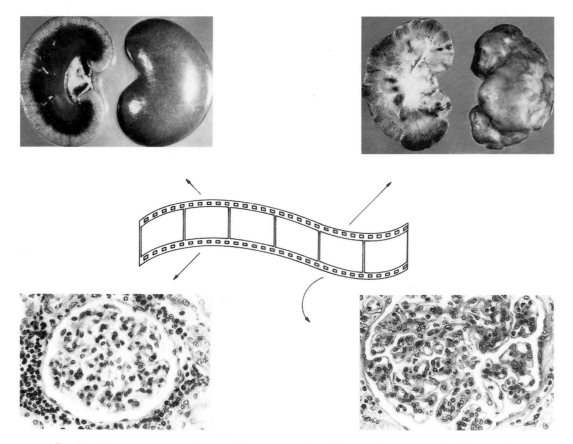

Fig. 1-8 Disease as a continuum. Diseases are dynamic, changing events. In this example, glomerulonephritis progresses from the acute stages to the chronic stages, and the disease looks different at different stages in its pathogenesis.

It is *not* just morbid anatomy, *not* just the recognition of lesions or the recognition of what the disease is. It is the *understanding* of disease processes, their morphological expression, and, most importantly, their functional expression and significance. To be good pathologists we must first become good biologists. To be students of pathology, we must be good students of biology. We must never forget that, whatever the disease, we are basically looking at normal processes functioning in an abnormal way.

An additional concept is worth introducing. We tend to be rather alert to any "new" diseases, such as the rapid appearance of canine parvovirus infections in the late 1970s, or more recently, Potomac horse fever, equine protozoal myelitis, and Lyme disease. But some of the "old" diseases have an annoying habit of never really going away, and we must be constantly vigilant. "Old" diseases such as tuberculosis in man and Johne's disease in cattle have assumed greater importance once again in recent years, and both veterinarians and physicians must be on the alert for resurgent as well as emergent diseases. The basic principles of pathology and medicine are equally applicable to the old and the new.

THE ROLE OF MOLECULAR AND CELLULAR BIOLOGY IN CONTEMPORARY PATHOLOGY

The concept of a cell summons forth varied images in various minds: a subunit of Hooke's sections of cork, blue-green algae floating in a saline sea, polygonal structures scraped from the belly of a frog, neurons as long as your arm, leukocytes packed with granules. All of these are highly specialized responders to external stimuli that carry from cell generation to cell generation a unique biological history. Tossed into a hostile environment by the pressures of evolution, the cell still struggles against disease. How do its secrets relate to present-day pathology? To disease?

Things used to be less complicated. In the not too distant past, cells enjoyed our relative ignorance and lived out their lives with little investigative intervention. We viewed their contents hazily, and speculated about their workings. As pathologists, we were often more concerned with lesions at the tissue level, and we spoke a language largely unfettered by molecular dialects. We tried to accumulate a common knowledge, and we probed disease mechanisms with rather uniform tools and beautifully simple techniques. Our purpose seemed to be the reproducible recognition of the altered state and the creation of explanatory dogma.

Disease no longer seems willing to settle for such historical innocence. We all have witnessed the emergence of a medical science of bewildering complexity. Disciplinary lines have blurred. Contemporary pathology now includes the disease-oriented aspects of what used to be the intellectual provinces of such diverse disciplines as immunology, cell and molecular biology, biochemistry, medicine, and physiology. Some of the old truths about disease pathogenesis seem so poorly applicable in the new world that they have become more a hindrance than an aid, not because the old truths have become false but because it is now clear that we do not fully understand them. They have become facts without a purpose. Observable phenomena without a palatable explanation.

Through it all, the cell has remained central. We have investigated the cells and they have repeatedly provided several new questions for each of our singular answers. We have been persistent. We have radiographed its surfaces and have cleaved its proteins; we have probed its cytoplasmic depths and simultaneously have probed our minds. Small wonder we are still sometimes confused. But we refuse, quite simply, to abandon the idea that an understanding of disease is within our reach. The *goal of pathology* here is explicit. It is simply to *understand life in the abnormal state* and thus to form a central bridge in the entire arch of medicine. Pathology is not "morbid anatomy," the science of lesions found in the dead. It exists largely because of its applicability to life. There is no limit to its scope, but its hallmark ultimately must continue to be the cell and its domains, its functions, and perhaps most importantly the controls over its behavior in the abnormal state.

It may be that the best way to mentally visualize the importance of the cell and its intracellular control mechanisms is to imagine what things would be like if no controls existed. The long list of successive chemical transformations that make up the metabolic pathways would proceed in an undirected and useless fashion, using too much here and leaving behind too little there. The machinery of biosynthesis and degradation would do its tricks oblivious to the real needs of the cell. The failure of these cooperative systems would lead to a greatly reduced ability to respond to adverse changes in the surrounding extracellular environment. In the end, these alterations in normal cellular control phenomena would lead to biochemical anarchy followed, in many cases, by the overthrow of the central governing systems. Cell death would be followed by tissue death. Lesions would occur.

Many of us are familiar with the analogy that the cell is something like a city. Surrounding it is a freeway (the cell membrane) with rather specific exit and entrance sites to and from the interior. City hall (the nucleus) houses the many administrative officials and is connected to the outlying freeway by a complicated maze of streets and roads (the cytoskeleton), which are difficult to map. Scattered along between streets are various buildings essential to the overall well-being of the metropolitan region: gas and electric company power plants (the mitochondria), various industrial factories for the manufacture of useful products (synthetic regions like the endoplasmic reticulum), sanitation engineering districts (detoxifying mechanisms), warehouses and storage sites (glycogen, lipids), and a post office for packaging and mailing (Golgi zone). In the city, food must be brought in and used, and then the resulting garbage and sewage must be removed. Products fabricated in specific parts of town must be transported throughout the city, and some things may even be packaged for exportation. A complicated communication system is needed to keep all this running smoothly. When communications break down, traffic jams are likely and robbery, smuggling, suicide, murder, and other illegal activities increase. Catastrophes can occur if the public transportation and sanitation workers go on strike, and life in the city becomes uncomfortable if not unbearable. The point is simple: the organism is dependent on tissue integrity, tissue integrity is linked ultimately to cellular integrity, and the cell is the functional sum of its parts, all of which must be perfectly integrated if homeostasis is to be maintained. We see diseases at the level of the whole organism, but we should not lose sight of the fact that *virtually all diseases are ultimately reflections of cellular biology gone wrong.*

If we wish therefore to learn how life begins and ends, we must study it at its greatest level of functional resolution. We must begin with the unit of life structure itself, the cell, and understand the environment in which it lives, its structure and function, and its control mechanisms and how its disturbances are expressed as disease. In its ultimate form, disease is merely a mirror that reflects to the outside changes in internal cellular function. We will therefore begin our study of disease by examining fundamental changes as they occur at the cellular level.

RECOMMENDED READING

Alberts B, Bray D, Lewis J, Raff M, Roberts K, Watson GAD: *Molecular biology of the cell,* ed 3, New York, 1999, Garland Publishing.

Banks WA: *Applied veterinary histology,* ed 3, St. Louis, 1993, Mosby.

Beers PC: Molecular genetic pathology: coming of age in the molecular world, *J Mol Diagn* 1:3-4, 1999.

Brown C: In situ hybridization with riboprobes: an overview for veterinary pathologists, *Vet Pathol* 35:159-167, 1998.

Cheville NC: *Introduction to veterinary pathology,* ed 2, Ames, Iowa, 1999, Iowa State University Press.

Cheville NC: *Ultrastructural pathology: an introduction to interpretation,* Ames, Iowa, 1994, Iowa State University Press.

Cheville NC: *Cell pathology,* ed 2, Ames, Iowa, 1983, Iowa State University Press.

Cohen MA: Resurgent and emergent disease in a changing world, *Br Med Bull* 54:523-532, 1998.

Collins F: Preparing health professions for the genetic revolution, *JAMA* 278:1285-1286, 1997.

Cotran RR, Camber V, Collins T: *Robbins' pathologic basis of disease,* ed 6, Philadelphia, 1999, Saunders.

Cross PC, Mercer CAL: *Cell and tissue ultrastructure: a functional perspective,* New York, 1995, Freeman.

Guyton AA, Hall SA: *Textbook of medical physiology,* ed 9, Philadelphia, 1996, Saunders.

Jones D, Fletcher CDM: How shall we apply the new biology to diagnostics in surgical pathology? *J Pathol* 187:147-154, 1999.

Jones TC, Hunt RD, King NW: *Veterinary pathology,* ed 6, Baltimore, 1997, Williams & Wilkins.

Jubb KVF, Kennedy PC, Palmer N: *Pathology of domestic animals,* ed 4, New York, 1994, Academic Press.

Kerr JB: *Atlas of functional histology,* St. Louis, 1999, Mosby.

Kumar V, Cotran R, Robbins SL: *Basic pathology,* ed 6, Philadelphia, 1997, Saunders.

Majno G, Joris I: *Cells, tissues, and disease: principles of general pathology,* Cambridge, Mass., 1996, Blackwell Science.

Majzoub JA, Muglia LJ: Knockout mice, *N Engl J Med* 334:904-907, 1996.

McGavin MD, Carlton WA, Zachary JF: *Thompson's special veterinary pathology,* ed 3, St. Louis, 2001, Mosby.

Naber SP: Molecular pathology: diagnosis of infectious disease, *N Engl J Med* 331:1212-1215, 1994.

Naber SP: Molecular pathology: detection of neoplasia, *N Engl J Med* 331:1508-1510, 1994.

O'Leary TJ, Becker RL, Frisman DM: *Advanced diagnostic methods in pathology: principles, practice and protocols,* Philadelphia, 2000, Saunders.

Rubin E, Farber JL: *Essential pathology,* ed 2, Philadelphia, 1995, Lippincott.

Singer AJ, Clark RAF: Mechanisms of disease: cutaneous wound healing, *N Engl J Med* 341:738-746, 1999.

Spurr N, Darvasi A, Terrett J, Jazwinska L: New technologies and DNA resources for high throughput biology, *Br Med Bull* 55(2):309-324, 1999.

Thomas L: *Lives of a cell: notes of a biology watcher,* New York, 1975, Bantam Books.

Williams TM (chairman): Special report: Goals and objectives for molecular pathology education in residency programs, *J Mol Diagn* 1:5-15, 1999.

Woolf N: *Cell, tissue and disease,* ed 3, London, 2000, Baillière Tindall.

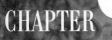

Disease at the
Cellular Level

Barry J. Cooper

To be able to understand disease in the whole animal, the level at which we usually study it as clinicians, it is important to realize that animals become diseased because some of their cells are not functioning normally. This might be stated in another way by saying that sick cells result in sick animals. Thus the present-day study of disease is an attempt to understand how cells react to injury and how this is manifested in the whole animal. We cannot claim, however, that this concept of the cellular basis of disease is a modern one. In fact, *cellular pathology* dates from the mid-nineteenth century and originated largely from the ideas of Rudolf Virchow. Relatively recently, however, we have acquired many sophisticated techniques that allow us to probe ever more deeply into the workings of the cell. As a result many diseases are now understood at the subcellular and, in more and more cases, at the molecular level. In this chapter we discuss the ways in which cells react to injury, providing a basis for subsequent chapters and, hopefully, for future clinical experience.

NORMAL CELLS AND CELLULAR ADAPTATION

Before describing how cells react to injury, we should briefly review the structure and function of the normal cell. Of course, differentiated cells differ from one another, depending on their specialized function, but almost all cells have in common the basic organelles necessary for synthesis of lipids, proteins and carbohydrates; for energy production; and for transport of ions and other substances (Fig. 2-1). Here we will concentrate on these shared features.

The Plasma Membrane

It is difficult to argue that any one organelle is more important to the well-being of the cell than any other but, from the point of view of cellular pathology, the plasma membrane occupies a special niche. It is critical to the functioning of the cell, and, as we shall see in this and in following chapters, interactions at the cell surface are of tremendous importance in disease processes. Physically the plasma membrane forms a barrier between the cell and its environment, and all the interactions of the cell with other cells, bacteria, viruses, hormones, and other substances involve the plasma membrane.

Ultrastructurally the plasma membrane has a trilaminar appearance, with two electron-dense layers separated by an electron-lucent layer. Chemically it is known to be composed predominantly of lipid and protein with some carbohydrate. It is easy, when one is viewing electron micrographs, to think of the plasma membrane as a rather static structure, but current evidence indicates that it is dynamic and

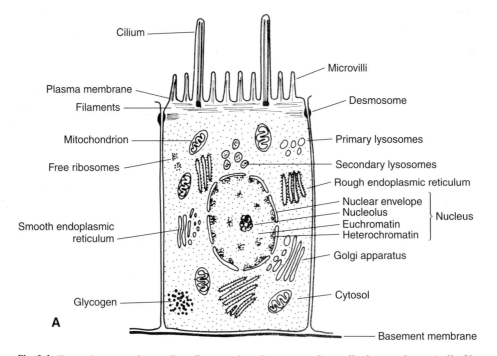

Fig. 2-1 Typical mammalian cell. *A,* Features found in mammalian cells shown schematically. Not all cells rest on a basement membrane, and desmosomes, cilia, and microvilli are surface specializations found on only some cells.

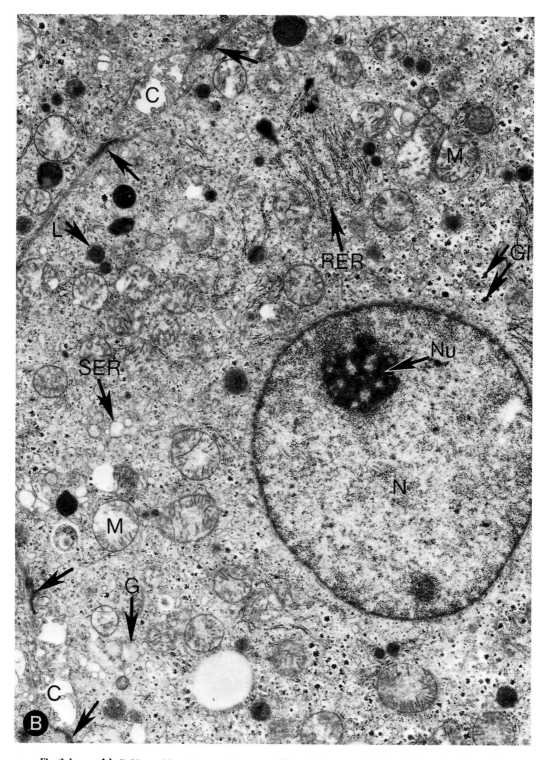

Fig. 2-1, cont'd *B,* Normal hepatocyte of a mouse. Most of the organelles found in mammalian cells can be identified. Desmosomes, *arrows,* are present on either side of the canaliculus, *C,* into which microvilli protrude. *G,* Golgi apparatus; *Gl,* glycogen; *L,* lysosomes; *M,* mitochondria; *N,* nucleus; *Nu,* nucleolus; *RER,* rough endoplasmic reticulum; *SER,* smooth endoplasmic reticulum.

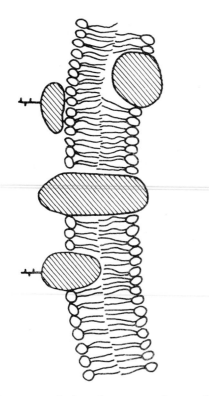

Fig. 2-2 Structure of the plasma membrane. Shown schematically is the lipid bilayer made up of lipid molecules with their hydrophilic ends in contact with the cytosol or the extracellular fluid. Embedded in the bilayer are peripheral and integral proteins. Some bear carbohydrate side chains that project from the cell surface and contribute to the glycocalyx.

can be modulated in response to a variety of stimuli. The modern concept of the structure of the plasma membrane, resulting from this knowledge, is known as the *fluid mosaic model*. In this model the membrane is considered to consist of a lipid bilayer in which are embedded various protein molecules and protein-carbohydrate complexes. The lipid molecules, predominantly phospholipids, are *amphipathic*. In other words, they have a polar and a nonpolar end. The polar ends of the molecules are hydrophilic, and the nonpolar ends are hydrophobic. As shown in Fig. 2-2, they are arranged in the membrane with their hydrophilic ends in contact with the aqueous phase of the cytoplasm or of the extracellular fluid.

Associated with the lipid bilayer is a variety of protein molecules (Fig. 2-2). These are mostly globular in conformation and are of two types. *Peripheral* membrane proteins are present on the external surface of the membrane and are fairly easily removed. *Integral* membrane proteins are embedded in the membrane but project from either the external or the cytoplasmic surfaces. These can be re-

moved only with difficulty. Currently no protein molecules are believed to be buried completely in the lipid bilayer. The protein molecules associated with the plasma membrane are believed to correspond to the tiny bumps that can be visualized when the membrane is examined *en face* in the electron microscope using the freeze fracture technique.

The lipid bilayer is believed to be fluid in the sense that both lipid and protein molecules embedded within it can move laterally but not throughout the depth of the membrane. In particular, proteins may move about on the surface of the cell so that their distribution may alter from diffuse to clustered or *vice versa*. However, this movement is regulated by the cell, and protein molecules can be immobilized or directed. A good example of this phenomenon is provided by the "capping" that is observed in lymphocytes allowed to contact specific antigen or treated with antibody against immunoglobulin. The immunoglobulin molecules on the surface of cells thus treated move to one pole of the cell to form a "patch," or cap. The plasma membrane therefore is a dynamic structure able to respond to a variety of stimuli and insults.

The plasma membrane has a variety of specialized functions too complex to more than summarize here. As already mentioned, it separates the interior of the cell from its environment. As such, it acts as a semipermeable membrane, critical to cell homeostasis, which allows passive diffusion of some molecules and energy-dependent active transport of others while completely preventing the entry of still others. Active transport processes are particularly important in maintaining differences in concentration of sodium, potassium, and other ions between the intracellular and extracellular fluids. As a consequence of this function, the content of cell water also is controlled. The fact that the cell membrane is central to the regulation of ionic homeostasis and that these phenomena are dependent on cellular energy is important in the pathogenesis of cell injury, as described later.

The proteins in and on the plasma membrane are important as cellular antigens, as receptors for hormones and other substances, and for cell-to-cell and cell-to-substrate interactions. Intercellular recognition and interaction is important in a variety of ways. For example, platelets and polymorphonuclear leukocytes interact with endothelial cells, B lymphocytes interact with T lymphocytes, and macrophages interact with lymphoid cells. In addition some cells, such as macrophages and sensitized lymphocytes, can recognize and interact with cells such as bacteria, parasites, or virus-infected cells. All these phenomena are believed to involve the cell surface. Changes in the plasma membrane therefore may be of great importance when we consider disease at the cellular level. Furthermore, as described in Chapter 6, alterations in the plasma membrane may be important in the pathogenesis of neoplasia where intercellular interactions and the control of growth are very abnormal.

Many cells are surrounded by a cell coat or *glycocalyx,* a carbohydrate-rich layer believed to be at least partly composed of the glycoprotein terminuses of membrane proteins. Many of the antigens and receptors already mentioned are in this layer. One particular surface protein, *fibronectin,* is believed to be important in the interaction of cells with one another and with connective tissue matrix components. Fibronectin binds to collagen, fibrinogen, actin, and glycosaminoglycans and is believed to be very important in the attachment of cells to the connective tissue substrate. It is also believed to be involved in wound healing (Chapter 4) and possibly plays a role in opsonizing material for phagocytosis (Chapter 4). There is some evidence, described in Chapter 6, that fibronectin binding is abnormal in cells that have undergone neoplastic transformation, which may be important in determining their ability to invade.

Finally, the plasma membrane may show a variety of morphological specializations. These include microvilli, interdigitations, caveolae, and myelin, all specializations related to specific functions of the cell bearing them. Many cells also show specialized intercellular attachments. These include tight junctions, gap junctions, and desmosomes.

The Nucleus

The nucleus might be thought of as the "brain" of the cell. It contains the genetic information that ultimately directs all the cell's activities. DNA is located and replicated in the nucleus, and RNA is synthesized there for transport to the cytoplasm. It is beyond the scope of this chapter to deal in detail with the functions of the nucleus. Instead, we concentrate on a discussion of its structure and the changes that it can undergo in response to alterations in cellular function.

The *nuclear envelope* surrounds the nucleus and separates the nuclear contents from the cytoplasm (Fig. 2-3). It is made up of a double membrane enclosing a space 10 to 15 nm wide called the *perinuclear cisterna.* A *fibrous lamina* is present immediately adjacent to the inner aspect of the nuclear envelope. This layer is made up of filamentous proteins (lamins and associated proteins) and is believed to be involved in nuclear organization as well as dif-

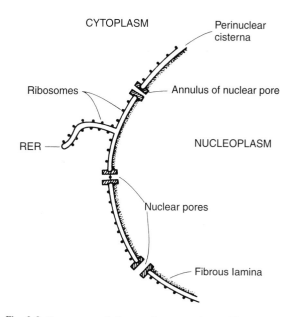

Fig. 2-3 Structure of the nuclear envelope. The arrangement of the nuclear envelope and its relationship to the endoplasmic reticulum are shown.

ferentiation and regulation of the cell cycle. The outer membrane of the nuclear envelope bears ribosomes on its outer surface and sometimes can be seen to be contiguous with the endoplasmic reticulum. For these reasons many people believe that the nuclear membranes and the perinuclear cisterna are a specialization of the endoplasmic reticulum. At regular intervals, the nuclear membranes are penetrated by *nuclear pores* 50 to 70 nm in diameter. Associated with the pore, a transmembrane cylindrical structure called an *annulus* also has been described, and across the pore a diaphragm sometimes can be visualized. Nuclear pores are believed to play a role in regulating the transfer of substances across the nuclear envelope, including transport of RNA molecules from the nucleus into the cytoplasm.

The characteristic blotchy appearance of the nucleus in stained histological or cytological preparations is attributable to its content of *chromatin,* which contains DNA and associated proteins. Two types of chromatin are recognized. *Heterochromatin* is condensed and intensely basophilic in light microscopic preparations. *Euchromatin* is dispersed and, as a result, stains relatively lightly. It is, however, the metabolically active form of the chromatin and therefore is prominent in cells that are actively synthesizing protein and RNA. This point is important in the recognition of rapidly dividing cells, as in neoplasia or hyperplasia. Recognition of unique changes in the distribution of chromatin is important in the identification microscopically of the process of apoptosis, described later in this chapter.

The *nucleolus* forms a roughly spherical substructure of the nucleus. It contains 5% to 10% RNA and a little DNA, the balance being mostly protein. The nucleolus is the site of synthesis of most of the components of ribosomal RNA, and cells that are actively synthesizing protein usually have one or more prominent nucleoli. Again this is of significance in interpreting lesions such as neoplasms.

Cytoplasmic Organelles

The cytoplasm of the cell is made up of many different organelles suspended in an aqueous gel called the *cytosol* (see Fig. 2-1). Cytosol is the fluid matrix of the cell and is itself a dynamic component. It contains many different soluble enzymes, transfer RNA, and other substances important in cell metabolism. The staining characteristics of the cytoplasm depend on the relative concentrations of protein and nucleic acids dissolved or suspended in the cytosol. The higher the concentration of nucleic acids, mainly present in ribosomes, the more basophilic is the appearance of the cytoplasm with conventional H&E stains.

Mitochondria

Through the process of oxidative phosphorylation, the mitochondria are the site of production of most of the ATP, the cell's source of energy. As such, they are critical to the normal function of the cell and, as discussed later in this chapter, they play a central role in apoptosis and cell injury. Drastic damage to the mitochondria usually heralds the death of the cell.

Mitochondria vary greatly in shape and size depending on the type of cell and, to some degree, on their functional status. As shown in Fig. 2-4 they are bounded by two membranes, the inner one of which is thrown into many folds called *cristae*. Two compartments are thus formed, the intermembranous compartment lying between the outer and inner membranes and the inner one (the mitochondrial matrix) inside the inner membrane. Electron-dense granules, which contain divalent cations and are called appropriately enough *mitochondrial dense granules*, also are located in the mitochondrial matrix.

There is a highly ordered structure-function relationship in mitochondria, with specific enzymes and proteins being localized in one or the other of the compartments or closely associated with one of the membranes (Table 2-1). The enzymes of the tricarboxylic acid cycle, except for succinate dehydrogenase, are located in the matrix, whereas those of the

TABLE 2-1	Distribution of Enzymes in Mitochondria
Outer membrane	Monoamine oxidase
	Fatty acyl CoA ligase
	Kynurenine hydroxylase
	Rotenone-insensitive NADH-cytochrome *c* reductase
Intermembranous compartment	Adenylate kinase
	Nucleoside diphospho-kinase
Inner membrane	ATP synthetase
	Succinate dehydrogenase
	Respiratory chain enzymes
	β-Hydroxybutyrate dehydrogenase
	Carnitine fatty acid acyltransferase
Matrix	Malate and isocitrate dehydrogenases
	Citrate synthetase
	Fumarase
	Aconitase
	α-Keto acid dehydrogenases
	β-Oxidation enzymes

respiratory chain and succinate dehydrogenase are located on the inner membrane. Other enzymes also are present in the mitochondria.

Mitochondria are dynamic structures, not only in terms of their metabolic activity but also in their size, shape, and numbers. They are able to replicate and are apparently continually destroyed and replaced in the cell. They may increase or decrease in numbers according to demands made on the cell. Mitochondria also contain a genome, which can be replicated locally, and they can synthesize RNA and protein. Mitochondria are not independent of nuclear genetic information, however, because many mitochondrial proteins are coded for by nuclear DNA.

The Endoplasmic Reticulum, Ribosomes, and Golgi Apparatus

The *endoplasmic reticulum* (ER) (Figs. 2-1 and 2-5) is an important membranous organelle system that is involved in various synthetic and metabolic processes. Two types of ER are recognized: rough, or granular, endoplasmic reticulum (RER) and smooth endoplasmic reticulum (SER).

In most cells the rough endoplasmic reticulum consists of a series of flattened, membranous sacs, known as cisternae, in which protein-rich material sometimes can be visualized. In some cells the ER

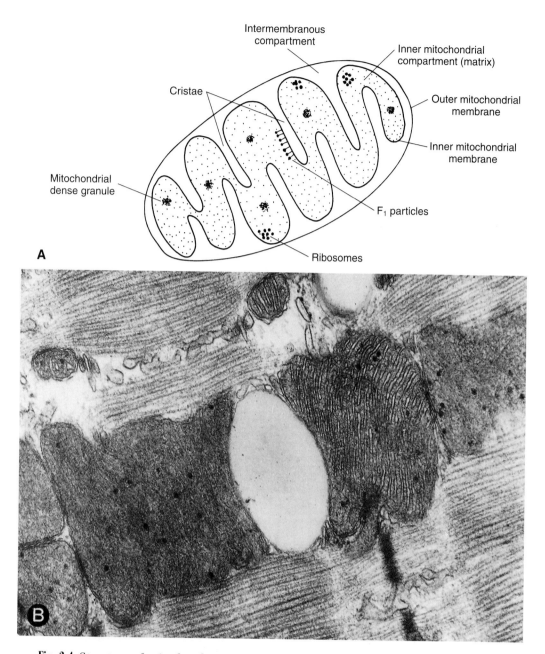

Fig. 2-4 Structure of mitochondria. *A,* Mitochondrion shown schematically. *B,* Mitochondria from a skeletal muscle fiber of a mouse. The outer membrane, the cristae, arising as infoldings of the inner membrane, and mitochondrial dense granules are clearly evident. A lipid droplet lies between two large mitochondria.

takes the form of tubules or small vesicles. Attached to the cytoplasmic surface of the RER, producing the granular ultrastructural appearance that gives it its name, are large numbers of *ribosomes.* Because both the RER and ribosomes are involved in the synthesis and secretion of protein, we will consider them together here.

Ribosomes are small (approximately 20 nm), dense granules that occur either free in the cytoplasm or, as already indicated, attached to the RER.

They usually are present as aggregates called *polysomes* and, on the RER, often are arranged in a spiral pattern. When examined by suitable ultrastructural techniques, they can be seen to be arranged along a "thread" believed to be mRNA. Ribosomes, of course, are rich in RNA and therefore impart basophilic staining properties. Cells that are actively synthesizing a lot of protein, then, tend to have relatively basophilic cytoplasm. Free cytoplasmic ribosomes as a general rule produce protein for use in

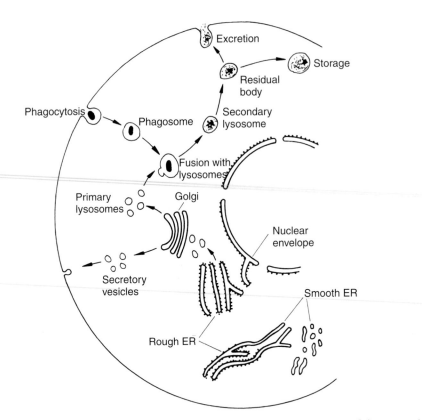

Fig. 2-5 Cytocavitary network. The relationships of the subcellular components of the cytocavitary network are illustrated (see text).

the cell, whereas ribosomes attached to the RER are involved in the synthesis of protein for export from the cell.

A series of experiments in the last few decades have clarified the role of the RER in the synthesis and packaging of secretory proteins. Polypeptide molecules are synthesized on the bound ribosomes and somehow are passed directly to the lumen of the RER where they often can be visualized in electron micrographs as finely granular material. The nascent peptide chains apparently pass through the membrane of the ER and serve a role in holding the polysome to the ER. Although in a few cases the secretory product is concentrated in the RER, it usually is transferred to the Golgi apparatus where final processing takes place.

The *Golgi apparatus* (see Fig. 2-5) is made up of a series of closely associated cisternae arranged something like a stack of coins. Associated with one face, the so-called forming face, is a series of small vacuoles or vesicles. Adjacent to the opposite face, the mature face, are somewhat larger vacuoles, often called "condensing vacuoles." The membranes of the Golgi apparatus are smooth, having no attached ribosomes but are frequently fenestrated near their edges and have many protrusions or irregularities,

which are believed to represent vacuoles in the process of fusion with the cisternal membrane.

The function of the Golgi apparatus is to modify, concentrate, package, and sort proteins destined for secretion. Many of these are glycoproteins, and although the initial carbohydrate moieties may be added in the RER, most carbohydrates are added in the Golgi apparatus. The general process of secretion is believed to involve the budding of vesicles from the RER, transport to the Golgi apparatus, and fusion with its cisternae. The product moves through the cisternae, where it is processed and eventually budded off as condensing vacuoles. In secretory cells these form secretory granules, the contents of which are released from the cell in response to the appropriate stimulus. Lysosomes, the structure and function of which are described below, are formed in a similar way.

The *smooth*, or *agranular*, *endoplasmic reticulum* is distinct from the RER in lacking attached ribosomes. Most commonly, it consists of a series of tubular or vesicular membranous structures. It varies greatly in amount depending on the type of cell. It is most abundant in hepatocytes and cells that secrete steroid hormones such as those of the adrenal cortex and the Leydig cells of the testis. The

SER sometimes can be seen to be connected to the RER, and it is believed that it is derived from the latter.

The SER has a variety of functions. In essence it acts as a membranous carrier on which are displayed enzymes that carry out biosynthetic or metabolic processes. In hepatocytes it is associated with enzymes that metabolize a variety of toxins and drugs. In steroid-secreting cells, many of the enzymes that synthesize the hormones are located on the membranes of the SER. Finally, we should mention that the amount of SER and its associated enzymes can vary depending on the demands made upon the cell. This has certain implications in the pathogenesis of some types of cell injury and is discussed in greater detail later in this chapter.

LYSOSOMES

Lysosomes (Figs. 2-5 and 2-6) are membrane-bound organelles that are important in the digestion of biological material within the cell. They contain a wide variety of enzymes capable of breaking down all types of cellular components including lipids, proteins, and nucleic acids. Lysosomal enzymes generally have their optimal activity at an acid pH and therefore are known as "acid hydrolases." Lysosomes are referred to by different terms depending on their functional state. *Primary lysosomes* are those that have not yet become involved in any digestive process, whereas *secondary lysosomes* are those that contain material undergoing active digestion. *Residual bodies* (Fig. 2-7) are the end point of the lysosomal digestive process. They contain remaining indigestible debris and little, if any, enzyme activity. Much of this material is lipid in nature and gives rise to the pigment *lipofuscin* sometimes found in aging or injured cells.

Generally, lysosomal enzymes are believed to be synthesized on the RER and finally packaged in the Golgi apparatus. Morphologically, lysosomes vary in appearance depending on the cell in which they are found and on their functional state. Primary lysosomes contain no ingested material and therefore often are difficult to distinguish from other membrane-bound vesicles. They can be demonstrated by means of histochemical stains that reveal their hydrolytic enzymes, the usual one used being acid phosphatase. Of course, once secondary lysosomes are formed, they can be recognized by their content of ingested material. Residual bodies sometimes contain whorled membrane-like material frequently referred to as "myelin bodies." In some cells, lysosomes are given special names. The best example is provided by the azurophilic granules of

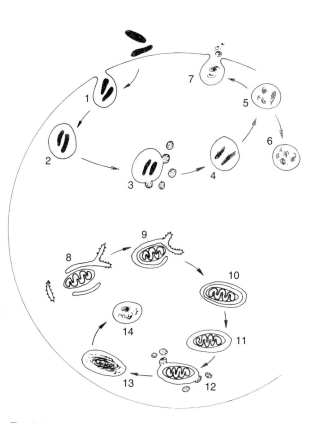

Fig. 2-6 Heterophagy and autophagy. In heterophagy, or phagocytosis, extracellular material is taken up by an infolding of the plasma membrane *(1)* to form a phagocytic vacuole *(2)*. The latter fuses with lysosomes *(3)* to produce a phagolysosome, or secondary lysosome, in which the contents are digested *(4, 5)*. The end products of digestion may be stored as residual bodies *(6)* or sometimes excreted from the cell *(7)*. In autophagy, effete or injured organelles are initially surrounded by a double membrane believed to be derived from endoplasmic reticulum, ER *(8, 9, 10)*. The inner of the two membranes is lost *(11)*, and the vacuole fuses with lysosomes to form a secondary lysosome *(12)*. The remainder of the digestive process is identical to heterophagy *(13, 14)*.

the neutrophil, which are in fact primary lysosomes (see Chapter 4).

The material that is digested by lysosomes can originate from within the cell or from material that the cell has ingested. *Autophagy* is the name given to the process by which part of the cell's own cytoplasm and organelles can be sequestered and digested. In this process the part to be digested is first surrounded by a membrane (see Fig. 2-6) that is believed to be derived from the endoplasmic reticulum. This vacuole then fuses with a primary or a secondary lysosome, the contents are exposed to the acid hydrolases, and digestion begins. Other studies have shown autophagic vacuoles to be formed directly from lysosomes in an energy-dependent process that apparently involves the participation of

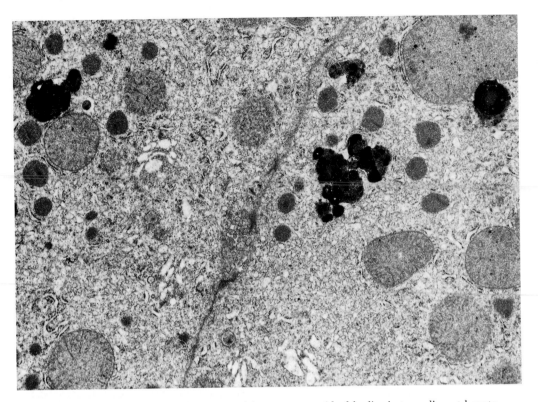

Fig. 2-7 Residual bodies. The dense material represents residual bodies in two adjacent hepato-cytes. *(Courtesy Dr. W.L. Castleman, Gainesville, Fla.)*

microfilaments. Autophagy is seen in degenerating cells, in cells treated with certain drugs, and in cells undergoing atrophy as well as in apparently healthy, active cells. It is presumed that autophagy is a mechanism by which damaged or otherwise effete organelles can be removed and by which normal turnover of organelles can occur. *Heterophagy* is the process by which material taken up from outside the cell is digested. Such material is ingested by the process known in general terms as *endocytosis*. It is first entrapped in an infolding of the plasma membrane, which is then pinched off to form a vacuole. Again the cytoskeleton is intimately involved in this process. Localized aggregation of microfilaments have been shown to occur shortly after the attachment of a particle to be phagocytosed. This process is also energy dependent and presumably is necessary for the local membrane movements required to form the pseudopodia that engulf the particle. When the material ingested is relatively large and particulate, the process is referred to as *phagocytosis*, and the vacuole formed is a *phagosome*. Fluid material, often containing solids in suspension, is taken up by *pinocytosis*. Despite the distinction made in naming these processes, they are mechanistically the same, differing only in the size of the vacuoles or vesicles formed. Pinocytotic vesicles are

relatively small. The subsequent steps of fusion with primary or secondary lysosomes are essentially identical to those already described for autophagy. A third mechanism for internalization of material from the exterior is called *receptor-mediated endocytosis*. This is a more specific mechanism in which the substance in question, such as a peptide hormone, interacts with receptors on the cell surface that are associated with coated pits. Coated pits are depressions in the cell membrane lined by electron-dense material in which a unique protein, *clathrin*, has been identified. Coated pits, with their bound material, are internalized as vesicles. Material internalized in this way appears to be able to follow a different route from that internalized by phagocytosis or pinocytosis. Instead of fusing with lysosomes, the material apparently may pass directly to elements of the Golgi apparatus or ER or to an intermediate compartment where the contents may be transferred for further transport. The contents of the vesicles and the membrane components can be separated, and the membrane, together with receptors, can be returned to the surface of the cell.

Phagocytosis is an important part of the defense armamentarium of the animal. Both neutrophils and macrophages are capable of recognizing foreign material, including invading organisms, and ingesting it. These cells add a special adaptation to the process by secreting additional enzymes, capable of killing organisms, into the phagosome. In the case of neutrophils, the enzymes are contained in the *specific granules,* which fuse with the phagosome along with lysosomes. The role of lysosomes in host defenses and in disease in general is further discussed later in this chapter and in Chapters 4 and 7.

THE CYTOSKELETON: MICROTUBULES AND CYTOPLASMIC FILAMENTS

It is now evident that the complex, dynamic, spatial organization of essentially all cells involves the interaction of three classes of filaments that collectively are referred to as the *cytoskeleton.* These are *microfilaments, microtubules,* and *intermediate filaments.* The cytoskeleton is considered to be important in the maintenance of cell shape and in cell movement.

Microfilaments are about 6 nm in diameter, are based on *actin,* and are most familiar as the classic thin filaments in muscle cells. However, nonmuscle cells also contain actin as well as numerous actin-associated proteins involved either in contraction and cell movement or in the regulation of microfilament formation. Microfilaments are involved in several distinct fiber systems. *Stress fibers* contain bundles of microfilaments and are believed to be involved in anchoring the cytoplasmic matrix to the substrate though they are also contractile. They are most commonly found in cultured cells and only rarely *in vivo,* though they have been found in certain pathological conditions, including in the endothelial cells of rats with experimental hypertension. Stress fiber–like filaments have also been described in the Schwann cells of dogs with an inherited demyelinating neuropathy. Microfilaments also form thinner bundles and meshlike arrangements that seem to be involved in maintaining the gel-like state of the cytoplasm. The microfilament system is complex from the molecular point of view. At least six molecular forms of actin are known, and actin exists in the cell either in its filamentous form, as F-actin, or as the monomeric, or globular, G-actin. There are many different regulatory proteins involved in the control of actin polymerization and the form that the resulting filaments adopt in the cell.

Microtubules are narrow cylinders, about 25 nm in diameter, formed by polymerization of the protein tubulin. They can be rapidly assembled and disassembled forming a dynamic component of the cytoskeleton. They are of variable length but may be quite long, perhaps 50 μm or more. Microtubules are also associated with other proteins, the so-called *microtubule-associated proteins,* which are believed in many cases to cross-link the microtubules to other cytoskeletal components. Microtubules are prominent components of flagella, cilia, and the mitotic spindle as well as of neurotubules in axons. However, they are present in all cells. They generally are considered to be important in the maintenance of cell shape, in the beating movement of flagella and cilia, and in the movement of chromosomes in cell division. They are important in the internal organization of the cell and the movement of cytoplasmic organelles and granules. For this reason they are intimately involved in the process of cellular secretion. Microtubules also are believed to play a role in cell movement by interacting with microfilaments. In particular, they seem to be important in coordinating directional movement. For example, if microtubules are destroyed (using the drug colchicine), the treated cells retain the ability to move but lose the ability to respond to directional stimuli. Microtubules are obviously important in the function of phagocytes such as neutrophils and are therefore important to the defense of the host. Defects in microtubules or their associated proteins are also known to cause abnormalities in the function of cilia in humans and in dogs. Because of the role of cilia in pulmonary clearance and defense (see Chapter 7), these defects commonly result in chronic respiratory infections.

Intermediate filaments form the third group of cytoskeletal filaments. They have a diameter of 7 to 11 nm and are believed to play a role in the maintenance of the cell's shape. There are five types of intermediate filaments made up of biochemically and antigenically related, yet distinct, proteins. The different intermediate filaments are tissue specific. *Cytokeratins,* which include the keratin of keratinizing stratified epithelia, are found in epithelial cells of all types and are the constitutional protein of the tonofilaments. Epithelia may even be subclassified based on the types of cytokeratins they contain. *Vimentin* is found in mesenchymal cells such as fibroblasts and certain other nonepithelial cells. *Desmin* is found in skeletal and cardiac muscle cells as well as in visceral smooth muscle and some vascular smooth muscle cells. Some vascular smooth muscle cells contain vimentin. *Glial fibrillary acidic protein* (GFAP) is found in astrocytes, in intestinal glial cells, and apparently in some Schwann cells. Astrocytes may co-express GFAP and vimentin. Finally, the triplet of *neurofilament proteins* are found in neuronal neurofilaments in the central and peripheral nervous systems. Using appropriate specific antibodies and immunocytochemistry one can identify the type of intermediate filament expressed in cell populations.

This is particularly important in the identification of neoplasms (see Chapter 6). For example, carcinomas arising from epithelial cells express cytokeratins, astrogliomas express GFAP, and tumors arising from muscle cells express desmin. Because tissue-specific intermediate filament type seems to be preserved even in many poorly differentiated neoplasms, intermediate filament proteins can act as *markers,* allowing classification of neoplasms that might be otherwise difficult to recognize.

The various components of the cytoskeleton are also linked to the plasma membrane and its proteins. They are believed to be important in the regulation of the movement of surface molecules, the stability of the plasma membrane, and such functions as phagocytosis. A defect in a cytoskeletal protein closely associated with the sarcolemma of skeletal muscle fibers leads to a severe form of muscular dystrophy in animals and humans.

PEROXISOMES

Peroxisomes are small roughly spherical organelles up to 1.5 μm in diameter. They are bounded by a single membrane and have a fairly homogeneous, moderately electron-dense internal structure. Morphologically peroxisomes, which apparently are derived from ER, resemble lysosomes but can be distinguished from the latter by their enzyme content. Also, they often contain a structure called a *nucleoid,* which is not found in lysosomes. Peroxisomes contain several enzymes related to the metabolism of hydrogen peroxide. Urate oxidase, D-amino acid oxidase, and α-hydroxy acid oxidase produce hydrogen peroxide, and catalase destroys it.

The role of peroxisomes in disease is not clear, but their enzyme content indicates that they may be involved in the destruction of hydrogen peroxide, a substance that may injure cells. They are potentially involved in cell injury caused by reactive oxygen metabolites, discussed below.

This review of the structure of the normal cell and the essential functions of its organelles is necessarily brief. The student who feels unfamiliar with this material is recommended to read a text in medical cell biology. It is a truism, but worth stating anyway, that we cannot appreciate the abnormal before we adequately understand the normal.

The Cytocavitary Network and Movement of Cell Membranes

Many of the membrane-bound cytoplasmic organelles that we have just discussed are considered to belong to a functionally contiguous system referred to as the *cytocavitary network.* This includes lysosomes, phagosomes, residual bodies, secretory granules, the Golgi apparatus, the endoplasmic reticulum (both SER and RER), peroxisomes, and the nuclear envelope (see Fig. 2-5).

These organelles are interconnected functionally by a series of membrane fusions and buddings, which provide directed traffic of membranes and contents of vesicles within the cell. For example, many proteins synthesized in the RER are transported to the Golgi for modification. This is accomplished by way of vesicles that bud from the ER and move to the Golgi, where they fuse. Similarly, phagosomes transport phagocytosed material to the lysosomes, and secretory vesicles transport material to the cell surface. There is now much evidence that the membrane involved in this traffic is recycled. For example, membrane that fuses with the plasma membrane in a secretory event is internalized and transported back to the Golgi for reuse. In this way the cell avoids a great deal of wastage. Both the Golgi apparatus and coated vesicles appear to play major roles in directing the movement of intracellular membrane traffic.

Presumably the cytoskeleton is important in providing direction to this membrane traffic. Integral proteins are limited in their lateral movement in the plasma membrane, and this seems to be attributable to connections with the cytoskeleton. It is believed that cytoskeletal elements can control the movement of membrane proteins, such as receptors, which would be important in phenomena such as capping and patching.

Dr. B.F. Trump and his colleagues introduced the terms *esotropy* and *exotropy* to describe the processes involved in fusion and budding of membranes. As shown in Fig. 2-8, esotropy involves the turning in of the membrane into the cell sap, followed by membrane fusion and the formation of a new membrane-bound vesicle. The inside of the vesicle is therefore topologically equivalent to the extracellular space. Exotropy involves the turning out of the membrane toward the extracellular space or the cytocavitary space followed by fusion to form a budded-off particle containing cell sap. Each of these processes can occur in either the forward or the reverse direction.

Forward esotropy includes such processes as pinocytosis and phagocytosis, the formation of vesicles from the ER for transport to the Golgi apparatus, and the formation of secretory granules from the Golgi. Reverse esotropy includes the fusion of secretory vesicles with the plasma membrane and the fusion of the phagosome with the lysosome. Examples of forward exotropy are autophagy, cell di-

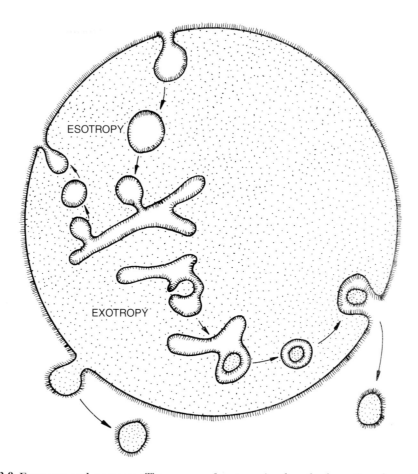

Fig. 2-8 Esotropy and exotropy. The process of esotropy involves the formation of membrane-bound structures in which the orientation of the membrane is reversed. The inside of such structures is equivalent to the extracellular surface of the plasma membrane. The process of exotropy maintains the orientation of the membrane and results in a structure containing cell sap. *(Adapted from Trump BF, McDowell EM, Arstila AU: Cellular reaction to injury. In Hill RB, LaVia MF, editors:* Principles of pathobiology, *New York, 1980, Oxford University Press.)*

vision, some forms of secretion (such as the secretion of lipid from mammary epithelial cells), and the budding of many enveloped viruses into the extracellular space or the cytocavitary space. Reverse exotropy is encountered in cell fusion as occurs in the formation of multinucleate giant cells from macrophages or in the formation of multinucleate skeletal muscle cells from myoblasts during embryogenesis or repair of skeletal muscle.

Cellular Adaptation

Cells normally exist and carry out their functions within a fairly narrow range of physicochemical conditions. Intracellular pH, the concentration of electrolytes, and a host of other factors are closely controlled by the cell. The maintenance of these conditions, that is, those compatible with cell survival and function, is called *homeostasis,* and serious de-

parture from the norm in some of them results in damage to the cell. In response to certain stimuli or altered demands, however, the cell can undergo adaptation. To accommodate these changed conditions, the cell establishes new levels of metabolic or other functional activity without impairment of its ability to survive. Usually these functional changes can be correlated with morphological alterations in the cell. Adaptive changes very often are seen as a response to altered work load. An example that is cited often is the increase in muscle mass that accompanies physical work such as weight lifting. This is a very obvious example, but many more subtle alterations may occur. The hepatocyte, for example, if subjected to increased need to detoxify drugs or toxins, as explained below, can increase its capacity to do so. The ability of the entire animal to respond to changes in its environment is therefore largely accounted for by the adaptive capacity of its constituent cells. Cells may respond by either increasing or decreasing their content of specific organelles.

ATROPHY

When a tissue or organ undergoes a reduction in mass, the process is known as "atrophy." Such a loss of substance can be caused by loss of cells (Fig. 2-9) or to reduction in size of individual cells (Fig. 2-10). In the latter case, atrophy is an adaptive response to altered demands on the cell, often a reduction in work load. In addition, loss of innervation or of hormonal stimulation, reduced blood supply or inadequate nutrition all can lead to atrophy of cells. Thus muscles that are denervated or are, for some reason, used less than usual will undergo atrophy accounted for by shrinkage of their constituent cells (see Fig. 2-10). The adrenal gland deprived of stimulation by ACTH will undergo adrenocortical atrophy, and the animal deprived of an adequate food supply will be thin, partly caused by atrophy of muscle cells. It is important to recognize that *atrophic cells are not dead* or really even injured. They have reduced functional capacity but retain the ability to control their internal environment and to pro-

duce sufficient energy to suit their new level of activity. Because they are still alive, they can adapt again if subjected at some later date to more normal functional demands. Therefore the muscles that have undergone atrophy as a result of immobilization will, given time, regain their normal bulk and strength when returned to use. This phrase "given time" is of considerable potential importance to the clinical consequences of some lesions involving atrophy. A common cause of adrenal cortical atrophy, for example, is excessive, prolonged treatment with corticosteroids. Because these drugs inhibit the release of ACTH from the adenohypophysis, the adrenal cortical cells are not stimulated as they normally would be and so undergo atrophy. It is very important to realize that the sudden withdrawal of the exogenous corticosteroids will produce a situation in which atrophic adrenal cortical cells suddenly are called upon to secrete sufficient cortisol to meet the needs of the animal, a demand that they simply may not be able to meet. The result may be acute adrenal cortical insufficiency, a potentially dangerous clinical syndrome known as "addisonian crisis." In contrast, gradual withdrawal of the drug will allow the adrenal glands to respond and adapt to progres-

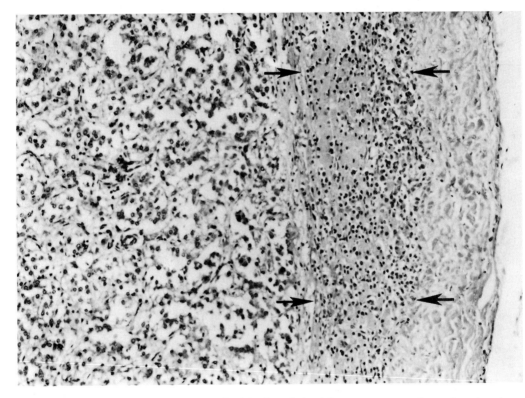

Fig. 2-9 Atrophy caused by necrosis. In this adrenal gland the cortex, *arrows*, is greatly reduced in thickness because of necrosis of adrenal cortical cells. The cells remaining are macrophages and a few infiltrating lymphocytes.

sively increasing functional demands thus avoiding a potentially lethal situation.

The mechanisms by which cells undergo atrophy, in particular the signals that trigger the process, are poorly understood. There is, however, actual loss of substance from the cell. In the case of muscle cells undergoing atrophy, for example, there is loss of myofilaments, mitochondria, and endoplasmic reticulum as well as reduced metabolic activity. In other words, catabolic processes exceed anabolic processes. One morphological manifestation of this process may be the formation of increased numbers of autophagic vacuoles, formed as the cell breaks down redundant organelles.

Finally, tissue atrophy may involve the death of cells. In many cases, especially in physiological circumstances, this involves the process of *apoptosis* (see below). In other cases loss of cells is a late stage event. For example, in denervated muscle, the long-term loss of the trophic influences of innervation eventually leads to actual loss of myocytes. Once that has happened, of course, it may be impossible to fully reverse the process. In other cases, atrophy may be reversed by the process of physiological hyperplasia.

HYPERTROPHY

When cells are subjected to increased functional demands, or increased work, they may enlarge, and, as a result, the whole organ or tissue mass also enlarges. Hypertrophy, then, is an adaptive response by which organs are increased in size as a result of an increase in cell size without cellular proliferation. The most striking example again occurs in skeletal muscle that is subjected to an unusual work load. We are all familiar with the increased muscle mass that results from weight lifting. A similar process can occur in the heart so that highly trained athletes may have hearts that are enlarged as a result of the increased physiological demands placed on them. Myocardial hypertrophy also, of course, can be attributable to pathological conditions that impose an abnormal work load on the heart. This is seen in stenotic valvular disease, in which the blood must be ejected through an abnormally narrow valvular opening. This requires more work by the myocardium, and hypertrophy results (Fig. 2-11).

Although the nature of the signal to the cell is poorly understood, hypertrophy involves an increase in total cellular proteins, including myofibrils in muscle cells as well as organelles such as mito-

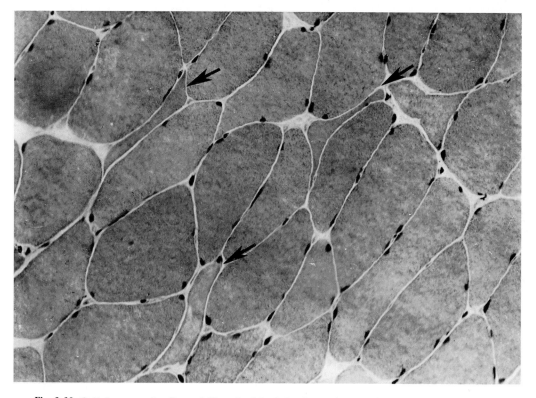

Fig. 2-10 Cellular atrophy. Several fibers in this skeletal muscle are reduced in diameter and angular in shape, *arrows*. Atrophy of muscle fibers in this case was attributable to denervation. The atrophic cells are still viable.

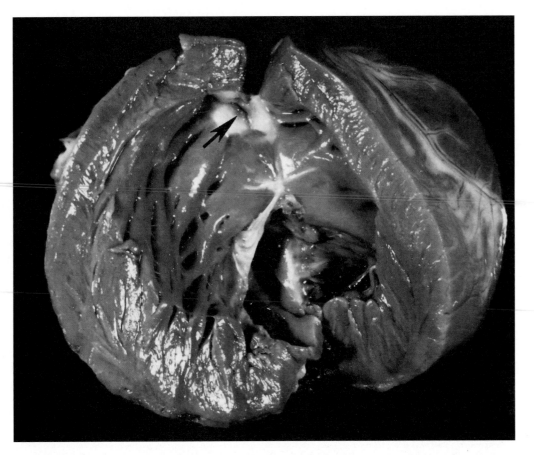

Fig. 2-11 Myocardial hypertrophy. Heart from a dog with pulmonic stenosis. The wall of the right ventricle, the cut surface of which is shown, is greatly thickened because of the increased work required to force blood through the stenotic pulmonary valve, *arrow*.

chondria and ER. There is increased synthesis of cellular constituents, and anabolic processes exceed catabolic ones.

Cellular hypertrophy may not always be to the advantage of the animal. In the case of the heart, in particular, there seems to be some limit beyond which hypertrophy cannot compensate for an underlying lesion or disease process. Hypertrophy may, in addition, produce conformational changes in the heart that lead to inefficient pumping. There is some evidence that, despite the increased numbers of mitochondria, the energy metabolism of hypertrophied myocytes is unable to meet the demands of the increased work load placed on the heart. All these factors can contribute to eventual heart failure despite the attempt of the individual cells to adapt to the altered circumstances.

In some cases there are more subtle changes in which cellular adaptation leads to hypertrophy of a specific organelle system. This is most dramatically illustrated in the liver by the induction, or hypertrophy, of smooth endoplasmic reticulum in animals treated with certain drugs or toxins. It was pointed out earlier in this chapter that the SER is associated with certain enzyme systems. These include a complex of enzymes, known as the *mixed-function oxidase* system, that is responsible for the metabolism of a variety of drugs and toxins. Over a period of time, exposure to a drug such as phenobarbital induces increased levels of these enzymes, a phenomenon manifested morphologically by a dramatic proliferation of the SER (Fig. 2-12). The inducing drug is more rapidly destroyed and, as a result, often has a more transient effect on the treated animal.

When proliferation of the SER occurs in response to a particular drug, there is also an enhanced capacity to detoxify other substances metabolized by the same system. This may be advantageous to the animal, but, when the intermediate products of metabolism are themselves highly toxic or when relatively high levels of reactive oxygen metabolites are produced, it can be extremely harmful. A classic example is the enhanced toxicity of carbon tetrachloride in animals pretreated with drugs such as phenobarbital. The toxicity of carbon tetrachloride is caused by free radicals produced as intermediate

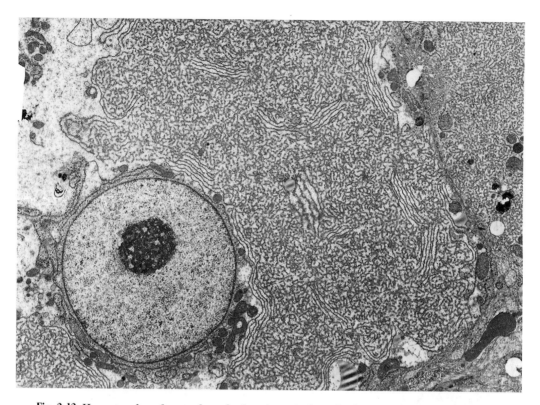

Fig. 2-12 Hypertrophy of smooth endoplasmic reticulum. In this liver cell most of the cytoplasm is occupied by smooth endoplasmic reticulum. This increase was induced by prolonged treatment of a dog with the drug primidone. *(Courtesy Dr. W.L. Castleman, Gainesville, Fla.)*

metabolites (see below), and the more rapid production of these in the animal with hypertrophy of the SER results in much more extensive hepatocellular damage

Hyperplasia and *metaplasia* also may be adaptive responses. Because they involve alterations in patterns of proliferation and differentiation, we have chosen to discuss them, together with other disorders of growth, in Chapter 6.

CELL INJURY AND CELL DEATH

So far, we have reviewed the structure and function of the normal cell and have seen how it can adapt, within limits, to changes in the demands made on it. When these demands reach the point at which there is impairment of the cell's overall functional capacity, the cell is said to be injured. Cell injury can be defined simply as any change that results in a loss of the ability to maintain the normal or adapted homeostasis or, in other words, loss of the ability to respond to appropriate functional demands. Injured cells therefore are unable to keep in balance all the processes that normally regulate their internal environment. As a result, a variety of morphological changes occur that we recognize as indications of cell injury.

The extent of injury to the cell can vary and depends on its severity, the cause, the type of cell involved, and its metabolic state at the time of the insult. In the case of sublethal injury, the changes in the cell may be relatively mild and are compatible with its continued survival. Such injury is reversible, and with removal of the stimulus the cell may revert to normal structure and function. The distinction between pronounced adaptation and mild injury therefore is difficult to define.

Reversible cell injury is sometimes referred to as *degeneration* and, traditionally, various manifestations of injury have been given specific names such as "cloudy swelling," "hydropic degeneration," and "fatty degeneration," according to the microscopic appearance of the affected cells. These terms will be clarified when we consider the morphological changes that occur in injured cells. For now, suffice it to say that current understanding of pathogenetic mechanisms indicates that they do not represent separate processes, and it is preferable to abandon these terms and use the simple term "cell injury."

The rate at which the changes in injured cells occur can vary widely. Acute injury produces rapid changes, which may be lethal to the cell if not quickly reversed, whereas chronic injury may persist for months or even years without the cell being killed.

If the insult is severe, injury may progress to the point where *irreversible cell injury* occurs, and the cell dies. Conceptually, cell death means that the changes in the injured cell can no longer be reversed. How cells die, either as the result of physiological or pathological processes, has been the subject of intense research interest in recent years and has led to the realization that cells can die in two ways (see Fig. 2-20): as a result of apoptosis, a process in which the cell actively participates, or as a result of nonapoptotic mechanisms, in which damage to cell membranes and organelles becomes lethal. The latter pathway is known as "necrosis." These processes are discussed in more detail later.

Morphology of Cell Injury
LIGHT MICROSCOPIC CHANGES

The most fundamental change in reversibly injured cells is swelling. *Cell swelling* is an early and almost universal manifestation of nonlethal injury. Re-

cently the term ~~oncosis~~ has been proposed to represent the process of cell injury with swelling, but the term has not yet gained great acceptance. In the light microscope, swollen cells are enlarged, which is particularly evident when they compress adjacent structures. In the liver, for example, hepatocellular swelling may compress sinusoids sufficiently to obliterate their lumens (Figs. 2-13 and 2-14). In mildly swollen cells the staining characteristics may be altered, producing a somewhat cloudy appearance. It is this lesion that used to be called "cloudy swelling." As the process progresses, vacuoles of variable size appear in the cytoplasm giving rise to the appearance sometimes called "hydropic degeneration," or "vacuolar degeneration."

Some caution should be exercised in making assumptions about the nature of vacuoles in injured cells. Commonly they represent distended organelles, most often distended ER, but in other cases they may be small lipid droplets or nonmembrane bound areas devoid of cytoplasmic organelles. Special techniques may be required to demonstrate the real nature of vacuoles. Special stains can identify lipids in vacuoles, and electron microscopy can identify distended organelles.

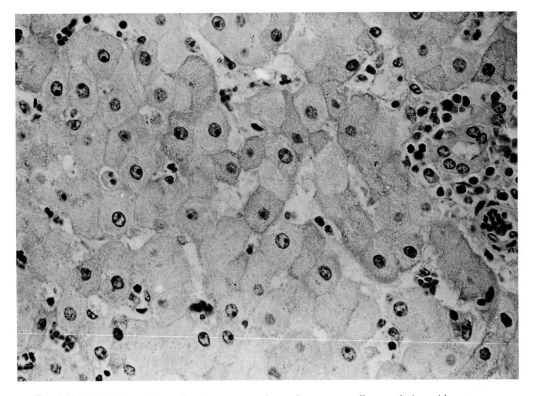

Fig. 2-13 Mild cell swelling. The hepatocytes shown here are swollen, and sinusoids are compressed. The cytoplasm of the cells is finely vacuolated. Such vacuoles usually represent dilated cisternae of the endoplasmic reticulum, but very small lipid droplets also might be present.

Cell swelling results from uptake of water caused by increased intracellular osmotic load and loss of the cell's normally precise control of movement of ions and water across the cell membrane. Increased osmotic load results from the generation of osmotically active molecules by continued cellular metabolism. These include breakdown products of ATP and creatine phosphate, as well as lactate. Cell swelling per se is not incompatible with survival of the cell. In fact, it often reflects relatively mild, reversible injury.

Cells that are so severely injured that they are destined to die also undergo swelling. Unfortunately it can be difficult to distinguish, at the light microscopic level, between a cell that is swollen because of reversible injury and one fortuitously fixed during its progression to cell death or even one fixed just after cell death has occurred. The alterations that occur in cells that make them microscopically recognizable as being dead actually represent degradative changes that take place after cell death, a process called *necrosis*. From the diagnostic viewpoint, however, the assessment of lesions in the light microscope is not quite so imprecise as this discussion might make it seem. In injured tissues, cells are usually present in various stages of injury.

If, for example, the majority of cells are swollen and many are actually necrotic, we would assume the injury to be more serious than one in which most cells are swollen without evidence of necrosis. The presence of necrotic cells, in other words, would indicate that many of the accompanying swollen, injured cells were dying or already dead (see Fig. 2-37).

Lipidosis, or fatty change, the accumulation of excessive intracellular lipid, is another common manifestation of reversible injury. It is seen most commonly in cells that normally metabolize a lot of fat. Lipidosis can affect renal tubular epithelial cells, cardiac myocytes, and especially hepatocytes. Morphologically it is characterized by the presence of lipid-filled vacuoles in the cytoplasm of affected cells (Fig. 2-15). Lipidosis is most easily recognized when the cytoplasm contains single, large, clearly demarcated vacuoles, but in some cases the vacuoles may be small and multiple. The presence of fat in vacuoles may be confirmed when frozen sections of the tissue are stained with an oil-soluble dye such as "oil red O." Frozen sections are necessary to avoid extraction of the fat by solvents used in conventional histological preparations. The pathogenetic mechanisms responsible for the accu-

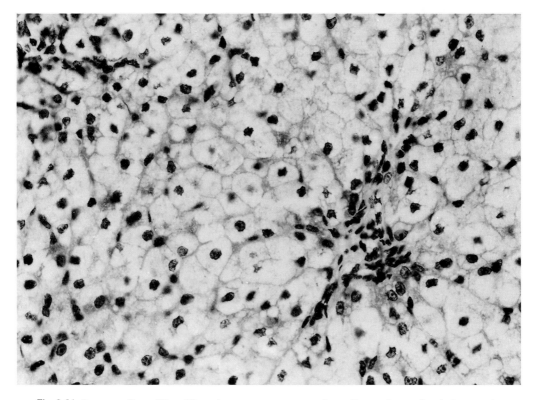

Fig. 2-14 Severe cell swelling. These hepatocytes are severely swollen and vacuolated. As a result, the sinusoids are obliterated. The vacuoles mostly reflect greatly distended cisternae of the endoplasmic reticulum, but an increase in lipid vacuoles contributes to this appearance.

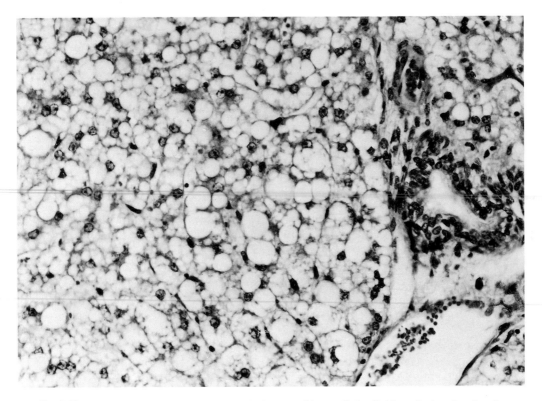

Fig. 2-15 Lipidosis. These hepatocytes contain increased intracellular lipid producing the sharply demarcated vacuoles seen here. Lipidosis may produce single large cytoplasmic vacuoles (macrovesicular) or multiple small vacuoles (microvesicular). Both types of vacuolation are present in this micrograph.

mulation of lipid in injured cells are considered in more detail later in this chapter.

Finally, injured cells may show alterations in nuclear morphology. In sublethal injury these changes are relatively subtle and consist in some clumping in the distribution of chromatin. Dramatic changes in nuclear morphology are usually indicative of cell death.

Ultrastructural Changes

The morphological changes that occur in injured cells can be appreciated at an earlier stage and can be better understood when their ultrastructure is studied. In the electron microscope changes can be detected in individual organelles, some being affected before others.

In the plasma membrane, the major change seen is the loss of surface specializations. Microvilli or cilia may be lost (Fig. 2-16), and intercellular attachments may break down. In addition, changes in cell outline, such as the formation of cytoplasmic blebs, may be seen.

Mitochondria commonly are altered in injured cells. Early in the process they may be condensed, with contraction of the inner mitochondrial com-

partment. This phase is transient, however, and they soon undergo swelling (Fig. 2-17) and even may rupture. Injured mitochondria lose their normal dense granules, but abnormal dense amorphous deposits may appear in the matrix. In addition, deposits of calcium salts may be formed in damaged mitochondria.

Another common change seen in injured cells and one that often accounts for the vacuolated appearance seen at the light microscopic level is dilatation of the endoplasmic reticulum (Fig. 2-18). Like cell swelling, it is presumably attributable to changes in the movement of ions and water across membranes, in this case those of the ER. In addition, ribosomes disaggregate and detach from the surface of the RER. Not surprisingly, this change is associated with impaired protein synthesis.

As injury progresses, the membranes of organelles may be disrupted and may lose phospholipids. Because of their amphipathic nature these molecules tend to reaggregate in the cytosol and spontaneously form membrane-like whorls often called *myelin figures* (Fig. 2-19).

As a fairly late change in cell injury, lysosomes also may be altered. They may swell and eventually rupture. Lysosomes tend to retain their functional

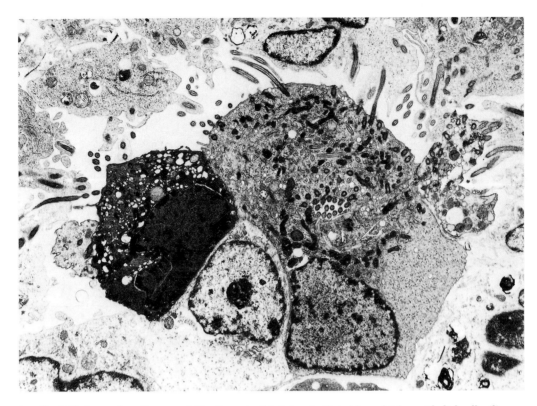

Fig. 2-16 Loss of surface specializations. In this injured ciliated bronchiolar epithelial cell, cilia have been lost by internalization. Cilia can be seen free in the cytoplasm. The very dark cell on the *left* is necrotic. Notice the cytoplasmic vacuolation. *(Courtesy Dr. W.L. Castleman, Gainesville, Fla.)*

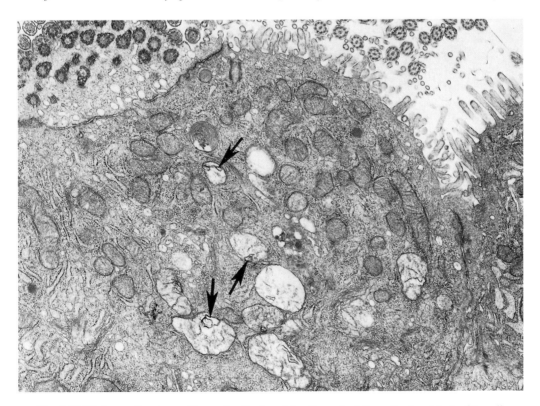

Fig. 2-17 High-amplitude swelling of mitochondria. Several of the mitochondria in this cell have undergone high-amplitude swelling. The presence of membranous arrays in some of them, *arrows*, is suggestive of damage to the inner mitochondrial membrane. *(Courtesy Dr. W.L. Castleman, Gainesville, Fla.)*

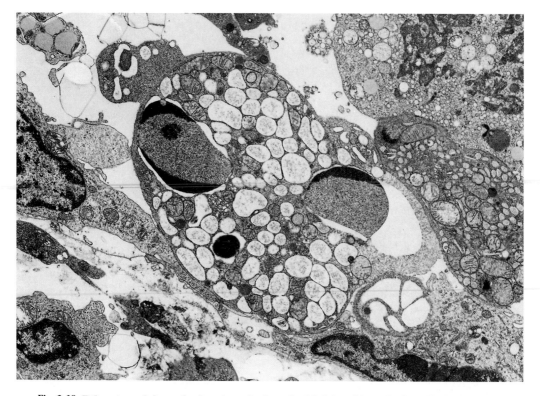

Fig. 2-18 Dilatation of the endoplasmic reticulum. In this injured bronchiolar cell, the cisternae of the rough endoplasmic reticulum are dilated. Notice the condensation of nuclear chromatin, characteristic of apoptosis. This cell therefore shows features of both apoptosis and necrotic injury. *(Courtesy Dr. W.L. Castleman, Gainesville, Fla.)*

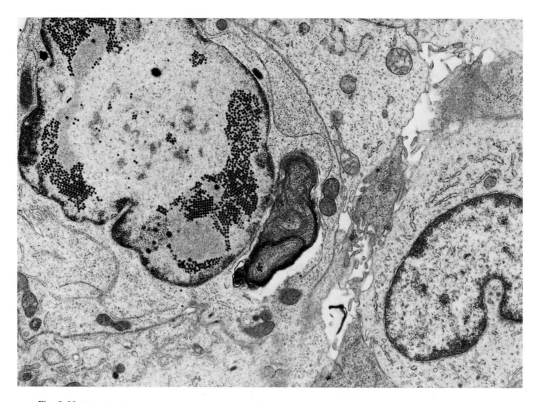

Fig. 2-19 Myelin figure. In this injured bronchiolar epithelial cell from a dog, a large myelin figure, with concentric swirls of membranous material, is present in the cytoplasm. Adenovirus particles can be seen in the nucleus. *(Courtesy Dr. W.L. Castleman, Gainesville, Fla.)*

capacity until late in the process of cell injury. As a result, they fuse with vacuoles containing the remains of injured cell organelles, and many autophagosomes may be found in injured cells. The enzymes released from damaged lysosomes are partly responsible for the breakdown of cell constituents that characterizes necrosis. However, it is generally believed that, in most forms of cell injury, by the time lysosomal enzymes escape into the cytoplasm, the cell is already dead. In certain cases, lysosomal enzymes may contribute actively to the injury to the cell.

Lethal Cell Injury: Apoptosis and Necrosis

As already mentioned, research in the last decade or so has led to the realization that there are two major pathways to cell death, namely, *apoptosis,* sometimes referred to as programmed cell death or cellular suicide, and cell death with *necrosis* (Fig. 2-20). Apoptosis is a process in which the cell actively participates in its own demise, whereas necrosis is a degradative process that occurs after nonapoptotic lethal cell injury. This terminology is somewhat unsatisfactory for many reasons. There is overlap between the two processes, and diverse injurious stimuli can lead to either apoptosis or necrosis, depending on prevailing conditions. For example, ischemia or hypoxia may initiate either apoptosis or necrosis depending in part on the severity of the insult. Furthermore, necrosis really refers to the degradative processes that occur after cell death and so is not really appropriate as a term describing a mechanism of cell death. To overcome this problem, the term *oncotic cell death,* to describe cell death accompanied by cell swelling, has been proposed. However, this term has not yet become widely accepted.

Apoptosis

A unique form of cellular destruction, termed "apoptosis," has long been recognized by pathologists because of its distinctive morphological appearance. Apoptosis is characterized by cell shrinkage, rapid condensation of nuclear chromatin and cytoplasm, convolution of the cell, and subsequent separation of fragments of the cell into *apoptotic bodies* (see Figs. 2-18, 2-21, and 2-22). Apoptotic bodies typically consist of nuclear fragments contained within a cytoplasmic mass in which organelle integrity is initially maintained, with all this enclosed within plasma membrane that is initially morphologically intact. The condensation of chromatin re-

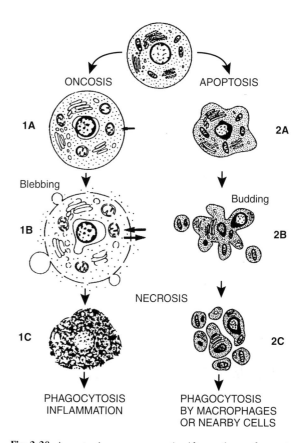

Fig. 2-20 Apoptosis versus oncosis. Alternative pathways to cell death are shown schematically. **1A,** Swelling. **1B,** Vacuolization, blebbing, and increased permeability. **1C,** Necrotic changes, that is, coagulation, shrinkage, and karyolysis. **2A,** Shrinkage and pyknosis. **2B,** Budding and karyorrhexis. **2C,** Breakup into a cluster of apoptotic bodies. *(Adapted from Majno G, Joris I: Am J Pathol 146:3-15, 1995.)*

sults in characteristic dense masses that abut the nuclear membrane (see Figs. 2-18 and 2-22). Apoptosis is a rapid process. Apoptotic bodies are phagocytosed by adjacent cells, both macrophages and tissue cells such as epithelial or neoplastic cells, and degraded within phagolysosomes. Because apoptotic cells do not release cellular constituents, they provoke essentially no inflammatory reaction. Although it is not always easy to distinguish apoptotic from nonapoptotic cell injury in conventional histopathological preparations, it is now clear that apoptosis and necrosis should be defined as distinct processes (Table 2-2).

Apoptosis can be induced by both physiological and pathological processes. It is seen in cells undergoing programmed cell death during development, in cells undergoing normal turnover in postnatal tissues, in physiological involution of tissues and in some forms of pathological tissue atrophy, in elimination of autoreactive lymphocytes, and in regression of hyperplasia. It is also commonly seen in malignant neoplasms, and in situations in which cell destruction is induced by cell-mediated immune reactions. For example, apoptosis has been observed in many diseases in which cell-mediated immunity is believed to be of pathogenetic importance in the destruction of tissues. Certain toxins, drugs, mild hyperthermia, hypoxia, and irradiation can also induce apoptosis.

Apoptosis is a coordinated process, often energy dependent. It involves the activation of a newly recognized group of cysteine proteases called *caspases* (cleaving at Cysteine-ASPartic residues, hence "cas-pase"). These enzymes are capable of cleaving cytoskeletal proteins and nuclear lamins, partly accounting for the morphological changes that accompany apoptosis, of activating one another, and of activating endonucleases involved in internucleosomal breakdown of DNA. Activation of caspases involves a complex cascade of events linking the initiating stimuli to the final destruction of the cell.

Our understanding of the mechanisms involved in apoptosis in mammalian cells has grown from an understanding of programmed cell death as it occurs during the development of the worm *Caenorhabditis elegans*, during which exactly 131

TABLE 2-2 Comparative Features of Apoptosis and Necrosis

FEATURE	APOPTOSIS	NECROSIS
Distribution	Usually single cells	Often contiguous cells
Cell size and shape	Shrinkage and convolution	Swelling
Nuclear morphology	Chromatin condensation; nuclear fragmentation	Lysis
Plasma membrane	Intact until phagocytosed	Damaged, leaky
Cytoplasm	Retained in apoptotic bodies	Contents released
Inflammation	Absent	Typically present

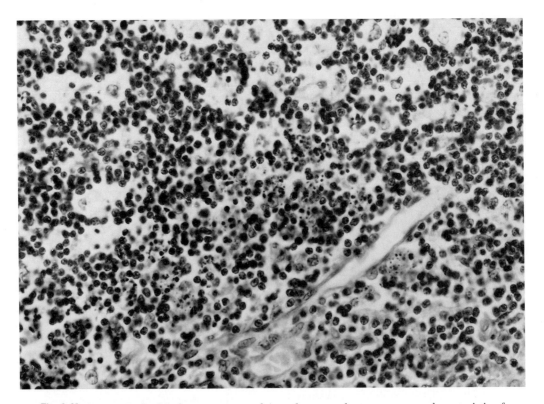

Fig. 2-21 Apoptosis. In this thymus many nuclei are fragmented, an appearance characteristic of apoptosis at the light microscopic level. The large pale cells are macrophages phagocytosing the apoptotic bodies. This appearance of nuclear fragmentation used to be referred to as "karyorrhexis."

cells die leaving 959 surviving cells. These numbers are unimportant except that they demonstrate the extraordinary accuracy and control in this system. In the worm, these events are now known to be controlled by a limited set of *ced* genes, which encode the CED proteins. In response to a death signal, CED-4 binds to an inactive precursor of CED-3, thus activating it. Together these proteins are responsible for the process of apoptosis. A membrane protein, CED-9 can bind to CED-4, preventing its activation of CED-3 and thus inhibiting the apoptotic pathway. Related genes and proteins involved in apoptosis have been discovered in mammalian cells. Although the mammalian system is much more complex (Fig. 2-23), the general scheme is similar. Death signals are transduced by so-called adaptor proteins, analogous to CED-4, which in turn transmit the signal to initiator caspases committing the cell to apoptosis. Additional enzymes known as executioner caspases, analogous to CED-3, are in turn activated leading to the morphological changes typical of apoptosis. Mammalian cells also have a complex system of positive and negative controls regulating apoptosis.

Death signals may be either extracellular, transmitted through the plasma membrane, or intracellular. Extracellular signals may be positive or negative. Positive signals include the interaction of ligands with receptors such as the tumor necrosis factor family of receptors (TNFR). Negative signals arise from interaction of receptors with hormones, growth factors, and other cytokines, which suppress apoptosis. Withdrawal of such factors leads to loss of suppression and results in apoptosis being activated. Examples of this loss of suppression are provided by tissue remodeling in response to the cycling of reproductive hormones. Intracellular signals include the response to a variety of injurious stimuli such as radiation, toxic insults, hyperthermia, and hypoxia.

Transduction of death signals is carried out by adaptor proteins, which link the death signal to activation of initiator caspases. A variety of regulatory proteins may be involved at this stage. These include Bcl-2, the mammalian homolog of CED-9, which can inhibit apoptosis, and Apaf-1, the homolog of CED-4, which promotes apoptosis. The mammalian Bcl-2 family is very complex, containing many related proteins, some of which are negative regulators of apoptosis and some of which are promoters. Mitochondria are also involved in the transduction of the apoptotic signals, which can activate the so-called mitochondrial permeability transition (PT), a pore that results in loss of mitochondrial membrane potential, deenergization, and mitochondrial swelling. Apoptotic signals can also cause the mitochondria to release cytochrome *c*, which is believed to be able to bind to Apaf-1, activating it, and triggering the initiator caspases. Bcl-2 is believed to regulate apoptosis by interfering with both of these steps.

Receptor-Mediated Apoptosis

Two important apoptotic pathways mediated by receptors in the plasma membrane have been identified. These are the Fas receptor, a transmembrane protein that is a member of the tumor necrosis factor (TNF) superfamily and the TNF (TNF-R1) receptor. Fas ligand (Fas-L) is also a membrane protein that induces apoptosis when it binds to Fas on a target cell. Fas and Fas-L are coexpressed in many tissues in which continuous cell turnover occurs. Fas and Fas-L are also known to be involved in deletion of autoreactive lymphocytes and in cell killing by cytotoxic T cells. For example, certain immune-privileged tissues express only Fas-L, the implication being that binding of an autoreactive lymphocyte bearing Fas to a cell bearing Fas-L would induce apoptosis in the lymphocyte.

Binding of Fas-L to Fas results in the binding of an adaptor protein, FADD (Fas-associated death

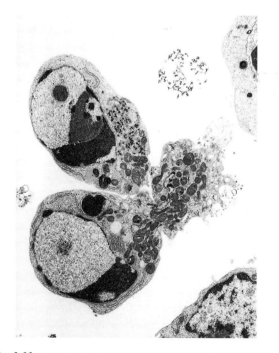

Fig. 2-22 Apoptosis. The process of apoptosis is shown in the NS-1 mouse myeloma cell line. Notice the constriction of the cell to form lobes containing organelles and nuclear fragments with characteristic dense chromatin masses. These lobes will bud off to form apoptotic bodies. *(Courtesy N.I. Walker et al:* Methods Achiev Exp Pathol *13:18-54, 1988.)*

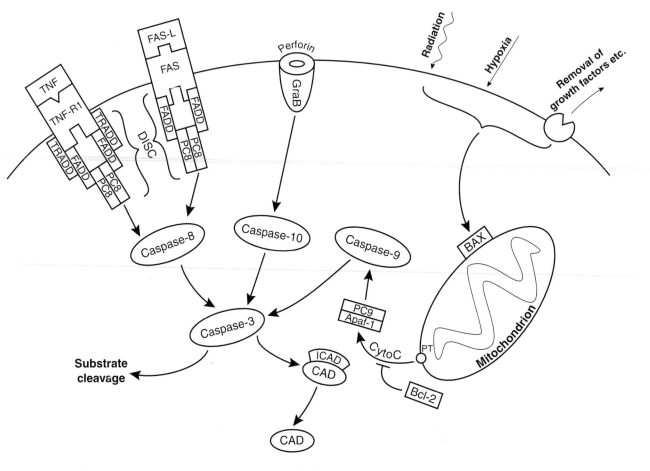

Fig. 2-23 Simplified diagram of some important pathways in apoptosis. Binding of the receptor FAS by FAS ligand (FAS-L) results in the recruitment of FADD and the activation of procaspase-8 (PC8) forming the DISC and generating the active enzyme, caspase-8. Similarly, binding of TNF to its membrane receptor, TNF-R1, recruits TRADD and FADD, again resulting in the activation of caspase-8. Insertion of granzyme B (GraB) by T cells by means of perforin results in the activation of caspase-10. Non−receptor mediated stimuli such as radiation or drugs, hypoxia, and removal of prosurvival stimuli such as growth factors can also lead to apoptosis. Pathways can include the association of Bax with the mitochondrial membrane and the release of cytochrome *c*. CytoC in turn binds to Apaf-1 and procaspase-9, forming the apoptosome and resulting in the generation of active caspase-9. Bcl-2 can inhibit this process. The initiator caspases caspase-8, -9, and -10 activate the executioner caspase, caspase-3, which can directly cleave cellular substrates. Caspase-3 also cleaves ICAD (inhibitor of CAD) from CAD (caspase-activated DNAse), which is then translocated to the nucleus where it cleaves DNA.

domain) to the intracellular death domain of Fas. This terminology can be a little confusing because both FADD and Fas have complementary death domains. FADD then associates with procaspase-8 by means of dimerization of the death effector domain (DED). This complex forms the so-called death-inducing signaling complex (DISC). Several other proteins may also be involved in the DISC, but they are not discussed in detail here.

The binding of TNF to TNF-R1 results in the binding of an adaptor protein TRADD (TNF receptor-associated death domain) with recruitment of FADD and another protein, RIP (receptor-interacting protein), and the activation of procaspase-8, thus assembling a similar DISC. In both cases the assembly of the DISC results in the activation of caspase-8 and the initiation of the caspase cascade, ultimately resulting in apoptosis.

Caspases

The caspases are a family of cysteine proteases with specificity for aspartate residues in their target substrates. They are present in the cell as proenzymes (zymogens) that are activated by proteolytic cleavage, often by other caspases, thus forming an activation cascade. They can also be autocatalytically activated. In many cases this is believed to be achieved when the molecules are brought into proximity through aggregation. The minimal enzymatic activity resident in the zymogen is then sufficient to cause cleavage. Some of the caspases, such as interleukin-1β–converting enzyme (ICE), are involved in proinflammatory events, but many of them are involved in apoptotic pathways.

The caspases can be classified into initiator and executioner groups. Caspase-3 is regarded as one of the most important of the executioner caspases, forming a final common pathway to cell destruction by proteolytically cleaving many important structural and functional proteins. There are several other executioner caspases. Caspase-3 can be activated by caspase-8, caspase-9, and caspase-10. Apaf-1, the mammalian homolog of CED-4, is one of a group of apoptotic protease-activating factors that seem to play a key role in the activation of downstream caspase-3. Apaf-1 is able to activate caspase-9, which then cleaves caspase-3. Caspase-10 is activated by granzyme B, which is inserted into target cells by cytotoxic T cells. In turn it can activate both caspase-3 and another executioner caspase, caspase-7. There is overlap and redundancy in these systems, allowing for alternative mechanisms for eliminating abnormal cells. For example, in the absence of caspase-10, granzyme B can activate other caspases, and it can even directly cleave other cellular substrates.

Caspases act on a wide variety of substrates including regulatory proteins, proteins involved in homeostatic and repair mechanisms, and structural elements such as cytoskeletal proteins and nuclear lamins, thus contributing to the morphological changes characteristic of apoptosis. In addition, caspases are responsible for the activation of the endonuclease that is responsible for the internucleosomal cleavage of DNA so characteristic of apoptosis. This enzyme, CAD (caspase-activated deoxyribonuclease) is present in the cytosol bound to an inhibitor ICAD. Caspase-3 cleaves the CAD-ICAD complex, freeing CAD to be relocated to the nucleus where it can act on DNA.

It should also be pointed out that inhibition of caspases does not necessarily prevent cell death after many types of apoptotic signals. The exception seems to be receptor-mediated apoptosis, where activation of caspases is required for completion of the process. These findings indicate that the commitment to cell death may occur upstream of caspase activation and that alternative pathways to cell death exist. These may involve alteration in mitochondrial function, as discussed below.

Role of Mitochondria in Apoptosis

As discussed elsewhere in this chapter, mitochondria are intimately involved in nonapoptotic cell injury (necrosis), where loss of ATP production may play an important pathogenetic role. It is now quite clear that mitochondria also play an active role in apoptosis and may even qualify as its primary regulator. To begin with, ATP appears to be required for some of the downstream events in apoptosis, indicating that some level of mitochondrial function may be necessary. In addition, many important reactants in apoptosis reside in the mitochondria. These include certain caspases and important regulatory proteins of the Bcl-2 family.

After many apoptotic stimuli, increased permeability of the outer mitochondrial membrane allows leakage of cytochrome c into the cytosol. Cytochrome c then associates with Apaf-1 and caspase-9 to form the so-called "apoptosome." As discussed above, activated caspase-9 in turn activates executioner caspases, leading to apoptosis. Furthermore, certain apoptotic stimuli, such as irradiation, induce loss of cytochrome c from mitochondria and cell death even when caspases are inactivated. Under these circumstances, these stimuli may result in conventional necrosis as a result of reduced ATP synthesis and generation of reactive oxygen metabolites such as O_2^-. Other proapoptotic factors are also released from mitochondria. These include caspase-2 and -9 and AIF (apoptosis-inducing factor). The latter is believed to be able to activate caspases and may itself be a caspase.

The mechanisms by which cytochrome c and other factors are released from the mitochondrial intermembranous space are still unclear. Many types of apoptotic signals result in the formation or opening of a mitochondrial permeability transition (PT) pore. The nature of the pore is not fully characterized, but it appears to include proteins from both the inner membrane (such as the adenine nucleotide translocator) and the outer membrane (such as the voltage-dependent anion channel, or VDAC) and probably forms at sites where the inner and outer membranes come into contact. The pore allows molecules up to 1.5 kD to pass and is thus insufficient to provide a passage for cytochrome c. However, it does allow the passage of ions, resulting in collapse of the mitochondrial membrane potential with loss of the H^+ gradient, uncoupling of the respiratory chain, and mitochondrial swelling. The importance of the PT is indicated by the fact that in many systems inhibitors of pore opening, such as cyclosporins and some cellular antiapoptotic proteins like Bcl-2, prevent apoptosis. Substances that promote pore opening, such as Bax, also promote apoptosis. Swelling of the mitochondrial matrix is believed to cause expansion of the matrical space and rupturing of the outer membrane, allowing the release of components of the intermembranous compartment. However, this theory is by no means proved and has some difficulties. For example, some forms of apoptosis appear to be independent of the opening of the PT. In addition, one of the features of apoptosis *in vivo* is the fact that mitochondria remain intact. Nevertheless, the fact that other components that are not participants in apoptotic pathways are also released is suggestive that the mechanism is nonspecific.

Regulators of Apoptosis

As might be expected, a process that can decide whether a cell lives or dies has multiple control mechanisms. Important among these is the Bcl-2 family of proteins. Bcl-2 itself corresponds to CED-9 of *Caenorhabditis elegans*. Interestingly and importantly, it was discovered in mammals as a protein that was constitutively activated by a chromosomal translocation in a particular form of lymphoma in humans. The resultant overactivity of Bcl-2, often coupled with the expression of other oncogenes, causes inhibition of the apoptosis, which should normally limit the growth of these cells, the result being neoplasia. Clearly then, neoplasia can result from disturbances of control of either proliferation or apoptosis, or both (see Chapter 6).

In mammals the Bcl-2 family is complex and contains a large number of proteins (15 at last count) that have both proapoptotic and antiapoptotic properties. All members are related through the presence of one or more of four Bcl-2 homology domains, BH1 through BH4. Although some proapoptotic members contain multiple BH domains, one group contains only the BH3 domain. The regulatory actions of these proteins seems to depend in part on their ability to heterodimerize via the BH3 domain. Thus the fate of the cell, that is, whether to undergo apoptosis or not, depends in part on the balance between antiapoptotic and proapoptotic proteins of the Bcl-2 family.

Bcl-2 and certain other antiapoptotic members of the family are present on the cytoplasmic face of the outer mitochondrial membrane as well as on the ER and nuclear envelope. In contrast, proapoptotic members of the family appear to be cytosolic in nonapoptotic cells. There are probably several mechanisms by which antiapoptotic members function. Some, including Bcl-X_L, appear to be able to bind to Apaf-1, preventing its association with and activation of caspase-9. Some proapoptotic members are believed to compete with Bcl-2 or Bcl-X_L, freeing Apaf-1 to interact with caspase-9. Bcl-2 and other antiapoptotic relatives also are able to inhibit the release of cytochrome *c* from mitochondria. This will also interfere with the formation of the apoptosome and the activation of caspase-9.

Several Bcl-2 family members have been sequenced, and their structure has been determined. This information has led to the realization that they resemble the pore-forming domains of certain bacterial toxins. This indicates that the Bcl-2 proteins may be able to form pores or channels in the membranes of mitochondria and other organelles, but how this property relates to apoptotic pathways is as yet unknown.

Although a detailed discussion is beyond the scope of this book, it should also be mentioned that the Bcl-2 family members are themselves under regulation. Certain cytokines can influence the levels of Bcl-2 proteins through transcriptional control, and other signals modify their activity through phosphorylation. Last, it would be inappropriate to leave this discussion without mentioning that apoptotic pathways can be modified by outside agents, in particular viruses, some of which encode inhibitors of apoptosis.

Role of Apoptosis in Disease

A complete picture of how apoptosis is involved in disease processes is still to emerge. However, it is clear that it can be involved in many diseases, including autoimmune diseases, through its role in eliminating autoreactive T cells; neurodegenerative diseases; aging; removal of cells damaged by irradiation, hypoxia, chemicals, and toxins; removal of cells infected by viruses; removal of excess myofibroblasts from granulation tissue; and in neoplasia. As we learn more about apoptosis, we should be able to manipulate the process to influence the outcomes of these diseases.

Necrosis

Necrosis is a long-established term traditionally used to describe the overall process that occurs when cells that are part of a living organism die. The morphological changes that we recognize microscopically as necrosis are, however, the result of *degradation* of the contents of the dead cell, which begins immediately after death of the cell. Most pathologists use the word "necrosis" (a little loosely) to include nonapoptotic cell death *and* the degradative changes that follow it. The initial degradative changes in the dead cell occur as a result of the action of endogenous enzymes derived largely from lysosomes. This is a process of *autolysis* (self-digestion). This term also is often used to describe the changes that occur in tissues after an animal has died. There is no real mechanistic difference between these processes, and the latter should be referred to as *postmortem autolysis* to distinguish it from the former.

Cells irreversibly injured by nonapoptotic pathways can exhibit all the changes already described, including swelling. Often necrosis involves locally extensive areas of tissue, as opposed to apoptosis, which usually involves single cells. At the light microscopic level, necrosis is characterized by increased eosinophilia of the cytoplasm as a result of enhanced binding of the stain eosin to altered proteins and to loss of ribosomes. The cytoplasm also may be hyalinized (having a homogeneous glassy appearance), or it may be vacuolated. Swollen mitochondria may be evident as eosinophilic cytoplasmic granules. As its contents are broken down, the cytoplasm becomes more vacuolated and "motheaten" in appearance. Under the right conditions, discussed below, the necrotic cells also may undergo calcification.

The nucleus also undergoes characteristic changes in the necrotic cell. Initially, in injured cells, the chromatin in the nucleus becomes clumped. In cells that have died, the nuclei initially shrink and become densely basophilic, a process called *pyknosis* (Fig. 2-24) or the nuclei may be lysed *(karyolysis)* (Figs. 2-24 and 2-26). Eventually the nucleus disappears. Lysis of the nucleus is a sure sign of necrosis and therefore of preceding cell death. Another term that is still seen is *karyorrhexis* (see Fig. 2-21), which means 'fragmentation of nuclei'. This was once interpreted as a manifestation of necrosis, but it is likely, in the light of modern understanding, that it indicates cell death by apoptosis. Nuclear pyknosis may also be seen as an early change in apoptotic cells.

Necrosis is sometimes appreciated only at the microscopic level, but we should mention that it may be discernable at the gross level as well. In other words, tissue necrosis is often visible to the naked eye. When locally extensive areas of tissue undergo necrosis, the lesion may be visible as tissue that is lighter in color than the surrounding normal tissue. This is attributable to coagulation of cytoplasmic proteins and frequently to reduced blood flow in the necrotic area. In this way infarcts, in the kidney for example, are often readily visible (Fig. 2-25). If there has been associated vascular injury, however,

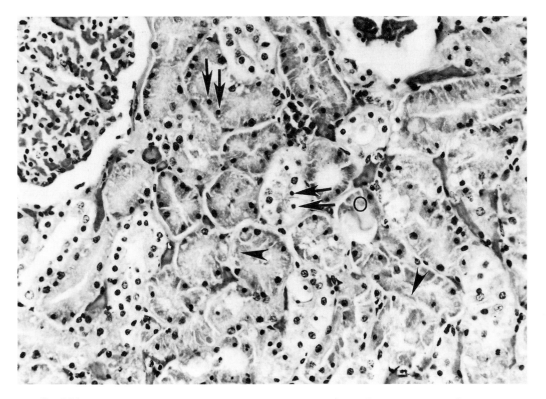

Fig. 2-24 Necrosis. Many of the renal tubular epithelial cells shown here are necrotic. Some contain small, dense nuclei (nuclear pyknosis, *arrows*). In others the nuclei have completely disappeared (karyolysis, *arrowheads*). This was a case of acute ethylene glycol poisoning in a cat. An oxalate crystal, *O*, is present.

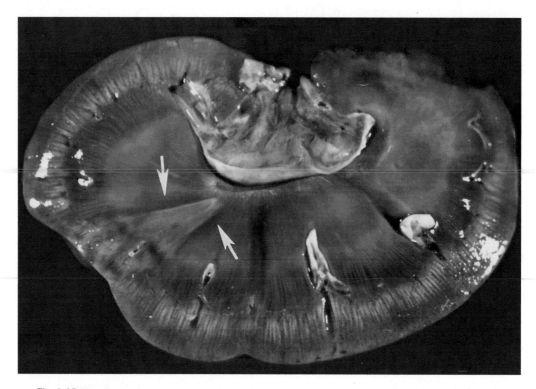

Fig. 2-25 Renal infarct. A wedge-shaped segment of pale necrotic tissue can be seen in this kidney from a dog. Its surface is depressed as a result of lysis and collapse of the tissue. The dark borders represent an inflammatory vascular response to the necrotic tissue, *arrows.*

necrotic tissue, including some infarcts, may be hemorrhagic. Necrotic tissue also may be swollen because of swelling of the individual cells, or it may be reduced in volume as a result of degradation, producing a depression on the surface of the organ. It also may be softer to the touch than the normal tissue, a change that is referred to as *malacia.* In addition, there may be a local reaction to the necrotic tissue that is apparent as a reddened zone of vascular congestion adjacent to the lesion (see Fig. 2-25). This represents an inflammatory reaction evoked by the necrotic tissue, and an influx of leukocytes may be appreciated microscopically in such areas. The ability to provoke an inflammatory reaction is one of the features that differentiates necrosis from apoptosis. Once one is able to recognize these changes it often is possible to detect the presence of necrosis during the gross postmortem examination or during surgery.

Classification of Necrotic Lesions

The gross and histological appearance of necrotic cells may vary somewhat depending on local conditions, in particular on how much fluid or blood flow is present in the lesion.

In the case of *coagulation necrosis* the dead cells take on the appearance of an eosinophilic

"shadow" of the original cells (Figs. 2-26 and 2-27). In other words, the original cellular shape and tissue organization are still apparent histologically, but cellular detail is lost, and the nucleus is usually lysed. This appearance often is seen when the blood supply is suddenly and completely cut off or when cytoplasmic proteins are denatured and resistant to digestion. Necrotic skeletal muscle fibers often show this coagulated appearance probably because the living cells contain relatively few lysosomes (see Fig. 2-27). Eventually these cells are phagocytosed by inflammatory cells derived from the circulation. The latter, mostly macrophages, release enzymes into the tissue that can digest the necrotic cellular debris. Once phagocytosed the remnants are digested in phagolysosomes.

In liquefaction necrosis, as the name implies, the affected tissue is liquefied. As a result, it is very soft and even may be quite fluid. It is seen frequently in inflammatory lesions containing a lot of neutrophils, such as an abscess. When an abscess is cut open, the contents often ooze out. The lysosomal enzymes derived from neutrophils as well as from autolytic digestion contribute to the process of liquefaction. Some tissues are more likely to show liquefaction necrosis than others. For example, the parenchyma of the central nervous system typically

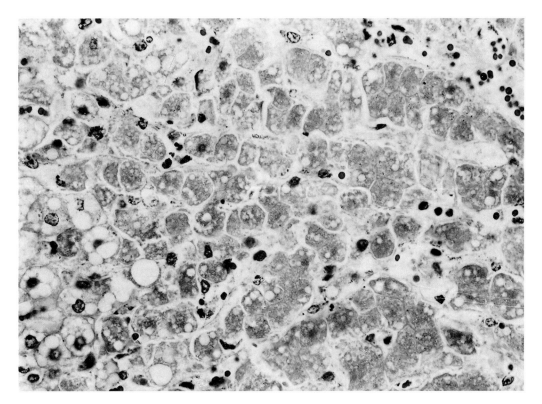

Fig. 2-26 Coagulation necrosis. Many of the cells shown in this micrograph lack nuclei and are obviously necrotic. They have retained their shape and are easily recognizable as liver cells. Even vacuoles of lipid that accumulated during the process of injury can still be recognized in their cytoplasm.

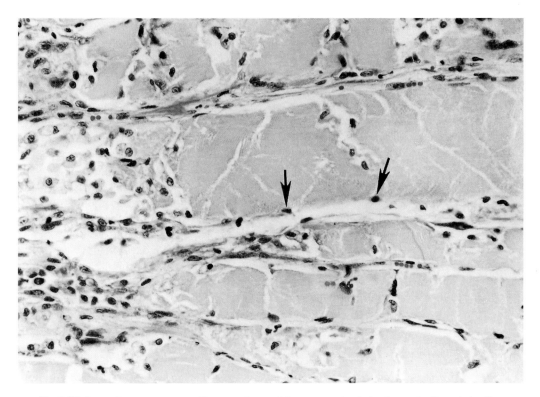

Fig. 2-27 Coagulation necrosis. The cytoplasm of these necrotic skeletal muscle fibers is hyalinized and fragmented. The cells lack muscle nuclei or have pyknotic nuclei, *arrows. On the left,* macrophages have invaded the tissue to phagocytose the necrotic cellular material. This is the typical appearance of necrotic muscle cells.

liquefies when necrotic. Such lesions are referred to as *encephalomalacia* in the brain and *myelomalacia* in the spinal cord. As already mentioned, malacia means softening and describes the gross appearance and consistency of the affected tissue.

Caseous necrosis is the term applied to describe necrotic tissue that, because of local conditions, is soft and pasty. In the past it was likened by some pathologists to cheese, with the name being derived from this comparison. This type of reaction is likely to be associated with certain bacterial infections. In some species, including man, it is seen in lesions caused by *Mycobacterium tuberculosis,* and in the sheep *Corynebacterium pseudotuberculosis* produces similar lesions. In the latter case the disease is even called *caseous lymphadenitis* because the infection commonly causes caseous necrosis in lymph nodes.

Gangrene is something of an archaic term applied to ischemic necrosis of extremities such as limbs, digits, or the tips of the ears (Fig. 2-28). From it the term *gangrenous necrosis* is derived. In reality, there is no distinction between this and either coagulation or liquefaction necrosis, depending again on local conditions. In the case of *dry gangrene* the histological appearance would be one of coagulation, whereas in *wet gangrene,* where the actions of bacterial enzymes may be important, it is one of liquefaction.

Especially when focal masses of tissue undergo necrosis, there is often a local response in the surrounding normal tissues. This may include vascular engorgement and congestion and, where there is vascular damage, hemorrhage. This vascular reaction gives rise to the red zone that often surrounds a necrotic lesion such as an infarct. In addition, the necrotic tissue can evoke an inflammatory response associated with which there is an infiltration of neutrophils and macrophages. As already explained, these cells contribute hydrolytic enzymes derived from lysosomes, which help to break down the dead tissue. They act as phagocytes, ingesting the necrotic debris, removing it from the tissue, and completing its digestion. This process paves the way for healing to occur. The defect left after the removal of dead tissue is repaired in one of a variety of ways depending on the tissue involved. In some the parenchyma can be replaced. In others a scar is formed. Mechanisms involved in the repair of injured tissues are discussed in detail in Chapter 4.

Consequences of Cell Injury

When injured cells are examined while alive, they show numerous abnormal functions. These are initially abnormal, violent cell movements, blebbing of

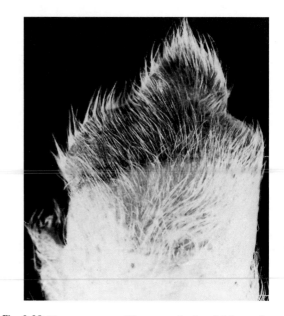

Fig. 2-28 Dry gangrene. The necrotic tip of this ear from a pig is dry and sharply demarcated from the viable tissue.

the plasma membrane, and, of course, cell swelling. These changes reflect loss of control of certain mechanisms by the cell. Abnormal cell shape and movement and blebbing of the plasma membrane presumably involve altered function of the cytoskeleton. Some of these changes are attributable to loss of cellular energy production and influx of calcium ions, but there are alterations in protein synthesis and other functions as well. Altered protein synthesis can lead to secondary changes in the cell such as the accumulation of lipids. These aspects are considered in more detail later. The importance of the injury to the animal as a whole partly depends on the tissue involved as well as the extent and the severity of the injury. If the myocardium is involved, for example, the consequences can be grave. On the other hand, if skeletal muscle is involved, a similar degree of tissue injury might be of little overall functional consequence. The *prognosis* (that is, the likely outcome of the disease process) is dependent on such factors, and the clinician needs to assess what tissues are involved and to what extent they are injured during the evaluation of the patient.

One result of cell injury that is useful in the establishment of a diagnosis and prognosis is the measurement of cellular enzymes in body fluids. When cells undergo necrosis, the plasma membrane becomes leaky, and, among other things, enzymes can escape into the circulation (Fig. 2-29). These can be measured by the clinician, and the study of serum enzymes forms a very important diagnostic aid. As an example, consider an animal that is sus-

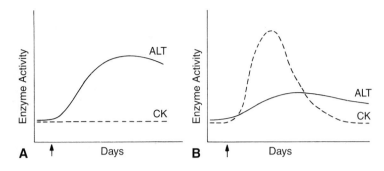

Fig. 2-29 Changes in serum enzymes after cell injury. After severe injury or necrosis to a tissue (indicated here by *arrows*) cellular enzymes may be released and appear in the serum. *A,* When liver cells, which are rich in alanine aminotransferase (ALT) and poor in creatine kinase (CK), are injured, much ALT but little CK appear in the serum. *B,* When muscle cells, which are rich in CK but have little ALT, are injured, much CK but little ALT appear in the serum. A knowledge of the tissue specificity of these and other enzymes makes serum enzymology a valuable diagnostic technique.

pected of having necrosis of skeletal muscle. If the clinician can measure the activity in the serum of an enzyme that usually is found only in skeletal muscle, this possibility can be confirmed (or denied). *Creatine kinase* (CK) is such an enzyme, found in quantity only in skeletal muscle, myocardium, and brain. An understanding of the relative amounts of certain enzymes in different tissues and the relative half-lives of the enzymes in the circulation therefore allows us to evaluate injury to a variety of tissues.

The Pathogenesis of Cell Injury

Having discussed the appearances of injured and necrotic cells and the consequences of such injury, we might now ask ourselves what mechanisms are involved. Why, for example, do injured cells swell? Why do some cells survive injury and others die? What are the critical changes that result in cell death? It soon will become clear that answers are available for only some of these questions. Analysis of the molecular events that occur in cell injury is difficult because they cannot be studied in isolation. The various biochemical changes that occur interact so that changes in one must be associated with changes in others. As a result it is extremely difficult to single out any one change and say, "That is the critical event in cell injury and cell death."

It is clear, however, that, despite the variety of tissues that may be involved and despite the plethora of potential causes, nonapoptotic cell injury is mediated by means of two main mechanisms. The first is interference with the energy supply of the cell, and the second is direct damage to cell membranes. Even this observation is an oversimplification because it is becoming clear that membrane damage is

a common factor in most, if not all, kinds of cellular injury, including anoxia.

CAUSES OF CELL INJURY

Cells can be damaged by a wide variety of agents too numerous to list in any detail here. However, we can consider certain groups into which most of these causes fall. They include hypoxia, chemical agents, physical agents including trauma, genetic abnormalities, biological agents, immune mechanisms, and nutritional abnormalities. As previously mentioned, some of these agents can also induce apoptosis, but in the discussion that follows we are referring to nonapoptotic cell injury.

Hypoxia is one of the most common causes of cell injury. It usually is associated with *ischemia,* or interruption of the supply of blood to the tissue. It also may be associated with reduced oxygen-carrying capacity of the blood or with interference with the respiratory chain. *Infarction,* or death of tissue caused by interruption of its blood supply, can result from a variety of vascular lesions, which are discussed in Chapter 3. Reduced oxygen-carrying capacity of the blood may occur whenever the effective levels of hemoglobin are reduced significantly. This may happen in severe anemia, in methemoglobinemia caused by nitrite poisoning, or in carboxyhemoglobinemia caused by carbon monoxide poisoning. The best known example of interference with the respiratory chain is cyanide poisoning. Cyanide inactivates cytochrome oxidase thus blocking the transfer of electrons on the respiratory chain. All these phenomena have the effect of interfering with the energy supply of the cell, and this probably occurs in many forms of cell injury.

Physical agents that can injure cells are diverse. They include direct trauma, such as lacerations or crush injuries, heat, cold, and radiation. The extent of such injuries may be increased by tissue hypoxia associated with local vascular damage. Radiation injury may be caused by x rays, radioactive isotope emissions, and most commonly ultraviolet (UV) radiation. Many of us have suffered cell injury caused by UV radiation, in the form of sunburn. Animals also may be sunburned, and those with unpigmented, poorly haired skin are particularly susceptible. In both animals and man, long-term exposure to UV and other forms of radiation also may cause cancer, a phenomenon discussed in Chapter 6.

Chemical agents are present in our environment in a bewildering variety, and many of them are more or less toxic. Even those that are essential for the health of our cells can paradoxically be injurious when present in excess. Examples include sodium chloride, selenium, copper and iron salts, and oxygen, to name only a few. Other chemicals are very potent toxins, minute quantities of which can injure cells and cause illness or death of the animal. Chemical toxins act in a wide variety of ways, but many either injure membranes directly (we include those that interact with receptors) or interfere with the energy metabolism of the cell.

Genetic abnormalities can produce a wide variety of disease entities. They are discussed together with injuries to DNA in Chapter 7.

Biological agents also may injure cells in numerous ways. The agents involved include viruses, bacteria, protozoa, fungi, and even algae. Viruses, for example, can alter the metabolism of host cells, bacteria can elaborate toxins (see Chapter 7), and many of these agents can cause cell injury mediated by the actions of the host's own immune response. The ways in which the immune response can cause cell injury are discussed in Chapter 5, but we can point out here that the mechanism usually involves damage to the cell membrane or hypoxia associated with vascular injury. The binding and activation of complement, for example, punches tiny "holes" in the plasma membrane of the target cell. The target cells may be bacteria, other organisms, or infected or otherwise abnormal host cells.

Malnutrition is a major cause of cell injury in many species. Deficiencies of protein, carbohydrate, or vitamins result in abnormal metabolic and synthetic processes. Overnutrition also can result in injury.

Because, as we have emphasized, membrane damage or interference with energy metabolism represent the major pathways of cell injury, they have been studied in some detail. Interference with energy metabolism has been most commonly studied using hypoxic cell injury produced by ischemia. In the case of membrane injury, models using chemical toxins have been used, one of the best characterized of which is injury to the liver by carbon tetrachloride. In the following section, the information obtained from these studies is discussed, with the emphasis being placed on the correlation of structural and functional changes.

HYPOXIC CELL INJURY

Injury as a result of hypoxia, in particular that associated with ischemia, is possibly the single most common cause of cell injury. Tissue cells vary in their susceptibility to hypoxia. Some can withstand relatively long periods of hypoxia without permanent injury, but others are lethally injured by brief periods of oxygen deprivation. In part, this is dependent on the capability of cells to utilize anaerobic glycolysis as a source of energy. Anaerobic glycolysis, however, is a relatively inefficient mechanism of energy production compared to oxidative phosphorylation and generates lactic acid, which, as we will see, can contribute to cell injury. Interference with the major energy supply of the cell has, of course, many functional consequences, and many biological processes fail. These vary in importance in terms of their contribution to cell injury. Here we will pay most attention to those that are significant in this regard.

The Sequence of Changes in the Injured Cell

During the progression of cell injury, alterations occur in many of the organelles. While changes are occurring in the mitochondria, for example, alterations also are occurring in the endoplasmic reticulum, the nucleus, the cytosol, and the plasma membrane. Some changes, however, are characteristic of early cell injury and others of the later stages.

In the cell deprived of oxygen there is rapid, severe impairment of oxidative phosphorylation. As a result, intracellular levels of ATP quickly fall, and the ADP:ATP ratio increases. As ATP is used and depleted, there is a concomitant rise in inorganic phosphate. This activates anaerobic glycolysis as an alternative source of energy. Therefore an early morphological manifestation of cell injury is depletion of glycogen. Associated with this, there is a fall in intracellular pH. These changes occur within 15 minutes of the beginning of hypoxia.

By about 15 minutes, early changes appear in the mitochondria. There is loss of mitochondrial matrix granules, and the mitochondria begin to undergo conformational changes. Initially the mitochondria have a condensed or contracted inner compartment and a relatively expanded outer compartment.

Between 15 and 30 minutes there is distortion of the outline of the plasma membrane with loss of specialized structures such as microvilli. The mitochondria continue to undergo condensation at this stage. At the same time, dilatation of the endoplasmic reticulum becomes apparent.

Between 30 minutes and 1 hour there is disaggregation and detachment of polyribosomes from the surface of the RER, the cytosol becomes pallid, and the cell swells. At the same time the mitochondria begin to swell. This change, called *high-amplitude swelling,* is characterized by distension of the inner mitochondrial compartment. Dense amorphous deposits also may begin to appear in the mitochondria.

From 2 to 4 hours after the onset of anoxia the mitochondria continue to swell and may be dramatically increased in volume. There are increased numbers of flocculent densities in the matrix, and breaks in the outer mitochondrial membrane may occur. Swelling of the endoplasmic reticulum continues, and it becomes fragmented. Breaks in the plasma membrane can occur. By this stage, the nuclear chromatin is severely clumped, and early karyolysis becomes evident.

From this time on, the changes continue to become more severe. Organelle membranes fragment, chromatin undergoes lysis (karyolysis), and myelin

figures derived from membrane components appear in the altered cytoplasm. During the later stages of cell injury lysosomes swell and release enzymes into the cytosol, and the process of autolysis begins. Soon the cell is recognizable in the light microscope as being necrotic.

The changes described above are those seen in cells subjected experimentally to sudden, complete anoxia. In real life, of course, the severity of the insult may vary, and the changes in the cell may be modified by local environmental conditions. The rate of progression of changes seen in individual cases therefore also varies. The general progression of acute lethal cell injury is, however, as we have described and is summarized in Fig. 2-30.

Mitochondria

Changes in mitochondrial structure and function are early indicators of hypoxic cell injury. Many of these changes are a direct consequence of altered mitochondrial function. The mitochondria themselves require ATP to continue to work. However, it is known that isolated mitochondria can withstand anoxia without permanent injury for longer periods than those subjected to anoxia *in vivo* can. The accelerated changes that occur in mitochondria *in vivo* are probably partly the result of altered intracellular environmental conditions such as changes

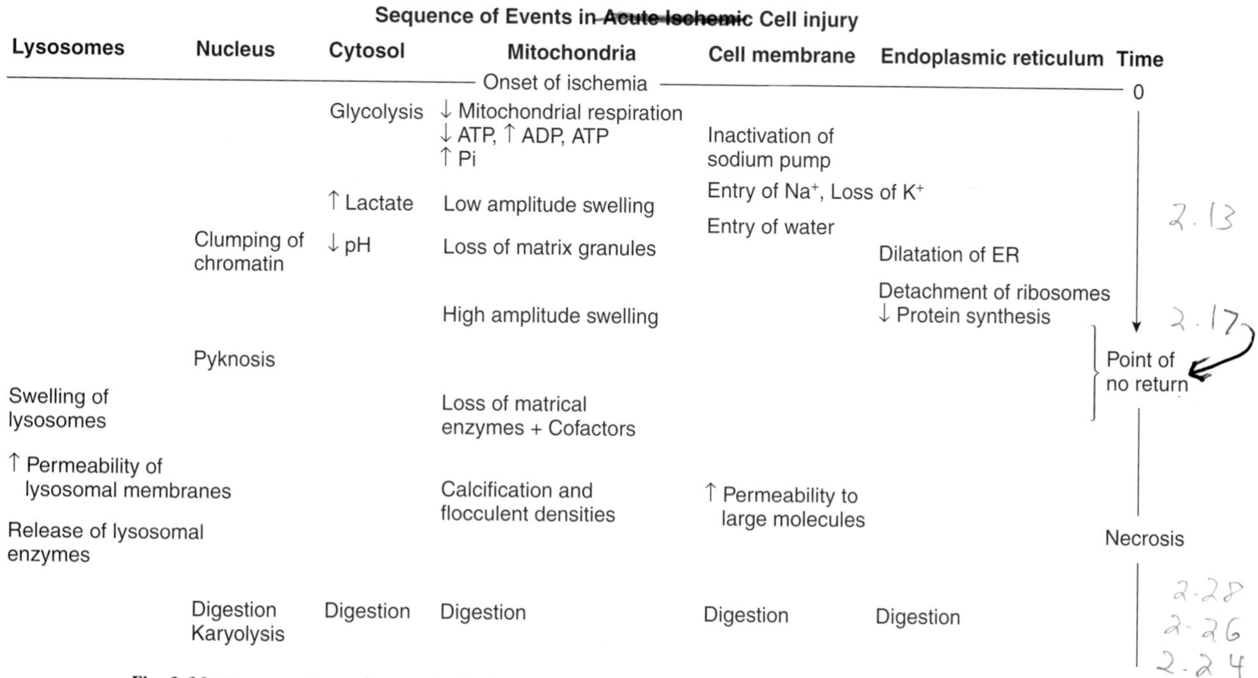

Lysosomes	Nucleus	Cytosol	Mitochondria	Cell membrane	Endoplasmic reticulum	Time
			Onset of ischemia			0
		Glycolysis	↓ Mitochondrial respiration ↓ ATP, ↑ ADP, ATP ↑ Pi	Inactivation of sodium pump		
		↑ Lactate	Low amplitude swelling	Entry of Na⁺, Loss of K⁺		
	Clumping of chromatin	↓ pH	Loss of matrix granules	Entry of water	Dilatation of ER	
			High amplitude swelling		Detachment of ribosomes ↓ Protein synthesis	
	Pyknosis					Point of no return
Swelling of lysosomes			Loss of matrical enzymes + Cofactors			
↑ Permeability of lysosomal membranes			Calcification and flocculent densities	↑ Permeability to large molecules		
Release of lysosomal enzymes						Necrosis
	Digestion Karyolysis	Digestion	Digestion	Digestion	Digestion	

Sequence of Events in ~~Acute Ischemic~~ Cell injury

Fig. 2-30 Progression of acute lethal anoxic cell injury. The cellular events that occur in injured cells are arranged here so that their temporal sequences and relationships to one another can be appreciated. (*Adapted from Scarpelli DG, Trump BF: Cell injury, Kalamazoo, Mich., 1971, Upjohn Co.*)

in concentrations of ions, particularly calcium ions. They may also relate to involvement of apoptotic mechanisms in altering mitochondrial function, such as opening of the permeability transition pore, even in cells that are destined to die by nonapoptotic mechanisms.

Initially mitochondria undergo condensation of the matrix (Fig. 2-31). This reaction is reversible and is essentially a physiological adaptation to altered levels of ADP and ATP in the cell. When the ADP:ATP ratio is increased, the mitochondria adopt this conformation. However, mitochondrial contraction depends on some ATP being present. When ATP is no longer available at all, the mitochondria begin to undergo high-amplitude swelling (see Figs. 2-17 and 2-31). This appears to be associated with damage to the inner mitochondrial membrane. Some ATP apparently is required to maintain the integrity of this membrane. Changes that occur include the loss of F_1 particles, believed to be the morphological correlate of magnesium-activated ATPase. These changes are associated with a loss of potassium and magnesium ions by the mitochondria and an in-

crease in sodium and calcium ions. Also, there is increased membrane permeability and uptake of water, accounting for the swelling that occurs.

Up to this point cell injury is usually still reversible. That is, cells containing significant numbers of mitochondria with early high-amplitude swelling still can recover if a source of oxygen is restored. In the mitochondria themselves, however, some functions may be lost whereas others are intact. In other words, the various functional systems in the mitochondria show a variable susceptibility to injury. Pyruvate kinase and α-ketoglutarate dehydrogenase, for example, are matrix enzymes that are drastically reduced in activity as an early event in mitochondrial injury. Oxidative phosphorylation also is greatly reduced early in the process. In contrast, succinate dehydrogenase, a tightly membrane-bound enzyme system, and the electron transport system are much more stable and persist even after the cell is irreversibly injured.

The susceptibility of matrix enzymes to early injury probably is attributable to their loss, together with cofactors such as NADH, by diffusion from

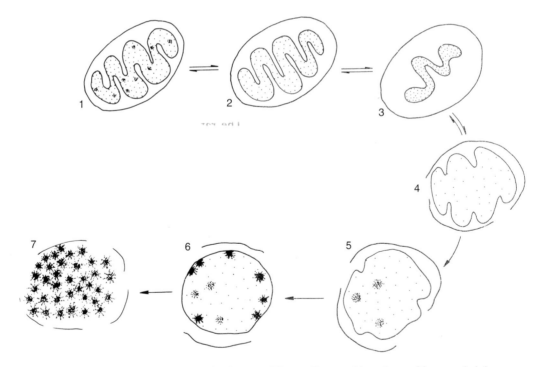

Fig. 2-31 Progression of mitochondrial injury. When cells are subjected to sudden anoxic injury, the mitochondria undergo a change from normal conformation *(1)* to the contracted conformation *(3)*. More or less at the same time, the mitochondrial-dense granules disappear *(2)*. With progression the mitochondria undergo high-amplitude swelling *(4)*, and defects in the outer membrane may appear. Up to this point and even when high-amplitude swelling has begun, the changes are reversible. As the injury progresses, the mitochondria continue to swell and develop matrical flocculent deposits *(5)* and changes in the inner mitochondrial membrane. Such changes are associated with loss of reversibility. Under some conditions the injured mitochondria may become calcified *(6, 7)*.

the mitochondria. Thus, as the capacity for oxidative phosphorylation is lost, the inner mitochondrial membrane is altered, ion and water shifts occur, and enzymes and their substrates and cofactors are lost as the mitochondria swell. *In vitro* studies have confirmed that mitochondria that undergo swelling do lose components from the matrix. Presumably, when these changes become severe enough, mitochondrial function cannot be restored even if a supply of oxygen is reestablished, but there are more important factors involved in the failure of mitochondria to recover from injury, as discussed later.

As high-amplitude swelling progresses, the matrix granules disappear, the matrix takes on a clarified appearance, and dense amorphous deposits of denatured proteins and lipoproteins form, corresponding to the flocculent densities described earlier. As already mentioned, calcium ions enter the injured mitochondria and under some conditions enough enter for the deposition of insoluble calcium salts to occur. This is most striking when the flow of blood to the injured tissue is at least partly preserved or when it is restored after a period of ischemia.

The Cell Membrane

Alterations of the plasma membrane are among the earliest changes to occur in the hypoxic cell. These are manifested morphologically as blebbing and loss of specialized structures. Such distortions may reflect abnormal cytoskeletal function as much as alterations in the plasma membrane because cytoskeletal components are dynamic and sensitive to changes in ion concentrations, especially that of calcium.

One of the fundamental properties of the cell membrane is the maintenance of ion and water homeostasis in the cell and through these processes the maintenance of cell volume. The sodium pump is an energy-dependent system located in the plasma membrane that is responsible for the active transport of sodium ions out of and potassium ions into the cell.

An early manifestation of hypoxia in the cell is the failure of this ion pump to operate. When this happens, the ions in the cytoplasm and in the extracellular fluid attempt to reach Gibbs-Donnan equilibrium. In other words, ions attempt to reach an equilibrium where the product of the ionic strengths inside and outside the cell (that is, on either side of a semipermeable membrane) are equal. The net result is that sodium ions enter the cell, potassium ions leak out, each moving along a concentration gradient, and the cell swells. The cell also tends to lose magnesium and accumulate calcium ions. Similar ion fluxes occur between compartments in the cell, as between the endoplasmic reticulum, or the mitochondria, and the cytosol.

It may at first not be clear why such free diffusion of ions into and out of the cell should cause the cell to swell. To understand this we must temporarily divert our attention to the way in which the sodium pump regulates cell volume. The basic problem is this: How can sodium chloride contribute to the osmotic effect that is responsible for maintaining cell volume if the cell membrane is permeable to it? The answer is that the colloid osmotic pressure of the protein molecules inside the cell is the critical element in this equilibrium. Protein is in higher concentration inside the cell than outside, and therefore there is a net positive colloid osmotic pressure inside the cell. To balance this, some osmotically active particles must be maintained in relative excess outside the cell. In a passive situation permeable ions could not accomplish this, but the sodium pump is able to maintain a high concentration of sodium ions outside the cell and a low concentration inside. In other words, as long as the sodium pump is working, sodium ions function as a nondiffusible external cation that balances the effect of the truly nondiffusible protein molecules inside the cell. When the pump stops, sodium ions enter the cell (accompanied by chloride) moving along their electrochemical gradient. This increases the internal osmotic pressure relative to the outside and draws water into the cell.

The rate of loss of potassium ions may initially exceed that of sodium loss, and the cell may transiently shrink. However, entry of sodium ions into the cell soon exceeds that of the potassium lost, and the cell swells. This again is exacerbated by the relatively high intracellular colloid osmotic pressure. As water is drawn into the cell, intracellular potassium is diluted, moving it closer to the equilibrium with the outside. Intracellular sodium also is diluted, but this moves it away from equilibrium with the outside and favors further entry of sodium ions; therefore the main driving force for cell swelling is, in fact, the gradient of colloid osmotic pressure that exists across the cell membrane. At least initially, the water that enters the cell is not distributed uniformly throughout the cytoplasm. Most of it seems to enter the cisternae of the endoplasmic reticulum producing the vacuolated appearance typical of cell injury at the light microscopic level.

The rate and degree to which the cell swells depends on many factors, including the relative permeability of the plasma membrane to the major ions sodium and potassium, the availability of extracellular water, and the degree of hypoxia and constraining viscoelastic forces provided by the supporting connective tissues. In complete ischemia there may be relatively little extracellular water available to be taken up by the cell, thus limiting swelling. The most explosive swelling usually is seen in ischemic tissue in which the blood flow is restored.

As the cell swells and injury progresses, physical damage to the cell membrane occurs, resulting in a large increase in its permeability. This serves only to exacerbate the process. Furthermore, the accumulation of cellular metabolites may contribute to the osmotic load inside the cell and thus to swelling. Early swelling may, in fact, be caused mostly by such metabolites. If such products accumulate during complete ischemia, they may contribute to the dramatic swelling that follows restoration of blood flow though reperfusion injury, discussed below, also may play a part.

Eventually the membrane becomes permeable to even large molecules, and enzymes and other proteins can leak out of (or into) the cell. This change forms the basis for dye exclusion tests as a means of determining cell viability *in vitro*. When isolated, severely injured cells are incubated in solutions of dyes such as trypan blue, their damaged cell membranes are permeable to the dye, and the cell is stained. Viable cells do not take up the dye and therefore are not stained.

Although cell swelling undoubtedly is a dependable marker for cell injury, its role in contributing to the death of the cell is less certain. Cell death can occur in the absence of appreciable cell swelling, depending on the factors already mentioned, and quite dramatic swelling can occur in reversibly injured cells. However, it is quite clear that prevention of cellular swelling can contribute to the survival of injured cells. This has been demonstrated in *in vivo*

studies as well as *in vitro*, usually with mannitol being used as a nonpermeable solute in the extracellular fluid. Even in cultured cells subjected to injury the prevention of cell swelling reduces the incidence of cell death. This may be attributable to a reduction in the distortion of the plasma membrane associated with swelling. On the other hand, mannitol is a known scavenger of the hydroxyl radical, and its action in alleviating cell swelling and cell death may be attributable instead to prevention of lipid peroxidation in ischemic cells, as discussed below. Whatever its mode of action, this principle is sometimes applied clinically in the intravenous administration of impermeant solutes such as mannitol to protect against cellular and tissue swelling.

The changes in ion permeability just described have profound effects on the function of excitable cells such as nerves, skeletal muscle cells, and myocardial cells. In the case of anoxic myocardial cell injury (a common enough event, especially in man), the injury can be detected by use of the electrocardiogram (Fig. 2-32). The changes that occur are a reflection of the altered electrophysiological functions that are associated with ionic shifts in these cells. In addition, products of abnormal lipid metabolism have been shown to be important in alterations of the electrophysiological function of the ischemic heart.

The Endoplasmic Reticulum

The endoplasmic reticulum undergoes dilatation (see Fig. 2-18) and fragmentation early in the progression of acute lethal injury caused by anoxia. In fact the ER seems to act as a reservoir in which much of the water initially taken up by the injured cell accumulates. Dilatation of the ER is associated with the movement of both water and sodium ions

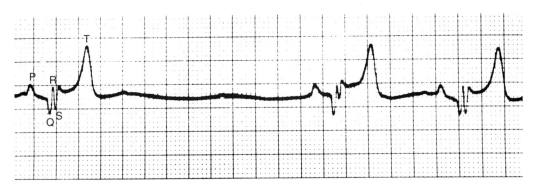

Fig. 2-32 Electrocardiographic changes in hypoxic myocardial injury. This lead II ECG is from a dog with aortic stenosis. There is elevation of the ST segment and an abnormally large T wave. The configuration of the QRS complex is abnormal, suggestive of a conduction disturbance. (Paper speed = 50 mm/sec, 1 cm = 1 mV) *(Courtesy the late Dr. Gary Bolton, Ithaca, N.Y.)*

across the membrane into the cisternal lumen. Associated with dilatation of the ER there is disaggregation and detachment of ribosomes from the surface of the RER. Early in the course of anoxic cell injury ribosomes are lost but apparently retain their membrane-binding capacity because the defect can be repaired by the addition of certain artificial polymers. Later this is not possible, an indication that, besides initial damage to the membranes of the ER, later changes in ribosomal proteins and nucleic acids take place. At any rate, as a consequence of ribosomal loss, protein synthesis is impaired. This can have important effects on the cell, typified by the development of lipidosis, the pathogenesis of which is discussed later in this chapter.

Lysosomes

Lysosomes contain a variety of potent hydrolytic enzymes that are capable of digesting essentially all components in the cytoplasm of the cell. It has long been argued, therefore, that the release of enzymes from damaged lysosomes in injured cells could be important in the pathogenesis of cell injury and might in fact be responsible for cell death. This concept of self-digestion is known as the "suicide-bag" hypothesis. Its validity has been vigorously debated over the years, but there is surprisingly little direct evidence that the intracellular release of lysosomal enzymes plays a direct role in causing or exacerbating cell injury.

Without doubt, lysosomes, like other cell organelles, undergo swelling in injured cells. This is presumed to be attributable to abnormal fluxes of ions and water and usually occurs before cell injury becomes irreversible. In addition, there is evidence that substrates normally excluded from the lysosome can enter it early in the process of cell injury. It has been difficult, however, to demonstrate *leakage of enzymes* from lysosomes into the cytosol before cell injury becomes irreversible. This is in contrast to the situation with respect to phagocytic cells such as the neutrophil and the macrophage, in which lysosomal enzymes can be released from living cells as a secretory event, contributing to injury of surrounding cells (see Chapter 4).

Against the suicide-bag hypothesis are the following observations: (1) In injured cells ultrastructural changes occur earlier in organelles such as mitochondria and the endoplasmic reticulum than in lysosomes. (2) If release of lysosomal enzymes were important, we might expect that changes in the cytoplasm and its organelles might be more severe near lysosomes. This expectation cannot be demonstrated. (3) If lysosomes are labeled with a phagocy-

tosed marker, such as ferritin, and the cell then is injured, release of the marker occurs late in the progression of injury.

On the other hand, there is some evidence that lysosomes can be injured as a primary event and that this does result in cell injury and cell death. If cells are allowed to phagocytose silica or sodium urate crystals, for example, the crystals enter lysosomes and directly damage them. Crystals can be seen free in the cytoplasm during the early stages of cell injury, and the treated cells die soon after. If phagocytosis is prevented, the exposed cell is not injured, an indication that the injury is attributable to lysosomal damage rather than a direct effect on the plasma membrane.

In conclusion, therefore, we cannot altogether rule out a role for release of lysosomal enzymes into the cytosol. It may be important in some forms of cell injury, and there is evidence that this may be so in some viral infections and in diseases involving abnormal copper metabolism, as discussed later. However, the overall evidence is that in most forms of cell injury, including hypoxia, the release of lysosomal enzymes is a relatively late event and apparently plays no part in causing cell injury. Lysosomal enzymes are eventually released, however, and after cell death has occurred, they play an important role in producing the changes that characterize necrosis.

Other Organelles

As we have already mentioned, injured cells initially may show abnormal cell motility, formation of surface blebs, and distortion of microvilli and other surface specializations. The basis of these changes is not well defined, but they may reflect altered function of the cytoskeleton associated with impaired energy metabolism, changes in concentration of calcium and other ions, and changes in pH.

In the cytosol, glycogen is depleted, and myelin figures may appear. The latter are believed to be derived from components of damaged cell membranes. In particular phospholipids "leached" from membranes may spontaneously reaggregate forming the laminar arrays that characterize myelin figures.

From our discussions so far, it is becoming clear that nonapoptotic cell injury caused by ischemia or anoxia revolves around damage to cellular membranes. There is evidence that paradoxically some of this damage is caused by reactive metabolites derived from oxygen itself. These products include free radicals and are discussed in more detail below. For now, suffice it to say that they can cause extensive damage to many cellular systems, among which membranes figure prominently.

CELL INJURY CAUSED BY MEMBRANE DAMAGE

Direct damage to cell membranes, both the plasma membrane and those of organelles, is the second major pathway through which cell injury can occur. In fact we will argue later that, in the final analysis, anoxic injury too is mediated through alteration of cell membranes. Thus it can be argued that there is a final common pathway through which cell injury occurs, regardless of its cause. It is not surprising to find that, regardless of cause, injured cells express very similar morphological and functional alterations. Despite the similarities, however, there are some differences in the morphological expression of cell injury caused by membrane damage and that caused by hypoxia. Here we will consider the changes seen in cells injured by damage to their membranes, stressing those lesions that are characteristic of this type of injury.

Causes of Membrane Damage

A great variety of agents cause injury to cells by damaging their membranes. They include irradiation, many chemical toxins and drugs, bacterial toxins such as the phospholipases produced by some species of *Clostridium* (see Chapter 7), and complement (an important immune and inflammatory effector mechanism; see Chapters 4 and 5). In addition some nutritional deficiencies, in particular deficiency of vitamin E or selenium, cause cell damage by increasing their susceptibility to membrane damage. Hepatocellular necrosis caused by intoxication by the solvent carbon tetrachloride (CCl_4) is one example of this type of injury that has been studied widely. We use this model as a basis for our discussion of injury to cell membranes, not because it is commonly encountered but because it is well characterized.

Mechanisms of Membrane Injury

Toxic agents injure membranes in various ways, commonly by direct interaction with them or by the formation of free radicals, which cause peroxidation of membrane lipids. Mercuric chloride, for example, is able to combine directly with sulfhydryl groups in the cell membranes, whereas CCl_4 acts through membrane lipid peroxidation. Regardless of the exact mechanism involved, the result is increased membrane permeability and loss of specialized membrane functions.

Carbon tetrachloride toxicity is a classic example of the way in which the metabolic activity of the host can produce intermediates that are potentially toxic to the cell. Carbon tetrachloride is metabolized by the mixed-function oxidase enzyme (P-450) system in the liver. During this process the free radicals CCl_3^- and Cl^- are produced. As pointed out earlier in this chapter, this enzyme complex is found in the SER. It can undergo dramatic hypertrophy as an adaptive response to repeated exposure to drugs metabolized by this system. Thus, an animal that has been treated with primidone, for example, would have hypertrophied SER and would be expected to metabolize CCl_4 more rapidly than usual. Consequently it would, at least transiently, produce high concentrations of toxic metabolites of CCl_4 and so enhance its toxicity. Because so many substances are metabolized by the mixed function oxidase system there is considerable potential for this sort of enhancement of toxicity. Another example worth mentioning, and one of more specific interest in clinical medicine, is intoxication by acetaminophen. This commonly used antipyretic and analgesic drug also is metabolized by the mixed function oxidase system. It, too, generates toxic intermediates that, if present in high enough concentrations, can cause lethal hepatocellular injury. Obviously patients who have been receiving drugs that can induce hypertrophy of the SER will be unusually susceptible to these toxic effects. The drugs whose toxic effects can be enhanced in this way are too numerous to list here but these observations hopefully should leave the prospective clinician with a healthy respect for the potential effects of drug interactions. The liver, being a major site of chemical modification of drugs and toxins, is peculiarly susceptible to drug and toxin-induced injury. It should also be mentioned that there can be major differences in capability for hepatic biotransformation between species leading to differences in their susceptibility to drug induced toxicity.

Lipid Peroxidation and Membrane Injury

The generation of free radicals is a fairly common mechanism of cell damage, and many toxic chemicals and drugs act this way. It is now believed that many compounds metabolized in the liver, for example, at least partially exert their effects through the production by the P-450 mixed function oxidase system of reactive oxygen species, some of which are free radicals. There are many other examples of tissue injury by reactive oxygen species including oxygen toxicity in the lung, damage induced by inflammatory cells such as neutrophils, and reperfusion injury. Reactive oxygen species are commonly derived from cellular oxidation-reduction reactions involving enzymes such as xanthine oxidase, aldehyde oxidase, flavine dehydrogenases, and peroxidases, or nonenzymatic reactions such as auto-oxidation reactions and "leakage" from the mitochondrial electron transport system. Cellular sources of free radicals are summarized in Fig. 2-33.

Important reactants in this context include superoxide anion (O_2^-), hydroxyl radical ($\cdot OH$), and hydrogen peroxide (H_2O_2). Hydrogen peroxide is not a free radical, but it can generate hydroxyl radicals through reaction with ferrous or cupric ions or by reaction with superoxide anion. The latter reaction is catalyzed by trace amounts of iron.

Free radicals are substances that have unpaired electrons and are therefore generally highly reactive. Because of this, most exist only briefly and in low concentrations and do not travel far from the site at which they are formed. Thus the initial reaction of a free radical in a biological system will be close to its site of formation. However, free radical chain reactions, such as lipid peroxidation, and the action of products of free radical reactions can produce cellular damage at some distance from the initial event. Free radicals are able to combine with unsaturated lipids in cell membranes, resulting in the formation of organic free radicals (lipid radicals). These in turn rearrange and combine with

oxygen to form lipid hydroperoxyl radical, which then undergoes further reaction to form another lipid radical and lipid peroxides, the whole process being called *lipid peroxidation*. The peroxides formed in this reaction are unstable and break down to produce aldehydes (including malondialdehyde) and other compounds as well as generating additional organic free radicals. This reaction, once started, is self-propagating, and limited interaction with the initiating free radicals has the potential to lead to rapid widespread membrane damage.

Associated with free radical reactions and lipid peroxidation there may be damage to DNA, enzymes, and structural proteins. Chemical changes can occur in amino acids, polypeptide chains can be cleaved, and, in particular, polymerization of protein molecules can occur. The product of lipid peroxidation responsible for the cross-linking that produces protein polymerization is believed to be malondialdehyde. Proteins containing sulfhydryl groups are more susceptible to damage by lipid peroxidation than others. Clearly the damage produced by lipid peroxidation can result in loss of function of enzymes and other proteins in cell membranes and can be devastating for the cell.

The major site of damage caused by lipid peroxi-

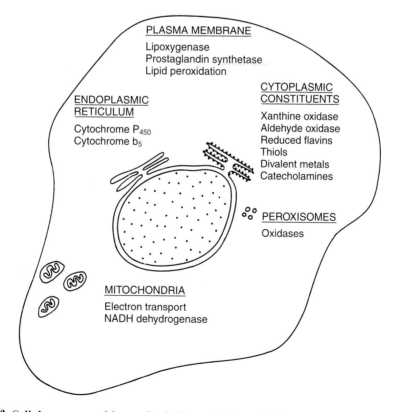

Fig. 2-33 Cellular sources of free radicals. Free radicals can be derived by means of many cellular metabolic functions.

dation is in membranes, especially those of subcellular organelles. The membranes of organelles, in particular those of mitochondria and endoplasmic reticulum, contain relatively high levels of unsaturated fatty acids making them very susceptible to lipid peroxidation. In addition, certain metals such as copper and iron, including iron-containing proteins, can act as catalysts for peroxidation reactions. In the mitochondria, therefore, the presence of cytochromes further enhances their susceptibility to damage by lipid peroxidation.

The membranes of lysosomes, in contrast, are relatively resistant to peroxidation, a consequence of their relatively low content of unsaturated fatty acids. As in hypoxia, lysosomal damage probably is a relatively late event in cell injury caused by membrane damage associated with lipid peroxidation. In one special case, however, lysosomal damage may be an important factor in causing cell injury. In Wilson's disease of humans and in a similar disease in some dog breeds, there is abnormal copper metabolism and storage of large amounts of copper in hepatocellular lysosomes. In these cases it is believed that the ability of copper to catalyze lipid peroxidation may cause primary lysosomal damage with release of enzymes and injury to the cell. This may be important in the pathogenesis of the extensive hepatocellular necrosis that can occur in these diseases. Massive liver necrosis also is common in chronic copper toxicity, another condition in which there is storage of copper in hepatocytes.

The consequence of all this membrane damage is of course abnormal membrane function. Most importantly, protein synthesis is disturbed because of damage to the RER, membrane permeability is disrupted, both in the plasma membrane and in organelles, and abnormal ion fluxes similar to those described in anoxic cell injury occur. Mitochondrial respiration is impaired because of membrane damage and to influx of calcium ions. Mitochondria provide an interesting example of a structure-linked enzyme activity, namely, oxidative phosphorylation. This is a closely membrane-associated system, and it has been shown that lipid peroxidation inhibits the coupling of phosphorylation to oxidation. The morphological and functional manifestations are enlarged upon below.

As would be expected, cells have mechanisms available to protect themselves against oxidative injury. In fact, the very presence of these defense mechanisms is evidence of the prevalence of free radical–generating reactions in biological systems. Important among these defenses are superoxide dismutases, which catalyze the conversion of superoxide anion to hydrogen peroxide, catalases, which break down hydrogen peroxide, and "endogenous antioxidants" such as vitamin E, glutathione, and ascorbate. Vitamin E, a lipid-soluble antioxidant that partitions into cellular membranes, and ascorbate, an aqueous-phase antioxidant, appear to be able to inactivate free radicals and prevent lipid peroxidation of membranes. Glutathione in its reduced form (GSH) reacts with hydrogen peroxide to form oxidized glutathione (GSSG). This reaction is catalyzed by the selenium-containing enzyme glutathione peroxidase. This enzyme also catalyzes the reduction of lipid peroxides by glutathione, thus preventing the propagation of lipid peroxidation reactions. Vitamin E and selenium can reduce the toxicity of some substances that act through free radical formation. Deficiency of either vitamin E or selenium, or both, is an important nutritional cause of disease in pigs, cattle, horses, sheep, chickens, and other animals. In all these species, necrosis of certain cell populations is a prominent feature of the disease. For example, selenium deficiency of cattle can cause muscle and myocardial necrosis, whereas vitamin E deficiency in horses has been implicated in motor neuron disease. Presumably the deficiency of vitamin E or selenium makes cell membranes unusually susceptible to oxidative injury and lipid peroxidation, which in turn result in cell injury.

It should also be mentioned that the toxic effects of reactive oxygen species have been very effectively exploited by phagocytic leukocytes as mechanisms for killing microorganisms. This phenomenon is believed to be mediated by superoxide and other radicals and is discussed in more detail in Chapters 4 and 7.

Functional and Morphological Consequences of Cell Membrane Injury

Not surprisingly, because both mechanisms of cell injury eventually produce membrane alterations, the morphological and functional changes that accompany cell injury caused by membrane damage do not differ substantially from those caused by anoxic cell injury. There are some differences that reflect differences in the most susceptible organelles in each case. The differences are stressed here rather than repeating the general features of cell injury that we already have discussed.

The earliest changes detectable in hepatocytes injured with CCl_4 are found in the RER. They appear as disaggregation and detachment of polysomes, presumably caused by lipid peroxidation of the membranes of the ER. There is evidence, however, that CCl_4 also can interfere directly with the interaction between ribosomes and mRNA.

Soon after this, there is disturbance of ion and water homeostasis that is first expressed as dilatation of the cisternae of the RER and eventually as cell swelling. As in hypoxic injury there is an influx of sodium ions and a loss of potassium. There also is an influx of calcium ions at about this time that occurs rapidly in this form of injury because of the ready supply of calcium ions from the blood. Calcium ions, being potent uncouplers of mitochondrial respiration, damage mitochondria and exacerbate the effects on the cell.

Because disaggregation of polysomes and their detachment from the RER occurs early in CCl_4 poisoning, reduction of protein synthesis can be detected within a few hours of onset of the injury. One consequence of this in the liver is a reduction in the availability of apolipoprotein, normally synthesized in hepatocytes. This protein is necessary for the export of triglycerides from the liver. Thus, lipids accumulate in hepatocytes injured in this way, and lipidosis is a characteristic of CCl_4 toxicity, though it certainly is not specific for it. In fact, accumulation of lipid is common is many forms of hepatocellular injury.

All the changes described above for CCl_4 intoxication are probably primarily the result of lipid peroxidation with subsequent membrane dysfunction. The features that distinguish this form of injury from anoxic cell injury are the early involvement of the RER and the relatively late involvement of the mitochondria. Once these initial changes have occurred, however, cell injury progresses in a manner comparable to that occurring in anoxia.

THE ROLE OF REACTIVE OXYGEN SPECIES IN ANOXIC CELL INJURY

Although it might seem rather paradoxical, there is now evidence that indicates that a significant amount of the damage occurring during ischemia or anoxia may be mediated by oxygen-derived free radicals. Most of the evidence for this comes from experimental models in which myocardial or intestinal ischemia is induced, often followed by reperfusion or reoxygenation. It is clear from numerous studies that the reestablishment of perfusion in ischemic tissue is followed by an exacerbation of cell injury. In the myocardium this is accompanied by the development of cell swelling and contraction bands. The concept that a transient period of ischemia causes the death of some cells has emerged. Others are "at risk" because of metabolic changes but are not yet dead and are, in fact, potentially able to be rescued. Reperfusion can rapidly induce cell death in a proportion of these

cells. This phenomenon has been termed *reperfusion injury*, and the generation of reactive oxygen species seems to be important in this setting.

The evidence for the involvement of oxygen-derived free radicals is both direct and indirect. Many studies in various species have shown that scavengers of these radicals, such as superoxide dismutase and catalase can reduce infarct size. It has also been shown that a sudden increase in free radical production and the formation of by-products of lipid peroxidation accompany reperfusion of ischemic tissue. Many potential sources of these radicals have been proposed, including the metabolism of catecholamines by monoamine oxidase, the "leakage" of oxygen free radicals from mitochondria, arachidonic acid metabolism, the action of the enzyme xanthine oxidase on hypoxanthine, and generation by leukocytes, primarily neutrophils, and macrophages, that infiltrate the ischemic lesion.

Xanthine oxidase is a potentially important source of oxygen-derived free radicals. The enzyme does not exist as such in normal tissues but is derived by sulfhydryl oxidation or limited proteolysis of xanthine dehydrogenase. It is hypothesized that activation of proteases by increased cytosolic calcium levels in ischemic cells leads to the conversion to the oxidase form of the enzyme. Evidence for this is that the reaction is irreversible, it occurs in the calcium paradox, and it can be inhibited by soybean trypsin inhibitor. This conversion can occur after only brief periods of ischemia. At the same time its substrate, hypoxanthine, is generated by the degradation of ATP. In the presence of molecular oxygen, xanthine oxidase acts on hypoxanthine to produce urate and superoxide anion (O_2^-). These interactions are summarized schematically in Fig. 2-34. It has been shown in numerous experimental models of myocardial or intestinal ischemia that infarction can be limited by treatment with allopurinol, an inhibitor of xanthine oxidase. Additionally the level of the xanthine oxidase form of the enzyme in ischemic myocardium has been shown to be about 300% of that in the normal tissue. There is therefore clear evidence for a role of xanthine oxidase in generating free radicals in ischemic tissue. However, this appears to be limited to certain species. For example, the enzyme, in either form, has been demonstrated to be present in tissues of dogs, cats, rats, and cattle but is absent from those of humans and rabbits.

Infiltrating leukocytes are an important source of reactive oxygen species in ischemic and reperfused tissue. As discussed in Chapter 4, macrophages and neutrophils, in particular the latter, generate abundant quantities of superoxide anion during phagocytosis. It has been shown that factors chemotactic

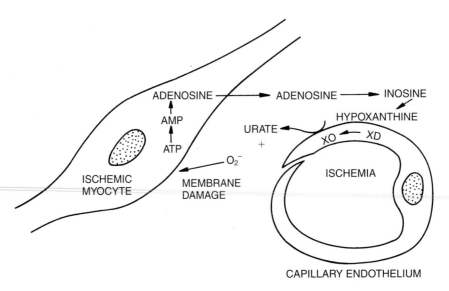

Fig. 2-34 Generation of superoxide radical by xanthine oxidase. Xanthine oxidase derived from xanthine dehydrogenase in endothelial cells acts on hypoxanthine to generate oxygen-derived free radicals.

for neutrophils, including cleavage products of complement, are generated in ischemic myocardial tissue, and there is a correlation between infarct size and the degree of neutrophil infiltration. Furthermore, depletion of neutrophils can reduce infarct size. Finally, drugs that inhibit the generation of superoxide anion by neutrophils have a similar effect.

REVERSIBILITY AND IRREVERSIBILITY

As cell injury progresses to its later stages, the changes in the various organelles remain qualitatively similar but become more severe. Eventually organelles break down, cytoplasmic proteins are denatured, and the organelles of the necrotic cell may be barely recognizable at the ultrastructural level. Without doubt such cells are dead, but what is the critical change in the cell that makes injury irreversible? Nobody can give an answer to that question. However, we can at least rule out some of the phenomena that we have discussed and suggest that others might be important.

Changes in the structure and function of the nucleus are probably not of primary importance. Certainly we know that erythrocytes live for over 100 days without a nucleus. Similarly, loss of the ability to synthesize protein caused by injury to the nucleus and RER are not immediately lethal. Agents that specifically block protein synthesis, for example, do not cause immediate cell death. Similarly, prevention of reduced intracellular pH does not prevent cell death. Indeed, there is now evidence that intracellular acidosis protects against or delays cell in-

jury probably by suppressing degradative enzymatic processes. It is believed that restoration of normal intracellular pH may be a factor in producing further cell death after reperfusion.

In hypoxic cells, reduction of cellular ATP is of more importance. If restored in time, transient reduction in ATP levels does not kill the cell, but prolonged reduction does. The important change therefore is likely to be some immediate consequence of sufficiently prolonged reduction in intracellular levels of energy. Some change follows severe reduction in ATP levels that apparently cannot be repaired. One event very likely to be of prime importance in the loss of reversibility and hence cell death is irreversible damage to mitochondria such that they cannot regenerate ATP. Such damage is associated with all the changes described above, and we know that after a certain period of anoxia and in the usual cellular milieu the mitochondria are unable to resume the production of energy even when oxygen again becomes available. As a result none of the energy-dependent functions of the cell can be reestablished. Thus it has been argued that anoxic cells die because a point is reached when the mitochondria are irreversibly damaged. It is presumably for this reason that severe ultrastructural changes in mitochondria correlate best with the onset of irreversible injury.

The Role of Calcium in Cell Injury

Much attention has been focused on the role of calcium ions in injured cells. As we have already pointed out, an increase in intracellular calcium ions is a consistent feature of necrosis, and necrotic cells may even contain deposits of calcium salts. This is attributable to redistribution from intracellular compartments such as the ER to the cytosol and to the influx of calcium ions that occurs as a result of membrane dysfunction. Of course, the presence of increased quantities of calcium in necrotic cells is not in itself proof that they are of importance in the pathogenesis of the injury. Certainly, though, we can say with confidence that calcified cells are dead cells.

The role of calcium ions in cell death has been extensively studied experimentally both *in vivo* and *in vitro,* and there is considerable evidence indicating that increased intracellular calcium levels can be involved. The most common systems that have been used are ischemic heart or liver. Such studies have confirmed that after a period of anoxia, the intracellular levels of energy stores, in particular ATP, fall dramatically and that when the tissue is reperfused, or reoxygenated, the mitochondria fail to regenerate ATP. In other words, the injury is irreversible, and many of the cells die. This is correlated with a large increase in mitochondrial content of calcium. The relationship of the latter to irreversibility of the injury has been tested in several ways. For example, when the overloading of the mitochondria with calcium is prevented, by initially reperfusion with a low-calcium solution, or by prior treatment with calcium-antagonist drugs, such as chlorpromazine or verapamil, the mitochondria are able to regain their functional capacity to generate ATP, and most of the cells recover. It is very interesting to note that such treatments do not prevent the occurrence of the ultrastructural changes that we have described as typical of irreversible cell injury, including high-amplitude swelling of mitochondria; thus even this morphological hallmark of irreversible injury is *not* necessarily irreversible, and such changes regress as the cell recovers.

If the influx of calcium into injured cells and their mitochondria is in fact of primary importance in determining irreversibility, it should be possible to test the hypothesis by causing increased entry of calcium as a primary event. This has been done by use of the so-called calcium paradox. If heart tissue, for example, is perfused first with a solution very low in calcium and then with one with normal levels of calcium, there is a massive influx of calcium ions into the cells. This leads to extensive mitochondrial uptake of calcium, loss of ATP-generating capacity, and depletion of cellular ATP. In this case, therefore, the disruption of mitochondrial function is the *result* of calcium influx, rather than the reverse.

Similar observations have been made *in vitro,* where the effects of both anoxia and toxic cell injury, in which there is direct attack on the cell membrane, have been tested. Such studies have shown that for many different drugs, cell death is dependent on the concentration of calcium ions in the external medium. In addition, treatment of cultured cells with calcium ionophores, which allow the influx of calcium ions into the cells, causes cell death. Calcium ionophores can also enhance the toxic effect of other drugs on cultured cells, presumably by amplifying the uptake of calcium ions.

Despite all this evidence, more recent studies have shown that, at least in some systems, increases in intracellular calcium concentrations cannot be linked to irreversible cell injury, and the role of calcium in cell death, as discussed below, is now rather controversial.

Relationship of Membrane Damage to Calcium and Cell Death

We have already discussed the fact that there is damage to cellular membranes in injured cells that results in altered mitochondrial function, increased permeability to ions, an influx of sodium and calcium ions, and a loss of potassium and magnesium ions. In addition, there is redistribution of ions within the cell, which, importantly, leads to a release of calcium ions from the sarcoplasmic reticulum and other cellular compartments into the cytoplasm. Calcium ions are known to be important as an intracellular messenger and are capable of modulating and activating many different cellular functions. Important among these are the calcium-activated ATPases, proteases, and the endogenous phospholipases. Activation of ATPases by increased levels of calcium ions serves only to further deplete cellular energy stores. Activation of phospholipases serves to further damage the already leaky cellular membranes, including the plasma membrane. There is clear evidence of loss of membrane phospholipids in ischemic liver and myocardium, reflecting membrane damage that affects both plasma membranes and those of the endoplasmic reticulum. Other factors are also apparently involved in producing membrane damage in anoxic cells. One of these is the accumulation of harmful metabolites in anoxic cells. We have already discussed the role of free radicals in ischemic cell injury and the fact that these can be generated by calcium-activated phospholipases and proteases. Long-chain acyl-CoA esters and long-chain acyl carnitine also accumulate in ischemic cells and have been proposed to have a detergent effect that can damage cellular membranes. In addition, there is evidence that lack of oxygen itself is important in contributing to the membrane damage in ischemic or anoxic cells. When cells are treated with metabolic poisons that block the synthesis of ATP, there is little effect on cell viability during the time scale in which actual anoxia produces extensive cell death. Thus the effects of anoxia involve more than just the depletion of cellular energy supplies. Oxygen is also utilized by many oxygenases, in particular the fatty acid desaturases, enzymes involved in the synthesis of polyunsaturated fatty acids required for the maintenance of cell membranes. These enzymes are blocked by cyanide, a metabolic poison that also blocks electron transport in the mitochondria and that does mimic the lethal effects of anoxia on cells. Inhibition of these enzymes therefore is another route by which membrane damage could result from anoxia. In addition, recent evidence has shown that exogenous glycine can protect cells depleted of ATP against membrane damage. When this is done, ATP-depleted cells can withstand high levels of calcium ions for long periods without losing viability.

As a consequence of all this it has been argued that the truly critical factor in producing irreversible cell injury is membrane damage. It is apparent that membrane damage is central to lethal cell injury whether it is attributable to anoxia or to direct attack on cell membranes. However, there is experimental evidence that membrane damage can also be repaired as long as influx of calcium is prevented. As membrane components are continually being turned over, it is reasonable to assume that a degree of damage to the cell membranes can be repaired as long as the necessary metabolic energy is supplied. This argument can become circular, with membrane damage leading to calcium influx and calcium influx contributing to membrane damage and mitochondrial dysfunction. In real disease situations membrane damage is a consistent and important factor, but the final outcome of the insult depends on the interactions of these various factors. The arguments that we have presented are summarized in Fig. 2-35.

Hepatic Lipidosis as a Model of Nonlethal Cell Injury

Cell injury, no matter what its cause, is not always lethal. Often, cells are injured and cannot adequately carry out their normal functions but are

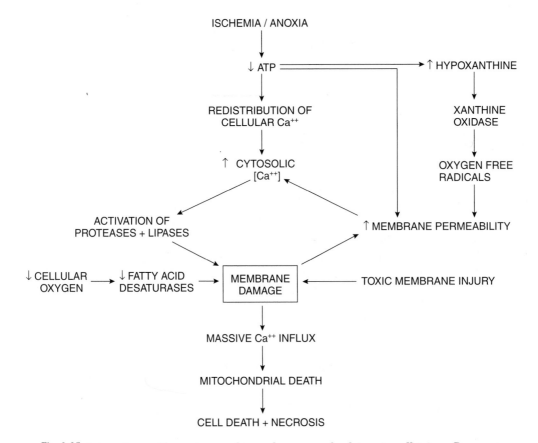

Fig. 2-35 Interactions of hypoxia, membrane damage, and calcium in cell injury. Damage to cell membranes is central to most forms of cell injury.

able to maintain homeostasis and stay alive. Lipidosis, or fatty change, the name given to abnormal accumulation of lipids in the cell, is a good example with which to illustrate this point. Lipidosis can occur in a variety of cells but is most often seen in the liver, renal tubular epithelium, and the myocardium. In the liver, which we consider in some detail here, it represents a common nonspecific response that may be seen in many diseases.

Grossly, lipidosis may impart a pale yellow color to the liver. If most cells are affected, the liver will be diffusely affected. If cells are affected in a zonal pattern, a reticular pattern will be seen grossly (Fig. 2-36). Histologically the lipid in the cells will be evident as vacuoles. Often these are evident as large, sharply demarcated single vacuoles, but at other times vacuoles are smaller and multiple (see Fig. 2-15). Although large, sharply demarcated single vacuoles are fairly distinctive and recognizable as lipidosis, not all cytoplasmic vacuoles contain fat. Vacuoles also may represent dilated cisternae of the ER, areas of the cytoplasm depleted of organelles or stored material in lysosomes. Special stains or electron microscopy may be required to identify their contents.

Lipidosis was, in the past, referred to as fatty degeneration or fatty infiltration. These terms are best not used because the presence of intracellular lipid does not necessarily indicate any degenerative change in the cell and the fat is not an infiltrate. Abnormal fat vacuoles do indicate an *increase in intracellular lipid* that may be attributable to abnormalities of synthesis or utilization or mobilization (export) of fat. Lipidosis is sometimes an expression of cell injury and, when it is, may be preceded or accompanied by cell swelling. In addition, lipidosis can occur as an expression of injury in cells that are destined to die. In the case of CCl_4 poisoning, for example, cells undergoing lipidosis may be observed adjacent to cells that are obviously necrotic. Presumably many of the cells containing lipid are severely injured and destined to die. A lesion of this type is shown in Fig. 2-37.

In the liver cell, which is particularly susceptible to lipidosis, numerous mechanisms may be involved in the accumulation of lipids. To understand them it is necessary to review briefly the normal metabolism of fats in the hepatocyte. This is summarized in Fig. 2-38. Briefly, lipids enter the liver cells as free fatty acids (FFA), which are mostly esterified to form triglycerides (TG). Some, however, are utilized in the synthesis of cholesterol esters or phospholipids, and some are degraded to produce ketone bodies. The hepatocyte is capable also of synthesizing some fatty

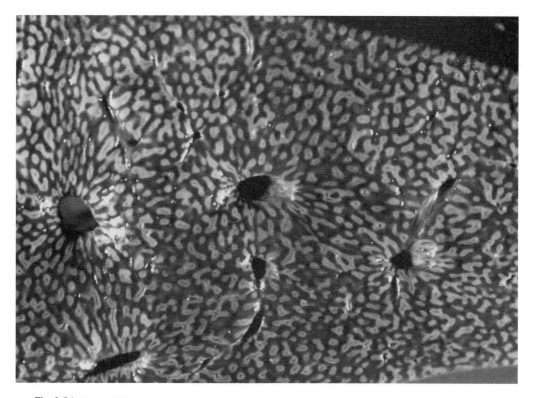

Fig. 2-36 Centrilobular hepatic lipidosis. The light areas represent parenchyma, adjacent to central veins, which has undergone lipidosis caused by hypoxia. They contrast with the darker normal tissue.

acids from acetate. To be exported from the hepatocyte, TG must be complexed with an apolipoprotein or lipid acceptor protein to form lipoproteins. In theory at least, accumulation of intracellular lipid can occur because of abnormalities in any of these steps.

Experimental models have shown that interference with the incorporation of FFA into phospholipids, impaired complexing of TG with apolipoprotein, or impaired export of the complex from the hepatocyte all can result in the accumulation of lipid in the liver

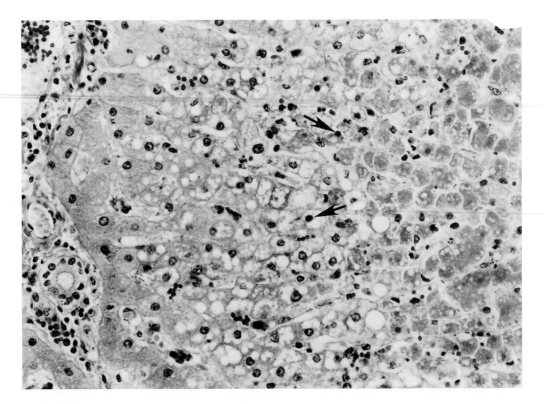

Fig. 2-37 Progression of cell injury. In this liver, the progression of cell injury can readily be appreciated. Near the portal area at *left* the hepatocytes show only mild cell swelling. Progressing toward the central vein (which is out of the picture to *right*), the cells show lipidosis and then more severe swelling with nuclear changes such as pyknosis, *arrows*, and eventually coagulation necrosis. This lesion was caused by hypoxia associated with methemoglobinemia. The hepatocytes near the central vein are more susceptible to such insults and thus are injured first, resulting in the sequence shown here.

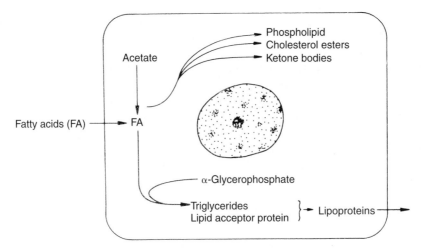

Fig. 2-38 Metabolism of fats in the hepatocyte. Fatty acids may be synthesized in the hepatocyte or be taken up from the blood. Some are converted to triglycerides. Lipid acceptor protein is essential for their export from the cell.

cell. In veterinary medicine two important mechanisms of lipidosis are commonly encountered. Excessive delivery of FFA to the liver when body fats are rapidly mobilized, as occurs, for example, in starvation, can overwhelm the capacity of the liver to export TG because packaging and export of lipoprotein is a rate-limiting step. Perhaps most relevant to our discussion of cell injury is the accumulation of TG because of reduced capacity to synthesize the apolipoprotein. The formation of lipoprotein is mandatory for the export of TG from the liver, and the protein moiety (the acceptor protein) is synthesized in the hepatocyte itself. Therefore any cell injury resulting in a reduction of protein synthesis will impair export of TG and result in lipidosis. As pointed out earlier, reduced protein synthesis is an early consequence of injury caused by membrane damage, and lipidosis is a characteristic finding in the liver injured by toxins, such as CCl₄ and phosphorus, and many other insults.

The reduction in protein synthesis and the accumulation of lipid are in themselves not lethal to the cell, and cells with lipidosis sometimes can survive for a long time. Obviously, as they survive, they can maintain at least minimal homeostatic mechanisms, but functions other than lipid acceptor protein synthesis also may be impaired. As a result, the animal may show signs of clinical illness.

PIGMENTS AND OTHER TISSUE DEPOSITS

Many pathological processes are accompanied by the accumulation, either inside cells or in the interstitium, of a variety of abnormal substances. These are known as *deposits* or, if colored, as *pigments*.

Intracellular Lipid Accumulation

One of the most common of such substances, namely, triglycerides, we have already discussed. Triglyceride lipids may accumulate in injured cells and are visible microscopically as clear vacuoles. Other lipids can accumulate producing a similar appearance. These include substances stored in the inherited storage diseases, the *lipidoses,* and phagocytosed lipids. When adipose tissue or the lipid-rich tissues of the central nervous system undergo necrosis, the lipid and other debris are phagocytosed by macrophages, imparting a vacuolated appearance to their cytoplasm. This appearance can be so dramatic that the cells are called "foam cells," or "foamy macrophages."

Cholesterol is another lipid substance that can accumulate in tissues. It deserves special mention because of its involvement in vascular disease in hu-

mans. Atherosclerosis is a lesion of arteries and arterioles in which cholesterol accumulates in smooth muscle cells in the walls of the vessels. The affected cells are vacuolated and appear foamy and may contain crystallized cholesterol, which produces a characteristic needle-like cleft in the tissue (Fig. 2-39, *A*). A comprehensive discussion of atherosclerosis is not appropriate here, but suffice it to say that it is a common lesion in humans that predisposes to other problems such as myocardial infarction. In dogs, atherosclerosis is sometimes seen as a complication of hypothyroidism. This condition is associated with hypercholesterolemia, or increased blood cholesterol levels, and affected animals often have widespread atherosclerotic lesions (Fig. 2-39, *B*). Atherosclerosis is, in general, much less important in animals than it is in man.

Occasionally adipose tissue infiltrates the interstitium of skeletal muscle, the myocardium, and other tissues. This process should be distinguished from intracellular lipid accumulation and is of considerably less importance. It is characterized by the presence of histologically normal adipose tissue in the interstitial connective tissue and is usually not associated with a functional disturbance.

Intracellular Protein Accumulation

Cells, of course, normally contain a great variety of proteins, but in a few circumstances unusual amounts of protein can be present and may be apparent histologically as eosinophilic droplets or bodies. In the kidney, protein lost into the ultrafiltrate as a result of glomerular disease is taken up to some extent by epithelial cells of the proximal tubules. This produces droplets in the cytoplasm of these cells, and such droplets represent protein in secondary lysosomes. In the case of plasma cells, the immunoglobulin proteins produced by these cells can accumulate in cisternae of the RER, again producing eosinophilic masses usually called, in this case, "Russell bodies." These changes are of little consequence in terms of cell injury.

The terms *hyaline* and *fibrinoid* are sometimes used to describe tissue deposits. These are descriptive terms coined by histopathologists and are really of limited use because they describe only the appearance of certain deposits rather than their true nature. Hyaline is the name given to any substance, intracellular or extracellular, that has a homogeneous, glassy, eosinophilic appearance. It does not represent a specific substance but often is protein in nature. For example, plasma proteins that leak through damaged endothelium may give the vessel wall a hyalinized appearance, thickened basement membranes may be hyalinized, and amyloid (dis-

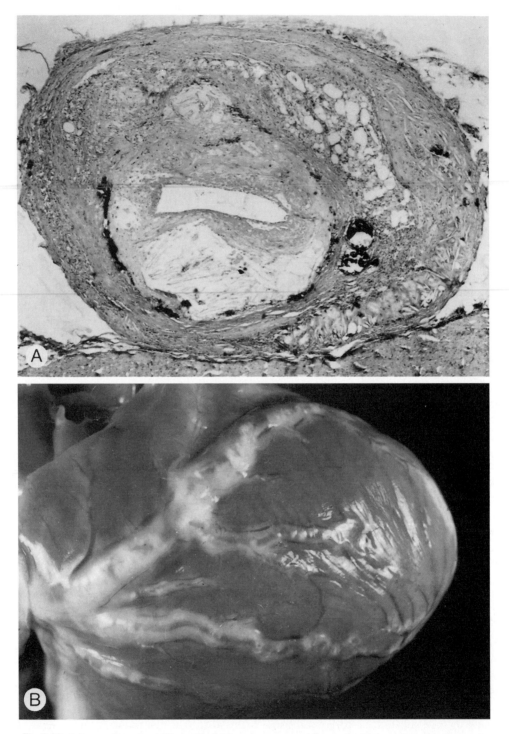

Fig. 2-39 Atherosclerosis. *A,* The wall of this coronary vessel is greatly thickened, and its lumen is reduced as a result of atherosclerosis. The light-colored vacuoles represent areas of lipid deposition, and the angular clefts, cholesterol deposition. The dark material is calcified tissue. *B,* In this heart the coronary vessels are prominent and light in color as a result of atherosclerosis. These lesions are from a dog with hypothyroidism.

cussed more fully below) also has this histological appearance. Fibrinoid is also a nonspecific term that indicates that the material present in the tissue has an appearance similar to that of fibrin. Like hyaline, fibrinoid material is variable in composition but is often protein in nature and may in fact contain fibrin or degradation products of fibrin.

Pigments

Pigments are substances that are inherently colored. A variety of pigments may accumulate in tissues, either inside or outside of cells. They are often subdivided into two groups, endogenous and exogenous pigments. *Endogenous pigments* originate in the affected animal, whereas *exogenous pigments* come from the external environment.

Exogenous pigments include carbon, soot, or other dusts. In special circumstances they may be predominantly silica dust or asbestos dust or other relatively homogeneous substances. These are often contaminants of the environment of people or animals. Silicosis, the deposition of silica dust in the lungs, is a special problem for miners, whereas anthracosis, the deposition of carbon particles, is a special problem of city dwellers. Such inhaled dust particles are found in macrophages in the lungs and draining lymph nodes. In the case of anthracosis, the pigment gives these tissues a black discoloration. Most pigments are relatively harmless, but, if present in the lung in large quantities, they may cause chronic injury leading to pulmonary fibrosis. Of course, the dust we inhale in large industrialized cities usually is accompanied by other substances that can be harmful. In particular, many of them are potential carcinogens (see Chapter 6) and may cause cancer.

Endogenous pigments include many substances that may be normal cell products or may result from the breakdown of normal substances. *Lipofuscin* already has been mentioned in our discussion of cell injury. In tissue sections it appears as a golden brown, finely granular, intracellular pigment (Fig. 2-40). It is derived chiefly from the breakdown

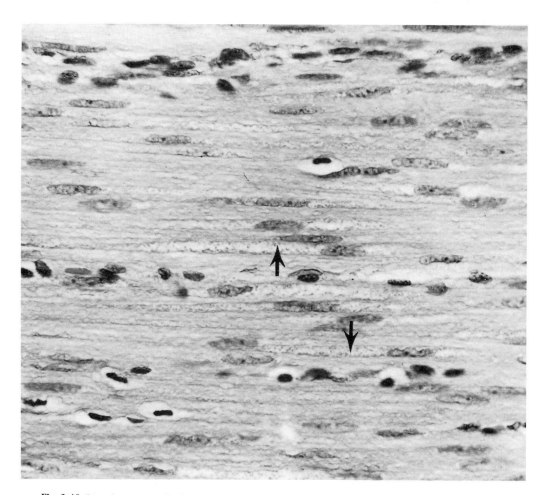

Fig. 2-40 Lipofuscinosis. In these smooth muscle cells, from the intestinal wall of a dog with vitamin E deficiency, there are accumulations of fine granular lipofuscin pigment, *arrows.*

products of lipids, usually those derived from cell membranes. Therefore it is found most commonly in aged cells, in particular, myocardial cells and neurons of old people or animals, or in chronically injured cells. It is in fact commonly referred to as "aging pigment" or "wear and tear" pigment. Because it is the result of breakdown of lipid-containing membranes in the lysosome, it essentially is the light microscopic equivalent of residual bodies.

Lipofuscin is increased in certain cells where there is increased turnover of organelles or increased membrane injury. In some species it is increased in amount as a consequence of vitamin E or selenium deficiency. In the dog, for example, such deficiencies lead to *lipofuscinosis* of the smooth muscle of the intestine, which imparts a grossly evident distinct yellow-brown discoloration to the organ. Lipofuscin also can be increased in amount when a diet rich in unsaturated fatty acids is fed.

Lipofuscin apparently consists of a complex of lipids, phospholipids, and some protein. It is somewhat variable in composition, presumably reflecting not only its variable origins but also the degree to which lysosomal substrates have been broken down. For this reason its staining characteristics are also variable. *Ceroid* is a variant of lipofuscin that is acid-fast and autofluorescent.

Melanin is a normal pigment that usually is found in melanocytes, in epidermal cells, and in the pigmented epithelial cells of the eye. Less commonly, other tissues such as the intestine, the kidney, or the leptomeninges contain melanin. Histologically it has a brown, finely granular, appearance. In the skin melanin is produced in melanocytes and transferred from these cells to basal cells of the epidermis where it provides some protection from ultraviolet rays. In some pathological conditions melanin also is found in macrophages. In these *melanophages* it is the result of phagocytosis of pigment derived from injured melanocytes or epithelial cells. *Pseudomelanosis* is a term used to describe an artifactual discoloration of tissues that produces an appearance similar to melanin pigmentation. It occurs as a postmortem event when hydrogen sulfide produced by bacteria reacts with iron in the tissues to produce iron sulfide.

Hemosiderin is an iron-containing yellow-brown granular pigment frequently observed in tissue sections. In cells, iron usually is stored, bound to the protein apoferritin, as *ferritin*. When large amounts of ferritin are present, aggregates form, producing the granules that we recognize histologically as hemosiderin. In sections, it is a yellow-gold, granular, intracellular pigment. Hemosiderin commonly is seen in areas of congestion or hemorrhage or where there is excessive breakdown of red blood cells. In almost any section of spleen, for example, it is possible to find at least some hemosiderin, typically in macrophages (Fig. 2-41). Hemosiderin also can be

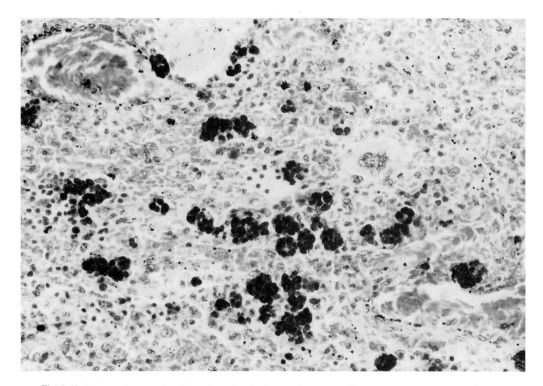

Fig. 2-41 Hemosiderosis. In this spleen the dark granular material represents hemosiderin. This is a common finding in the spleen.

found in macrophages in other tissues. In animals with congestive heart failure it is commonly found in alveolar macrophages in the congested lung (see Fig. 3-3) and grossly may impart a light brown color to the tissue. In most cases hemosiderin causes no damage to the cell.

Less commonly, copper may be stored in tissues, particularly in hepatocytes. This is seen in animals with chronic copper poisoning, most commonly in sheep, in some dog breeds that have an inherited defect in copper metabolism, and sometimes as a consequence of chronic liver disease. Storage of large amounts of copper is potentially toxic to the hepatocyte, and affected animals often have relatively sudden onset of acute hepatocellular necrosis. What precipitates this event is not clearly understood. Like iron, copper is capable of catalyzing lipid peroxidation, and damage to lysosomal membranes may be involved in this form of hepatocellular injury.

Bile pigments, including *bilirubin,* are normal products of the breakdown of the heme portion of hemoglobin. Because red blood cells are continually being destroyed and replaced, there is continual production of bilirubin. It is conjugated in the hepatocyte to its glucuronide, which makes it soluble in water, and then excreted into the bile. Bilirubin may accumulate in the blood or in tissues when there is increased breakdown of erythrocytes, as in hemolytic diseases, or when there is hepatic disease. In the latter case it may accumulate because of failure of conjugation, failure of excretion, or cholestasis. Accumulation of bilirubin in the blood produces a generalized yellow discoloration of the tissue known clinically as "jaundice," or "icterus." In sections, bilirubin is a green-brown to yellow-brown pigment. It may be observed in bile canaliculi in cholestasis, in hepatocytes, and in renal tubular epithelium. In the latter it is believed to be toxic, producing the so-called bile nephrosis, or renal tubular necrosis, sometimes seen in icteric animals. Occasionally, at sites of previous hemorrhage, a yellow-brown pigment called *hematoidin* accumulates. It is believed to be locally precipitated bilirubin and, unlike hemosiderin, is negative in special stains for iron.

It is clear from this discussion that several pigments, namely, hemosiderin, bile pigments, copper, melanin, and lipofuscin, have a similar appearance in tissues. In practice it often is necessary to use special staining procedures to identify them. In addition, pigment-like material may be deposited as an artifact of preparation. Most troublesome among these is *acid hematin,* a derivative of hemoglobin produced in tissues fixed in improperly buffered formalin. Superficially it resembles hemosiderin but usually can be seen to overlie cells instead of being them.

Calcification

As we have already discussed, calcification is a common manifestation of lethal cell injury, but it is sometimes also seen when there is no apparent preceding cell death. When calcification occurs in injured tissues, it is said to be *dystrophic,* and when it occurs in apparently normal tissues, it is said to be *metastatic.*

Dystrophic calcification is not associated with hypercalcemia or other disturbances of calcium homeostasis. It occurs in cells injured in a variety of ways including vascular, toxic, metabolic, or inflammatory causes, but, as already mentioned, it is most prominent when a functional blood supply is present in the injured tissue. In sections stained with hematoxylin and eosin, the calcium deposits have a finely granular appearance and are basophilic (Fig. 2-42). In necrotic fat cells, calcium often is deposited in the form of insoluble calcium soaps derived from the interaction of calcium ions and fatty acids produced in the necrotic cells.

The pathogenesis of dystrophic calcification is poorly understood. However, like its physiological counterpart, the process may involve the deposition of calcium on or in so-called *matrix vesicles.* These are membranous vesicles probably derived, in physiological situations, by budding of the plasma membrane and, in pathological processes, as products of cellular disintegration. Acidic phospholipids in these membranous vesicles, in particular phosphatidylserine, may serve as binding sites for calcium. As we have already discussed in this chapter, calcium can be taken up by injured cells, and mitochondria may serve as foci for calcium deposition in injured cells.

Metastatic calcification commonly is associated with hypercalcemia or disturbances of calcium metabolism. For example, it may be seen in hyperparathyroidism, hypervitaminosis D, renal failure (renal secondary hyperparathyroidism), and certain neoplastic diseases. The calcium salts may be deposited in many sites but are commonly seen in the gastric and intestinal mucosa, the interstitium of blood vessel walls, the lung, and the kidney. Very often they are deposited along basement membranes (Fig. 2-43). Why these sites are more susceptible than others to metastatic calcification is poorly understood.

Amyloid and Amyloidosis

One of the most important of all tissue deposits is amyloid, so named by Virchow because he believed it to be of polysaccharide, or starchlike, composition. Actually it is now known to be protein in nature.

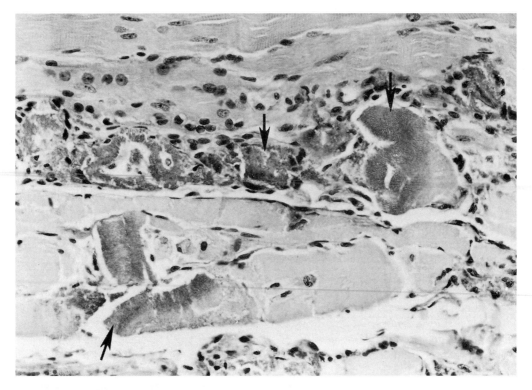

Fig. 2-42 Dystrophic calcification. In this skeletal muscle the dark material, *arrows*, represents calcification of necrotic fibers. The striated appearance seen in some areas is attributable to the orientation of the mitochondria, the primary site of calcium deposition, with the sarcomeres.

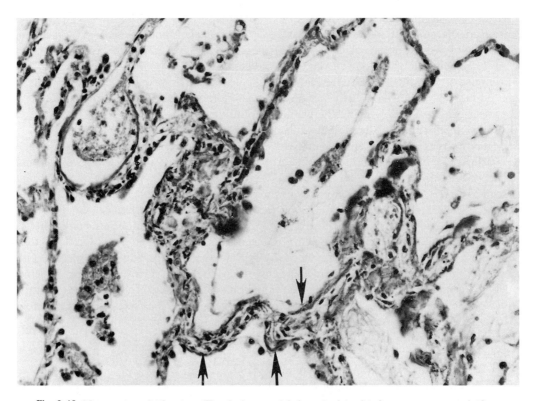

Fig. 2-43 Metastatic calcification. The dark material deposited in this lung represents calcification in a case of chronic renal failure in a cat. This type of calcification often shows a predilection for basement membranes. This can be appreciated here in a blood vessel, *upper left*, and in some alveolar septa, *arrows*.

Amyloid may be deposited locally or systemically, and a disease process resulting from deposition of this material is known as *amyloidosis*. Histologically amyloid is a lightly eosinophilic, amorphous, hyaline material that is deposited extracellularly. Frequently it is present in or around the walls of blood vessels. At other times it may be more diffuse in its distribution. When extensive, amyloid deposits may compress or distort adjacent tissues and cause dysfunction. A common example is amyloidosis of the renal glomeruli. In this case the amyloid is deposited within the walls of glomerular capillaries (Figs. 2-44, *A*, and 2-45) leading to leakage of proteins from the plasma into the urine.

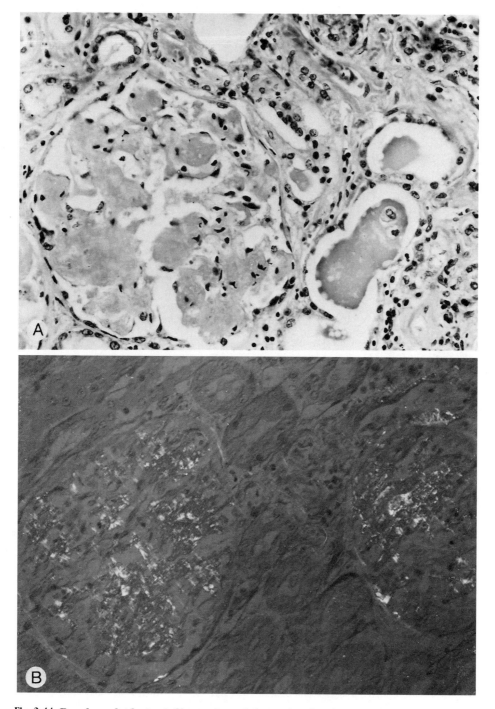

Fig. 2-44 Renal amyloidosis. *A*, Glomerulus at *left* contains abundant amorphous hyaline material typical of amyloid. Two tubules to the *right* contain proteinaceous material reflecting the loss of protein, mostly albumin, through the affected glomeruli. *B*, Under polarized light, affected glomeruli stained with Congo red are birefringent and appear light in this photomicrograph.

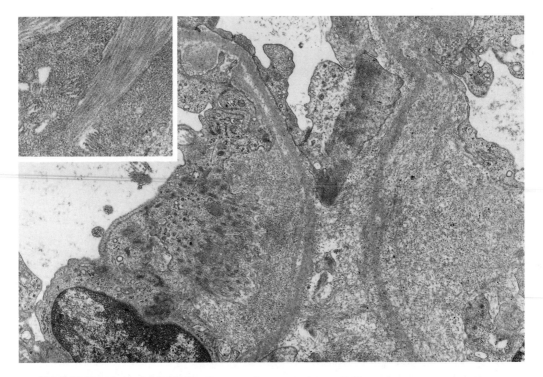

Fig. 2-45 Renal amyloidosis. By electron microscopy the amyloid can be seen to separate endothelial cells from their basement membrane. In the *inset* the filamentous nature of the amyloid can be appreciated.

Amyloid is distinguished from other deposits of similar appearance by the use of special stains. The most commonly used is *Congo red*, which stains amyloid orange red and renders it birefringent under polarized light (Fig. 2-44, *B*). Ultrastructurally amyloid is made up of masses of linear, nonbranching fibrils 7.5 to 10 nm in diameter (see Fig. 2-45).

The deposition of amyloid is a rather ubiquitous response to a variety of pathological conditions. It may be associated with chronic inflammatory disease, and it may be found associated with certain neoplasms, especially those of endocrine origin. At other times amyloid is deposited in the absence of an identifiable predisposing cause. Traditionally the latter is referred to as *primary amyloidosis* (most commonly seen in humans), whereas the form associated with other diseases is known as *secondary amyloidosis.*

Amyloid now is known not to be a specific chemical substance. Rather, the characteristic appearance and staining reactions of amyloid are attributable to a particular conformation of the constituent polypeptides known as the β-*pleated sheet*. Therefore any polypeptide molecules that can adopt this conformation can produce fibrils that, although chemically variable, are in fact amyloid. Because of this, the complex of syndromes involving amyloid deposition have been referred to as the β-*fibrilloses*. This peculiar conformation confers the tinctorial properties of amyloid and makes it rather resistant to enzymatic degradation. Even pure amyloid fibrils created *in vitro* share these staining characteristics. Although amyloid seems to persist in tissues for a long time, its stability has never been rigorously proved.

Although amyloid can be derived from a variety of different proteins (at least 18 in humans), two forms are most important. One form is composed of immunoglobulin light chains and is referred to as *amyloid protein AL*. The other form contains a protein called *amyloid protein AA*. The primary form of amyloidosis is associated with deposition of amyloid of the AL type. This protein also is deposited in amyloidosis associated with multiple myeloma (plasma cell neoplasia), and it appears that most patients with primary amyloidosis have plasma cell dyscrasias. Amyloid protein of the AL type apparently is composed of homogeneous light chains, of the lambda or kappa type, with or without their N-terminal fragments. In addition, circulating proteins that are immunologically cross-reactive with the amyloid deposits often can be demonstrated.

Primary amyloidosis, at least in humans, therefore appears to be associated with abnormalities of plasma cells, or plasma cell dyscrasias, associated with which is the production of free light chains or fragments of them. Fragments derived from some such light chains apparently have the capacity to adopt the β-pleated sheet conformation, which is the primary prerequisite for amyloid formation.

Secondary amyloidosis is associated with the deposition of amyloid protein AA. In contrast to AL, AA proteins have a rather similar amino acid sequence at their N-terminus, and AA proteins are highly conserved in different species. These proteins are not completely uniform, however, and a variety of AA proteins apparently exist. Secondary amyloidosis in a variety of animal species has been associated with the deposition of AA protein.

A group of circulating serum proteins antigenically related to AA protein and designated *serum amyloid A (SAA)* has been described in mice with experimental amyloidosis and in humans with amyloidosis of the AA type. These are high-molecular-weight proteins containing sequences found in AA protein. SAAs appear to be acute-phase proteins associated with the inflammatory reaction. They are synthesized in the liver in response to induction by *interleukin 1* and probably other cytokines.

Current evidence indicates that amyloid proteins may be derived by partial proteolytic degradation of parent proteins. The evidence for this includes the generation of amyloid fibrils *in vitro*, sequence relationships between amyloid proteins and suspected parent proteins, immunological cross reactivity between amyloids and parent proteins, and the apparent initial association of amyloid fibrils with lysosomes of macrophages. Some forms of amyloidosis in humans are associated with mutant precursor proteins.

A second protein, *amyloid-enhancing factor* (AEF) has been associated with persistent inflammation and with the deposition of amyloid. AEF has the ability to dramatically shorten the time required for the deposition of amyloid in experimental models. It is a glycoprotein that apparently alters the metabolism of SAA and appears to be essential for the deposition of AA amyloid, at least in experimental models. Additional events are probably also required for the deposition of amyloid, however, because the induction of SAA by interleukin 1 in the presence of AEF is insufficient to produce the disease.

There are also forms of amyloid other than those we have described. In humans and animals there are familial forms of amyloidosis. Familial forms of amyloidosis occur in the shar-pei dog and the Abyssinian cat. The amyloid that is sometimes deposited in endocrine tumors apparently is derived from the polypeptide hormones or prohormones that the neoplastic cells may produce. Amyloidosis of the pancreatic islets is fairly common in cats, in which it can cause diabetes mellitus. It has been shown that this particular form of amyloid is derived from a hormone produced by islet cells, islet amyloid polypeptide.

It should also be pointed out that amyloid contains components other than the fibril proteins. These include glycosaminoglycans (GAGs) and so-called *amyloid P component* (AP). The latter is related to a serum protein, also synthesized in the liver, which appears to behave as an acute-phase reactant in most species. The almost constant association of AP with various different forms of amyloid indicates that it plays a significant role in the development of amyloid deposits, but this role is so far not understood. Certain apolipoproteins, in particular apolipoprotein E (apoE), are also consistently associated with amyloid deposition. It has been suggested recently that apoE is involved in the formation of several different forms of amyloid.

Finally, although amyloid is usually regarded as a relatively stable deposit, resistant to degradation, there is some evidence that serum factors, probably serine proteases, can degrade it. In humans serum degradative activity may be inversely correlated with the deposition of amyloid. It is possible, therefore, that abnormalities in the degradation of AA may play a role in the pathogenesis of amyloidosis.

CELLULAR PATHOLOGY IN PERSPECTIVE

In concluding this chapter we would like to emphasize once more the fact that all disease is a consequence of abnormal cell function or, in other words, cell injury, be it morphologically apparent or not. Cellular pathology is the study of how cells are injured and how they react to injury. As such, it forms a keystone on which a knowledge of disease can be based. Amazingly, cell injury in all seems rather simple; only a few basic mechanisms are involved in injuring cells. Why then is disease so difficult to understand? The answer lies in recognizing the complexity of normal cellular functions and how abnormalities of function in different kinds of cells affect the tissues and the host. At this point we have largely ignored the *interaction* of host cells with one another, with mediators released by various cells, and with exogenous agents such as microorganisms. In subsequent chapters we will explore the role of such interactions as causes and consequences of cell injury and disease.

RECOMMENDED READING

Braughler JM: Calcium and lipid peroxidation. In Halliwell B: *Oxygen radicals and tissue injury,* Bethesda, Md., 1988, Federation of American Societies for Experimental Biology.

Campbell AK: Intracellular calcium: friend or foe? *Clin Sci* 72:1-10, 1987.

Carden DL, Granger DN: Pathophysiology of ischemia-reperfusion injury, *J Pathol* 190:255-266, 2000.

Cheung JY, Bonventre JV, Malis CD, Leaf A: Calcium and ischemic injury, *N Engl J Med* 314:1670-1676, 1986.

Clark IA: Tissue damage caused by free oxygen radicals, *Pathology* 18:181-186, 1986.

Cohen AS, Connors LH: The pathogenesis and biochemistry of amyloidosis, *J Pathol* 151:1-10, 1987.

Comporti M: Lipid peroxidation and cellular damage in toxic liver injury, *Lab Invest* 53:599-623, 1985.

Cotran RS, Kumar V, Collins T: *Robbins pathologic basis of disease,* ed 6, Philadelphia, 1999, Saunders.

De Groot H, Littauer A: Hypoxia, reactive oxygen, and cell injury, *Free Radic Biol Med* 6:541-551, 1989.

Dong Z, Saikumar P, Griess GA, Weinberg JM, Venkatachalam MA: Intracellular Ca^{2+} thresholds that determine survival or death of energy-deprived cells, *Am J Pathol* 152:231-240, 1998.

Downey JM, Hearse DJ, Yellon DM: The role of xanthine oxidase during myocardial ischemia in several species including man, *J Mol Cell Cardiol* 20(suppl 3):55-63, 1988.

Ericsson JLE, Brunk UT: Alterations in lysosomal membranes as related to disease processes. In Trump BF, Arstila AU: *Pathobiology of cell membranes,* vol 1, New York, 1975, Academic Press.

Falk RH, Comenzo RL, Skinner M: The systemic amyloidoses, *N Engl J Med* 337:898-909, 1997.

Farber JL: Membrane injury and calcium homeostasis in the pathogenesis of coagulative necrosis, *Lab Invest* 47:114-123, 1982.

Farber JL, Chien KR, Mittnacht S: The pathogenesis of irreversible cell injury in ischemia, *Am J Pathol* 102:271-281, 1981.

Farber JL, Gerson RJ: Mechanisms of cell injury with hepatotoxic chemicals, *Pharmacol Rev* 36:71-75, 1984.

Farber JL, Kyle ME, Coleman JB: Mechanisms of cell injury by activated oxygen species, *Lab Invest* 62:670-679, 1990.

Ferrari R, Ceconi C, Curello S, Cargnoni A, Medici D: Oxygen free radicals and reperfusion injury; the effect of ischemia and reperfusion on the cellular ability to neutralise oxygen toxicity, *J Mol Cell Cardiol* 18:4-67, 1986.

Flaherty JT, Weisfeldt ML: Reperfusion injury, *Free Radic Biol Med* 5:409-419, 1988.

Freeman BA, Crapo JD: Free radicals and tissue injury, *Lab Invest* 47:412-426, 1982.

Glenner GG: Amyloid deposits and amyloidosis: the β-fibrilloses, *N Engl J Med* 302:1283-1292, 1980.

Gorevic PD, Buhles WC: Amyloidosis, *Annu Rev Med* 32:261-271, 1981.

Green DR: Apoptotic pathways: the roads to ruin, *Cell* 94:695-698, 1998.

Gross A, McDonnell JM, Korsmeyer SJ: BCL-2 family members and the mitochondria in apoptosis, *Genes Dev* 13:1899-1911, 1999.

Gutteridge JMC: Lipid peroxidation: some problems and concepts. In Halliwell B: *Oxygen radicals and tissue injury,* Bethesda, Md., 1988, Federation of American Societies for Experimental Biology.

Halliwell B: Oxidants and human disease: some new concepts, *FASEB J* 1:358-364, 1987.

Hawkins HK: Reactions of lysosomes to cell injury. In Trump BF, Arstila AU: *Pathobiology of cell membranes,* vol 2, New York, 1980, Academic Press.

Hess ML, Manson NH: Molecular oxygen: friend and foe. The role of the oxygen free radical system in the calcium paradox, the oxygen paradox and ischemia/reperfusion injury, *J Mol Cell Cardiol* 16:969-985, 1984.

Jennings RB, Ganote CE, Reimer KA: Ischemic tissue injury, *Am J Pathol* 81:179-198, 1975.

Jennings RB, Reimer KA: Lethal myocardial ischemic injury, *Am J Pathol* 102:241-255, 1981.

Jennings RB, Reimer KA: The cell biology of acute myocardial ischemia, *Annu Rev Med* 42:225-246, 1991.

Jolly RD, Walkley SU: Lysosomal storage diseases of animals: an essay in comparative pathology, *Vet Pathol* 34:549-556, 1997.

Kaplowitz N: Mechanisms of liver cell injury, *J Hepatol* 32(suppl 1):39-47, 2000.

Kehrer JP, Jones DP, LeMasters JJ, Farber JL, Jaeschke H: Mechanisms of hypoxic cell injury. Summary of the symposium presented at the 1990 annual meeting of the Society of Toxicology, *Toxicol Appl Pharmacol* 106:165-178, 1990.

Kim KM: Pathological calcification. In Trump BF, Arstila AU: *Pathobiology of cell membranes,* vol 3, New York, 1983, Academic Press.

Kisilevsky R: Amyloidosis: a familiar problem in the light of current pathogenetic developments, *Lab Invest* 49:381-390, 1983.

Macknight ADC: Cellular response to injury. In Staub NC, Taylor AE: *Edema,* New York, 1984, Raven Press.

Majno G, Joris I: Apoptosis, oncosis, and necrosis: an overview of cell death, *Am J Pathol* 146:3-15, 1995.

Marzella L, Ahlberg J, Glaumann H: Autophagy, heterophagy, microautophagy and crinophagy as the means for intracellular degradation, *Virchows Arch [Cell Pathol]* 36:219-234, 1981.

McCord JM: Oxygen-derived free radicals in postischemic tissue injury, *N Engl J Med* 312:159-163, 1985.

McCord JM: Superoxide radical: a likely link between reperfusion injury and inflammation, *Free Radic Biol Med* 2:325-345, 1986.

McCord JM: Free radicals and myocardial ischemia: overview and outlook, *Free Radic Biol Med* 4:9-14, 1988.

McNutt NS, Hoffstein S: Membranes and cytoskeleton: role in pathologic processes, *Fed Proc* 40:206-213, 1981.

Minotti G: Metals and membrane lipid damage by oxyradicals, *Ann NY Acad Sci* 551:34-46, 1988.

Moll R, Franke WW: Intermediate filaments and their interaction with membranes, *Pathol Res Pract* 175:146-161, 1982.

Naylor WG: The role of calcium in the ischemic myocardium, *Am J Pathol* 102:262-270, 1981.

Nayler WG, Panagiotopoulos S, Elz JS, Daly MJ: Calcium-mediated damage during post-ischaemic reperfusion, *J Mol Cell Cardiol* 20(suppl 3):41-54, 1988.

Naylor WG: Calcium and cell death, *Eur Heart J* 4:33-41, 1983.

Naylor WG, Poole-Wilson PA, Williams A: Hypoxia and calcium, *J Mol Cell Cardiol* 11:683-706, 1979.

Robinson JR: Colloid osmotic pressure as a cause of pathological swelling of cells. In Trump BF, Arstila AU: *Pathobiology of cell membranes,* vol 1, New York, 1975, Academic Press, p 173.

Rungger-Brandle E, Gabbiani G: The role of cytoskeletal and cytocontractile elements in pathologic processes, *Am J Pathol* 100:361-392, 1983.

Saikumar P, Dhong Z, Mikhailov V, Denton M, Weinberg JM, Venkatachalam MA: Apoptosis: definition, mechanisms, and relevance to disease, *Am J Med* 107:489-506, 1999.

Scarpelli DG, Trump BF: *Cell injury,* Kalamazoo, Mich., 1971, Upjohn Co.

Schafer KA: The cell cycle: a review, *Vet Pathol* 35:461-478, 1998.

Shine KI: Ionic events in ischemia and anoxia, *Am J Pathol* 102:256-261, 1981.

Simpson PJ: Myocardial ischemia and reperfusion injury: oxygen radicals and the role of the neutrophil. In Halliwell B: *Oxygen radicals and tissue injury,* Bethesda, Md., 1988.63, Federation of American Societies for Experimental Biology.

Simpson PJ, Lucchesi BR: Free radicals and myocardial ischemia and reperfusion injury, *J Lab Clin Med* 110:13-30, 1987.

Smuckler EA, James JL: Irreversible cell injury, *Pharmacol Rev* 36:77-91, 1984.

Southorn PA, Powis G: Free radicals in medicine. I. Chemical nature and biologic reactions, *Mayo Clin Proc* 63:381-389, 1988.

Southorn PA, Powis G: Free radicals in medicine. II. Involvement in human disease, *Mayo Clin Proc* 63:390-408, 1988.

Tappel AL: Lipid peroxidation and fluorescent molecular damage to membranes. In Trump BF, Arstila AU: *Pathobiology of cell membranes,* vol 1, New York, 1975, Academic Press.

Trump BF, Arstila AU: Cell membranes and disease processes. In Trump BF, Arstila AU: *Pathobiology of cell membranes,* vol 1, New York, 1975, Academic Press.

Trump BF, Berezesky IK, Chang SH, Phelps PC: The pathways of cell death: oncosis, apoptosis and necrosis, *Toxicol Pathol* 25:82-88 1997.

Trump BF, McDowell EM, Arstila AU: Cellular reaction to injury. In Hill RB, LaVia MF: *Principles of pathobiology,* ed 3, New York, 1980, Oxford University Press.

Walker NI, Harmon BV, Gobé GC, Kerr JFR: Patterns of cell death, *Methods Achiev Exp Pathol* 13:18-54, 1988.

Ward PA: Role of toxic oxygen products from phagocytic cells in tissue injury, *Adv Shock Res* 10:27-34, 1983.

Waterhouse NJ, Green DR: Mitochondria and apoptosis: HQ or high-security prison? *J Clin Immunol* 19:378-387, 1999.

Weinberg JM: The cell biology of ischemic renal injury, *Kidney Int* 39:476-500, 1991.

Weiss SJ: Tissue destruction by neutrophils, *N Engl J Med* 320:365-376, 1989.

Werns SW, Lucchesi BR: Leukocytes, oxygen radicals, and myocardial injury due to ischemia and reperfusion, *Free Radic Biol Med* 4:31-38, 1988.

Westermarl P: The pathogenesis of amyloidosis: understanding general principles, *Am J Pathol* 152:1125-1126, 1998.

CHAPTER 3

Disturbances of Blood Flow and Circulation

David O. Slauson

OUTLINE

All the cells and tissues of the body are quite explicit about their requirements for a normal blood supply and an adequate fluid milieu in which to bathe. A wide variety of disease settings, unfortunately, disturb these critical support systems. Imbalances of the fluid microenvironment or of the microvasculature itself can cause shifts in the location of normally intravascular water, electrolytes, and plasma proteins. Such abnormalities are commonplace and result in the accumulation of fluids in the extracellular space and other extravascular sites. This is known as *edema*. The blood is an essential and important tissue critical to normal homeostasis but can cause severe clinical problems when it forms unnecessary blood clots or fails to remain within the conduit profiles of the vascular system. In a large number of clinical settings, blood escapes from the vascular system and enters the tissues or the outside world as *hemorrhage*.

Even while still within the vascular system, blood responds to various physiological and pathological cardiovascular alterations with the result that too much blood is actively or passively forced into different tissue sites, a condition known as *hyperemia*. The delicately balanced hemostatic mechanism responsible for the lifesaving blood clot sometimes assumes major pathological importance when intravascular coagulation, or *thrombosis,* occurs. When formed, such thrombi sometimes break off from their initial point of formation to sail downstream as *emboli* to lodge in a smaller, distant vascular site. These intravascular coagula not only produce major local hemodynamic changes but can also occlude the blood supply to vital tissues and produce *ischemic necrosis,* or *infarction.*

Such changes rarely qualify as diseases in their own right. More commonly they are *manifestations* of some underlying disease process. As such, the kinds of pathological alterations to be discussed here are basic expressions of disease mechanisms that have broad application to a wide variety of clinical settings.

HYPEREMIA AND CONGESTION

Hyperemia literally means 'too much blood'. This refers to a volume and flow change, however, and should not be confused with *polycythemia,* 'too many red blood cells'. The terms "hyperemia" and "congestion" are basically synonymous, though they often are used to imply different mechanistic and anatomical information. *Hyperemia* commonly is used to imply an active, arteriole-mediated engorgement of the vascular bed, whereas *congestion* commonly is used to indicate a passive, venous engorgement. Both terms, however, indicate an excess of blood in the vessels of a given tissue or tissue site. Our purpose here is to discuss the mechanisms of hyperemia, and therefore we will use "passive hyperemia" to indicate congestion. Our discussion is therefore predicated on the idea that hyperemia can basically occur only in two ways: either too much blood is being brought in through the arterioles (active hyperemia) or too little blood is being removed through the venules (passive hyperemia).

It is important to make a clear distinction between hyperemia and hemorrhage. Although some hemorrhage can occur because of a slow dribbling of a small number of red blood cells through the vessel walls into tissues *(hemorrhage by diapedesis)* during hyperemia, the two phenomena are, by definition, different in that hyperemia implies that the blood is still *within* the vascular system whereas hemorrhage implies that blood has escaped to extravascular sites.

Types of Hyperemia

Although all forms of hyperemia are basically similar in that there is vascular engorgement of the affected tissue, it is useful to dissect the various kinds of hyperemia into categories that have different pathophysiological backgrounds.

PHYSIOLOGICAL HYPEREMIA

Not all hyperemia is pathological. The increase in blood flow to the stomach and intestines during digestion is a form of physiological hyperemia. The red faces on many members of the jogging fraternity represent an increased blood flow to the skin in an effort to augment cutaneous heat loss by escalating the rate and volume of blood flow to exposed, cooler surface sites. Similar active increases in perfusion occur in the muscles of athletes during exercise. Blushing as a manifestation of acute embarrassment or nervousness is basically a form of neurovascular hyperemia. These and other physiological forms of hyperemia are interesting but are less germane to our focus than the pathological forms of hyperemia.

PATHOLOGICAL HYPEREMIA

Other than the types of physiological changes mentioned above, all forms of hyperemia are pathological. In virtually all situations, hyperemia is only a *manifestation* of some alteration in blood flow characteristics. It is not the *cause* but rather the *result* of some underlying pathological process. It is useful in sorting out the various kinds of hyperemia to consider three factors: the *duration* of the hyperemia, the *extent* of hyperemia within the tissue or within the body as a whole, and the *mechanism* by which the hyperemia occurred (Box 3-1).

The duration of hyperemia can be simply divided into *acute* and *chronic*. Acute hyperemia implies an abrupt onset and a fairly rapid development. Chronic hyperemia indicates either that the lesion has been present for a longer period or has been slow to develop, or both. It is similarly convenient to divide the hyperemias into *local* hyperemia or *generalized* hyperemia, based on the extent of tissue involvement. Local hyperemia implies that the change is confined to a discrete area and is localized or limited in extent. Generalized hyperemia implies a somewhat different picture. Generally it is used to indicate systemic changes (as in the generalized passive hyperemia of heart failure), but it can also mean that the hyperemia is generalized within an organ. For example, if the entire lung is hyperemic, there is generalized pulmonary hyperemia, even though the change may be restricted to the lungs.

A simple view of the mechanisms behind hyperemia already has been given. If the hyperemia is attributable to increased arteriolar flow, it is *active* hyperemia. If the hyperemia is attributable to impaired venous drainage, it is *passive* hyperemia. With this background, it is possible to construct an anatomical and mechanistic classification scheme for the hyperemias that can be useful clinically (see Box 3-1). It should be noted that not all combinations and permutations theoretically possible based on this scheme occur in real life. For example, chronic generalized active hyperemia is an impossible situation. There is simply not enough blood in the vascular system to produce active arteriolar hyperemia at all sites simultaneously. Indeed, there are basically only four patterns of hyperemia that are sufficiently repeatable to warrant our attention.

Acute Local Active Hyperemia

As the name implies, acute local active hyperemia is an engorgement of the vascular bed caused by increased arteriolar blood flow into the area. As we will learn in the next chapter, *redness* (along with heat, swelling, and pain) is one of the cardinal signs of inflammation. Acute local active hyperemia is the *hyperemia of inflammation* (Fig. 3-1). The redness and heat we associate with acute inflammatory reactions is attributable to the active hyperemia that occurs. The increased rate of blood flow to the area and the increased *volume* of blood in the region at any one time form the basis for the redness and warmth. Increased arteriolar flow opens new capillary beds, and the newly dilated small vessels extend the arteriolar blood pressure into smaller vascular radicles. It is sometimes even possible to feel a pulse over acutely inflamed areas because of the arteriolar dilatation and increased blood flow. Acute local active hyperemia is an event fairly specific to inflammation. It is a chemically mediated response of the microvasculature to histamine, bradykinin, and other vasoactive substances in acute inflammatory reactions.

Acute Local Passive Hyperemia

When local obstruction to venous drainage occurs, there is passive engorgement of the drainage area served by the obstructed vessel. Blood backs up into the microvascular bed, and local venous engorgement occurs. In contrast to the situation in acute local active hyperemia, the involved tissues here are dark red in color, rather than being bright red because they are engorged with poorly oxygenated venous blood instead of well-oxygenated arterial blood. Additionally it is unlikely that any pulse wave would be palpable because of the lower blood pressure in the venous system and because the arteriolar flow here is normal. Such hyperemic changes may be seen in the service area of thrombosed or

---

BOX 3-1 Classification of Hyperemia

DURATION
Acute: abrupt onset, rapid development
Chronic: slowly developing, present for long time

EXTENT
General: generalized, systemic, or throughout an organ or system
Local: confined to a discrete area, localized, limited

MECHANISM
Active: increased arteriolar inflow
Passive: engorgement of vascular bed, venous impedance

EXAMPLES IN USE
Acute local active hyperemia: the hyperemia of inflammation
Acute local passive hyperemia: engorgement of bowel in a torsion
Chronic local passive hyperemia: engorgement behind progressive obstruction; tumor, abscess, etc.
Chronic general passive hyperemia: as in congestive heart failure

otherwise acutely obstructed veins. Acute local passive hyperemia may reach its maximal levels in situations where torsion of a viscus has occurred. In this situation, the venous drainage is seriously impaired, but the thicker-walled arteries remain functional, and so the interposed microvascular bed becomes extremely engorged with blood. Lesions such as this form the basis for one form of equine colic.

Chronic Local Passive Hyperemia

The only major difference between acute and chronic forms of local passive hyperemia is the time frame required for their development. Lesions such as extravascular tumors or abscesses that slowly enlarge and eventually compress adjacent veins can produce passive hyperemia. Because the development of the venous obstruction is slow, the vascular system often has an opportunity to adjust to the progressing obstruction, and channels of collateral flow gradually are opened to provide alternative routes of venous drainage. If this adaptive mechanism is successful, hyperemia may not develop at all.

Sometimes chronic local passive hyperemia can occur when organs or organ systems develop chronic inflammatory lesions, which can then progress to fibrosis and hence to obstruction of that tissue's venous system. A reasonable example of this can be drawn from hepatic *cirrhosis* in which the progressive loss of hepatic lobular structural architecture by fibrosis eventually leads to portal hypertension. In addition to developing ascites (edema fluid in the peritoneal cavity), such patients often develop substantial collateral venous channels and intrahepatic arteriovenous anastomoses. The normal route of blood flow may be reversed in such situations, and so portal blood is shunted to the esophageal veins and thence into the azygos system. The greatly heightened pressure in the esophageal plexus produces dilated tortuous vessels called *varices*. In man, where advanced cirrhosis is more common than in other animals, approximately two thirds of all cirrhotic patients have esophageal varices that sometimes rupture and produce life-threatening episodes of hemorrhage. As in other forms of chronic local passive hyperemia, the clinical signs and the vascular engorgement itself are related to changes away from the actual causative lesion. In other words, the effects of local, passive hyperemia are always *upstream* from the location of the underlying lesion.

Chronic Generalized Passive Hyperemia

It is a useful rule of thumb that *all* generalized passive hyperemias (congestions) involve either the

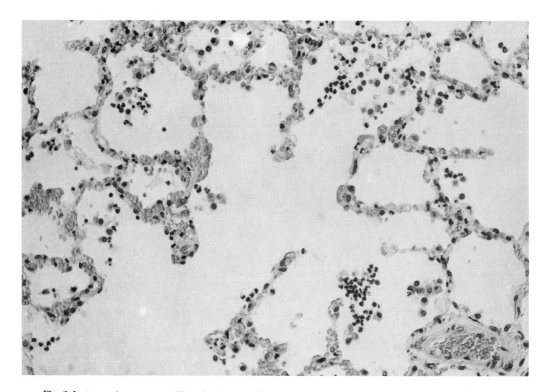

Fig. 3-1 Acute hyperemia. The alveolar capillaries in this dog lung are engorged with red blood cells. A few leukocytes have emigrated into alveolar spaces.

heart or the lungs as the major site of underlying pathological change. If the heart is the source of the problem, the chronic generalized passive hyperemia that results is usually referred to as *congestive heart failure*. Most often the underlying lesion is a valvular one. Depending on the nature of the lesion and its location within the heart, the primary tissue target for chronic passive hyperemia may be either the liver or the lungs. This makes sense if you merely reconstruct the routes of blood flow through the heart (Fig. 3-2). In the case of *pulmonic stenosis* (narrowing of the pulmonary valve), insufficient right ventricular emptying during right ventricular systole backs blood up into the right atrium and the vena cava system, and the primary target for the venous engorgement would be the liver. The same situation would prevail in *tricuspid insufficiency,* in which blood is ejected through the insufficient tricuspid valve during right ventricular systole and eventually backs up through the right atrium and vena cava system to the liver. Hence, pulmonic stenosis and tricuspid insufficiency produce chronic passive hyperemia of the liver as the initial vascular bed to experience the engorgement.

On the left side of the heart, *aortic stenosis* tends to produce chronic passive hyperemia that first involves the lungs as blood is backed up through the left atrium and pulmonary veins because of insufficient left ventricular ejection through the narrowed aortic orifice during left ventricular systole. By the same token, dogs with *mitral insufficiency,* a fairly common acquired valvular lesion, often first show a chronic nonproductive cough that is related to chronic passive hyperemia and edema of the lungs. Here the insufficient mitral valve allows blood to be ejected back into the left atrium and pulmonary veins during left ventricular systole. Congestive heart failure tends to be a progressive disorder, and, although the organ distributions described above hold true initially, generalized hyperemia involving both

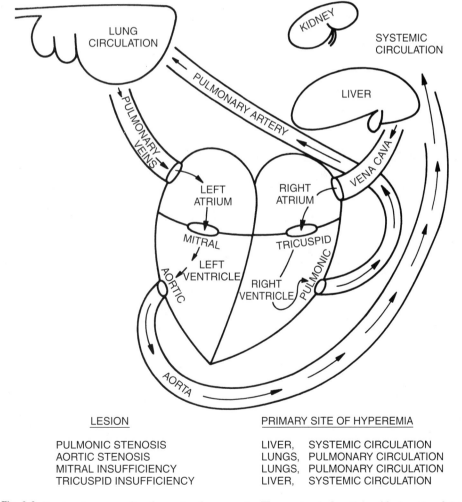

LESION	PRIMARY SITE OF HYPEREMIA	
PULMONIC STENOSIS	LIVER,	SYSTEMIC CIRCULATION
AORTIC STENOSIS	LUNGS,	PULMONARY CIRCULATION
MITRAL INSUFFICIENCY	LUNGS,	PULMONARY CIRCULATION
TRICUSPID INSUFFICIENCY	LIVER,	SYSTEMIC CIRCULATION

Fig. 3-2 Routes to generalized passive hyperemia. The anatomic location of lesions involving cardiac valves is a major determinant of the primary site of passive hyperemia in other tissues.

the lungs and the liver eventually may be seen as the cardiac decompensation becomes more advanced.

Chronic generalized passive hyperemia also may accompany certain types of primary pulmonary disease in which there is progressive loss of the pulmonary vascular bed and consequent *pulmonary hypertension*. When heart failure occurs secondary to primary pulmonary disease, the syndrome is referred to as *cor pulmonale*. As pressure becomes greatly elevated in the normally low-pressure pulmonary arterial system, blood is backed up through the right side of the heart, and ascites and chronic passive hyperemia of the liver can result.

APPEARANCE OF HYPEREMIA

If a cut were made through a hyperemic tissue examined at necropsy, the cut surface would be excessively bloody. The reasons for this are obvious. It also is likely that edema would be encountered because the congestion of capillary beds is closely allied with the development of edema. Hyperemia and edema are often found concurrently. This is particularly true in the case of the acute local active hyperemia of inflammation in which edema is almost always seen.

In chronic hyperemias, the engorgement of the tissues by poorly oxygenated venous blood often leads to a degree of chronic local hypoxia that can produce degeneration or even necrosis of the relatively delicate cells of parenchymal organs. Because the lungs and liver are the most common targets for chronic passive hyperemia, we examine the characteristic changes in these tissues in more detail.

In chronic passive hyperemia of the *lungs*, the alveolar capillaries become engorged with blood, dilated, and sometimes tortuous. Many such small capillaries may rupture, and so minute intraalveolar hemorrhages occur. These extravascular red blood cells become the targets of the alveolar macrophages, which phagocytize and break down the red blood cells to eventually become laden with the hemoglobin-breakdown pigment called *hemosiderin*. Indeed, the appearance of these hemosiderin-laden macrophages is so characteristic of chronic passive hyperemia of the lungs that they have become widely known as simply *"heart-failure cells"* (Fig. 3-3). In severe forms of chronic passive pulmonary hyperemia, the alveolar walls themselves become widened both by edema fluid and by the dilated and engorged alveolar capillaries. Such edematous and hyperemic alveolar septa eventually can become fibrotic.

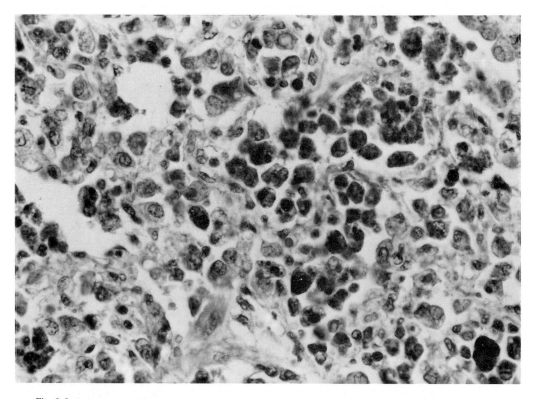

Fig. 3-3 Pulmonary chronic passive hyperemia. The persistent hyperemia and diapedesis of red blood cells lead to phagocytic degradation of the red blood cells to produce these dark-staining "heart-failure cells," or macrophages full of hemosiderin.

In chronic passive hyperemia of the *liver,* there is initially an overall increase in hepatic size as a result of the volume and mass of added blood. Eventually the chronic low-grade hypoxia and the pressure of the added blood in the widely dilated sinusoids will produce atrophy and loss of hepatic cord cells (Fig. 3-4). Such livers often exhibit a characteristically mottled gross appearance referred to as *"nutmeg liver"* as a result of the dark red appearance of the zones around the central veins and the yellow-brown appearance of the less-affected parenchyma around the portal areas (Fig. 3-5). Hemosiderin-filled fixed macrophages (Kupffer's cells) may be found in such livers for the same reasons they are found in chronically hyperemic lungs. If sufficient time passes, there may be fibrous thickenings around the central veins in response to the increased blood pressure to which the area is being subjected. This fibrous tissue sometimes can extend even into the surrounding lobule creating a fairly distinctive pattern sometimes referred to as *"cardiac cirrhosis."*

It must again be stressed that, in both the liver and the lung in chronic passive hyperemia, the real underlying lesion is not located in these tissues. Rather, the lung and liver end up expressing major pathological changes because they bear the brunt of the pressure alterations created elsewhere, usually in the heart. The astute clinician or pathologist who encounters chronic passive hyperemia of the liver or lungs always conducts a thorough examination of the heart as the most likely underlying source of the problem.

HEMORRHAGE

The escape of blood from the cardiovascular system is known as *hemorrhage.* In the event that a substantial rent or tear is present in the blood vessel (or heart), the flow of blood from the defect is substantial and is known as *hemorrhage by rhexis.* If only a small defect is present or if red blood cells merely pass through vascular structures in the process of, for example, hyperemia or inflammation, the event is known as *hemorrhage by diapedesis.* Obviously there are considerably different outcomes to these two events, and the clinical significance is similarly varied.

In either event, the escaped blood may accumulate within tissues or within tissue spaces to produce a three-dimensional extravascular clot known as a *hematoma* (Fig. 3-6). Small hematomas often result from simple venipuncture procedures and are

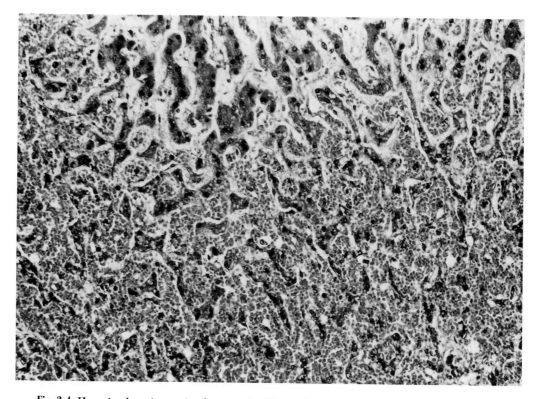

Fig. 3-4 Hepatic chronic passive hyperemia. The prolonged hyperemia and low-grade hypoxia has led to significant dilatation of hepatic sinusoids and atrophy of hepatic epithelial cells. Hepatic cords are reduced to thin wispy rows of cells.

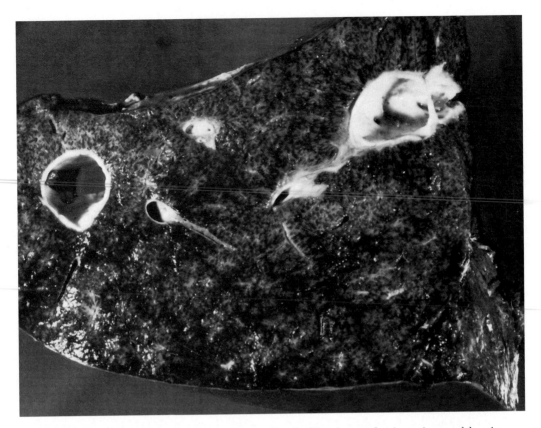

Fig. 3-5 Hepatic chronic passive hyperemia. Greatly dilated central vein regions and less involved portal areas give this cow's liver a distinctly mottled pattern called "nutmeg liver."

especially common whenever blood is drawn from or injections are given into the arteries. Hematomas are also frequently seen after trauma, where much of the visible lesion seen clinically is related to hemorrhage into tissue. The *significance* of this type of hemorrhage depends largely on the *site* of its accumulation, the *rate* of accumulation of the hemorrhage itself, and the total *volume* of blood lost, which will determine the size of the hematoma. A substantial subcutaneous or intramuscular hematoma may be awkward and painful but carries no great life-threatening significance. A much smaller subdural hematoma, on the other hand, may produce a comatose state as a result of the pressure it exerts on the brain within the bony anatomical confines of the calvaria.

The same processes that produce hematomas in tissue or in tissue spaces may lead to hemorrhage, which is named differently in different anatomical locations. For example, if blood escapes into a serous cavity, it is referred to as *hemopericardium,* *hemothorax,* or *hemoperitoneum.* Blood within the joint spaces is called *hemarthrosis,* and the coughing up of blood clots from the trachea and bronchi is called *hemoptysis.* Bleeding from the nose is *epistaxis.* Most of these terms are really only re-

gional derivatives useful to a particular organ or organ system. In all cases they basically represent hemorrhage, or *extravasation* of blood from vessels into extravascular sites.

Hemorrhages often are named by their size. For example, *petechial* hemorrhages (or *petechiae*) are minute, pinpoint foci of hemorrhage up to a range of 1 to 2 mm in diameter (Fig 3-7). *Ecchymotic* hemorrhages *(ecchymoses)* are larger than petechiae and are usually blotchy or irregular areas up to 2 or 3 cm in size (Fig. 3-8). Extensive hemorrhage within the substance of a tissue is sometimes referred to as simply "extravasation" (Fig. 3-9). Sometimes hemorrhages are more linear or streaked in appearance, particularly on serosal or mucosal surfaces, and look as through a brush dipped in red paint was hastily splashed across the tissue. These hemorrhages are appropriately referred to as *paint-brush* hemorrhages. When petechiae, ecchymoses, and even larger areas of hemorrhage are scattered on many body surfaces, the lesion is said to represent *purpura.* Many of these terms are useful for communication purposes if nothing else. When the pathologist tells the clinician that there were many petechiae and ecchymoses found on the capsular surfaces of the kidneys of a patient recently necrop-

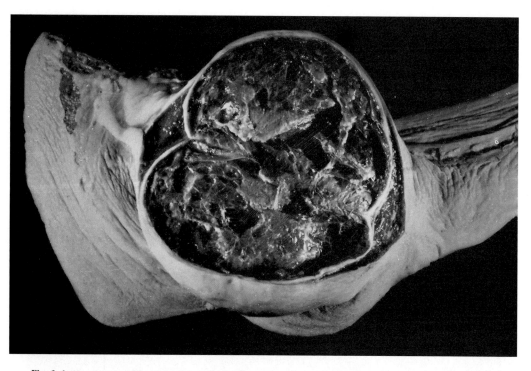

Fig. 3-6 Hematoma. The prominent three-dimensional mass of hemorrhage in this equine spleen is a hematoma. The hematoma is beginning to organize.

sied, the terms bring to mind a specific image of what the tissue looked like.

Causes of Hemorrhage

There are many kinds of disease backgrounds that can lead to hemorrhage. In domestic animals surely the most common cause is *trauma*. In general, hemorrhage is a nonspecific lesion; it indicates only that vascular injury of some kind may have occurred. Despite its lack of specificity, there are some useful and repeatable patterns that can be helpful to the practicing pathologist and clinician.

Widespread petechiae and ecchymoses often are suggestive of a septicemic, viremic, or toxemic condition in which systemic damage to many small vascular radicles has occurred. Hemoperitoneum, on the other hand, would be caused by local blood loss into the abdominal cavity, and the underlying cause most likely would be located in proximity to that cavity itself. Subcutaneous or intramuscular hemorrhage is often a manifestation of trauma.

Hemorrhage often is associated with a variety of disorders of the coagulation mechanism. Prothrombin deficiency may be encountered as an acquired condition in vitamin K deficiency or in some diffuse liver diseases. Several of the clotting factors are vitamin K dependent. Synthesis by the liver of Christmas factor (IX), proconvertin (VII), Stuart-Prower

factor (X), and prothrombin (II) depend on the availability of vitamin K. Vitamin K is required for the transformation of protein precursors into the structure of these clotting factors. Cattle fed *dicumarol* (or *dicoumarin*) (which is abundant in lush sweet clover) can develop a devastating hemorrhagic disorder associated with prolongation of the clotting time and actually attributable to prothrombin (II) deficiency. Dicumarol and the related *warfarin* (a widely used rat poison) have structural similarities to vitamin K and presumably exert their effect by competitive inhibition.

Hereditary deficiencies of coagulation factors, such as *hemophilia*, often become clinically significant as a result of hemorrhage. Similarly, thrombocytopenia leads to abnormal bleeding tendencies because there are too few platelets to aggregate and form the initial hemostatic plug as a nidus for clot formation. In many of these situations, defects in the clotting mechanism predispose the patient to the development of substantial hemorrhage from relatively trivial trauma to small vessels. This increased tendency toward hemorrhage in the clotting deficiency syndromes is responsible for their being grouped under the name *hemorrhagic diatheses*. Because the various specific etiological factors related to hemorrhage are more properly the domain of special pathology, we do not detail them here. Of greater concern to us from the standpoint of disease

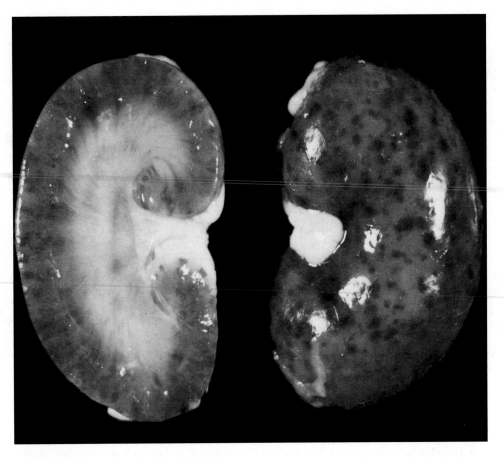

Fig. 3-7 Petechiae. The multiple small hemorrhages on the kidney of this pup that died of herpesvirus infection are petechial hemorrhages.

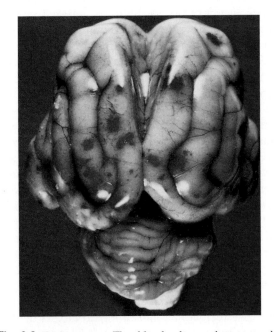

Fig. 3-8 Ecchymoses. The blotchy hemorrhages on the brain of this cat are larger than petechiae and are called "ecchymoses."

mechanisms is to develop an understanding of the potential significance of hemorrhage and the ways in which extravascular blood is handled by the body.

Clinical Significance and Outcome of Hemorrhage

As we mentioned above, the clinical significance of hemorrhage depends largely on three things: *where*, *how fast*, and *how much*.

The *location* of hemorrhage by itself and independent of volume considerations narrows our view to two critical sites: the central nervous system and the heart. Even a small amount of hemorrhage into the brain parenchyma can have a disastrous outcome if it interrupts or interferes with vital functions. This might be especially true of hemorrhage into the brainstem or medulla. The all-too-common *stroke*, or *cerebrovascular accident*, in man produces clinical signs not by virtue of the underlying vascular disease but because hemorrhage (and sometimes infarction) has occurred in the brain. Similarly, extracerebral but intracranial hemor-

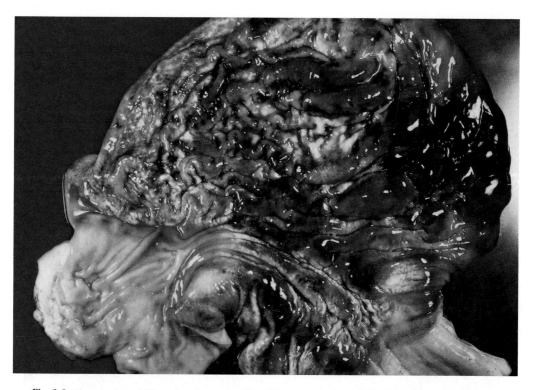

Fig. 3-9 Hemorrhage. There has been considerable extravasation of blood in the gastric mucosa of this dog with renal failure (uremic gastritis).

rhage is always potentially dangerous because of the space limitations of the calvaria. *Subdural hematomas* thus can produce the same sort of clinical signs as an abscess or a neoplasm that compresses the brain from without might cause.

The heart is similarly vulnerable because intramyocardial hemorrhage may weaken or destroy vital cardiac muscle tissue or may interrupt important conduction pathways. In like fashion, hemopericardium (which is the heart's answer to the brain's subdural hematoma) can be serious because of *pressure* on the heart from without that impairs diastolic filling and therefore adversely affects cardiac output. *Cardiac tamponade* refers to a specific syndrome of acute cardiac failure that is often caused by massive hemopericardium (Fig. 3-10).

In contrast to the situation in the central nervous system and the heart, most tissues can tolerate some hemorrhage without undue loss of function. When substantial hemorrhage occurs in any tissue, however, clinical disease may result. Thus the *volume* of blood lost becomes important, not only to the potential effects on the tissues where the hemorrhage occurred, but also to the body as a whole should sufficient blood be lost to lead to the syndrome of *hemorrhagic shock*. This form of shock occurs when blood loss has been sufficient to result in an impairment of peripheral perfusion. The critical

volume of blood loss necessary to produce shock varies with the rate of hemorrhage, but it is generally in the neighborhood of 20% to 40% of the total blood volume. Because this syndrome is based on blood loss, it is often referred to as *hypovolemic shock* to reflect the underlying problem. The more rapid the hemorrhage, the less will be the total volume required to produce shock.

Shock has so many variable features and so many pathophysiological implications and pathogenetic sequences that it is difficult to construct a meaningful brief definition. It is basically a clinical term meaning *peripheral circulatory failure*. This results in inadequate perfusion of tissue cells with a resultant imbalance between the available vascular supply and the metabolic needs of the cells and tissues. Cellular hypoxia results and leads to a decline in aerobic glycolysis and an increase in anaerobic glycolysis. This in turn leads to increased production of lactic acid, and the resultant metabolic acidosis further perpetuates cellular injury (see also Chapter 2). This vicious circle eventually leads to peripheral vascular collapse, visceral pooling of blood, and inadequate central perfusion, which ultimately can be fatal. It is beyond our scope here to discuss the fascinating subject of shock in detail. Readers seeking additional information should consult the recommended reading list at the end of the chapter.

We have mentioned previously that the *rate* of hemorrhage may play an important role in determining the outcome of bleeding. Extremely slow blood loss, as might occur through a chronic inflammatory lesion in the stomach, is probably of less significance than the underlying lesion actually responsible for producing the hemorrhage. On the other hand, an acute gastric ulcer may hemorrhage profusely into the lumen of the stomach and intestinal tract, and the patient may in fact die of shock before a single indication of blood has appeared in the feces. In these two situations, the *amount* of blood lost may be similar. That is, over a period of months the chronic gastric inflammatory lesion may produce a volume of blood loss by diapedesis equal to that lost by rhexis in the acutely fatal gastric ulcer. The volume is the same, but the clinical significance is different because the *rate* of blood loss is clearly different.

It is also worth noting that in clinical settings where a small amount of blood is lost over a long period of time, such as the gastric inflammatory lesion mentioned previously, the host has time to invoke different adaptive responses such as increased blood production *(hematopoiesis)*. These adaptive responses usually take time to occur and help to further explain why different clinical outcomes attend different *rates* of blood loss.

Resolution of Hemorrhage

After hemorrhage has occurred, the problem for the patient is a simple one. What now happens to the blood? Assuming that the hemorrhage has not been fatal and that the bleeding has been arrested, there are really only two options open for the resolution of hemorrhage into tissue spaces. It is either *reabsorbed*, or it must be *organized*. Which of these options actually occurs depends on several factors, and in many situations probably both apply.

Because extravascular blood tends to clot, the opportunity for reabsorption of fluid blood is usually limited. As the clot contracts, there may be local plasma, which has been expressed from the clot, to reabsorb. Usually, however, much of the blood lost to hemorrhage must be handled by the processes of phagocytosis and organization. In an *organizing hematoma* (see Fig. 3-6), the mass of fibrin and red blood cells are surrounded by vascular connective tissue, which supplies the nutritive and supporting structures necessary to sustain the phagocytes that leave the bloodstream and enter the hematoma. Here they phagocytose and degrade both the fibrin and the red blood cells themselves. Such phagocytes often become laden with *hemosiderin*, a breakdown product of hemoglobin that often is abundant in sites of old hemorrhage. The process of organization of a hematoma is very similar to the organiza-

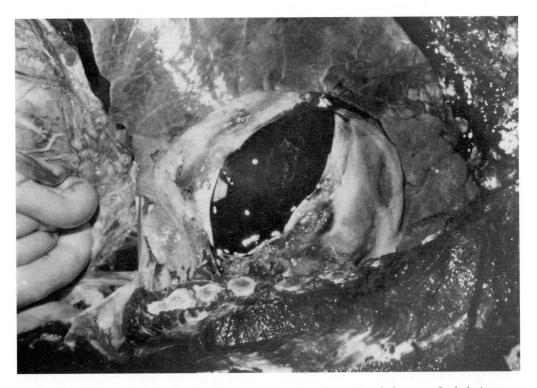

Fig. 3-10 Hemopericardium. Massive hemorrhage into the pericardial space. Such lesions compress the heart and produce "cardiac tamponade."

tion of a thrombus, which we discuss in a later section.

THROMBOSIS
General Background

Blood is normally a flowing fluid within the vascular conduits of the cardiovascular system. When a solid mass is formed within the blood vessels or the heart from the constituents of the blood, the process is called *thrombosis*, and the resultant mass is called a *thrombus*. If several are formed, they are called *thrombi*. If pieces of a thrombus break off from the original mass and sail downstream in the flowing bloodstream to lodge at a distant site, that process is called *embolism* and the mass that broke off and lodged at the distant site is called an *embolus*. If several of these are present, they are *emboli*.

It is difficult to make a clear definitional distinction between a *thrombus* and a *blood clot* because the two are clearly related. A thrombus is essentially a pathological type of blood clot that is formed *intravascularly,* that is, within the vascular system. A blood clot, on the other hand, differs from a thrombus, since *blood coagulation* is a physiological necessity whereas *thrombosis* is a pathological manifestation of blood coagulation. The classical definition of a thrombus also states that it is attached to the vessel wall. Such attachments are not always easy to find. Perhaps the simplest way to solve this definitional problem is to consider thrombi as a special subset of blood clots formed under pathological conditions. The *chicken-fat clot* commonly seen at necropsy in horses is really a plasma clot that develops because of spontaneous erythrocyte *rouleaux* formation and the rapid sedimentation rate of red blood cells in equine blood; this type of postmortem clot therefore is gelatinous in appearance and contains relatively few red blood cells. Chicken-fat clots are intravascular, but they are not thrombi because they are not pathological.

Normal blood coagulation often takes place largely extravascularly, as in the arrest of hemorrhage, and is often referred to as *hemostasis* to distinguish it from the process of *thrombosis*, or *thrombogenesis*. Both hemostasis and thrombosis involve *coagulation of the blood*. Hemostasis, or clotting of the blood, is a vital physiological process necessary to life; thrombosis is a pathological event.

With the recent rapid advances in the field of coagulation and thrombosis research, it is difficult to present the subject in a relevant and contemporary factual manner without losing sight of the classical pathology of thrombosis that is essential to an understanding of the process. We hope here to provide a contemporary synopsis of the pathogenesis of thrombosis, one that presents it as a dynamic process involving the interplay of many factors and forces present in the blood and the living blood vessels. In this context, thrombosis may be viewed as an abnormal or exaggerated expression of the hemostatic mechanism and often involves underlying vascular damage. A good example of this is the thrombosis that can occur after coronary artery disease in man. Thrombosis also often involves hemodynamic adjustments. Nonetheless, the cornerstone of the process of thrombosis is the coagulation of the blood, and we begin our study of thrombosis by reviewing the mechanisms by which this fascinating biological phenomenon occurs.

Overview of Blood Coagulation

Scientists have long marveled at the curious way in which fluid blood becomes transformed into a solid coagulum when it leaves the vascular system. Indeed, curiosity about the coagulation of the blood can be traced to antiquity. Blood coagulation involves a delicate interplay between the vascular tissues themselves and the blood cells and plasma. After injury, the vessel walls have the unique ability to constrict and to provide a variety of platelet and plasma protein activators and inhibitors. The platelets, by the processes of adhesion and aggregation, provide the initial means of arresting blood loss. The plasma protein constituents of the coagulation process serve to provide local fibrin formation to impart structural solidity to the platelet plug at the site of injury and to ultimately contribute to the tissue-repair process. As in many other complicated biological events, a variety of chemical signals, which initiate and terminate different stages of the process, serve to amplify and dampen the coagulation events with a built-in system of checks and balances. Many of these initiation and control events are carefully coordinated enzymatic reactions. Things that disturb this delicate balance disturb the entire system, and the result is usually a pathological manifestation of the coagulation process: either too much at the wrong time and place (thrombosis) or too little when needed the most (hemorrhage). These abnormalities of the coagulation mechanism can be either localized or can be disseminated.

One model for understanding the intricacies of blood coagulation, hemostasis, and thrombosis would indicate that three separate anatomic and physiological compartments may pertain: (1) the *plasma proteins,* such as the coagulation factors and cofactors, procoagulants, anticoagulants, and fibrinolytic proteins and zymogens, (2) the *blood platelets,* in normal numbers and function, and (3) the *blood vessels* and specifically the *endothelial cells* that line them. The various cellular and biochemical components of these three compartments and their intricate interactions have been studied extensively.

To appreciate abnormalities that can result from defective function of the coagulation mechanism it is necessary for us to understand the various coagulation factor interactions that ultimately produce the fibrin clot. It is not our intention to review *ad nauseam* the incredible amount of biochemical detail available regarding blood coagulation. We do believe strongly, however, that students with a good grasp for the players in this drama and their various interactions have a much better chance to actually understand the process of thrombosis. Those seeking information beyond what is provided here are referred to the recommended reading list at the end of this chapter.

Mechanisms of Blood Coagulation

An explanatory note regarding terminology seems like an appropriate beginning to this discussion. Most clotting factors are enzymes (proteins) or coenzymes that are synthesized independently. They are generally present in the plasma in an inactive *zymogen* form and must be "activated" to become biologically functional in the clotting mechanism. This activation is accomplished either by the activated form of the clotting factor's predecessor or, more often, by a complex composed of activated and nonactivated components. Much of the activation process takes place on surfaces of one kind or another. In the presently accepted nomenclature (Table 3-1), roman numerals refer to the *inactive precursor* state (zymogen) of the various clotting factors, whereas the *active form* is designated by the letter "a" after the roman numeral. The coagulation factors also have names. Indeed, they often have several names as a natural outgrowth of the sequence of discovery, and recent advances in our un-

TABLE 3-1 Coagulation Factors

FACTOR	NAME	PROPERTIES AND FUNCTIONS
I	Fibrinogen	M_r 340,000; six disulfide-linked peptide chains; converted by thrombin to fibrin monomer
II	Prothrombin	M_r 72,500; single-chain glycoprotein; circulating precursor converted to thrombin by factor Xa proteinase
III	Tissue thromboplastin	Several biochemical identities; greatly shortens clotting time; initiates extrinsic system; tissue factor
IV	Divalent calcium	Cofactor in several activation steps; forms molecular bridges
V	Proaccelerin	M_r 350,000; glycoprotein; participates with factor Xa in prothrombin activation
VI	(There is no factor VI in current terminology)	
VII	Proconvertin	M_r about 50,000; single polypeptide chain glycoprotein; precursor of proteinase that activates factor X
VIII	Antihemophiliac factor	Ambiguity in molecular weight; accessory protein with factor IXa in intrinsic activation of factor X
IX	Christmas factor	M_r 56,000; single polypeptide chain glycoprotein; participates in intrinsic activation of factor X
X	Stuart-Prower factor	M_r 56,000; two polypeptide chain glycoprotein, precursor of proteinase that converts prothrombin to thrombin
XI	Plasma thromboplastin antecedent	M_r 124,000 (bovine); two equal polypeptide chains in disulfide linkage; precursor of factor XIA, which converts IX to IXa; Hageman factor substrate
XII	Hageman factor	M_r 80,000; single polypeptide chain glycoprotein; initiates intrinsic (contact) coagulation system
XIII	Fibrin stabilizing factor	M_r 320,000; four different peptide chains; precursor of transglutaminase, which covalently crosslinks fibrin monomers to fibrin polymer
(None)	Prekallikrein (Fletcher factor)	M_r 88,000; single polypeptide chain; precursor of proteinase kallikrein; participates in cleavage of XII to form XIIa
(None)	High-molecular-weight kininogen (Fitzgerald factor)	M_r 76,000 (bovine); single polypeptide chain glycoprotein; accessory protein in factor XII–factor XI activation scheme

derstanding of coagulation have lengthened the list of participating coagulation factors.

In our discussions here, we have tried to utilize the most commonly used names as well as their roman numerals. Thus we refer to prothrombin (II), thrombin (IIa), plasma thromboplastin antecedent (XI), and activated Hageman factor (XIIa) by both name and numeral. You will notice that not all the coagulation factors have roman numerals. For example, prekallikrein and high-molecular-weight kininogen are not numbered though they are important to the activation of Hageman factor (XII). Von Willebrand factor and protein C also did not make the numbered list. In like fashion, the number list does not include platelets though they are clearly of critical importance in coagulation. Other cofactors, such as divalent calcium (IV), however, are both named and numbered. To round things out, there is no factor VI. It is almost inevitable that some confusion will result from this complex terminology. In this regard, we can only suggest that "familiarity breeds contentment."

At a simplistic level, clot formation consists in the conversion of a soluble plasma protein called *fibrinogen* (I) into an insoluble polymer called *fibrin* by the action of an enzyme called *thrombin* (IIa). To accomplish this involves the sequential interaction of a large number of plasma proteins as well as some derived from tissue cells, phospholipid membrane surfaces derived largely from platelets, divalent calcium (IV), a variety of other full-time and part-time reactants, and an equally complicated system of control mechanisms.

It must be stressed that much of our understanding of blood coagulation has been acquired primarily in the test tube and not in living animals. We must recall, however, that hemostasis as it occurs in the living animal involves phenomena that take place on the surfaces of biological membranes, not the walls of test tubes, and that *in vitro* systems may only partly reflect the processes by which hemostasis and thrombosis are triggered in living tissues. There are few laboratory containers in which normal blood will *not* clot unless anticoagulants are added; thus there is a fundamental difference between the fluidity of the blood in clotting tubes and that in the circulation. The key issue, it seems to us, is *not* to explain why blood clots in a tube but to understand why it does *not* clot *in vivo*. This issue is much easier to raise than to resolve. Nonetheless, the disease states in which one or more of the clotting proteins or regulatory molecules are deficient generally have confirmed or extended what was discerned based on test tube data. In addition, many of the coagulation proteins and regulatory molecules

were, in fact, discovered through the study of living patients with hemostatic problems. These "experiments of nature" have proved to be invaluable in validating the scientific data that has come from the laboratory. Examples are scattered throughout our discussion, and we briefly highlight three examples here to illustrate the value of a contemporary biochemical understanding of disease *before* our discussion of coagulation in the hope of making the entire business more *real* for students.

1. It has long been known that fibrinogen is essential for platelet aggregation and that platelet aggregation is a crucial step in normal hemostasis. *Glanzmann's thrombasthenia* is a rare congenital hemorrhagic disorder in which the platelets have defective aggregation responses. Platelets from such patients do not bind fibrinogen, and two major platelet membrane glycoproteins, the *GP IIb-IIIa complex,* are greatly diminished or absent in such patients. As a result, such patients have bleeding tendencies and poor clot retraction. Glanzmann's patients have allowed the demonstration that the GP IIb-IIIa complex is in fact the platelet fibrinogen receptor, and the clotting defect in these patients has thus been explained in molecular terms. Beyond that, such patients have contributed much to our understanding of platelet function in normal hemostasis.

2. The *von Willebrand factor complex* is a noncovalent association of two biologically important and distinct proteins; one, antihemophilic factor (VIII), is a procoagulant cofactor that is deficient in *hemophilia A,* and the other, *von Willebrand factor* (vWF), is a large multimeric glycoprotein with an essential role in primary hemostasis after small vessel injury. It is deficient or dysfunctional in *von Willebrand disease.* Patients with this disease have recurrent episodes of mucocutaneous bleeding, bruising, epistaxis, and gingival hemorrhage. Von Willebrand factor is present both in plasma and in platelets and mediates platelet attachment to exposed tissues through multiple functional domains and is essential for platelet adhesion to subendothelial collagen that is exposed by vessel wall damage. It is synthesized and secreted by endothelial cells and binds to subendothelial type I and type III collagen. When vascular damage occurs, the initial platelet adhesion to the damaged site is mediated by platelets binding to this collagen-bound vWF by means of specific surface receptors on platelets. Von Willebrand disease has been extensively studied in swine. Pigs homozygous for the defect have a hemophilia-like

condition and exhibit the same impairments of primary hemostasis noted in the severe form of the disease in man: serious hemorrhagic tendencies, a prolonged bleeding time, reduced platelet adhesion, very low (3% of normal) levels of vWF, and reduced levels of antihemophilic factor (VIII) coagulant activity. Such pigs have also stimulated investigations into the role of platelets in coronary atherosclerosis and thrombosis, since the absence of vWF may be responsible, in part, for the impaired platelet–arterial wall interactions and resistance to atherosclerosis and thrombosis found in these animals.

3. Unlike most of the coagulation factors, *protein C* was discovered and its basic biological functions determined by a combination of biochemical and physiological experiments before its clinical relevance was understood. Only recently has clinical information been obtained linking protein C to thrombotic disease. Protein C interacts with thrombin (IIa) bound to a specific endothelial cell receptor *(thrombomodulin)*, and such an interaction results in the activation of protein C (see Fig. 3-17). The activated protein C subsequently serves a regulatory role in hemostasis by inactivating proaccelerin (V) and antihemophilic factor (VIII). All the biochemical data from the laboratory indicated that protein C was likely an important regulatory molecule and that a deficiency in protein C would be associated with thrombotic tendencies. A screening program was initiated, and such patients were subsequently identified. Protein C deficiency was found to be associated with recurrent thrombotic tendencies in the heterozygote and early, lethal thrombosis in the homozygote. Once again, the biochemical and clinical data correlated well.

These few examples are taken from many and serve to collectively emphasize that an understanding of coagulation at the molecular level has very real clinical significance. We reiterate this point again because students sometimes feel overwhelmed by the abundant detail inherent in blood coagulation. All complexity is, however, relative. Anyone who has survived calculus and organic chemistry, as many of our students have, should find the level of detail presented here to be quite refreshing.

For our purposes, we divide the clotting process into four major steps of importance rather than paying specific attention to all the intricacies of the coagulation scheme. We consider (1) the activation process and the early steps in coagulation, (2) the formation of the enzyme called "activated Stuart-Prower factor (Xa)" as a central character around which the intrinsic and extrinsic coagulation systems meet, (3) the formation of the enzyme thrombin (IIa), and (4) the formation of fibrin.

THE ACTIVATION PROCESS AND EARLY STEPS IN COAGULATION

Traditionally the clotting system has been divided into two pathways (Fig. 3-11). The *intrinsic* pathway involves components normally present in the circulation, and the *extrinsic* pathway involves a "tissue factor" in addition to blood components. These alternative activation mechanisms are reflected in the main screening tests used in the clinical pathology laboratory to examine the coagulation cascade: *prothrombin time* (PT) and *activated partial thromboplastin time* (APTT); PT reflects extrinsic system activation and APTT reflects intrinsic system activation. The two activation systems merge around the activation of Stuart-Prower factor (X) into a final common pathway leading to fibrin formation (Fig. 3-12).

In the *intrinsic* pathway, or "contact" system, activation revolves around the cleavage of *Hageman factor* (XII). Hageman factor (XII) is a surface-sensitive single polypeptide chain protein with a M_r (relative molecular mass) of about 80,000. Native Hageman factor (XII) is converted to activated Hageman factor (XIIa) by cleavage of one or more internal peptide bonds to yield two chains linked by disulfide bridges. The amino terminus of the heavy chain contains surface *binding* sites, whereas the COOH-terminus of the lighter chain contains the active *proteolytic* site. The cleavage of Hageman factor (XII) can occur in several ways and usually involves activation on a negatively charged surface. Collagen (particularly types I and III) exposed upon vascular injury presumably forms the usual *in vivo* substrate upon which activation takes place, but other surfaces also suffice.

Factor XIIa becomes bound to the negatively charged surface by means of the surface binding sites on its heavy chain and, once bound, has the ability to activate *prekallikrein* and *plasma thromboplastin antecedent* (PTA, XI), using the proteolytic sites on its light chain. These activities are enhanced by *high-molecular-weight kininogen* (HMW kininogen), which acts as an important cofactor. This is not a simple affair. At least four proteins seem to be involved in this set of activation reactions: Hageman factor (XII) itself, prekallikrein, plasma thromboplastin antecedent (XI), and HMW kininogen, and the precise sequence of biochemical reactions that take place and ultimately result in the cleavage of PTA (XI) is still not entirely

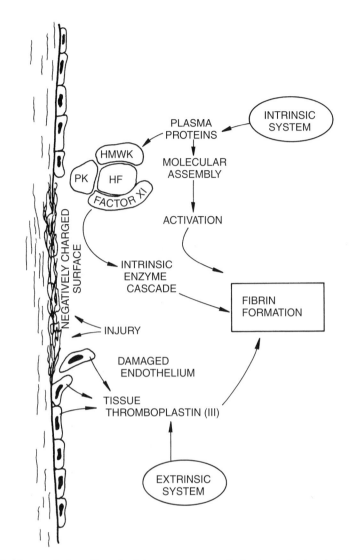

Fig. 3-11 Blood coagulation. Vascular injury exposes negatively charged subendothelial structures upon which the contact activation (intrinsic) system can be assembled and activated, and extrinsic activation proceeds with expression of tissue thromboplastin (III) by injured endothelium. *HF,* Hageman factor (XII); *HMWK,* high-molecular-weight kininogen; *PK,* prekallikrein.

clear. It appears that Hageman factor (XII), prekallikrein, and HMW kininogen are assembled when plasma contacts a negatively charged surface, and the resultant activity can cleave PTA (XI) to initiate the "cascade" of intrinsic coagulation.

The major regulator of this system appears to be the same molecule as the inhibitor of activated complement component C1 (C1 esterase inhibitor, *C1 INH*), the deficiency of which is not manifested in blood coagulation but as *hereditary angioedema.* C1 INH contributes about 90% of the inhibitory activity in normal plasma toward activated Hageman factor (XIIa). In the intrinsic system, most of the components exist in plasma in precursor form and become sequentially activated through cleavage by an active enzyme generated during the previous

step (see Fig. 3-11). Thus activated Hageman factor (XIIa) cleaves PTA (XI) to produce a proteinase (XIa), which functions as a proteolytic enzyme to activate *Christmas factor* (IX). Activated Christmas factor (IXa) then combines with *antihemophilic factor* (VIII), which along with *proaccelerin* (V), phospholipids, and divalent calcium (IV) activate the *Stuart-Prower factor* (X).

The relative importance of the "contact," or intrinsic, system to normal blood coagulation is unclear because patients with Hageman factor (XII), prekallikrein, or HMW kininogen deficiency do not exhibit bleeding tendencies or deficiencies in the inflammatory response. Only PTA (XI) deficiency is associated with a mild bleeding state. The Hageman factor (XII) pathways, however, may be

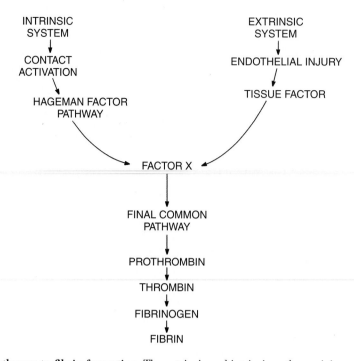

Fig. 3-12 Pathways to fibrin formation. The extrinsic and intrinsic pathways join around factor X activation into a final common pathway leading to fibrin formation. (The coagulation factor numbers are defined in Table 3-2.)

more important in a broader setting in the inflammatory response, since they link together other plasma proteolytic pathways capable of generating inflammatory mediators like bradykinin as well as fibrinolytic activity (see Chapter 4). The relative importance of such basic processes as inflammation, blood coagulation, and fibrinolysis is underscored by the extreme redundancy of available initiating pathways.

The *extrinsic* system is so named because its major initiator, "tissue factor," "thromboplastin," or the term we will use, *tissue thromboplastin* (III), is found in tissue rather than in blood. Tissue thromboplastin (III) is an integral membrane glycoprotein that is found in most tissues and apparently comes largely from endothelial cells, with some coming apparently from fibroblasts, smooth muscle cells, or injured cells of other types. Its structural identity is less secure than most of the other factors, and efforts to elucidate the molecular nature of "tissue factor" have spanned most of this century. It apparently exists as a membrane-bound glycoprotein that forms a stable complex with lipid and has a M_r of around 52,000. The structural similarities of many human and bovine coagulation proteins and the activity of human tissue thromboplastin (III) with bovine enzymes allow prediction that the basic features of tissue thromboplastin (III) action will be similar in many species.

The extrinsic system begins with tissue thromboplastin (III) existing in a sort of protected state

within the plasma membrane. Upon endothelial injury, it can be released into the circulation to form a complex with *proconvertin* (VII) in the presence of divalent calcium (IV). Proconvertin (VII) is a vitamin K–dependent protein. The activity of the complex of tissue thromboplastin (III) and proconvertin (VII) seems to be largely dependent on the concentration of tissue thromboplastin (III), though the subsequent enzymatic activity generated and the proteolytic activation of Stuart-Prower factor (X) by this extrinsic pathway resides in the activated proconvertin (VIIa) molecule. It is clear, however, that proconvertin (VII) and its activated form (VIIa) have an obligate requirement for tissue thromboplastin (III) to interact with their substrate proteins.

FORMATION OF ACTIVATED STUART-PROWER FACTOR (XA)

As we have just indicated, the active enzyme Xa can be derived from the inactive glycoprotein precursor Stuart-Prower factor (X) by both the intrinsic and extrinsic coagulation pathways (Fig. 3-13). In the extrinsic pathway, released tissue thromboplastin (III) in a complex with proconvertin (VII) and in the presence of divalent calcium (IV) forms a molecular complex that can generate the active enzyme Xa from native Stuart-Prower factor (X). Clot formation by means of the extrinsic system is remarkably more rapid than it is by the intrinsic pathway. In-

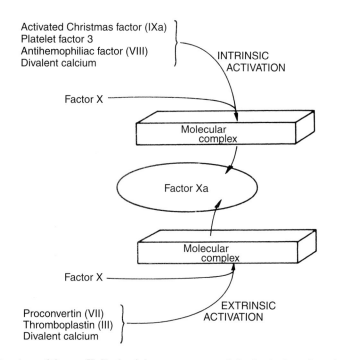

Fig. 3-13 Activation of factor X. Each of the components of the intrinsic and extrinsic pathways forms a molecular complex with Stuart-Prower factor (X), resulting in its cleavage to form activated Xa.

deed, clotting tests that may take several minutes in intrinsic system assays are accelerated to about 10 to 15 seconds when tissue thromboplastin (III) is added to initiate activation of the extrinsic system. The reason for this is not entirely clear, but it appears to be attributable to the increased activation of Stuart-Prower factor (X) by means of the extrinsic system in a reaction catalyzed by proconvertin (VII). In short, this is essentially a single-step reaction in the extrinsic system, whereas several sequential steps are required to activate Stuart-Prower factor (X) by the intrinsic pathways (see Fig. 3-11). Recent evidence has accumulated to indicate that proconvertin (VII) can also attack Christmas factor (IX) to produce activated Christmas factor (IXa), thus providing yet another link between the extrinsic and intrinsic coagulation pathways. This story will no doubt continue to unfold.

The intrinsic pathway to Stuart-Prower factor (X) activation involves the participation of activated Christmas factor (IXa), antihemophilic factor (VIII), phospholipids (platelet factor 3), and divalent calcium (IV). These various factors again form a complex, and it is the complex that generates the enzyme Xa from native Stuart-Prower factor (X). In this reaction it is believed that antihemophilic factor (VIII) plays a regulatory role whereas activated Christmas factor (IXa) serves as the cleaving enzyme. Indeed, activated Christmas factor (IXa) alone can cleave Stuart-Prower factor (X) to Xa, but the reaction is greatly accelerated in the presence of the other components. Antihemophilic factor (VIII) in this setting appears somehow altered, probably by thrombin, and this alteration seems to be required for its functioning in the complex. Activated Stuart-Prower factor (Xa) can also appropriately alter antihemophilic factor (VIII) for this purpose. Thus, intrinsic activation of Stuart-Prower factor (X) is greatly aided by prior cleavage of Stuart-Prower factor (X) by means of extrinsic activation to provide Xa, or by thrombin (II) generation to suitably "alter" antihemophilic factor (VIII) for its participation in the intrinsic activation of Stuart-Prower factor (X). Given these subtleties, it is not surprising that the extrinsic system is much more rapid.

The actual activation of Stuart-Prower factor (X) to Xa is a proteolytic process in which the native molecule is cleaved to release one or more polypeptide fragments, one of which becomes the active enzyme Xa, which figures prominently in the activation of prothrombin (II) to form the enzyme thrombin (IIa).

FORMATION OF THROMBIN

The active enzyme *thrombin* (IIa) is derived from its inactive precursor protein prothrombin (II). *Prothrombin* (II) is a constituent of normal plasma where it circulates as a single polypeptide chain glycoprotein with a M_r about 70,000. Prothrombin (II) is a vitamin K–dependent factor synthesized in the liver. Thrombin (IIa) itself is about half the size of prothrombin (II) and usually has two polypeptide chains linked by a disulfide bridge.

The conversion of prothrombin (II) to thrombin (IIa) occurs in several steps. Activated Stuart-Prower factor (Xa) is the enzyme basically responsible for cleaving two essential peptide bonds in prothrombin (II) to produce thrombin (IIa). Although factor Xa can cleave prothrombin (II) by itself, it functions optimally when linked with proaccelerin (V), divalent calcium (IV), and phospholipids derived primarily from platelets (platelet factor 3; phosphatidylinositol and phosphatidyl-L-serine). Thus a molecular complex of all five components is formed, and under these conditions optimal thrombin (IIa) generation occurs (Fig. 3-14). If any one of the five components that compose the complex is reduced in concentration, there is a corresponding reduction in the rate and amount of thrombin (IIa) generation. Thus, despite the delicacy and complexity of the reaction, a precise relative quantitative relationship seems to be essential. Thrombin (IIa) attacks only the amino terminal region of specific chains within the fibrinogen (I) molecule where it breaks only specific arginyl-glycine peptide bonds. Its activity in the production of fibrin is explained more fully in the next section.

FORMATION OF FIBRIN

Although we might consider the penultimate stage in the coagulation process to be the critical conversion of prothrombin (II) to thrombin (IIa), it is the formation of *fibrin* that is the final visible end point of all the preceding biochemical intricacies. It is easier to understand the events associated with fibrin formation if we dissect the process into three distinct phases: (1) the proteolysis of fibrinogen (I), (2) the polymerization of fibrin monomers, and (3) the stabilization, or cross-linking, of fibrin (Fig. 3-15).

Proteolysis of Fibrinogen

It will facilitate our understanding of this process if we first take a look at the fibrinogen (I) molecule (Fig. 3-16). It consists of three pairs of disulfide-linked polypeptide chains, which are designated $(A_\alpha)_2$, $(B_\beta)_2$, and γ_2. In the proteolytic phase of fibrin formation, the enzyme thrombin (IIa) attacks the amino terminal region of the A_α and B_β chains and splits specific arginyl-glycine peptide bonds to release a pair of peptides from the native fibrinogen (I) molecule. These are called *fibrinopeptides* A and B. The γ chains of the native fibrinogen (I) molecule are not involved in this process, and the resultant molecule (consisting of fibrinogen minus the fi-

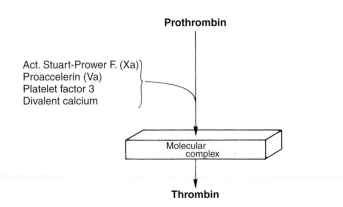

Fig. 3-14 Formation of thrombin. The cleavage of prothrombin (II) requires phospholipids (platelet factor 3) as a surface upon which the enzyme Xa, the determiner (factor V), and the substrate (prothrombin II) interact in a complex mediated by divalent calcium (IV).

brinopeptides A and B) is called *fibrin monomer.* Because of the specificity of thrombin (IIa) for arginyl-glycine peptide bonds in the A_α and B_β chains of fibrinogen (I), the COOH-terminal amino acid of the fibrinopeptides A and B is always arginine.

Polymerization of Fibrin Monomers

During the polymerization phase of fibrin formation, various fibrin monomer molecules are assembled into a structure known as *fibrin polymer.* This is basically a spontaneous nonenzymatic self-assembly process whereby end-to-end and side-to-side aggregation of individual fibrin monomer molecules takes place. Although this is a self-assembly process, it is no mere casual gathering together of pieces of fibrinogen (I). The formation of fibrin polymers results from the exposure of sets of *polymerization domains* in the fibrinogen (I) molecule, after thrombin (IIa) cleavage, which are responsible for the local conformational changes associated with fibrin polymer formation. One set of such domains appears to govern end-to-end assembly, whereas a second set is responsible for side-to-side assembly. The resulting aggregate (fibrin polymer) remains soluble in such solutions as 5 M urea and hence is sometimes referred to as *soluble fibrin polymer.* It is only after specific cross-linking of the polymerized fibrin network that the final product, insoluble fibrin, is created.

Stabilization and Cross-linking of Fibrin

The stabilization of fibrin occurs through the process of *cross-linking*, in which covalent bonds are introduced into the already polymerized fibrin network. This process is the result of the activity of activated

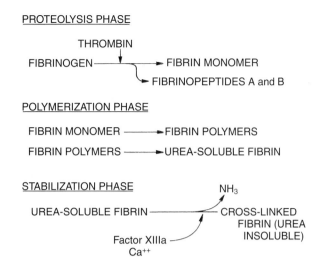

Fig. 3-15 Phases of fibrin formation. Fibrinogen is acted on by thrombin (IIa) to produce fibrin monomers, which are first spontaneously polymerized and then stabilized by factor XIIIa.

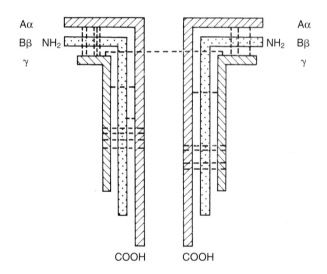

Fig. 3-16 Fibrinogen molecule. Three pairs of disulfide-linked peptide chains designated A_α, B_β, and γ make up the native molecule. This is a dimeric molecule, as shown, and the *dashed lines* indicate the disulfide bonds. The cleavage site by thrombin (IIa) is located near the N-terminus of both subunits of the A_α and B_β chains.

fibrin-stabilizing factor (XIIIa). This enzyme exists in plasma (and in platelets) as an inactive precursor (factor XIII) that is a tetramer of about M_r 320,000. It is activated to XIIIa by the enzymes thrombin (IIa) and activated Stuart-Prower factor (Xa) in a reaction that requires divalent calcium (IV). The active molecule of fibrin-stabilizing factor (XIIIa) functions as a unique transpeptidase that, in the presence of divalent calcium (IV), can introduce isopeptide bonds between the amino groups of lysine residues and the carboxyamide groups of glutamine residues.

The cross-linking process produces the kind of fibrin that forms in the normal plasma clot. It is structurally more solid than soluble fibrin polymers and is more elastic and less susceptible to lysis by various fibrinolytic agents. Interesting enough, plasminogen is also incorporated into the clot (see section on Fibrinolysis and Thrombolysis, p. 114). Thus, through the series of reactions outlined above, the soluble molecule fibrinogen (I) is converted into the insoluble gel called "fibrin."

REGULATORY MECHANISMS IN HEMOSTASIS AND THROMBOSIS

One would expect that any system as complicated as blood coagulation would have equally complicated regulatory controls to keep the system in balance. This is, in fact, true. Living animals are continually subjected to various minor traumatic episodes that trigger local hemostasis, yet the clotting mechanism rarely proceeds uncontrolled. What are the mechanisms by which the body contains thrombosis and prevents the propagation of clots? It is beyond our scope to detail the biochemical intricacies of the various control mechanisms, but recent studies that have added to our understanding of the diversity of regulatory mechanisms involved in maintaining hemostatic balance are worthy of our attention. We address three major regulatory mechanisms that control the activity of the coagulation system (Fig. 3-17); (1) the *antithrombin III system,* in which the proteases of the coagulation cascade are directly inhibited by proteinase inhibitors, (2) the *protein C system,* in which control involves regulation of the cofactors, and (3) *fibrinolysis.* Each of these control systems acts on different aspects of the coagulation mechanism, and each appears essential for effective control of clot formation. That is, if any one of these three regulatory systems is faulty, the entire control system is faulty.

Antithrombin III

The large family of glycoprotein serine proteases includes several important inhibitors such as the C1-esterase inhibitor, alpha$_1$-antitrypsin (also known as alpha$_1$-antiproteinase to better reflect its broad substrate activity), alpha$_2$-antiplasmin, and *antithrombin III* (AT III). Many of these inhibitors exhibit a considerable degree of functional cross-reactivity and even sequence homology. AT III is the major physiological inhibitor of thrombin (IIa) as well as activated Stuart-Prower factor (Xa), two of the most important enzymes of the entire coagulation cascade, and additionally can inhibit several other coagulation factors.

The precise mechanisms by which AT III interacts with thrombin (IIa) in the circulation is not yet clear, but it appears that neutralization of thrombin (IIa) actually occurs on the surfaces of endothelial cells (see Fig. 3-17); thrombin (IIa) rapidly binds to the surfaces of endothelial cells and can be neutralized by AT III there. Heparin and heparin-like glycosaminoglycans (heparan sulfate) at the endothelial surface catalyze the inactivation of thrombin by antithrombin III. AT III serves as a substrate for thrombin (IIa) and Stuart-Prower factor (Xa), and the resultant cleavage of AT III forms very stable bonds between the substrate (AT III) and the enzyme that resist denaturation. The enzyme thus is linked to AT III in a 1:1 molar complex, the active site of the enzyme is bound into the complex, and

the enzyme is thus effectively neutralized. It seems likely that the AT III–enzyme complex does not remain bound to the endothelium but is released back into the circulation where it is apparently eventually removed by means of specific receptors in the liver. Patients with antithrombin III deficiency have an increased tendency for the development of thrombosis. There has been increasing interest in identifying such patients in veterinary clinical medicine in recent years.

Protein C

Current evidence strongly indicates that the protein C anticoagulation pathway may be one of the major regulatory mechanisms responsible for the control of coagulation through the selective inactivation of the cofactors proaccelerin (V) and antihemophilic factor (VIII). Protein C is a vitamin K–dependent proenzyme that is normally present in plasma, and the activated form (protein Ca) actually degrades proaccelerin (V) and antihemophilic factor (VIII). Protein C activation is a unique process initially involving the interaction of thrombin (IIa) with an endothelial cell thrombin (IIa) surface receptor called *thrombomodulin.* When thrombin (IIa) binds to thrombomodulin, a rapid alteration in enzyme reactivity occurs; it can no longer either activate proaccelerin (V) or cleave fibrinogen (I), but the thrombin-thrombomodulin complex can rapidly activate protein C to protein Ca (Fig. 3-18). Once activated, protein Ca is released to the circulation where it expresses its considerable anticoagulant activity by selective proteolytic inactivation of proaccelerin (V) and antihemophilic factor (VIII). It should be noted, however, that activated protein Ca has an almost total dependence of the availability of a cofactor called *protein S,* also a regulatory protein of the complement system, to express its anticoagulant activity.

Recent work additionally suggests that protein Ca also interfaces with the fibrinolytic system through its ability to neutralize a circulating inhibitor of the tissue type of plasminogen activator (t-PA). By shifting the balance between t-PA and its inhibitor in the direction of increased activation of circulating t-PA, protein Ca accelerates the conversion of plasminogen to plasmin and hence facilitates fibrinolysis. These fibrinolytic reactions are more fully explained later.

Fibrinolysis

In addition to the regulatory coagulation controls available by the antithrombin III and protein C sys-

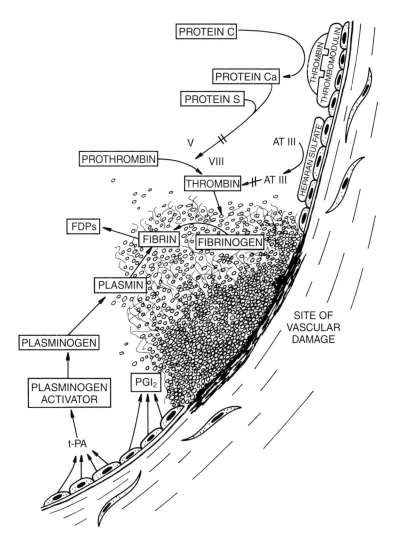

Fig. 3-17 Regulatory mechanisms in thrombosis and hemostasis. The actions of activated protein C (Ca), antithrombin III (AT III), and fibrinolysis obtained by means of the tissue type of plasminogen activator (t-PA) assist in local regulation of the developing clot. Prostacyclin (PGI$_2$) from endothelial cells also contributes.

tems, fibrin deposition and clot removal is effected by the fibrinolytic systems. These are not really regulatory systems for hemostasis, since they function only after fibrin has been formed, but they are clearly linked to the overall control of blood coagulation. (See section on Fibrinolysis and Thrombolysis, p. 114.)

PERSPECTIVES ON COAGULATION

It is easy to get lost in the biochemical complexities of the coagulation pathways. The terminology and the numbering system for the various components seem awkward and difficult to relate to. The reactions are complicated, and we sometimes find ourselves falling prone to memorization for the sake of memorization and because routine cerebrations often fail to place things into proper perspective for us.

These are the prices that we all, as students of disease, must pay for medical progress. How much simpler it must have been for Galen, who could only marvel at the way in which fluid blood became transformed magically into a jelly-like mass. The payoff for us is that an understanding of the basic mechanisms behind the coagulation process allows us to appreciate how blood loss occurs, how thrombosis is achieved, and how we might be able to intervene in a therapeutic sense. Galen did not have such luxuries.

Pathogenesis of Thrombosis

A major turning point in our understanding of the pathogenesis of thrombosis came around 1845 when a young German pathologist delivered a lecture on his views of the mechanisms of

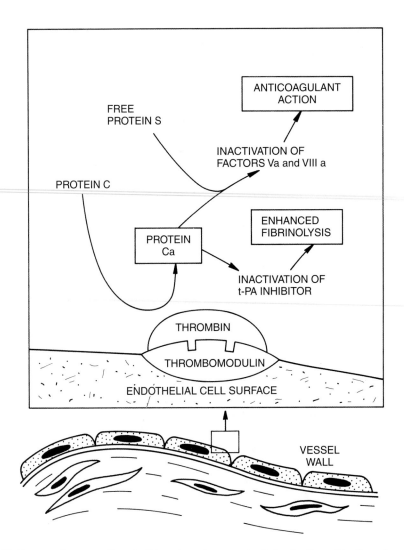

Fig. 3-18 Protein C system. Protein C is activated to protein Ca by the thrombin-thrombomodulin complex on the endothelial surface. Protein Ca with cofactor protein S inactivates Va and VIIIa and neutralizes a circulating t-PA inhibitor.

thrombogenesis. In this lecture, Dr. Rudolf Virchow (who was then only 23 years old) presented a conceptual framework for the pathogenesis of thrombosis that has stood the test of time. Virchow envisioned that thrombosis basically involved three related but distinct mechanisms: (1) changes in the vessel wall or surface, (2) changes in the hemodynamics of blood flow or stasis, and (3) changes in the blood itself and its coagulability. This has become known as "Virchow's triad" (Fig. 3-19) and remains an extremely useful way to approach an understanding of the pathogenesis of thrombosis.

Thrombosis is a common and often catastrophic complication of a wide variety of disease states and as such contributes to the natural history of many pathological processes. It remains one of the central remaining enigmas of modern medicine, and many of the readers (and perhaps the authors) of this book will succumb to it. Despite intensive study, its precise cause remains obscure, its diagnosis is difficult and often inaccurate, its prophylaxis of unproved efficacy, and its treatment largely empirical. The pathogenesis of this important process involves an interplay between vessel walls and the blood clotting system and cellular elements in blood. The initiation of thrombosis is still not well understood, but it appears to be triggered most often by an *injury* of some sort to the vessel wall and by alterations in the blood itself. The local characteristics of the thrombus that forms are determined, at least in part, by the character of local blood flow and is greatly influenced by hemodynamic alterations.

Virchow's triad remains a useful way to approach an understanding of the pathogenesis of thrombosis, and we direct our attention here to (1) changes in the vessel wall or its surface, (2) changes in the

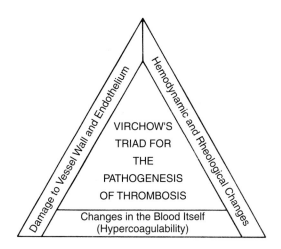

Fig. 3-19 Virchow's triad. The three major determinants in the pathogenesis of thrombosis are grouped as Virchow's triad.

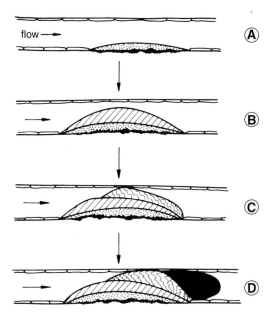

Fig. 3-20 Thrombus propagation. A thrombus grows by layering, particularly where blood flow is rapid. Intimal damage leads to deposition of a layer of platelets, *A*, which is followed by the deposition of fibrin and white blood cells, *B*, and later by further fibrin deposition, *C*. A tail of clotted whole blood, *D*, may become attached in the area immediately downstream from the thrombus.

hemodynamics of blood flow or stasis, and (3) changes in the blood itself.

VASCULAR MECHANISMS IN THROMBOSIS

Injury to the vessel wall in general and to the endothelial lining specifically may be the major event that precipitates the thrombotic process. It is known that platelets, white blood cells, and fibrin itself rarely adhere to normal intact endothelium. In direct opposition to the thromboresistant properties of the endothelial lining, however, are the thrombogenic properties of the deeper portions of the vessel wall, particularly the collagenous supporting structures. Much of this relates to type III collagen in the surrounding tissues; the basement membrane contains mostly type IV collagen, which is not particularly thrombogenic. If a vessel is injured, the injured vessel wall along with platelets, circulating coagulation factors, and, finally, fibrinolytic factors combine in a series of interlacing reactions resulting in vasoconstriction and the formation of a coagulum consisting of platelets and fibrin. These plugs form within the lumen of the vessel, and the thrombus tends to enlarge by additional coagulation occurring on its surface, propagating the thrombus in the direction of blood flow (Fig. 3-20).

Numerous studies have documented that if the vessel wall is injured platelet thrombi occur only where the endothelium is detached and the underlying connective tissue is exposed. The earliest morphological expressions of endothelial injury are generally visible only with the electron microscope and include a separation of endothelial cells from basement membrane, disappearance of certain organelles, and swelling of the mitochondria and en-

doplasmic reticulum. Vacuoles may appear in the cytoplasm, and the cells appear to "round up," or contract, to expose underlying structures. Eventually, partial detachment leads to complete detachment as the injured endothelial cells are lost and swept downstream.

There is a large number of ways in which such thrombogenic endothelial injury can occur. One obvious method is by direct physical force (trauma), but electrical damage, chemical injury, infection, inflammation, drugs such as epinephrine, and even high doses of vitamin D can produce the necessary endothelial injury to initiate thrombogenesis. Bacterial endotoxins also have been shown to produce endothelial injury, which may be widespread and of importance in the pathogenesis of the "consumption coagulopathy," or *disseminated intravascular coagulation* (DIC) syndrome that can accompany gram-negative sepsis (see Chapter 7).

Inflammation of vessels certainly can produce the necessary endothelial injury. This may include *vasculitis* (inflammation of blood vessels) in a general sense or be restricted to *arteritis* (inflammation of the arteries) or *phlebitis* (inflammation of the veins). Phlebitis can be a particular problem because the blood flow is slower in veins and hence favors interaction of the blood components with the injured endothelium.

As the propagating thrombus develops, leukocytes and platelets often become trapped in the fibrin mesh. On aggregation, platelets have been shown to release serotonin, acid hydrolases, ADP, an elastolytic factor, thromboxane A_2, permeability factors, and other reactive chemicals. The products released from platelets can additionally influence other cell types. Leukocytes, particularly the neutrophils, are similarly endowed with an impressive battery of chemicals, which can be released locally. Thus, further endothelial damage may occur once the platelet and leukocyte-release reactions have occurred. In addition, the disturbance to local blood flow may produce a local hypoxemia, which also is damaging to the endothelial cells.

Whatever the specific etiological background, it is clear that in most clinical conditions in which thrombosis occurs, vascular injury with disruption of endothelial continuity occurs. Minor degrees of injury do not necessarily result in thrombosis, but, even here, the opportunity is enhanced over the situation in normal vessels. The more usual situation, however, is that before large-vessel thrombosis can occur, it is necessary for areas of endothelial sloughing to occur to expose large zones of underlying basement membrane and supporting connective tissue. The bottom line in this story continues to relate to the need for *endothelial continuity* if normal blood flow is to be maintained. As such, the endothelial cells themselves are worthy of our consideration.

ROLE OF THE ENDOTHELIAL CELL

One of the fundamental properties of normal, intact, nonactivated endothelial cells is that they do not promote activation of either the extrinsic or intrinsic coagulation pathways nor the adherence of unstimulated platelets and leukocytes. These nonthrombogenic properties of the lining of vessel walls have been known since the days of Virchow. For a long time, at least part of the reason for this phenomenon has been attributed to the carbohydrate-rich cell coat, or *glycocalyx*. Biochemically the glycocalyx is a composite of intrinsic membrane glycoproteins and glycolipids as well as membrane-associated polysaccharides and glycosaminoglycans. Heparan sulfate in the glycocalyx has similarities to the anticoagulant heparin. In addition, alpha$_2$-macroglobulin, which is a potent antiprotease, is associated with the vascular lining and can serve to inhibit activation of some of the clotting factors.

It also is possible that the *surface negativity* of endothelial cells (and the leukocytes and platelets with which endothelium might interact) leads to a sort of mutual electrostatic repulsion between the two sets of negatively charged cells and that this repulsion in part prevents the platelets and leukocytes from adhering to the endothelial surface. This point recently has been challenged, however, by data that indicate that thrombogenic substrates such as collagen and elastin may have charge densities similar to that of the endothelial surface. Both the "glycocalyx" theory and the "surface negativity" theory are still widely debated. Both concepts place the endothelial cells in a somewhat passive role; it just lies there, and its thromboresistant properties are related to surface modifications in charge and in chemical characteristics.

It is now clear that this limited view of the endothelium is far too restrictive. There is abundant evidence that the endothelial cell is not merely a passive lining for the blood vessels that lies there and lets things pass over it. Indeed, endothelial cells are emerging from their previous role as passive participants and are now known to be metabolically active cells that influence both the plasma coagulation system and platelet function. Endothelial cells have been shown to actively metabolize some of the prostaglandins, serotonin, adenine nucleotides, bradykinin, and angiotensin I, all of which promote platelet aggregation. They are rich sources of tissue thromboplastin (III). Endothelial cells also apparently can bind thrombin (IIa) and other coagulation components and can secrete both the tissue type and the urokinase type of plasminogen activator for entry into the fibrinolytic schemes.

Because of their location and contact with the flowing bloodstream, endothelial cells are perfectly positioned to modulate the various biological systems in blood, particularly the coagulation system. A contemporary view of these flattened cells lining our blood vessels must therefore recognize their active involvement in the coagulation process. In addition, these cells play both sides of the game; they have procoagulant and anticoagulant properties (Box 3-2).

Endothelial Procoagulant Properties

One of the first visible components of a developing thrombus is a layer of platelets deposited where endothelial damage has occurred to expose subendothelial structures. Platelets bind not to the endothelial cells themselves but to subendothelial collagen where they aggregate and release their constituents, including *thromboxane A_2 (TXA$_2$)* to promote further platelet aggregation. Adhesion of platelets to the subendothelium is dependent on *von Willebrand factor (vWF)*, which is synthesized and

BOX 3-2 **Procoagulant and Anticoagulant**
Properties of the Endothelium

PROCOAGULANT PROPERTIES

Synthesis, storage, and release of von Willebrand
factor
Major tissue thromboplastin (III) source
Plasminogen activator inhibitors
Platelet-activating factor source

ANTICOAGULANT PROPERTIES

Barrier between blood and thrombogenic
subendothelium
Endothelial cell surface properties (heparan
sulfate, alpha$_2$-macroglobulin)
Surface inactivation of thrombin (IIa) by
antithrombin III
Thrombin-thrombomodulin complex and protein
Ca
Prostacyclin (PGI$_2$)
Conversion of ADP to nonaggregating nucleotides

---

stored in the so-called *Weibel-Palade bodies* of
the endothelial cells for later secretion. Released
vWF subsequently binds to subendothelial collagen.
Platelets bind to the subendothelial collagen-bound
vWF by means of membrane receptors for vWF
(Fig. 3-21). Endothelial cells can express tissue
thromboplastin (III) on their surface to promote proconvertin (VIIa)-mediated activation of cell-bound
Christmas factor (IX) and Stuart-Prower factor (X).
They can also modulate certain "antithrombogenic"
activities, for example, by producing plasminogen
activator inhibitors. Last, endothelial cells can release platelet-activating factor (PAF), a very potent
platelet-aggregating agent.

Endothelial Anticoagulant Properties

In addition to the surface properties of endothelial
cells mentioned previously, normal endothelium
contributes to the inhibition of thrombosis by the
inactivation of thrombin, fibrinolysis, and the inhibition of platelet aggregation. As we have mentioned, endothelial cells can bind thrombin (IIa) and
other coagulation factors. Heparin-like glycosaminoglycans (heparan sulfate) at the cell surface
catalyze the inactivation of bound thrombin by
antithrombin III. Thrombin also binds to thrombomodulin receptors, where it is involved in the
cleavage of protein C to release the activated anticoagulant protein Ca (see section on Regulatory
Mechanisms in Hemostasis, p. 97, and Fig. 3-18).
Endothelial cells are also rich sources of the tissue

type of plasminogen activator (t-PA) and hence assist in controlling thrombosis by local fibrinolysis.

Endothelial cells have the capacity to convert the
strongly proaggregating substance ADP released
from platelets to adenine nucleotide platelet inhibitors. Endothelial cells also downregulate thrombotic events by inhibiting platelet aggregation in
another way. A novel cyclooxygenase-produced derivative of membrane-esterified arachidonic acid
called *prostacyclin (PGI$_2$)* is released at low levels
even by resting endothelial cells, and increased release can be stimulated by a variety of stimuli including interleukin-1, thrombin (II), endotoxin, and
TNF (tumor necrosis factor, cachectin). This discovery considerably altered thinking about endothelial
cell and platelet physiology. Through the local release of adenosine diphosphate (ADP) and the generation of prostaglandin endoperoxides and thromboxane A$_2$ (TXA$_2$), adherent platelets form the
initial primary hemostatic plug and promote local
vasoconstriction.

Thromboxane A$_2$ is a potent platelet-aggregating
agent and additionally promotes vasoconstriction.
It seems reasonable, then, that if endothelial cells
are to be truly thromboresistant they should somehow be able to counteract the potent thrombogenic
activities generated during the formation of the initial hemostatic platelet plug. This in fact occurs
through the endothelial synthesis and release of
PGI$_2$, which converts the released platelet endoperoxides and thromboxanes to unstable structures,
which can prevent or reverse platelet aggregation
and relax several kinds of blood vessels. It has been
suggested that the ability of the endothelial cells to
produce PGI$_2$ is a basic thromboresistant mechanism characteristic of the lining of the vasculature.
It is currently envisioned that when the endothelial
cells are injured there would be a lack of PGI$_2$ synthesis and release and local clot formation would
occur. In other settings, an interplay presumably
takes place between the TXA$_2$ in the platelets, with
its strong platelet-aggregating and vasoconstrictive
properties, and the PGI$_2$ in the endothelium, with
its potent antiaggregating activity and vasodilator
functions. A powerful set of checks and balances is
thus visualized.

It is also interesting to note that the PGI$_2$ synthetic enzymes in the endothelial cells can apparently use platelet-derived endoperoxides as a substrate. Hence a novel surveillance system exists to
prevent or counteract any overzealous platelet activation. It must, however, be stated that PGI$_2$-TXA$_2$
interaction is certainly not the only control mechanism available, since incubation of endothelial
cells with cyclooxygenase inhibitors (preventing

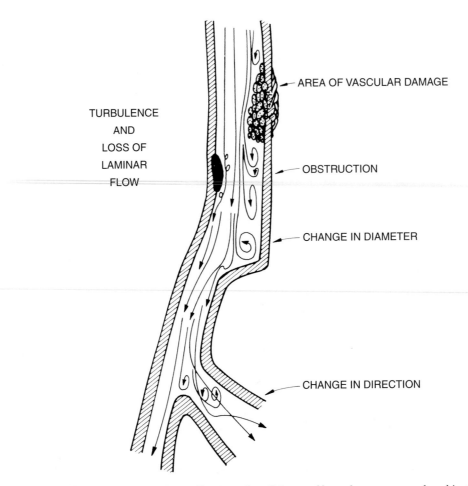

TURBULENCE
AND
LOSS OF
LAMINAR
FLOW

AREA OF VASCULAR DAMAGE

OBSTRUCTION

CHANGE IN DIAMETER

CHANGE IN DIRECTION

Fig. 3-21 Turbulence and loss of laminar flow. Schema of how changes are produced in the normal axial streaming of flowing blood by vessel lesions, changes in lumen size, or flow direction. Such changes increase the opportunity for thrombi to form.

synthesis of PGI_2) does not completely remove the "nonthrombogenic" properties of endothelial cells. The discovery of these unstable but very active products of arachidonic acid metabolism has, however, allowed fresh insight into the control of hemostasis and possible prevention of thrombosis.

RHEOLOGICAL AND HEMODYNAMIC MECHANISMS OF THROMBOSIS

The thrombogenic contributions of decreased blood flow and vascular stasis have also been recognized since Virchow's time. Venous stasis may occur in a wide variety of pathological and physiological conditions including immobilization, pregnancy, shock, and heart failure or even during anesthesia. The rheological properties of blood are such that a drop in flow rate results in increased viscosity. It appears that altered rheological properties augment the thrombotic process largely in two ways: by creating altered turbulence to accelerate the cellular and enzymatic

reactions important in thrombogenesis and also by producing further injury to the vessel wall itself.

Blood flow in arteries and veins is normally *laminar*. This means that the blood tends to flow as a series of concentric fluid cylinders with the innermost stream moving forward at the fastest rate and with each "layer" moving successively slower as one moves toward the wall of the blood vessel. Immediately adjacent to the endothelium is a thin layer of plasma. In areas of hydraulic stress such as sharp bends, valves, and branches, there is a natural tendency for turbulence to occur, which tends to disturb the laminar flow of the blood (Fig. 3-22). Indeed, such areas of turbulence are more prone to develop thrombi than other sites.

In areas where vascular injury has taken place, the disruption of the endothelium and the local hemostatic plug that develops also create turbulence and disrupt laminar flow. A vicious circle can thus become established where local platelet clumping at a site of endothelial discontinuity causes turbulence

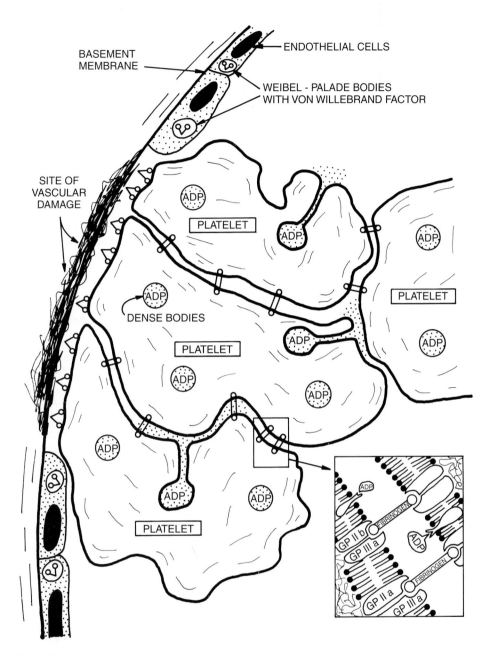

Fig. 3-22 Mechanisms of platelet adhesion and aggregation. Platelets are anchored to subendothelium by receptors for collagen-bound von Willebrand factor (vWF). vWF is synthesized and stored in granules (Weibel-Palade bodies) in the endothelial cell and released upon injury. Platelets bind to each other by fibrinogen linking at the GP IIb–GP IIIa receptor site in an ADP-catalyzed reaction. *(Adapted from Hawiger J:* Hum Pathol *18:111-122, 1987.)*

and the turbulence thus created increases thrombus formation to accelerate and aggravate the process. Turbulence also occurs in the slower-flowing venous system, as around the venous valves.

In addition to turbulence, slowing of the blood flow and stasis increase the probability for thrombosis, though stasis alone probably does not cause thrombosis unless accompanied by endothelial damage or a hypercoagulable state of the plasma. Pre

cisely how stasis contributes to thrombosis is not entirely clear. At a mechanistic level, the increased viscosity of the blood and the loss of laminar flow disturb the relationships of cellular and plasma elements in the blood and favor the interaction of coagulable proteins and platelets with the endothelium. It also may be that stasis reduces the removal of activated clotting factors by delaying their clearance into the liver and reticuloendothelial system. It would also presumably delay the dilution of activated clotting factors and slow their inactivation by naturally-occurring inhibitors. It also has been suggested that the slowing of blood flow and stasis are sufficient to produce local hypoxemia and that one endothelial response to hypoxemia is to release tissue thromboplastin (III) to initiate extrinsic coagulation.

Although the precise reasons why the rheological properties of blood are so important to thrombosis are as yet not clear, it would appear that at least certain hemodynamic alterations such as turbulence, loss of laminar flow characteristics, and increased blood viscosity increase the likelihood of thrombosis. The opportunity for thrombosis to occur in the face of any or all of these hemodynamic changes is greatly increased by damage to the endothelial lining of the blood vessels or by changes in the blood itself that may lead to a hypercoagulable state.

BASIC MECHANISMS IN THE BLOOD RELATED TO THROMBOSIS

There are three major biological contributions or functions of the blood that may become activated or altered to participate in the pathogenesis of thrombosis. These are the formation of the fibrin coagulum by the intrinsic and extrinsic coagulation pathways, the phenomenon of platelet aggregation and adhesion, and fibrinolysis. We have previously discussed the first two points, and the third one is covered in some detail in a later section.

Most of the plasma clotting factors were discovered during investigations of clinical patients in which abnormalities of coagulation were diagnosed. Many of these patients had bleeding tendencies or a hemorrhagic diathesis. It is still reasoned by some that if a deficiency of the coagulation factors leads to hemorrhagic tendencies then thrombosis might be promoted if an increased concentration of the clotting factors was present. There is very little experimental proof for this concept, however, though increased concentrations of some clotting factors are found in certain thrombotic conditions. This situation is sometimes referred to as a *"hypercoagulable state,"* which we might attempt to define as an altered state of the circulating blood that requires a smaller quantity of clot-inducing substance to produce intravascular coagulation than is required to produce comparable thrombosis in a normal subject.

During pregnancy there are often elevated levels of fibrinogen (I) as well as antihemophilic factor (VIII), proconvertin (VII), and Stuart-Prower factor (X). In the immediate postpartum period and after some surgical operations, where the risk of deep vein thrombosis is elevated, increased plasma concentrations of coagulation factors can be demonstrated. It is equally possible, however, that hypercoagulability could result from deficiencies in control mechanisms; rather than more procoagulants, there could be a decrease in inhibitors. For example, patients deficient in antithrombin III or protein C have an increased incidence of thrombosis.

There also seems to be an increased tendency to thrombosis associated with the nephrotic syndrome (protein-losing renal failure), diabetes mellitus, cardiac failure, valvular heart disease, severe trauma or burns, disseminated cancer, prolonged immobilization during severe illness or after surgery, and virtually all chronic debilitating diseases. Despite these situations, it has been very difficult to draw any solid conclusions with respect to a definite cause-and-effect relationship. That is, although we are quite aware of the many situations that may predispose to thrombosis, we are still relatively unable to adequately *define* hypercoagulability and its relationship to thrombotic events. This is, in part, because thrombosis is usually studied after the fact, since we lack truly useful diagnostic tests to identify patients at risk in a prospective way. Much current research is directed at this precise problem.

As in other areas of science, more attention has been directed to the forward activation phase of blood coagulation than to the inhibitory mechanisms that keep the system in check. It is reasonable at the outset, however, to consider that a disturbance in the levels of natural inhibitors of the coagulation process also might predispose to thrombosis. In short, a hypercoagulable state theoretically might result from either increased activation of the clotting system or from decreased inhibitory activity. Clinicians have identified patients that support both possibilities. With respect to blood coagulation, several major groups of inhibitors have been defined (see section on Regulatory Mechanisms in Hemostasis).

Although we have added many details since the times of Virchow, his triad remains the best overall explanation of the various factors that participate in the pathogenesis of thrombosis. It should hardly be necessary for us to point out that any predisposition to the development of thrombosis is magnified by any increase in the number or intensity of various predisposing influences in any one individual. Of Virchow's triad, probably only endothelial injury itself can stand alone in inducing thrombosis. When all three are present, the risk is clearly higher, but any two of the three corners of the triad may suffice. Thus a patient with vessels roughened by arteriosclerosis or atherosclerosis who because of persistent proteinuria caused by the nephrotic syndrome is deficient in antithrombin III would be a prime candidate for the development of thrombosis.

ROLE AND PROPERTIES OF PLATELETS IN HEMOSTASIS AND THROMBOSIS

The platelets are important components of blood that circulate as anucleate bits of cellular cytoplasm derived from the megakaryocytes in the bone marrow and other hematopoietic tissues. The past two decades have given rise to remarkable advances in our understanding of blood platelets and their interactions with the vessel wall.

The physiological integrity of the circulation depends on continuous monitoring of the vessel wall by circulating platelets. This is quantitatively no small chore. During each minute of transit time within the circulation, 10^{12} platelets survey thousands of square meters of capillary surface carpeted with 7×10^{11} endothelial cells. If the platelets detect a break in the continuity of the vessel wall, they immediately respond by contacting the area of injury, spreading out and adhering to the injured zone, and clumping. Such platelets become activated, and their surfaces are transformed into batteries of receptors. Their interiors receive an influx of Ca^{++} and become metabolic furnaces for the enzymatic oxidation of arachidonic acid into endoperoxides, which are subsequently converted to powerful thromboxanes, which are potent vasoconstrictors and platelet aggregators. The storage granules of the platelets are discharged into the local environment, where they are targeted toward other platelets as well as cells of the vessel wall such as smooth muscle. The platelets are remarkable, hair-trigger surveillance instruments; unfortunately they participate with equal fervor in covert pathological operations such as thrombosis.

Although the platelets that circulate in the blood do not normally adhere to each other or to normal endothelium, a primary function of platelets is adhesion. *Adhesion* in this context refers to sticking to a nonplatelet surface and is distinct from *aggregation,* which refers to the sticking of platelets to each other. When the endothelium is stripped from the inner aspect of the blood vessels, platelets adhere to the subendothelial extracellular matrix. When platelets are exposed to collagen (especially types I and III), microfibrils, elastin, smooth muscle cells, or fibroblasts, they adhere to these structures rapidly and become activated. Part of the activation process involves platelet aggregation, which leads to what is known as the *platelet release reaction.*

This is a nonlytic secretory reaction whereby platelets release their stores of active chemicals, form thromboxane A_2, participate in activation of the blood coagulation system, and cause further platelet aggregation.

The biological role of platelets in hemostasis and thrombosis is well established though probably not completely understood (Box 3-3). Primary arrest of bleeding in small vessels is achieved initially by the formation of a platelet plug at the severed end of the vessel. Platelets provide critical phospholipids such as platelet factor 3 to promote clot formation. By restoring a covering over areas of vessels denuded of endothelium, they also assist in reducing the exposure of plasma to the clot-promoting subendothelial surfaces. They also participate in inflammatory reactions (see Chapter 4).

Unfortunately the platelet properties of adhesion, aggregation, and secretion, which make them so useful in the hemostatic mechanism, also allow them to participate in thrombogenesis. We can perhaps best appreciate the functions of platelets in hemostasis and thrombosis if we briefly consider the three critical functions of platelets in these processes: adhesion, aggregation, and secretion, or the platelet release reaction.

Platelet Adhesion

As we mentioned before, adhesion refers to the ability of platelets to stick to nonplatelet surfaces. With respect to the vascular system, several subendothelial surface components promote such adhesion: collagen, elastin, basement membrane, microfila-

BOX 3-3 Biological Properties of Platelets with Respect to Hemostasis and Thrombosis

HEMOSTASIS
Adhesion to subendothelium (collagen)
Primary arrest of bleeding
Formation of initial platelet plug
Furnishing of phospholipids for coagulation
Enhancement of blood coagulation
Helping in covering areas of stripped endothelium

THROMBOSIS
Rapid response to vascular injury
Platelet factors accelerate thrombogenesis
Platelet plug promotes turbulence
Enzymes can further damage endothelium
Generation of thromboxane A_2
Promotion of thrombus propagation

ments, fibronectin, and even amorphous ground substances. Platelets have been observed microscopically to adhere to all these substrates. Hence, in an injured blood vessel where endothelial cells have been lost, abundant opportunities for platelet adhesion are created by the exposure of subendothelial connective tissue components. Prominent among these is *collagen* (types I and III) because of its ability to bind von Willebrand factor, as previously discussed. Other formed elements of the blood seem to participate in this process. Erythrocytes, for example, may be important to the process of platelet adhesion both by virtue of their rheological properties and because they are an important source of ADP, which can precipitate platelet aggregation and the release reaction. The adhesion of platelets to the subendothelium also seems to require divalent calcium (IV) for successful adhesion to occur.

The biochemical and biophysical basis for platelet adhesion has been clarified in recent years. The factor VIII/von Willebrand factor complex appears to be the major adhesive cofactor for platelet adhesion to subendothelium (see Fig. 3-22). Normally, vWF does not bind to circulating platelets; however, it binds "on demand" when released from the Weibel-Palade bodies of injured endothelial cells when platelets need to be anchored to the break in the continuity of the vessel wall. The binding of vWF to platelets is stimulated by ADP. A long list of other agents may activate platelets and promote their receptor mediated interaction with the vessel wall including epinephrine, thrombin, certain prostaglandins (TXA$_2$), and platelet-activating factor (PAF). It is likely that *in vivo* many of these various stimuli can effect increased platelet adhesiveness, and the length of the list is only a reflection of the need for redundancy in a system so critical to formation of the initial hemostatic plug.

Platelet Aggregation

If collagen is added to a suspension of platelets in plasma, some of the platelets will stick to the collagen (adhesion), but after a short delay the remaining platelets begin to swell, adopt considerable conformational changes, and stick to each other. This is platelet aggregation. Pseudopodia protrude from the platelet surface, the platelet organelles are centralized within the platelet, and the overall shape changes from that of a somewhat flattened disk to a rotund sphere. Such conformational changes appear necessary to reorganize platelet surface membrane components to expose the clot-promoting phospholipids called "platelet factor 3." Numerous biological stimuli can induce platelet aggregation

and thus can predispose to thrombus formation. This long list includes ADP, thrombin, collagen, arachidonic acid, TXA$_2$, epinephrine, immune complexes, and platelet-activating factor (PAF).

Recent studies have confirmed that certain components of plasma are essential to the platelet-aggregation process. Platelet aggregation is diminished in patients with *congenital afibrinogenemia,* and *in vitro* studies have documented that fibrinogen (I) is an essential cofactor for platelet aggregation. Similar evidence can be cited for patients with antihemophilic factor (VIII) or with von Willebrand factor deficiency. Platelet aggregation has been extensively studied, and the physiological basis for this important event can now be understood at a molecular level.

It is useful to break platelet aggregation down into two phases: a primary reversible phase and a secondary irreversible phase. In primary *reversible* aggregation, platelets undergo shape change with pseudopod formation. In resting platelets, the GP IIb-IIIa membrane glycoprotein complex that constitutes the fibrinogen receptor is distributed uniformly over the platelet membrane. After stimulation, however, large clusters of GP IIb-IIIa collocalize with fibrinogen on the developing pseudopods and between adherent platelets, and such a process initiates the secondary *irreversible* phase of aggregation with recruitment of additional platelets and the release of platelet granule proteins (see Fig. 3-22).

The triggering event for platelets to form aggregates is ADP-catalyzed exposure of binding sites for fibrinogen on the platelet membrane. As a result, fibrinogen links two platelets together, which are rapidly joined by others through a "snowball effect" to produce a platelet aggregate. It is now believed that the primary role of agonists like ADP is to induce exposure of binding sites for fibrinogen. This is no small affair; ADP induces approximately 40,000 to 50,000 binding sites for fibrinogen on a single platelet. In addition to other constituents, the platelet α-granules contain four major adhesion proteins; fibrinogen, von Willebrand factor, thrombospondin, and fibronectin.

Thrombospondin is secreted by platelet α-granules and binds to the activated platelet surface where it interacts with bound fibrinogen and other components to function as a sort of agglutinin to stabilize platelet aggregates and support the conversion of microaggregates into macroaggregates. The release of these various granule contents during platelet aggregation allows them to achieve high local concentrations and play an important role in irreversible aggregation and the secretion phase of aggregation. Irrespective of the various contributory forces behind platelet aggregation, once it occurs the platelets change their shape radically, develop secretory channels to the outside, and progress through a series of events known as the "platelet release reaction."

Platelet Secretory Events: The Platelet Release Reaction

Platelets are secretory cells; as a consequence of aggregation, platelet constituents are released into the local environment. This release reaction has basically two stages (Fig. 3-23). At first, a variety of intense cytoplasmic activity can be detected, and it culminates with the extrusion of the contents of the cytoplasmic dense bodies or storage granules into the surrounding medium. This phase places dense body contents such as adenine nucleotides and serotonin into the local environment. Sometimes the reaction stops here, but if the stimulus for aggregation is strong enough, there occurs a second phase of release in which the contents of the lysosomal granules are discharged. At this time, hydrolytic enzymes such as β-glucuronidase, acid cathepsins, and β-N-acetylglucosaminidase are released. After the release reaction, most of the cytoplasmic organelles of the platelet are gone. The platelet itself usually is not lysed, as documented by the fact that cytoplasmic enzymes such as lactic dehydrogenase (LDH) are not released. The released ADP is a major stimulus for the formation of additional platelet aggregates. Platelets stimulated to aggregate also produce thromboxane A_2 (TXA_2), the most potent platelet-aggregating agent known. It may well be that the generation and release of TXA_2 is even more important than ADP in promoting additional platelet aggregation.

During the conformational changes that accompany platelet aggregation, platelet factor 3 (PF3) is made available on the platelet cell membrane as mentioned previously. PF3 is an important procoagulant molecule that appears to participate in the formation of thrombin (IIa) in at least two

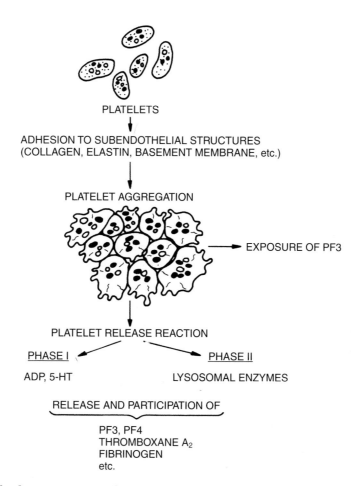

PLATELETS

↓

ADHESION TO SUBENDOTHELIAL STRUCTURES
(COLLAGEN, ELASTIN, BASEMENT MEMBRANE, etc.)

↓

PLATELET AGGREGATION

→ EXPOSURE OF PF3

↓

PLATELET RELEASE REACTION

<u>PHASE I</u>   <u>PHASE II</u>

ADP, 5-HT   LYSOSOMAL ENZYMES

<u>RELEASE AND PARTICIPATION OF</u>

PF3, PF4
THROMBOXANE A_2
FIBRINOGEN
etc.

Fig. 3-23 Platelet aggregation and release. The exposure of platelets to appropriate stimuli produces platelet aggregation first and then the platelet release reaction with its two characteristic phases. *ADP,* Adenosine diphosphate; *5-HT,* 5-hydroxytryptamine (serotonin); *PF,* platelet factor.

reactions: the activation of factor VIII and the cleavage of prothrombin (II). Precisely how it contributes is not yet totally understood. Platelets also release platelet factor 4, a basic polypeptide that can function to inhibit the prolongation of clotting time produced by heparin. It also can neutralize the anticoagulant properties of some of the fibrin degradation products (FDPs), may alter the surface properties of the platelet membranes to expose more PF3, and apparently can assist in the polymerization of soluble fibrin monomers.

The mechanism by which products stored in the secretory granules of platelets are released to the exterior has been the subject of considerable interest. In human platelets, an extensive *cytocavitary network* known as the *open canalicular system* (OCS) communicates directly with the surrounding medium through uninterrupted openings to the plasma membrane. After platelet activation, the various secretory granules in human platelets become centrally concentrated within the platelets and then fuse their membranes with the cytoplasmic OCS, which serves as a conduit for the release of secretory products to the exterior. Interestingly enough, *bovine platelets* lack the OCS found in human platelets, and, after activation, secretory granules remain more peripheral within the cytoplasm, and secretion occurs by direct fusion of the granule membranes with the plasma membrane. The basis for these species variations in platelet structure that result in different routes for secretion of granule contents remains unknown.

It is increasingly clear that platelets are intimately linked to the hemostatic mechanism and to the pathogenesis of thrombosis. This is a two-way street: platelets promote blood coagulation, and blood coagulation promotes platelet aggregation and its attendant effects.

Morphology and Morphogenesis of Thrombi

Thrombi can occur anywhere within the cardiovascular system. When they occur within the vascular system, they are *vascular thrombi,* which can be in arteries *(arteriothromboses)* or within veins *(phlebothromboses).* They also can occur within the heart itself *(cardiac thrombosis),* where they can involve either the cardiac valves *(valvular thrombosis)* or the walls of the chambers of the heart *(mural thrombosis).* When thrombi build up on the cardiac valves, they are commonly referred to as *vegetations,* or *vegetative valvular thromboses,* because of their appearance.

Thrombi vary widely in their appearance and composition because of local factors that affect their formation. One of the most important determinants of the size and structure of a thrombus is the rate of blood flow in the area in which they are formed. Thrombi formed in a rapidly flowing bloodstream (arterial thrombi) differ in appearance from thrombi arising in a sluggish blood flow (venous thrombi).

ARTERIAL THROMBOSIS

In most of the arterial system, blood flows at a high rate under normal conditions. If endothelial injury occurs in an artery or arteriole, a fairly predictable type of thrombus will develop. The rapid blood flow and high pressure are sufficient to sweep away all but the most tenacious of the clotting contributors, and the typical arterial thrombus is a pale gray-tan mass that consists of nearly concentric layers of alternating bands of fibrin and platelets mixed with rather scanty amounts of darker red coagulated blood (Fig. 3-24). The laminated appearance of such thrombi relates to their underlying pathogenesis. As the rapid flow sweeps away many of the components of blood, currents conducive to activation and accumulation of clotting factors are found only in the peripheral recesses of the developing low-profile thrombus. They are rarely occlusive thrombi at first but require a slower buildup of components.

The flow of blood over the developing thrombus contributes to its gradual increase in size, a phenomenon referred to as *propagation* of the thrombus. A platelet layer that may be deposited first by adhesion to the damaged endothelium is followed by local platelet aggregation. Gradually fibrin forms to stabilize the platelet mass. The flow of blood deposits more platelets onto the growing mass, which is then followed by more fibrin deposition. It is this layering effect, largely caused by alternating zones of platelets and fibrin with scant amounts of blood, that produces the laminations known as the *lines of Zahn.* Because such thrombi are composed largely of platelets and fibrin, they are often called *"white"* or *"pale"* thrombi.

Although the flow of blood in the arterial system usually prevents these thrombi from being occlusive initially, eventually the thrombus formed on the damaged arterial wall propagates to form an *"occlusive"* thrombus. In such situations, the *head* of the thrombus tends to receive accumulations of fibrin and platelets because of its exposure to the flowing bloodstream and hence remains pale, whereas the *tail* of the thrombus accumulates coagulated blood from the stagnant downstream flow

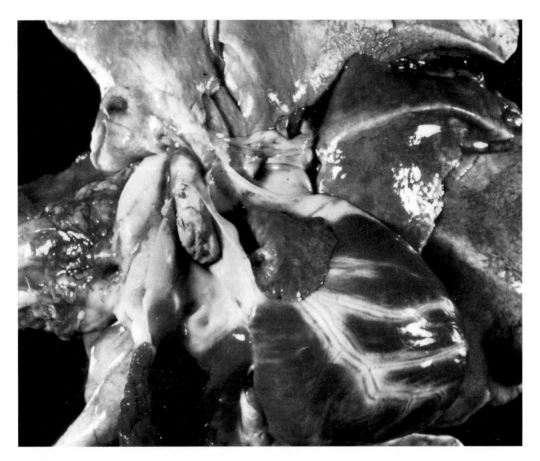

Fig. 3-24 Pulmonary thrombosis. A large thrombus is present in the main branch pulmonary artery of this dog with renal amyloidosis and the nephrotic syndrome.

and the turbulence of the blood on the leeward side of the propagating thrombus. The tail of such thrombi thus tends to be dark red because of its accumulation of coagulated blood (see Fig. 3-20). Not all of the thrombus may be attached to the vessel wall. The distal or downstream segment may be more or less suspended in the flowing blood as a sort of undulating tail. Such segments often break off and as such are a common source of emboli (Fig. 3-25).

VENOUS THROMBOSIS

Blood flow in the venous system is often slow. This is especially true in larger distal veins in which gravity works against the system. Indeed, it has been shown that the blood flow can virtually stop under conditions where prolonged periods of inactivity are present.

Much of the ability to move blood in the larger distal veins is tied to the pumping actions of the skeletal muscles through which the veins run. Hence, muscular activity is necessary to keep the venous system flowing properly and flow rates decline greatly during inactivity. Thrombi developing within the deep veins tend to resemble an intravascular clot of whole blood, much as one might expect if blood were drawn into a glass tube. They are dark red in color and more moist or gelatinous than arterial thrombi and sometimes are referred to as "*red*" thrombi, "*stasis*" thrombi, or "*coagulation*" thrombi. Such thrombi can be difficult to distinguish from *postmortem thrombi,* which result from coagulation of the blood within vessels after death. They differ from postmortem thrombi by having a point of attachment to the vessel wall and by virtue of the fact that they usually have some tangled strands of fibrin mixed within their substance. They are easily separated by their appearance from the so-called *chicken-fat clot* so commonly seen as a postmortem event, particularly in horses. Here, the rapid sedimentation rate for equine red blood cells allows separation of the blood before postmortem coagulation, and the result is a moist golden yellow plasma clot attached to a dark red blood clot.

Venous thrombi, unlike arterial thrombi, are rarely mural. The slow blood flow in the veins permits total blood coagulation, and so all the cellular

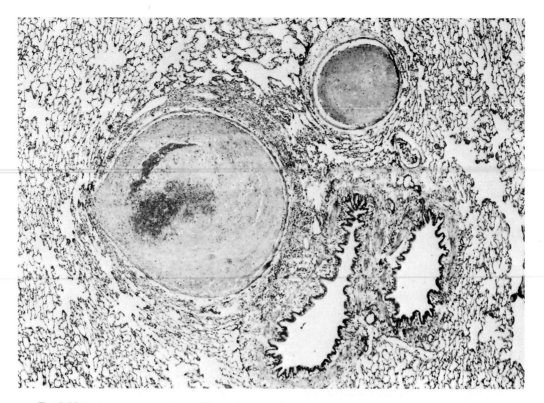

Fig. 3-25 Pulmonary embolism. Two pulmonary branch arteries contain recent emboli. Notice that the surrounding lung tissue is normal (not infarcted) because of the rich collateral blood supply to the lung.

elements become trapped in the thrombus rather than being swept away as they are by the higher flow rates on the arterial side. Because of this, venous thrombi tend to be occlusive and often resemble nearly perfect casts of the lumen of the vessel in which they are found.

In a venous thrombus, the distribution of the formed elements of blood is more or less random, as it is in normal whole blood, and so few, if any, of the structural or architectural features of the arterial pale thrombus can be identified. An additional difference relates to the tenacity of the attachment to the underlying vessel wall. Since venous thrombi are formed in a slow-flowing system, they do not usually generate points of attachment to the vessel wall nearly so tenaciously as arterial thrombi do. Therefore the venous thrombus is in many ways easier to dislodge, and some impressive emboli can result when this occurs. Such emboli can be a serious clinical problem in man where sudden activity such as walking or merely standing up after prolonged bed rest or inactivity may be sufficient to dislodge a poorly attached venous thrombus in a deep leg vein and send it sailing toward the heart and lungs (pulmonary embolism), where the results can be catastrophic.

Fate of Thrombi

After a thrombus has formed, what then? Much of the answer to this question lies in the nature of the local collateral vascular supply to the tissue supplied by the thrombosed vessel. That is, if there is abundant collateral circulation, the service area of the thrombosed vessel may not be sufficiently altered to result in clinical signs.

There are basically only four different evolutionary pathways that a thrombus can follow (Fig. 3-26). Either the thrombus will be (1) *propagated*, become larger, and eventually produce obstruction, or it will be (2) fragmented to result in *embolism* of distal tissues, or it will be (3) removed by *fibrinolysis* (thrombolysis) by either the plasma-derived fibrinolytic systems or phagocytes, or it will be (4) *organized* into the vessel wall. There is a degree of mechanistic overlap in some of these options, but they do basically represent divergent outcomes.

Propagation of Thrombi

We already have touched briefly on the means by which thrombi are propagated. The basic outcome is an overall increase in size of the thrombus itself.

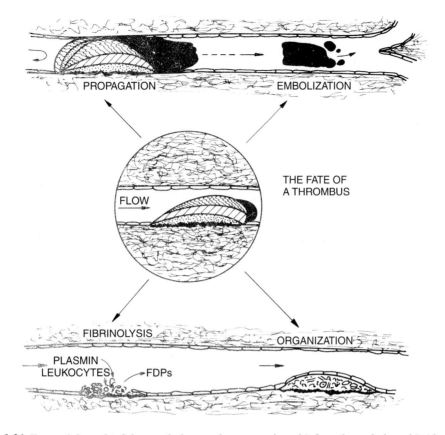

Fig. 3-26 Fates of thrombi. Schema of what can happen to thrombi. Once formed, thrombi either propagate, embolize, undergo fibrinolysis, or organize. *FDP*, Fibrin degradation products.

Because of the nature of blood flow in the arterial and venous divisions of the vascular system, propagation differs in much the same way that thrombus formation differs. Basically, thrombus propagation in both systems refers to the overall enlargement of the thrombotic mass as a result of progressive clot formation. Usually this elongates the mass in the direction of the heart. It is possible, particularly in the venous system, for such propagating thrombi to become extremely large. A thrombus originating, for example, in a branch of the femoral vein may become locally occlusive and subsequently propagate until it protrudes into the lumen of the femoral vein itself. Occasionally, further propagation occurs, and the thrombus may even extend into the iliac vein or caudal vena cava. Propagation of thrombi is one of the major events underlying embolism, since the growing, advancing tail of the thrombus is particularly susceptible to fragmentation and subsequent embolism. As the advancing tail of the thrombus reaches a bifurcation, rapidly flowing blood sweeps past the thrombus to cause dislodgment of part of the thrombus and give rise to an embolus.

EMBOLISM

An *embolus* is a detached physical mass carried in the bloodstream from its site of origin to a more distant site. As an embolus moves downstream, it eventually encounters a blood vessel smaller than the diameter of the embolus and partial or complete occlusion of the vessel then occurs. Although most emboli originate from thrombi, there are other less common types of emboli including fat, air bubbles, tumor cell clumps, aggregates of bacteria or other parasites, and even amniotic fluid. After extensive trauma with fractures, bone marrow embolism may even occur. Most commonly, however, emboli originate from intravascular thrombi. As such, they are most common at sites downstream from the most common sites for thrombosis.

In man, approximately 95% of all venous emboli arise from thrombi within the deep leg veins. Although this can occur in animals, it is unusual because most animals are active and hence use their leg muscles constantly. As we have mentioned previously, activity of this kind tends to prevent venous thrombosis through the continual accessory pumping action of the skeletal muscles. In domestic animals, it is more common for thrombosis to occur in the heart and on its valves than anywhere else; hence emboli and their sites of arrest are determined by the specific location of the thrombi in the heart. Valvular thrombosis involving the left side of the heart usually produces emboli in the systemic circulation, whereas right-sided cardiac thrombosis more often produces pulmonary embolism. Cattle sometimes develop liver abscesses that can erode into the vena cava and initiate local thrombosis. Emboli arising from such caval thrombi usually are arrested in the lungs. Thrombosis of the vena cava is not, of course, limited to cattle and can in fact occur in any species (Fig. 3-27). Cats with primary cardiomyopathy often develop left atrial thrombi, and embolism of the iliac bifurcation is a common sequel. Such iliac emboli often lie directly at the bifurcation and extend into the right and left main branches. They are often referred to as "saddle emboli" (Fig. 3-28).

Once an embolus has arrived at an appropriately sized vessel, it usually becomes attached to the underlying vessel wall and may begin to propagate locally much as a thrombus forming at the same site would. Indeed, it can be extremely difficult to discern, in many cases, whether one is dealing with an attached and propagating embolus or if the mass is in fact a thrombus that originated locally. For this

reason, the term *thromboembolism* is sometimes used to avoid having to make an arbitrary distinction. From our standpoint, it is clear that the *processes* of thrombosis and embolism are different and that the two terms describe quite different events.

The eventual outcome of embolism is much the same as thrombosis, for emboli also can propagate, form more emboli, undergo fibrinolysis, or become organized. They also can produce ischemic necrosis or infarction of the tissues served by the vessels they occlude, as we discuss shortly.

FIBRINOLYSIS AND THROMBOLYSIS

The systems responsible for clot resolution and fibrinolysis form an integral part of the physiological mechanism by which any fibrin, formed extravascularly as well as intravascularly, is removed. As such, *fibrinolysis* functions not only in the resolution of thrombi but also in the degradation of fibrin deposited in inflammatory reactions and in healing and repair processes (see Chapter 4). Fibrin that is formed at sites of thrombosis or tissue inflammation must be removed if normal tissue structure and function is to be restored. The fibrinolytic system is the principal effector of clot removal and controls

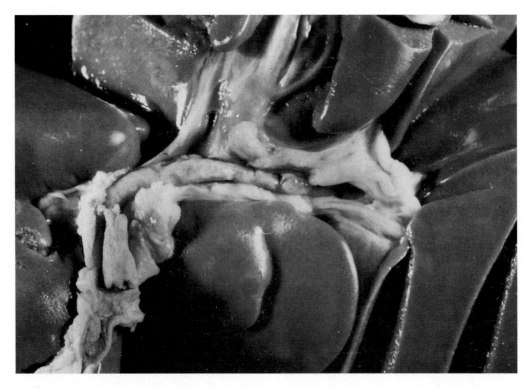

Fig. 3-27 Vena cava thrombosis in dog. A large thrombus is present in the vena cava and portal vein. Notice that the liver here appears normal. This thrombus is more pale than many caval thrombi.

the enzymatic degradation of fibrin. Its action is controlled by the coordinated interaction of inactive precursors *(zymogens),* their activators, specific inhibitors, and active enzymes to provide local control at sites of fibrin deposition.

The proteolytic degradation of fibrin clots *(fibrinolysis)* is mediated by the enzyme *plasmin*, a trypsin-like endopeptidase that can hydrolyze susceptible arginine and lysine bonds in fibrinogen and fibrin. Plasmin is formed from the inactive precursor *plasminogen*, a normal constituent protein of plasma as well as being present in most body fluids including saliva, tears, and milk, by cleavage of a single peptide bond through limited proteolytic action of *plasminogen activators,* serine proteases with a high specificity for their substrate plasminogen.

There are many different plasminogen activators, all apparently serine proteases, and some of them function in such diverse processes as ovulation and spermatogenesis, embryonic development, mammary gland involution, prohormone processing, and keratinocyte differentiation as well as fibrinolysis. Plasminogen activator secretion thus appears to be a general cellular mechanism for inducing localized extracellular proteolysis. Like many other biologically relevant biochemical schemes, the activation of plasminogen is a complex process that is apparently regulated at several levels. Nonactive proactivators first require activation. In addition, the "active" activator can be bound by specific inhibitors, and the substrate, plasminogen, is itself modulated during the activation process. Fibrin itself can modulate the activity of some types of plasminogen activators. The active enzyme plasmin also creates a positive feedback mechanism through its ability to activate additional proactivator and convert plasminogen to plasmin. Plasmin itself is inhibitable by a variety of protease inhibitors. As is so often the case in biological responses, the outcome of any fibrinolytic process represents a functional summary of the relative contributions of different inhibitory and activation pathways.

It is also interesting to note that this is not strictly a host-derived defense system because several activators of plasminogen have been described in microorganisms such as β-hemolytic streptococci (streptokinase), staphylococci (staphylokinase), and certain fungi (brinase). Since the activation of plasminogen is a key step in the production of fibrinolytic activity (and hence thrombolysis), we briefly describe some of the means by which plasminogen activator generation can occur. Some of the various means of generating activity capable of cleaving plasminogen are shown in Fig. 3-29.

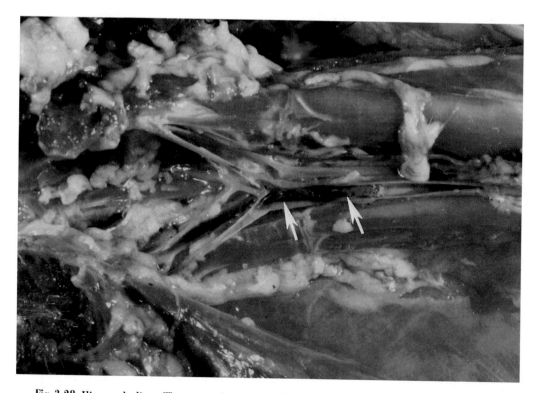

Fig. 3-28 Iliac embolism. The terminal aorta and iliac bifurcation, *arrows*, contain a "saddle embolus" in this cat with hypertrophic cardiomyopathy.

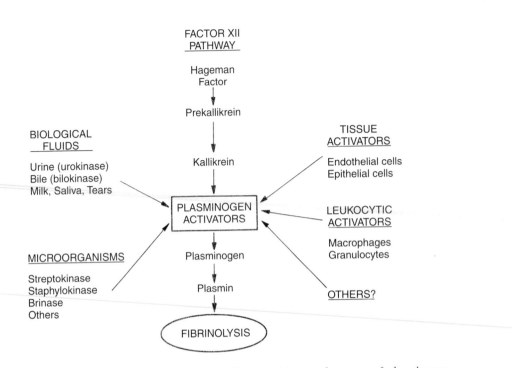

Fig. 3-29 Plasminogen activation. A variety of cellular and humoral sources of plasminogen activators provides multiple entry points to the fibrinolytic system.

Fibrinolysis: The Activation of Plasminogen

Mammalian plasminogens can be identified and isolated from plasma and serum and are single-chain monomeric proteins with multiple molecular isoelectric forms. Most forms have an M_r of about 85,000. The mechanism of activation of plasminogen to the active enzyme *plasmin* involves the cleavage of one or more specific peptide bonds in the native plasminogen molecule. Different methods of activation of plasminogen appear to involve slightly different bond cleavages, but by all pathways of plasminogen activation the fibrinolytic product generated from the cleavage of plasminogen is an active enzyme called "plasmin."

Plasmin has general proteolytic activity and is able to hydrolyze a wide variety of proteins. Plasmin resembles trypsin and thrombin in the sense that it splits only lysyl and arginyl bonds in proteins. As indicated in Fig. 3-29, there are many ways of generating plasminogen-cleaving activity (plasminogen activators) and hence gaining access to the biologically important fibrinolytic process. It is useful to divide the plasminogen activators into the *intrinsic* activators, derived from activation of the Hageman factor–dependent pathways, and the *extrinsic* activators, derived from most tissues and body fluids.

Hageman Factor–Dependent Activity. Shortly after the discovery of coagulation factor XII (Hageman factor), it was found that the surface-dependent activation of Hageman factor (XII) also resulted in the generation of fibrinolytic activity (see Fig. 4-38). It is now known that at least four proteins participate in the generation of fibrinolytic activity in this system: Hageman factor (XII) itself, prekallikrein, high-molecular-weight kininogen, and plasminogen. These first three are the same molecules responsible for initiating intrinsic coagulation (see Fig. 3-11). Activation involves molecular assembly of the various components to result in limited proteolytic cleavage of the native molecule into one or more active fragments. These fragments then activate prekallikrein to kallikrein, which in turn activates plasminogen to plasmin.

Little or no plasmin generation occurs in plasma that is deficient in prekallikrein, high-molecular-weight kininogen, or Hageman factor, but the physiological importance of this fibrinolytic system remains uncertain. No clearly identifiable pathological state attributable to impaired fibrinolysis has been identified in patients with profound defects in components of the Hageman factor system, though the original Hageman factor–deficient patient (John Hageman) died of pulmonary embolism. In addition, Hageman factor pathway–derived plasminogen activators appear to have one ten-thousandth to one forty-thousandth the plasminogen-activating activity of, for example, urokinase. It is interesting to note, however, that at least two products of this activation scheme, kallikrein and plasmin, can cleave additional native Hageman factor (XII), thus providing a means for cyclical activation of the system for continuing mediator production (see Fig. 4-38).

Extrinsic Plasminogen Activators. The plasminogen activators important to fibrinolysis that are present in most tissues and fluids can be divided into two major types, one related to the activator found in tissues and referred to as *tissue-type plasminogen activator* (t-PA) and the other related to the activator found in urine *(urokinase)* and referred to as *urokinase-type plasminogen activator* (u-PA).

These two types of plasminogen activators have somewhat different biochemical and functional characteristics. The t-PAs consist of a single polypeptide chain and have the properties of binding avidly to fibrin and expressing greater enzymatic activity in the presence of fibrin. Molecular sites responsible for the affinity of t-PA for fibrin reside in the so-called "kringle" structures of t-PA, which are similar to the fibrin-binding "finger" domains of the important extracellular matrix glycoprotein and cell adhesion molecule *fibronectin.* The t-PA binds to lysine residues in fibrin that are not exposed in the native fibrinogen molecule. Thus the binding of t-PA to fibrin is specific. In addition, native plasminogen binds to the same lysine residues in fibrin and, as a result, becomes both localized and rendered tenfold more susceptible to conversion to plasmin by t-PA. There are many inhibitors of t-PA, but as long as t-PA remains bound to fibrin, it is resistant to inhibition because the inhibitors also use the lysine binding site of t-PA as their own binding site.

The production of fibrin therefore has built-in mechanisms for inducing its own degradation in a localized manner. Fibrin binds t-PA as well as plasminogen and thereby greatly increases the local production of plasmin. Plasmin degrades the fibrin and in so doing is eventually released. The freed enzymes are then susceptible to rapid inhibition by inhibitors. These unique characteristics both localize t-PA activity and enhance its fibrinolytic activity at sites of fibrin deposition.

Because *thrombosis* represents intravascular coagulation, it stands to reason that *vascular* sites for fibrinolysis would be important. Indeed, the vascular endothelium is a rich source of plasminogen ac-

tivator (t-PA type), which probably mediates much of the clot removal within the circulation by local vascular fibrinolysis. t-PA activity is downregulated by plasma plasminogen activator-inhibitors that form stable covalent complexes with t-PA to provide a viable local control mechanism.

The structure and properties of u-PAs are different from t-PAs in that they generally contain two polypeptide chains and apparently lack the fibronectin-like "finger" domains for high-affinity binding to fibrin and do not exhibit enhanced plasminogen activator activity in the presence of fibrin. Very small amounts of u-PA activity can be detected in plasma and certain molecular forms of u-PA (single-chain urokinase type of plasminogen activator, *scu-PA*) may also be involved with t-PA in intravascular thrombolysis, though they seem not to be so important in this regard as t-PA. u-PA may, however, be very important to certain types of *tissue fibrinolysis.*

Whereas t-PA is secreted primarily by endothelial cells to provide enzymatic activity largely restricted to the circulation, the biochemically and functionally distinct u-PA is secreted by many cell and tissue types, including tissue macrophages. Urokinase has the unique property of functioning in a cell-associated form and of being less reactive to the protease inhibitors of plasma. This has considerable implications for active tissue fibrinolysis, since the inhibitor-activator balance would be shifted toward activation. As an example of the importance of u-PA in tissue fibrinolysis, fibrin-rich alveolar exudates in the lung are handled primarily by u-PA of alveolar macrophage origin rather than t-PA of vascular origin. Investigations of pulmonary fibrinolytic activity in lung-lavage fluids has shown that the bulk of the plasminogen activation is associated with u-PA of macrophage origin.

Macrophages have unique capabilities relative to coagulation and fibrinolysis. They can degrade fibrin through secretion of soluble u-PA or by direct contact of plasminogen incorporated in the fibrin clot with macrophage membrane-bound u-PA, the latter having the unique advantage of being relatively protected from soluble proteinase inhibitors. Macrophage production of u-PA, modulated by specific plasminogen activator-inhibitors, may play a key role in macrophage migration through inflamed tissue and in the removal of fibrinous deposits from sites of inflammation. Macrophages apparently have considerable procoagulant activity as well and can synthesize and express the coagulation factors VII and tissue factor (III) as well as others on their cell surface. It thus appears that macrophage-mediated formation and degradation of fibrin results from the coordinated expression of procoagulant and fibrinolytic functions.

At the present time, it is thus envisioned that two quite distinct fibrinolytic schemes exist; the *t-PA system*, which functions largely within the circulation, and the *u-PA system*, which functions largely at tissue sites. It is also probable that some interaction between these two systems occurs. Finally, for students of disease, it is worth noting that these advances in the molecular definition of plasminogen activation are *not* merely exercises in biochemical verbosity but also hold very real promise for direct clinical application. Indeed, the first clinical trials with recombinant t-PA indicate that effective thrombolysis can be obtained under certain conditions. Further developments in this field can be expected.

Degradation of Fibrinogen and Fibrin Clots

THE FIBRINOLYTIC PROCESS. The biochemical details of the action of plasmin on fibrinogen/fibrin substrates have been extensively detailed, and interested readers are referred to the reading list given at the end of this chapter. We only briefly review the essential features of the process here. The proteolysis of fibrin (or fibrinogen) by plasmin involves essentially the same steps (Fig. 3-30). The initial cleavage liberates the carboxy-terminal polar appendage of the A_α chain and also a peptide from the N-terminal portion of the B_β chain producing a

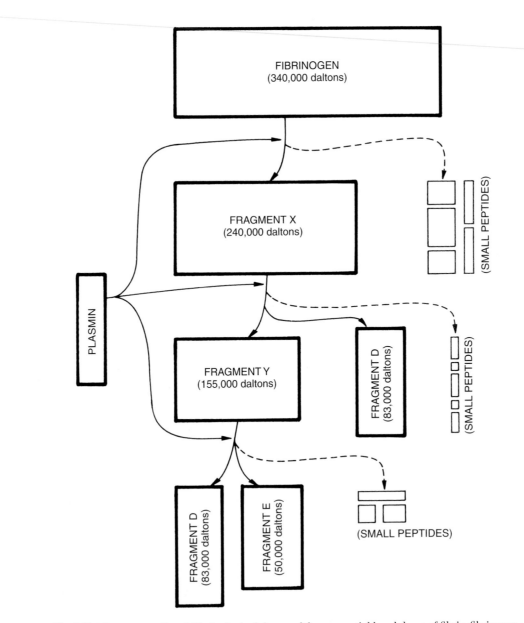

Fig. 3-30 Plasmin-mediated fibrinolysis. Schema of the sequential breakdown of fibrin-fibrinogen by plasmin to yield the FDPs (fibrin degradation products, fragments X, Y, D, and E).

fragment termed *fragment X*, which has a molecular size of about 240,000 daltons. Fibrinogen itself, we must recall, is the plasma precursor of insoluble fibrin and circulates as a plasma protein with a molecular weight of around 340,000 daltons.

After initial cleavage by plasmin, subsequent proteolysis of fragment X results in the formation of *fragment Y*, which has a molecular weight of around 155,000 daltons, and a smaller piece (called *fragment D*), which has a molecular size of about 83,000 daltons. The final stage of fibrinogen/fibrin fragmentation involves the breakdown of fragment Y into a second fragment D and another piece of smaller size (50,000 daltons) called *fragment E*. Plasmin degradation of non–cross linked fibrin is essentially identical to that of fibrinogen in both the kinetics of the reaction and the structure of the derivative fragments. This supports the concept that there is little structural change in the fibrin monomer unit during polymerization. On the other hand, cross-linked fibrin is degraded more slowly by plasmin, and the derivative fragments released during solubilization are distinct. These unique degradation products are the result of prior crosslinking of fibrin monomer by factor XIII, not of a unique proteolytic attack by plasmin.

The details of the proteolytic attack of plasmin on fibrin clots are not just an impractical recitation on the making of biological alphabet soup (fragments X, Y, D, E, and so on), for the breakdown products of fibrinogen/fibrin (called *fibrin degradation products,* FDPs) have considerable relevance to our focus on the pathogenetic mechanisms of disease. The most pronounced biological activity of the FDPs is their anticoagulant activities through competitive inhibition of the clotting action of thrombin on fibrinogen substrates. In addition, the smaller FDPs impair platelet adhesiveness, aggregation, and release reactions, whereas the larger ones may have an opposite effect. Some of the fragments also can cause smooth muscle contraction, increase capillary permeability, and induce the chemotaxis of granulocytes.

Although the plasmin-mediated lysis of both fibrin and fibrinogen produces FDPs, which can be measured in routine clinical assays, it is only the degradation of fibrin that produces the product called "D-dimers," suggestive of fibrin-specific lysis. Because of their biological importance, it is common to measure the circulating levels of FDPs. Elevated levels of FDPs in the circulation are used as an indication of clinically important states of elevated fibrinolysis such as disseminated intravascular coagulation (DIC) after gram-negative sepsis, surgical trauma, shock, and different infectious and neoplastic disease states (see also Chapter 7). Lastly, we should not fail to mention that although enzymatic degradation of fibrin/fibrinogen by plasmin proteolysis constitutes an important means of fibrinolysis and thrombolysis, phagocytic degradation also occurs, with intracellular digestion of the coagulum taking place within phagocytic vacuoles of the neutrophils and macrophages. This is of particular importance to the process of organization (see also Chapter 4).

ORGANIZATION OF THROMBI

Recent thrombi usually are dissolved by the actions of the plasma-derived fibrinolytic scheme just described. This system is so efficient that it is often difficult, in experimental settings, to preserve an intravascular clot long enough to properly study it. Thrombi of clinical significance, however, are usually large enough to produce a delay in resolution by the plasmin system. In addition, the local hemodynamic alterations caused by the thrombus and the potential local hypoxia often lead to additional damage to the vessel wall, and so a kind of inflammatory reaction ensues. It can, in fact, become rather difficult to differentiate between an inflamed vessel in which thrombosis has occurred and a thrombosed vessel in which inflammation has occurred. In time, thrombi not resolved by the plasma fibrinolytic system undergo a process called *organization* (Fig. 3-31). This basically refers to a sequence of events in which the thrombus is reduced in size and becomes ultimately converted into a fibrous connective tissue thickening within the wall of the vessel itself.

Thrombi become organized by processes that are remarkably similar to those that occur in wound healing and repair. The adjacent endothelium begins to grow over the surfaces of the thrombus, acting to insulate it from the circulating blood and hence diminish the possibility for continued propagation of the thrombus. Sometimes the thrombus itself becomes invested with small growing vessels, which restore some order of blood flow by the process of *recanalization* (Fig. 3-32). It seems clear that both the regrowth of endothelium over the surface of a thrombus and the growth through the thrombus of restored vascular channels originates from preexisting endothelium at the margins of the thrombus itself at its attachment point to the vessel wall. Neither reendothelialization of the surface of the thrombus or recanalization of its mass can occur unless the thrombus is attached. Hence, for organization of a thrombus to occur, attachment to the vessel wall is an absolute prerequisite.

As the surface of the thrombus is being covered by endothelium, growth of small capillaries into the

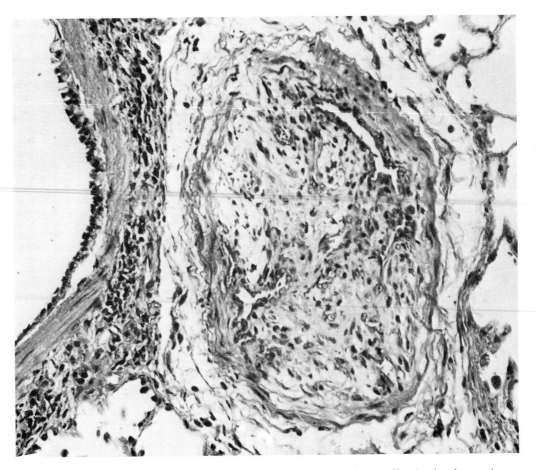

Fig. 3-31 Organization of a thrombus. This pulmonary thrombus shows infiltration by phagocytic cells, several areas of firm attachment to the vessel wall, and peripheral recanalization.

thrombotic mass occurs from the base at its attachment point to the denuded vessel wall. These capillaries provide the nutrient supply for the phagocytic cells that soon emerge from the neocapillaries to enter the thrombus itself. Their job is to phagocytose, degrade, and remove the clotted blood (Fig. 3-33). This is primarily a job for the macrophages, but granulocytes also contribute in the clearing of debris from the organizing thrombus. Macrophages ingest the fragments of red blood cells and platelets present in the thrombus and assist in the fibrinolytic breakdown of the fibrin meshwork that the cellular elements have invaded (see Fig. 3-33). Ultimately, fibroblasts invest the area and lay down collagen so that the thrombus eventually can become completely converted into fibrous connective tissue and incorporated into the structure of the wall of the preexisting vessel. Such structures may produce a narrowing of the lumen of the vessel, but either by circumferential flow or by recanalization it often is possible for an adequate nutritive blood supply to become reestablished. The success of this process often is serendipitously confirmed when old orga-

nized or recanalized thrombi are discovered as totally incidental findings in a necropsy. Such events indicate that organization and recanalization can be highly useful biological means of dealing with thrombi.

INFARCTION

An *infarct* is a localized area of ischemic necrosis in a tissue or organ. It can be produced by either occlusion of the arterial supply or venous drainage of the tissue, but by far the most common cause is occlusive arterial obstruction. The all-too-common "heart attack" that awaits many members of civilized Western society is, in fact, acute myocardial infarction caused by occlusive coronary arterial thrombosis. Emboli can, of course, produce the same effect, though there are often mechanistic differences that relate to the processes whereby thrombi form in arteries and veins. Venous infarction usually is related to direct intravascular venous thrombosis without embolization. Arterial infarction, on the other hand, is more often embolic in na-

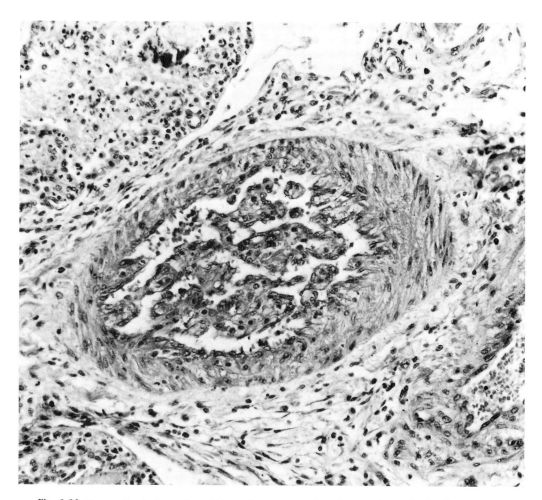

Fig. 3-32 Recanalized thrombus. This pulmonary arteriole from a dog with dirofilariasis was thrombosed some time ago, and the thrombus has now been invested with endothelium-lined channels to permit some blood flow through the area.

ture, though direct thrombotic infarction certainly can occur.

We must again stress that arterial infarction is far more common than venous infarction. The reasons for this are largely anatomical. There are greater numbers of vascular collaterals on the venous side than on the arterial side, and so occlusion may produce only sufficient stasis and backpressure to open anastomotic channels. Infarcts vary somewhat in appearance depending on their pathogenesis and the time after infarction when the tissue is examined. Venous infarcts are usually intensely hemorrhagic as blood backs up into the affected tissue behind the obstruction. Arterial infarcts vary in appearance but are often initially hemorrhagic and later become pale as the area of coagulation necrosis becomes evident. There may be later hemorrhage into the necrotic tissue, however (Fig. 3-34).

There are also some variations depending on the involved tissue. Solid parenchymatous organs, such as the heart and kidneys, tend to have pale infarcts. The spleen also sometimes has pale infarcts, but they clearly can be hemorrhagic (Fig. 3-34). Arterial infarcts in "loose" tissues such as the lung are usually hemorrhagic, however. All infarcts tend to be shaped according to the service area of the vessel whose occlusion was responsible for the development of infarction. Hence, many infarcts are wedge shaped with their apex directed toward the area of vascular occlusion (see Fig. 2-22).

The typical appearance of infarcted tissues is that of *ischemic coagulation necrosis* of the affected cells. The morphological and biochemical alterations that characterize coagulation necrosis have been detailed in Chapter 2 and are not reiterated here. We focus instead on certain characteristics of various tissues that are important in determining the outcome of an episode of occlusive thrombosis or embolism. These include features related to the cardiovascular system as a whole as well as the

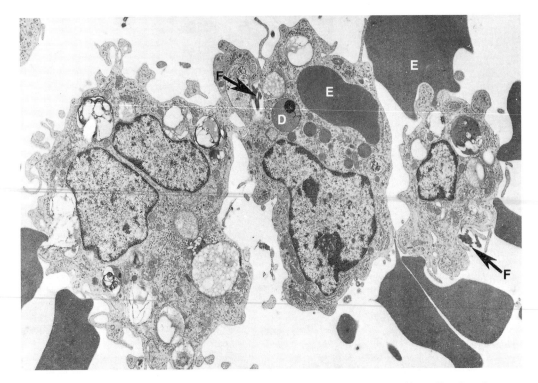

Fig. 3-33 Phagocytic cells in a thrombus. These macrophages are ingesting fibrin, *F*, and erythrocytes, *E*, in a thrombus. Several degraded red blood cells also are seen in the cells, *D*. (Micrograph courtesy Dr. W.L. Castleman, Gainesville, Fla.)

specific vascular anatomy of a tissue and its general vulnerability to ischemia.

Determinants of Infarction

ISCHEMIC SUSCEPTIBILITY

Not all tissues respond equally to ischemia. Since ischemic injury is basically anoxic injury, another way to state the problem is to note that there are wide variations in the tissue responses to anoxia. Possibly the most sensitive are the cells of the central nervous system, which will tolerate total anoxia for only a few minutes before undergoing irreversible degenerative changes and necrosis. Renal tubular epithelium is also extremely sensitive to anoxia. Most parenchymal cells and tissues are, in fact, quite susceptible to ischemic necrosis because of their intolerance of anoxia. Indeed, renal tubular epithelial cells do not even like hypoxia, much less anoxia. The metabolically and physiologically active myocardial cells also are susceptible to ischemia and usually respond by dying.

It is not coincidental, therefore, that the brain, the kidneys, and the heart are rather common sites for infarction. An additional reason for this lies in the nature of the blood supply to these tissues, as

described later. In contrast to the situation in the brain, the heart, the kidneys, and most parenchymal tissues, mesenchymal cells such as fibroblasts are relatively resistant to anoxic injury. This is an extremely useful distinction because the preservation of these stromal supporting elements often allows survival of the *framework* of a tissue even though the more sensitive parenchymal elements have succumbed. As described in Chapter 4, the maintenance of the stromal supporting framework is an essential prerequisite for the reconstruction of injured tissue, by regeneration, in those tissues composed of labile or stable cell populations capable of controlled cell proliferation as a repair mechanism.

ANATOMY OF THE VASCULATURE

Most tissues of the body have one of three basic patterns of vascular supply. Many tissues and organs are limited to a blood supply that arrives through a *single vessel* that then ramifies into smaller and smaller radicles within the tissue or organ. Vessels of this type often are referred to as "functional end arteries" and are typified by the kind of vasculature that serves the spleen and the kidneys. Thrombotic or embolic occlusion of such end arteries almost invariably leads to infarction

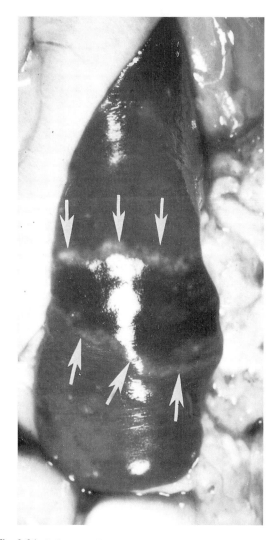

Fig. 3-34 Splenic infarct. The area of infarction, *arrows*, is well delineated from the surrounding parenchyma in this spleen from a cat with calicivirus infection. A pale border of leukocytes is present.

unless the occluded vessel is an extremely small one. To a large extent the cerebral and coronary vessels are also functional end arteries.

Some organs and tissues receive their blood supply through separate but functionally *parallel systems*, which often have substantial numbers of functional or anatomic anastomotic channels. Thrombosis rarely produces infarction of skeletal muscles for this reason. Similarly the arterial supply to the tubular viscera includes many plexiform anastomotic networks near the mesenteric border of the intestines. When such vessels are occluded by thrombi or emboli, infarction rarely results because the circulation at the level of the tissue cells may be largely unaffected. We should point out, however, that if one of the larger mesenteric vessels becomes occluded near its origin at the abdominal aorta, in-

farction certainly can occur. This forms the basis for what is known clinically as "thromboembolic colic" in horses. In this disease, verminous arteritis and thrombotic occlusion of the cranial mesenteric artery and embolism of smaller vessels occurs after vascular damage caused by larval stages of the helminth *Strongylus vulgaris* (Fig. 3-35).

Only a few tissues have a truly *dual blood supply.* The lungs are perfused by both the pulmonary arterial system and the bronchial arterial system. The liver also receives blood through two distinct circulatory systems, the portal vein and the hepatic artery. In most instances, occlusion of one of these blood supplies is usually without significant effect because tissue remains perfused through the other. Thus hepatic and pulmonary infarction is an uncommon event provided that the overall cardiovascular function of the host is normal. If, however, changes, such as chronic passive congestion from cardiac failure or severe anemia, are present, infarction can occur in the liver or lungs because the dual blood supply system is compromised. It is a useful rule of thumb for clinicians and pathologists alike that pulmonary infarction is unusual unless the lung already has chronic passive congestion. The same might be said for the liver.

OVERALL CARDIOVASCULAR FUNCTION

As we have suggested in the preceding paragraphs, the overall cardiovascular and hematological health of the individual can play a deciding role in determining the outcome of an episode of occlusive thrombosis. Anything that reduces the oxygen-carrying capacity of the blood predisposes to infarction as a sequel to thrombosis. Similarly, significant alterations in the velocity of blood flow or of blood volume actually can favor the development of ischemic infarction. Severe anemia, by virtue of the overall reduction in blood oxygenation, predisposes to thrombosis. It has been shown experimentally that even partial coronary occlusion leads to myocardial infarction in severely anemic subjects whereas control subjects with normal red blood cell counts rarely develop myocardial infarction. It is also a well-known clinical observation that aged humans with severe coronary arteriosclerosis may develop myocardial infarction after episodes of anemia or acute blood loss. It stands to reason that generalized circulatory conditions such as shock or congestive heart failure impair the circulation and hence the oxygenation of all tissues, and therefore such conditions predispose to the development of infarction should thrombosis or embolism occur.

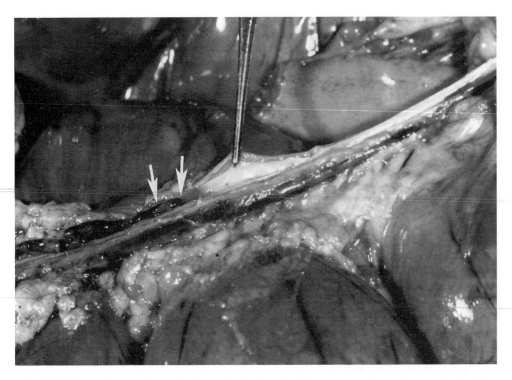

Fig. 3-35 Thromboembolic colic. The colonic artery in this horse contains a large embolus, arrows, that originated from a thrombus at the cranial mesenteric artery where verminous arteritis was present.

CLINICAL SIGNIFICANCE OF INFARCTION

As a cause of tissue destruction and acute clinical disease with considerable morbidity and mortality, infarction ranks equally with the various infectious diseases and malignancies as a major pathological process in man. It is a grim statistical prospect indeed to realize that some 20% of *all* human deaths from *all* causes in the United States are attributable to myocardial infarction. When the reaper comes, he may well arrive disguised as a thrombus designed with malice aforethought to steal in and occlude our coronary arteries (Fig. 3-36).

The situation in most other animal species is, happily, not quite so bad. Infarction of the heart or the brain or even the lungs are occasional causes of death in any species, but there is no one single syndrome in any species that assumes the magnitude of importance that myocardial infarction does in man. Often, infarcts may be associated with other underlying disease problems such as vegetative valvular endocarditis with embolism of a variety of distant sites. The clinical significance of infarction depends on *where* it occurs and upon the *size* of the infarct. In this regard it is somewhat similar to hemorrhage as a pathological event. A small cerebral infarct may have considerable clinical importance and be a much more ominous development than, for example, an infarct in the spleen that was twice as large

would be. Myocardial infarcts similarly are usually serious pathological changes. Fatality from infarction thus depends to a large extent on the site where the infarction occurred, with the brain and the heart being the least tolerant. Substantial infarcts of any tissue can be serious, and certainly pulmonary infarction can lead to fatality.

In many tissues and particularly in the case of smaller infarcts, only transient clinical signs or none at all may be apparent. The frequency with which healed infarcts are discovered as incidental findings in routine necropsy specimens bears this out. Usually such infarcts have healed by fibrosis, but the compensatory functional capacity of the affected tissues is often sufficient to circumvent lasting clinical effects. This in no way should be construed to indicate that ischemic necrosis secondary to infarction is not an important pathological process. Virtually all pathologists and clinicians have seen infarction cause death often enough to hold it in considerable respect as a significant mechanism of disease.

EDEMA

Edema is the accumulation of excessive amounts of extracellular water in the interstitial fluid space, that is, outside of the vascular fluid compartment

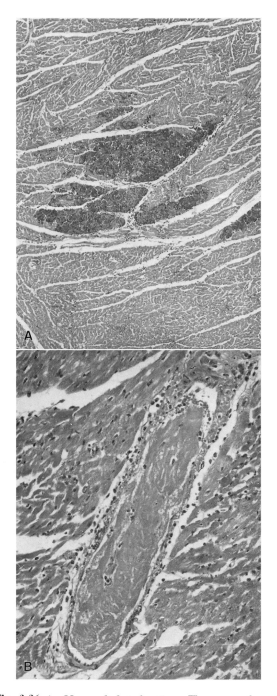

Fig. 3-36 A, Myocardial infarction. The area of acute ischemic necrosis and hemorrhage is clearly visible in this section of heart. **B, Coronary thrombosis.** This section is from an area adjacent to the infarct in A. The small coronary arteriole contains a recent thrombus.

is often a reflection of cellular injury with sufficient damage to the cell membrane and its functions that alterations in water and electrolyte fluxes across that membrane are produced. Cell swelling also can occur as a consequence of decreased osmolality of the extracellular water or increased osmolality of the intracellular water. Such changes are more properly discussed as functions of cellular injury (see Chapter 2), and we will direct our attention here to *tissue edema*, or the accumulation of excessive interstitial or extracellular fluid. To understand the pathogenesis of edema, it will be helpful if we briefly review the structure and physiology of the terminal vascular bed, the interstitial space, and the extracellular matrix.

The Interstitium and the Extracellular Matrix

What is the *interstitium?* This is a reasonable question and a good place to begin. The interstitium is the space between tissue compartments and binds most cellular and structural elements into discrete organs and tissues. At a simplistic level, it is what is left over after you remove all the blood and lymphatic vessels, nerves, and parenchymal cells from a tissue. It is the place where tissue edema fluid accumulates. The interstitium is not acellular but contains both cellular and extracellular elements. It consists mainly of various fibers and fibrils and connective tissue cells like fibroblasts, but it is the *extracellular matrix* (ECM) itself that is of particular interest (Table 3-2). Until recently, the ECM was believed to be largely a relatively inert structural scaffolding that stabilized the physical structure of tissues. It is now clear that the ECM plays a far more active and complex role in regulating the behavior of the cells that contact it, and the water-attracting property of glycosaminoglycans is particularly germane to our discussion of edema.

The ECM consists of various glycoproteins, proteoglycans, and glycosaminoglycans that are secreted by cells and assembled locally into an organized network. The metabolism of the cells embedded in the ECM, such as fibroblasts, is particularly concerned with the biosynthesis and secretion of matrix material. For convenience, the ECM may be viewed as consisting of an *insoluble* fibrous phase, containing proteins like collagen, tissue fibronectin, elastin, and other structural glycoproteins, and a *soluble* gel phase, largely protein polysaccharides (or proteoglycans), which fill the space between the insoluble fibers and fibrils. Thus the ECM consists primarily of fibrous proteins embedded in a hydrated protein polysaccharide gel. Connective tissue cells are completely surrounded by the ECM,

and outside of the cellular fluid compartment. It does not imply anything about the plasma volume or about the volume of cells themselves. Indeed, the plasma volume may or may not be increased at all, and cellular fluid volumes are usually normal. It is possible, however, to get an increase in the fluid volume of cells. This usually produces cell swelling and

TABLE 3-2 Composition of the Extracellular Matrix

COMPONENT	STRUCTURE	FEATURES
Collagens	Triple helix, fibrils, fibers	Several types, present in all tissues
Elastic fibers	Cross-linked network of elastin	Can stretch and recoil
Fibronectin	Large fiber-forming glycoprotein	Promotes cell adhesion etc.
Laminin	Large glycoprotein, two subunits	Found in all basal laminae, diverse functions
Glycosaminoglycans (GAGs)	Unbranched chains of polysaccharides	Bound to protein in ECM, attract water
Proteoglycans	Protein spine with attached GAGs	Form hydrated gels, large aggregates with link proteins

whereas other types of epithelial, endothelial, and muscle cells are separated from it by a specialized sheet of ECM known as the *basal lamina* (basement membrane) (see also Chapter 2).

The biochemical composition of the ECM varies among tissues, but the two main classes of extracellular macromolecules are the *collagens* and the polysaccharide *glycosaminoglycans* (GAGs), which are usually covalently linked to protein to form *proteoglycans*. The GAGs and proteoglycan molecules form a highly hydrated, gel-like "ground substance" in which the collagen fibers are embedded. In many areas, fibers of *elastin* are also present and contribute to the resiliency of the ECM. In addition, two high-molecular-weight glycoproteins are among the major components of the ECM: tissue *fibronectin*, which is widely distributed in connective tissues, and *laminin*, which is found largely in basement membranes.

The *collagens* are the most abundant of the ECM components and are so abundant that they constitute about 33% of the total protein mass of most animals. A central feature of all collagens is their stiff, triple-stranded helical structure. Three collagen polypeptide chains are wound around each other in a regular helix to form the ropelike collagen molecule. After being secreted into the extracellular space, the collagen molecules are assembled into ordered polymers called collagen *fibrils*, which are usually grouped together into larger bundles called collagen *fibers*, which can be seen in the light microscope. Many different types of *collagen* have been identified; they vary in the composition of the chains in the triple helix and in tissue distribution. Type I collagen, for example, is widely distributed in skin, tendon, and bone, whereas type IV collagen is the main type in basement membranes. The collagens serve a wide variety of structural and mechanical functions.

Certain tissues that require greater elasticity (skin, blood vessels, lung) have an extensive network of *elastic fibers*. The main component of elas-

tic fibers is *elastin*, a M_r 70,000 protein that is secreted into the ECM where filaments and broad sheets are formed in which the individual elastin molecules are highly cross-linked to each other to form an extensive network. These unique molecules remain unfolded such that random coils are formed. It is this cross-linked, random-coil structure of the elastic fiber network that allows it to stretch and recoil like a rubber band. Collagen fibers interwoven with the elastic fibers limit the extent of stretching and prevent tissue tearing.

The noncollagen glycoproteins of the ECM have been relatively ignored until recent years. *Fibronectin* first attracted attention when it was found to be present in greatly reduced amounts on the surface of malignant fibroblasts as compared to normal fibroblasts. Fibronectin is now known to be a member of a growing family of ECM glycoproteins with dramatic effects on cell migration, differentiation, morphology, and metabolic activities. It is probably the best characterized of the ECM *cell adhesion molecules* and has the ability to interact specifically with a large number of other biologically important molecules. Fibronectin is a large, fiber-forming glycoprotein composed of two disulfide-bonded subunits of about M_r 250,000 each and exists in the ECM as large filaments and aggregates. It functions in a wide variety of activities, many of which are associated with cell-to-substrate adhesion and migration, and has been recently implicated in embryonic differentiation. Fibronectin is perhaps best viewed as a multifunctional molecule with a series of specialized binding sites that mediate its functions. In addition to binding to the surfaces of most eukaryotic cells, fibronectin binds to collagen, fibrin and fibrinogen, heparin and heparan sulfate, actin, DNA, and the C1q component of complement. The potential range of functions mediated by this molecule is thus as long as the list of its major binding activities.

The *basal lamina* (basement membranes) are the thin sheets of specialized ECM that underly all epithelial cell sheets and tubes and surround certain individual cells such as muscle cells and Schwann cells, separating them from the underlying or surrounding connective tissue matrix. There is increasing evidence, however, that the basal laminae serve more than a simple structural and filtering role; they can induce cell differentiation, influence cell metabolism, and serve to direct specific cell migration. The basal lamina is synthesized by the cells that rest on it and hence has a somewhat different chemical composition at different sites. In addition to type IV collagen, the basal lamina contains proteoglycans, fibronectin, hyaluronic acid molecules, and the large glycoprotein *laminin*, which has been shown to be a major component of all basal laminae studied to date. Laminin consists of at least two large subunits (M_r 220,000 and 440,000) that are disulfide bonded.

It is interesting to note that recent sequencing data has shown considerable homology in the cell surface receptors for fibronectin, laminin, the platelet membrane glycoproteins GP IIb–GP IIIa, and the leukocyte adhesion complex LFA-1/Mac-1/p150,95. Many of these receptors recognize sites that include the tripeptide arg-gly-asp *(the RGD sequence)*, suggestive of a common genetic background. This family of cell surface receptors has been called the *integrins* and participates in a variety of cell-matrix and cell-cell adhesion events important to embryological development, wound healing, and immune and nonimmune host defenses as well as hemostasis and thrombosis.

Glycosaminoglycans (GAGs), formerly known as "mucopolysaccharides," are long, unbranched polysaccharide chains with repeating disaccharide units and are perhaps the most important constituents of the ECM with respect to their potential role in edema. The name "glycosaminoglycans" comes from the fact that one of the two sugar residues in the repeating disaccharide unit is always an amino sugar (either *N*-acetylglucosamine or *N*-acetylgalactosamine). Like the collagens, there are several different types of GAGs (dermatan sulfate, chondroitin sulfate, heparan sulfate, and so on) that differ chemically and in tissue location.

All the GAGs are covalently linked to a protein core to form a *proteoglycan*. Sometimes there are formed giant aggregates of proteoglycans in which many proteoglycan monomers are noncovalently bound to a central core through special *link proteins*. These large molecules are folded and refolded every few thousand nanometers so that, instead of a long linear fibril, they actually form jumbled, folded, random coils. In the interstitial space, there are truly millions of these coiled, springlike molecules. They entangle and compress each other and restrict each other's movement. They also can interact with dissolved substances in the interstitial fluid and can hold other molecules by electrostatic charges. It is this tangled mass of proteoglycans that gives the interstitium its gel-like characteristic. The GAG chains thus form extended, random-coil conformations that occupy a huge volume relative to their mass. They effectively *fill* the extracellular space even though by weight the GAGs constitute less than 10% of the contribution of the fibrous proteins like collagen and elastin. The proteoglycans attract large amounts of water and are *hydrated gels* even at low concentrations, a tendency greatly enhanced by their high density of negative charges. Their porous and hydrated organization allows them to participate in the diffusion of water and water-soluble molecules in the extracellular space and is likewise responsible for the pressure (turgor) of the ECM.

Most of the interstitial fluid is water. Since molecular coils of the proteoglycans are of appropriate molecular dimensions, they offer tremendous viscous resistance to the flow of water molecules through their substance. Water thus moves through the interstitial space largely by diffusion rather than by convectional flow. The gelled interstitial fluid exhibits the phenomenon of *thixotropy*. This means that if the interstitial fluids are somehow stirred up so that the entangled proteoglycan coils become separated, the interstitium takes on more fluid characteristics. An additional example of this phenomenon comes from the fluids of the synovial, pleural, pericardial, and peritoneal cavities, all of which contain molecules similar to the interstitial fluid. However, these fluids are constantly "stirred up" by the motions of the tissues they bathe and hence have a much more fluid state than normal interstitial fluid does. Even so, such fluids are highly viscous, almost like an oil in the case of synovial fluid, and perform an important lubricating function in their respective cavities.

The proteoglycans and GAGs in the interstitium behave as giant polyelectrolytes in that they can undergo sensitive changes in conformation with changes in the local environment; when the ionic strength is lowered, as might be expected with the addition of low protein-content edema fluid, the polysaccharide backbone structures have a greater tendency to repel one another, and the molecules take on an extended conformation. There is also evidence that the polymer chain formations are affected in concentrated solutions; when the concentration increases, as might be expected with the addition of protein-rich edema fluid, the molecules collapse into more compact coils.

It is currently envisioned that this molecular compression is an osmotic effect of competition between neighboring molecules for water with the result that water is withdrawn from the hydrated domain of the molecules. Thus the old explanation that "connective tissue substances bind edema fluid" has been given a potentially useful molecular definition. It has been theorized that there is a two-phase system consisting of a gel-like phase composed of proteoglycans associated with a fluid volume from which the protein content of the fluid is excluded and, between the proteoglycans, a free-fluid phase containing the plasma proteins. Fluxes of fluid between these two phases would depend on the relative concentrations of protein and polysaccharide in the various compartments. With increased molecular definition of the composition and function of the ECM, particularly the proteoglycans and GAGs, a better understanding of edematous states can be envisioned for the future.

Our consideration of the interstitial space where edema fluid accumulates would not be complete without a consideration of *interstitial fluid pressure.* Interstitial pressure is important in the determination of edema in that it can determine in part where and to what extent fluid can move. It is made up of several components including interstitial osmotic pressure, interstitial hydrostatic pressure, and pressure exerted by the elasticity of the gel matrix itself. Interstitial pressure helps to determine whether fluids can leak from the vascular to the interstitial compartment and helps the movement of fluid from the interstitial compartment into lymphatics. It will play an important role in our discussion of the physiology of fluid movements at the terminal vascular bed and their functions in the pathogenesis of edema.

Microvascular Physiology

The details of capillary exchange and tissue fluid convection are fascinating subjects in their own right and have attracted and stimulated a large number of physiologists. Our interest is more directed, and we are concerned here only with those features of the structure and function of the terminal vascular bed that relate to body fluid homeostasis and its alteration in the edematous state. In short, we will deal only with those factors (forces) that function to control the net balance between the outward and inward movement of fluid at the capillary membrane.

In a typical capillary bed, an arteriole gives rise to numerous capillaries, which then coalesce to form venules. True capillaries arise from either a *terminal arteriole* or a *meta-arteriole,* which is a sort of structural intermediary between arterioles and capillaries. At the point where the capillaries emerge, there is usually a smooth muscle fiber wrapped around the mouth of the capillary and called the *precapillary sphincter.* This structure functions to help control flow conditions within the capillary network. The structure of a typical terminal vascular bed is shown in Fig. 3-37.

It is across the capillary wall itself that filtration actually takes place. If we examined a typical capillary, we would find an endothelial lining resting on a thin basement membrane and little else (see Fig. 4-12). The interendothelial junctions are not true tight junctions, and they can open to allow communication between the intravascular and extravascular fluid compartments.

There are basically three major physical factors that normally are operative in regulating the exchange of water and electrolytes between the vascular compartment and the interstitial compartment. These are (1) an intact, functioning circulatory system, (2) a normal, functioning lymphatic system, and (3) the concentration of albumin in the serum. If one or more of these factors is significantly altered, water and electrolytes may escape from the circulation faster than they return, and edema results.

To understand edema it is necessary to review the concept of *Starling equilibrium,* which describes the relationships between the various forces at work at the level of the microcirculatory bed (Fig. 3-38). Starling equilibrium is achieved by the balance of filtration pressures and absorption pressures exerted across the filtering membranes of the terminal vascular bed. The *net filtration pressure* is represented by the differences in hydrostatic and colloidal osmotic pressures between the plasma and tissue interstitial compartment at the arterial end of the capillary vascular bed, and the *net absorption pressure* is determined by differences in hydrostatic and colloidal osmotic pressures between the plasma and tissue interstitial compartment at the venous end of the capillary vascular bed. Basically, at the *arteriolar end* of the microvascular bed, we have a plasma hydrostatic pressure of about 30 mm Hg that is offset by a tissue hydrostatic pressure of about 8 mm Hg, leaving a balance of a 22 mm Hg pressure (30 minus 8), which favors filtration. Operating against the hydrostatic pressure favoring filtration at the arterial end of the bed is the colloidal osmotic pressure of plasma, which acts as a force to keep fluid within the vascular lumen. This colloidal osmotic pressure of plasma (about 25 mm Hg) must work against a tissue colloidal osmotic pressure of about 10 mm Hg, which tends to "pull" fluid towards the interstitium. Hence there results an os-

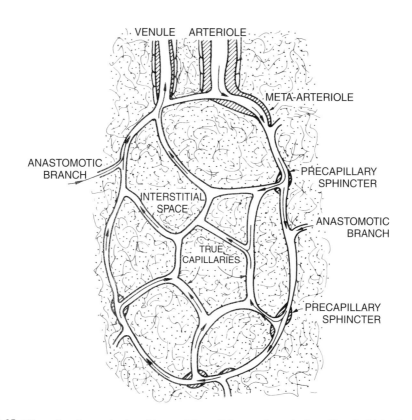

Fig. 3-37 Microcirculatory bed and interstitium. Schema of a typical capillary bed lying between the terminal arteriole and the collecting venule. The interstice lies between the anastomotic branches of the capillary bed.

motic pressure differential of 15 mm Hg (25 minus 10), which basically is the difference between the osmotic pressure of plasma and that of tissue and acts to keep fluid in the cardiovascular compartment. The net filtration pressure at the arteriolar end of the microvascular bed then is about 7 mm Hg and represents the difference between the hydrostatic pressure difference (22 mm Hg) favoring filtration and the osmotic pressure difference (15 mm Hg) working to keep fluid in the vascular compartment.

At the *venular end* of the system, the plasma hydrostatic pressure is lower (about 17 mm Hg), but the other pressure relationships remain similar to that encountered at the arteriolar end. Hence, a plasma-tissue hydrostatic pressure difference of 9 mm Hg (17 minus 8) favoring filtration is offset by a plasma-tissue colloidal osmotic pressure difference of 15 mm Hg (25 minus 10), which leaves a net absorption pressure at the venular end of about 6 mm Hg. As you will recall, the net filtration pressure at the arteriolar end was about 7 mm Hg. With an arteriolar input to the interstitial space of 7 mm Hg and a net absorption pressure of only 6 mm Hg, edema would gradually develop. What happens to the extra 1 mm of pressure? This is where the lymphatics enter

the picture. The lymphatics are basically a very low pressure system that can operate to maintain fluid homeostasis at the level of the microvascular bed by taking care of this 1 mm of pressure by absorption. With the lymphatic system functioning normally, the system is then in equilibrium.

It is likely that the Starling equilibrium hypothesis is a gross oversimplification even though it is widely accepted as the explanation for water and small-molecule transfer in the terminal vascular bed. Certainly it is reasonable not to attach too much specific significance to the actual numbers associated with the various forces at work (see Fig. 3-38). These undoubtedly vary from species to species and from region to region within the body. For our purposes, however, Starling equilibrium provides an extremely useful way to look at the pathogenesis of edema. Indeed, *virtually all clinical forms of edema can be traced to some alteration in Starling equilibrium or to increased vascular permeability, which disturbs Starling equilibrium.*

Pathophysiology of Edema

Most animals are about 60% water by mass, divided into intracellular and extracellular compart-

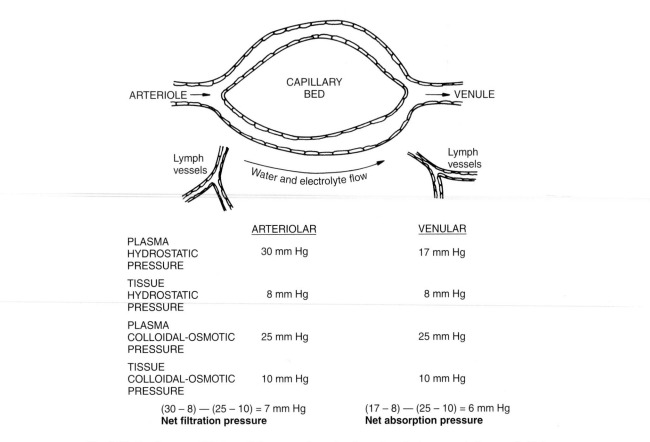

	ARTERIOLAR	VENULAR
PLASMA HYDROSTATIC PRESSURE	30 mm Hg	17 mm Hg
TISSUE HYDROSTATIC PRESSURE	8 mm Hg	8 mm Hg
PLASMA COLLOIDAL-OSMOTIC PRESSURE	25 mm Hg	25 mm Hg
TISSUE COLLOIDAL-OSMOTIC PRESSURE	10 mm Hg	10 mm Hg
	(30 − 8) — (25 − 10) = 7 mm Hg **Net filtration pressure**	(17 − 8) — (25 − 10) = 6 mm Hg **Net absorption pressure**

Fig. 3-38 Starling equilibrium. Schema to show the interplay of plasma and tissue colloidal-osmotic and hydrostatic forces that determine filtration and absorption across the microvascular bed.

ments, the latter consisting of plasma water and interstitial water. In the final analysis, edema basically is nothing more than an expansion of the interstitial fluid compartment. As we have discussed above, the interchange of water between the vascular and interstitial compartments is governed by the forces responsible for Starling equilibrium, the plasma and tissue hydrostatic and osmotic pressures, and the contribution of interstitial lymphatics. Although they are not actively a part of the forces at play in Starling equilibrium, it should be obvious that the entire system is ultimately dependent on the normal integrity of the endothelial barrier lining the vascular bed in which the fluid exchange takes place. In the normal animal, there is almost certainly a continual balancing of these various factors to maintain fluid homeostasis. Edema results only when the balancing ability of the various forces at play is disturbed to the point where equilibrium is lost in favor of accumulation of fluid in the interstitial compartment.

Theoretically any disturbance of Starling equilibrium could lead to edema, but from a practical standpoint, there are basically only four dynamic mechanisms that can underlie the development of

edema: (1) decreased plasma colloidal-osmotic pressure, (2) increased blood hydrostatic pressure, (3) lymphatic obstruction, and (4) increased vascular permeability. The location and extent of edema formation depends in part on which of these mechanisms is operative. For example, a decrease in plasma colloidal-osmotic pressure would tend to produce a generalized effect; increased plasma hydrostatic pressure might induce either local or systemic effects depending on the pathogenesis of the increase, whereas lymphatic obstruction and vascular permeability increases are almost always localized effects producing localized edema. Let us examine these four major mechanisms of edema in somewhat more detail.

DECREASED PLASMA COLLOIDAL-OSMOTIC PRESSURE

Colloid osmotic pressure refers to the effect of colloidal solutes on the chemical potential of water molecules. The largest and most important group of colloids in body fluids such as plasma are the proteins. In plasma, proteins function as a sort of giant "polyelectrolytes" by virtue of the fact they

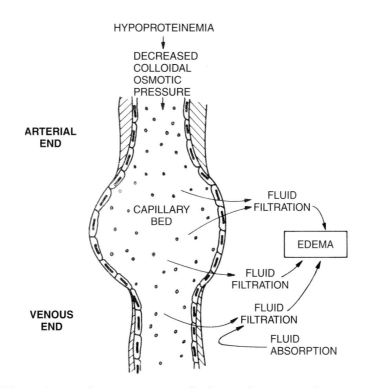

Fig. 3-39 Edema–decreased osmotic pressure. Decline in plasma protein levels, *small open circles*, decreases the colloidal-osmotic pressure of plasma and upsets Starling equilibrium to result in edema.

are generally negatively charged, and the pH of most body fluids is well off the isoelectric point of the proteins. Proteins normally are present in plasma in concentrations of 60 to 70 g/liter and exert their full effective osmotic pressure across the capillary membrane to oppose the flow of liquid to the interstitial compartment under the force of hydrostatic pressure in the capillary bed. As the most abundant of the plasma proteins and having a relatively low M_r (68,000), albumin is the most important of the plasma proteins with respect to edema formation because it exerts the major portion of the plasma colloid osmotic effect. Hence, decreases in plasma colloid osmotic pressure reflect a decrease in total plasma proteins, but this is largely attributable to decreases in albumin concentration because globulins are only about 25% as effective in maintaining colloid osmotic pressure as albumin is. Therefore edema as the result of a decrease in plasma colloid osmotic pressure usually has its basis in hypoalbuminemia.

Returning to the concept of Starling equilibrium (see Fig. 3-38), a 50% drop in the albumin concentration in plasma would produce a corresponding decline in the plasma colloid osmotic pressure to a value, to use our previous numbers, of about 12.5 mm Hg. This would so disturb the system that the

net filtration pressure on the arteriolar side would be about 19.5 mm Hg. Although the decline in plasma colloid osmotic pressure also would affect the venular side of the equation, the change would be less dramatic because of the lower plasma hydrostatic pressure on the venous side. Nonetheless, if you work through the numbers, you will find that rather than having a net absorption pressure on the venous side, a decline in albumin levels of this magnitude would in fact produce a net positive filtration pressure of about 6.5 mm Hg, even on the absorptive end of the capillary bed. In such a situation, lymphatic flow would no doubt be increased, but the net result would be the accumulation of fluid in the interstitial space because the lymphatics could not effectively deal with a total net filtration pressure across the vascular bed of some 26 mm Hg. Edema would result (Fig. 3-39).

Decreases in the albumin concentration can, at a simplistic level, result from basically only two mechanisms: either not enough albumin is being synthesized to keep up with its normal rate of catabolism, or albumin is being normally synthesized and delivered to the plasma but is being lost at a rate greatly exceeding normal. Decreases in albumin synthesis can occur in starvation syndromes where a protein-deficient diet fails to provide sufficient material for albumin synthesis. As albumin is synthesized in the liver, some forms of liver disease also are accompanied by hypoalbuminemia as a result of a decrease in hepatic albumin synthesis. Albumin can be lost from the body largely by two routes: renal and gastrointestinal. The dog described in the case study in Chapter 5 was losing protein through damage to the glomerular ultrafiltration system because of diffuse glomerulonephritis. This is one form of protein-losing renal disease, and edema is often a part of the clinical picture. Gastrointestinal loss can occur in various infectious enteric diseases, in the various protein-losing enteropathy syndromes, and when whole blood is lost by the gastrointestinal tract in some kinds of parasitism such as haemonchosis (from *Haemonchus* nematodes). Regardless of the specific etiological background, all these forms of clinical edema have their basis in decreased plasma colloid osmotic pressure caused by hypoalbuminemia.

INCREASED BLOOD HYDROSTATIC PRESSURE

The hydrostatic pressure of the blood is the force that acts to overcome the colloid osmotic pressure of the plasma and acts normally to allow the passage of nutritive fluids into the tissues. If it is in-

creased, edema can result. We must recall that the pressure at the level of the capillary bed is influenced mostly by the venous pressure and not the arterial pressure. Thus, although arterial hypertension might seem to be a likely background for the development of edema, this is in fact a rather unusual occurrence. A far more important group of causes are things that increase capillary pressure by raising the venous pressure. To return to our model of Starling equilibrium, envision what might occur if the blood hydrostatic pressure were raised to about 30 mm Hg, or the same as it is at the arterial end of the microvascular bed. This would be an approximate doubling of the hydrostatic pressure at the venous end of the capillary bed. Now, if you do the arithmetic, you will discover that rather than having a net absorption pressure of 6 mm Hg at the venous end of the capillary bed, you have a net filtration pressure of some 7 mm Hg. Thus the increase in venous back pressure negates the absorptive function of the venous bed and, in fact, fluid filtered at the arterial end fails to return to the circulation. The result is edema (Fig. 3-40).

This process can occur at both the localized and the generalized levels. At a local level, the most common background to increased hydrostatic pressure involves *local obstructions* to venous flow,

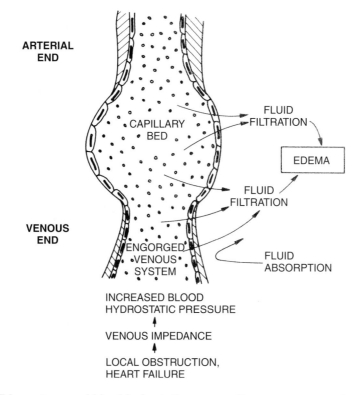

Fig. 3-40 Edema—increased blood hydrostatic pressure. Venous engorgement from raised hydrostatic pressure dilates the venules (passive hyperemia) and disturbs Starling equilibrium to result in edema. *Small open circles,* Protein.

which, naturally enough, raise pressure behind the obstruction. This can be related to occlusion of a vein by an intravascular thrombus or a tumor or can occur if the vessel becomes obstructed from without as might occur with pressure on a vessel by a tumor or an abscess. The gravid uterus sometimes can exert enough pressure on iliac veins to cause increased venous pressure and edema in the posterior limbs. An additional example of this phenomenon can be drawn from equine medicine and surgery where a 180-degree or 360-degree rotational torsion of the abdominal viscera sometimes occurs around the root of the mesenteric vasculature. In this situation, the more easily collapsed veins become totally obstructed, whereas the thicker-walled arteries remain at least partially operative. The result is an extremely edematous and congested intestine, one that often produces severe colic and death.

Cardiac failure is the most important cause of a generalized increase in venous pressure. Because the anatomic cause of the problem here is such that a generalized elevation in blood pressure occurs at the venous end of the capillary bed, the edema also tends to be more generalized than would result from a locally obstructive lesion. In cardiac failure, the venous pressure rises considerably, and the stretching and dilatation of the venules and capillaries may render them more permeable as well. This excessive venous pressure that occurs in cardiac failure is by no means the only mechanism by which heart failure causes edema. An increase in aldosterone production leading to increased sodium retention also contributes to the process.

Lymphatic Obstruction

If we return to our model of Starling equilibrium once again, the effects of a functional removal of lymphatic drainage should be clear. Recall that in the normal state, the difference between the 7 mm Hg net filtration pressure and the 6 mm Hg net absorption pressure is made up by lymphatic absorption. When the lymphatics are obstructed by any lesion that impedes normal lymph flow or absorption, excess tissue fluid accumulates in the interstitial space, and edema results (Fig. 3-41). The lesion need not be within the lymphatic channels themselves because lesions at the level of the lymph nodes that impede lymphatic flow also may cause edema. Thus damage to or obstruction of the lymphatics by trauma, surgical intervention, or inflammatory or neoplastic disease can result in edema. This form of edema is particularly common in association with certain kinds of malignant tumors that grow into and obstruct lymphatic drainage. A striking cause of this form of edema is the inflammatory obstruction of lymphatics that occurs in certain filarial infections of man such as that caused by *Wuchereria bancrofti* (elephantiasis). Here, massive lymphatic obstruction and striking local edema are clinical highlights.

In lymphatic obstruction, the edema that results almost always is localized because the lesion almost always is localized. There are virtually no acquired forms of generalized lymphatic edema, and even in elephantiasis the edema is usually localized.

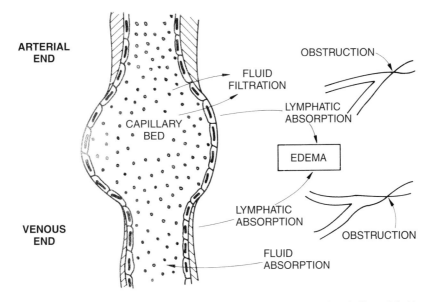

Fig. 3-41 Edema—lymphatic blockade. Failure of lymphatic vessels to absorb filtered fluid causes accumulation of that fluid in the interstices and edema results. *Small open circles,* Protein.

INCREASED VASCULAR PERMEABILITY

As mentioned previously, the success of Starling equilibrium is dependent on the structural integrity of the microvascular bed. When endothelial integrity is compromised, edema results. This can occur in a generalized way with certain potent toxins or chemicals, but for the most part, the edema resulting from increased capillary permeability is a localized phenomenon. This, in fact, is the *edema of inflammation*. A critical feature of the evolving inflammatory reaction is the opening of interendothelial gaps to permit plasma proteins and circulating leukocytes to enter the tissue to perform their critical defensive functions (see Chapter 4). Anyone who has experienced a bee sting has experienced this form of edema. In this example, part of the edema is probably a direct result of damage to the endothelium from toxins in the bee venom, and part of the edema is a result of chemically mediated increases in local vascular permeability caused by local histamine release from tissue mast cells. We explore this phenomenon in greater detail in the next chapter.

An additional feature of inflammatory edema that sets it apart from most other forms of edema is the *high protein content* of the fluid leaving the vasculature and entering the tissues. In most forms of edema, the fluid itself remains an ultrafiltrate of plasma consisting largely of water and dissolved electrolytes. In inflammatory edema, however, the integrity of the microfilter is lost because of endothelial damage and chemically mediated permeability alterations, and so, in addition to water

and dissolved electrolytes, significant amounts of protein are found in the fluid (Fig. 3-42).

Appearance of Edema

It should be obvious that the changes produced by edema in the tissues will reflect the severity, rapidity of onset, extent, anatomic location of the edema, and the underlying cause. In generalized edema, fluid tends to collect in the lowermost portions of the body such as the ventral abdomen and the limbs, a pattern referred to as *dependent edema*. When such edema is severe and generalized, it produces a diffuse noticeable swelling of the subcutaneous tissues. Because the swelling represents an expansion of the interstitial fluid space, it often is possible to push a finger against such edematous tissues and actually produce a dent in the tissue. Such edematous changes are known as *pitting edema*. When edema is severe and generalized and causes diffuse swelling of all tissues and organs in the body, particularly noticeable in the subcutaneous tissues, it is called *anasarca*.

Although edema fluid often accumulates in tissue interstitial compartments, it may be prominent in body cavities as well. The collection of edema fluid in the peritoneal cavity is known as *ascites*, in the pleural cavity as *hydrothorax*, and in the pericardial sac as *hydropericardium*, or *pericardial effusion*.

Edema is often easier to detect grossly than microscopically. At the gross level, the accumulation of edema fluid can be recognized by the excess clear fluid within a body cavity or a tissue. This is most

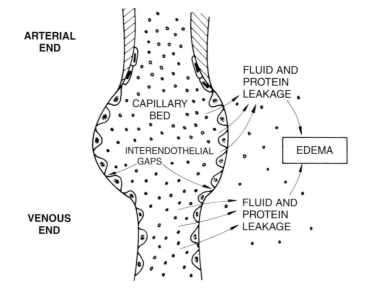

Fig. 3-42 Edema—increased vascular permeability. The edema of inflammation involves changes in endothelial cells that permit not only water and electrolytes but also protein, *small open circles*, to accumulate as edema fluid.

easily visualized in a loosely organized tissue with much interstitium where the edema fluid physically pushes apart the normal tissue structures (Fig. 3-43). The tissues are wet, shiny or glistening, and heavy because of the added component of water. It is sometimes more difficult to detect edema in a solid parenchymatous organ such as the liver or kidney where the only visible manifestation may be an overall increase in size and weight.

Edema fluid varies in its microscopic appearance. If the fluid is largely composed of water and electrolytes (a transudate), there is nothing to take up a stain, and the presence of edema may be detected only by its *dilutional effect* on normal tissue components. Water as a substance is invisible microscopically; hence its presence must be assumed by the spreading apart of normal tissue components and the *dilatation of lymphatics* in the tissue. If inflammatory edema is present, the protein content of the fluid will allow easier visualization of the lesion because the protein will be stained *pink* in hematoxylin and eosin preparations making it easily visible (Fig. 3-44).

Clinical Significance of Edema

The significance to clinical medicine of edema depends largely on its extent, its location, and its du-
ration. In the brain and lungs, for example, edema may have serious or fatal consequences, whereas edema of the subcutis may have little functional significance. Cerebral edema is a justifiably feared consequence of various forms of brain injury and can have a fatal outcome. In addition to the violent headaches, projectile vomiting, and convulsive seizures that may accompany cerebral edema, herniation of the brainstem or cerebellar tonsils into the foramen magnum can occur as a result of the greatly raised intracranial pressure. In pulmonary edema, we are presented with the unique situation of "drowning from within." As fluid fills the alveoli and terminal bronchioles, the gas-exchange function of the lungs can become so compromised that it produces sufficient hypoxia to be fatal. In addition, the accumulation of fluid in the lungs is accompanied by an increased opportunity for secondary infections to become established. With the possible exceptions of cerebral and pulmonary edema, where direct intervention may be needed to prevent a fatality, one usually approaches edema by attempting to sort out the ultimate cause and pathogenesis and then to treat it accordingly. This is as it should be, and an understanding of the basic mechanisms underlying the development of edema make the process of therapy a good deal easier.

From a clinical standpoint, edema often is classi-

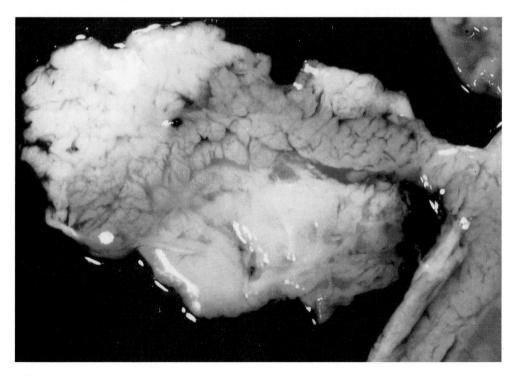

Fig. 3-43 Edema. The wet, glassy appearance of this edematous dog pancreas is caused by edema fluid. Notice that the fluid has dissected the pancreas into visible lobulations and arborizations not normally seen.

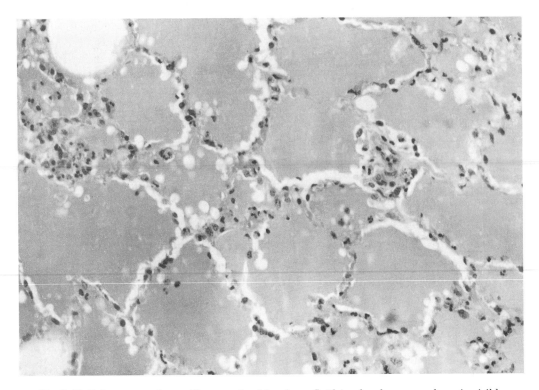

Fig. 3-44 Pulmonary edema. The protein-rich edema fluid in alveolar spaces here is visible because of the staining properties of the protein present in the fluid.

TABLE 3-3 Mechanistic View of Seven Clinical Forms of Edema

NAME	CLINICAL FEATURE	BASIC PROBLEM	DISTURBANCE OF STARLING EQUILIBRIUM
Renal edema	Proteinuria	Hypoproteinemia	Decreased plasma colloidal osmotic pressure
Cardiac edema	Generalized edema	Venous impedance	Increased blood hydrostatic pressure
Nutritional edema	Decreased protein intake	Hypoproteinemia	Decreased plasma colloidal osmotic pressure
Parasitic edema	Loss of whole blood in gastrointestinal tract	Hypoproteinemia	Decreased plasma colloidal osmotic pressure
Hepatic edema	Loss of hepatic albumin synthesis	Hypoproteinemia	Decreased plasma colloidal osmotic pressure
Inflammatory edema	Direct or indirect microvascular injury	Leaky vessels	Increased vascular permeability
Lymphatic edema	Lymphatic obstruction	Raised lymphatic pressure	Increased tissue hydrostatic pressure

fied according to the nature of the disease that produced the edema. Hence you will read about "renal edema," "cardiac edema," "nutritional edema," "parasitic edema," and so on. Implicit in such terms is an understanding of the basic mechanisms that underlie the development of edema in these various disease states. It is beyond our scope to enter into a detailed discussion of clinical edema, but Table 3-3 should help in documenting that most common clinical forms of edema obey the rules we have set out here. They all involve a disturbance of one or more of the critical variables responsible for maintaining homeostasis by Starling equilibrium at the level of the microcirculation.

RECOMMENDED READING

Albelda SM, Karnovsky MJ, Fishman AP: Perspectives in endothelial cell biology, *J Appl Physiol* 62:1345-1348, 1987.

Alving BM: The hypercoagulable states, *Hosp Pract* 28:109-121, 1993.

Andersson B: Regulation of body fluids, *Annu Rev Physiol* 39:185-200, 1977.

Asch AS, Nachman RL: Thrombospondin: phenomenology to function, *Prog Hemost Thromb* 9:157-176, 1989.

Badylak SF: Coagulation disorders and liver disease, *Vet Clin North Am Small Anim Pract* 18:87-93, 1988.

Bell WR: The pathophysiology of disseminated intravascular coagulation, *Semin Hematol* 31(suppl 1):19-24, 1994.

Beutler E, Lichtman MA, Coller BS, Kipps TJ: *Williams' hematology*, ed 5, New York, 1995, McGraw-Hill.

Bick RL: Hypercoagulability and thrombosis, *Med Clin North Am* 78:635-665, 1994.

Bick RL, Murano G: Physiology of hemostasis, *Clin Lab Med* 14:677-707, 1994.

Blasi F, Vassalli J-D, Dano K: Urokinase-type plasminogen activator: proenzyme, receptor, and inhibitors, *J Cell Biol* 104:801-804, 1987.

Boudreaux MK: Platelets and coagulation: an update, *Vet Clin North Am Small Anim Pract* 26:1065-1088, 1996.

Brandt JT: Current concepts of coagulation, *Clin Obstet Gynecol* 28:3-14, 1985.

Brigham KL, Staub NC: Pulmonary edema and acute lung injury research, *Am J Respir Crit Care Med* 147(4 pt 2):S109-S113, 1998.

Broze JB Jr.: Tissue factor pathway inhibitor and the revised theory of coagulation, *Annu Rev Med* 46:103-112, 1995.

Bruijn JA, Hogendoorn PCW, Hoedemaeker PJ, Fleuren GJ: The extracellular matrix in pathology, *J Lab Clin Med* 111:140-149, 1988.

Car BD, Slauson DO, Suyemoto MM, Doré M, Neilsen NR: The expression and kinetics of induced procoagulant activity in bovine pulmonary alveolar macrophages, *Exp Lung Res* 17:939-957, 1991.

Car BD, Suyemoto MM, Neilsen NR, Slauson DO: The role of leukocytes in the pathogenesis of fibrin deposition in bovine acute lung injury, *Am J Pathol* 138:1191-1198, 1991.

Carmeliet P: Mechanisms of angiogenesis and arteriogenesis, *Nat Med* 6(4):389-396, 2000.

Carson SD: Tissue factor-initiated blood coagulation, *Prog Clin Pathol* 9:1-14, 1984.

Carson SD, Brozna JP: The role of tissue factor in the production of thrombin, *Blood Coagul Fibrinolysis* 4:281-292, 1993.

Carson SD, Johnson SR, Tracy SM: Tissue factor and the extrinsic pathway of coagulation during infection and vascular inflammation, *Eur Heart J* (suppl K):98-104, 1993.

Clouse LH, Comp PC: The regulation of hemostasis: the protein C system, *N Engl J Med* 314:1298-1304, 1986.

Cokelet GR: Rheology and hemodynamics, *Annu Rev Physiol* 42:311-324, 1980.

Collen D, Stump DC, Gold HK: Thrombolytic therapy, *Annu Rev Med* 39:405-424, 1988.

Colman RW: Surface-mediated defense reactions: the plasma contact activation system, *J Clin Invest* 73:1249-1253, 1984.

Colman RW: Disseminated intravascular coagulation due to sepsis, *Semin Hematol* 31(suppl 1):10-17, 1994.

Colman RW: Biological activities of the contact factors in vivo: potentiation of hypotension, inflammation, and fibrinolysis, and inhibition of cell adhesion, angiogenesis, and thrombosis, *Thromb Haemost* 82:1568-1577, 1999.

Colman RW, Schmaier AH: Contact system: a vascular biology modulator with anticoagulant, profibrinolytic, antiadhesive, and proinflammatory attributes, *Blood* 90:3819-3843, 1997.

Comp PC: Hereditary disorders predisposing to thrombosis, *Prog Hemost Thromb* 8:71-102, 1986.

Coughlin SR: Molecular mechanisms of thrombin signalling, *Semin Hematol* 31:270-277, 1994.

Coutre S, Leung L: Novel antithrombotic therapeutics targeted against platelet glycoprotein IIb/IIIa, *Annu Rev Med* 46:68-75, 1995.

Dahlback B: Blood coagulation, *Lancet* 355:1627-1632, 2000.

Doolittle RF: Fibrinogen and fibrin, *Annu Rev Biochem* 53:195-229, 1984.

Ebert BL, Bunn HF: Regulation of the erythropoietin gene, *Blood* 94:1864-1877, 1999.

Erickson LA, Schleef RR, Ny T, Loskutoff DJ: The fibrinolytic system of the vascular wall, *Clin Hematol* 14:513-530, 1985.

Esmon CT: Cell-mediated events that control blood coagulation and vascular injury, *Annu Rev Cell Biol* 9:1-26, 1993.

Esmon CT: The regulation of natural anticoagulant pathways, *Science* 235:1348-1352, 1987.

Francis CW, Marder VJ: Concepts of clot lysis, *Annu Rev Med* 37:187-204, 1986.

Francis CW, Marder VJ: Physiologic regulation and pathologic disorders of fibrinolysis, *Hum Pathol* 18:263-274, 1987.

Furie B, Furie BC: The molecular basis of blood coagulation, *Cell* 53:505-518, 1988.

Furie B, Furie BC: Molecular and cellular biology of blood coagulation, *N Engl J Med* 326:800-806, 1992.

Fuster V, Griggs TR: Porcine von Willebrand disease: implications for the pathophysiology of atherosclerosis and thrombosis, *Prog Thromb Hemost* 8:159-184, 1986.

Gallo R, Badimon JJ, Fuster V: Pathobiology of coronary ischemic events: clinical implications, *Adv Intern Med* 43:203-232, 1998.

Gillis S, Furie BC, Furie B: Interactions of neutrophils and coagulation proteins, *Semin Hematol* 34:336-342, 1997.

Goldhaber SZ: Thrombolytic therapy, *Adv Intern Med* 44:311-325, 1999.

Green RA: Clinical implications of antithrombin III deficiency in animal diseases, *Compend Cont Ed* 6:537-545, 1984.

Green RA: Pathophysiology of antithrombin III deficiency, *Vet Clin North Am Small Anim Pract* 18:95-104, 1988.

Haines ST, Bussey HI: Thrombosis and the pharmacology of antithrombotic agents, *Ann Pharmacother* 29:892-905, 1995.

Hajjar KA: Changing concepts in fibrinolysis, *Curr Opin Hematol* 2:345-350, 1995.

Hajjar KA, Nachman RL: The role of lipoprotein A in atherogenesis and thrombosis, *Annu Rev Med* 47:121-131, 1996.

Hawiger J: Formation and regulation of platelet and fibrin hemostatic plug, *Hum Pathol* 18:111-122, 1987.

Hawiger J: Mechanisms involved in platelet vessel wall interaction, *Thromb Haemost* 74:369-372, 1995.

Hibbetts K, Hines B, Williams D: An overview of proteinase inhibitors, *J Vet Intern Med* 13:302-308, 1999.

Hoffbrand AV, Lewis SM, Tuddenham EGD: *Postgraduate haematology,* ed 4, Oxford, 1999, Butterworth-Heinemann.

Hooper WC, Evatt BL: The role of activated protein C resistance in the pathogenesis of venous thrombosis, *Am J Med Sci* 31:120-128, 1998.

Hormia M, Virtanen I: Endothelium: an organized monolayer of highly specialized cells, *Med Biol* 64:247-266, 1986.

Jaffe EA: Cell biology of endothelial cells, *Hum Pathol* 18:234-239, 1987.

Johnson LR, Lappin MR, Baker DC: Pulmonary thromboembolism in 29 dogs, *J Vet Intern Med* 13:338-345, 1998.

Kane KK: Fibrinolysis—a review, *Ann Clin Lab Sci* 14:443-449, 1984.

Kaplan AP, Silverberg M: The coagulation-kinin pathway of human plasma, *Blood* 70:1-15, 1987.

Kaushansky K: Thrombopoietin: understanding and manipulating platelet production, *Annu Rev Med* 48:1-12, 1997.

Kluft C, Dooijewaard G, Emeis J: Role of the contact system in fibrinolysis, *Semin Thromb Hemost* 13:50-68, 1987.

Ku DN: Blood flow in arteries, *Annu Rev Fluid Mechanics* 29:112-121, 1997.

Lämme B, Griffin JH: Formation of the fibrin clot: the balance of procoagulant and inhibitory factors, *Clin Haematol* 14:281-341, 1985.

Lane DA, Grant PJ: Role of hemostatic gene polymorphisms in venous and arterial thrombotic disease, *Blood* 95(5):1517-1537, 2000.

Lee GR, Foerster J, Lukens J, Paraskevas F, Greer J, Rodgers GM: *Wintrobe's clinical hematology,* ed 10, Baltimore, 1999, Williams & Wilkins.

Leung L, Nachman RN: Molecular mechanisms of platelet aggregation, *Annu Rev Med* 37:179-186, 1986.

Levi M, ten Cate H: Disseminated intravascular coagulation, *N Engl J Med* 341:586-592, 1999.

Lijnen HR, Collen D: Mechanisms of plasminogen activation by mammalian plasminogen activators, *Enzyme* 40:90-96, 1988.

Longenecker GL: *The platelets: physiology and pharmacology,* New York, 1985, Academic Press.

Lorenzet R, Napoleone E, Celi A, Pelegrini G, Di Santo A: Cell-cell interaction and tissue factor expression, *Blood Coagul Fibrinolysis* 9(suppl 1):S49-S59, 1998.

Luscher TF, Barton M: Biology of the endothelium, *Clin Cardiol* 20(suppl 2):II-3-10, 1997.

Mann KG: Membrane-bound enzyme complexes in blood coagulation, *Prog Hemost Thromb* 7:1-24, 1984.

Mannucci PM: Drug therapy: hemostatic drugs, *N Engl J Med* 339:121-134, 1998.

Marcus AJ: Thrombosis and inflammation as multicellular processes: significance of cell-cell interactions, *Semin Hematol* 31:261-269, 1994.

Mayne R: Collagenous proteins of blood vessels, *Arteriosclerosis* 6:585-593, 1986.

Meyer D, Baumgartner HR: Interactions of platelets with the vessel wall, *Adv Inflamm Res* 10:85-98, 1986.

Meyers KM: Pathobiology of animal platelets, *Adv Vet Sci Comp Med* 30:131-166, 1985.

Moroose R, Hoyer LW: Von Willebrand factor and platelet function, *Annu Rev Med* 37:157-164, 1986.

Mosler DF: Physiology of fibronectin, *Annu Rev Med* 35:561-576, 1984.

Narayanan S, Hamasaki N: Current concepts of coagulation and fibrinolysis, *Adv Clin Chem* 33:133-168, 1999.

Nawroth PP, Stern DM: Endothelial cell procoagulant properties and the host response, *Semin Thromb Hemost* 13:391-397, 1987.

Noris M, Remuzzi G: Uremic bleeding: closing the circle after 30 years of controversies, *Blood* 94:2569-2574, 1999.

Oates JA, Hawiger J, Ross R: *Interaction of platelets with the vessel wall,* Bethesda, Md., 1985, American Physiological Society.

Ogletree ML: Overview of physiological and pathophysiological effects of thromboxane A_2, *Fed Proc* 46:133-138, 1987.

Osterud B: Tissue factor expression by monocytes: regulation and pathophysiological roles, *Blood Coagul Fibrinolysis* 9(suppl 1):S9-S14, 1998.

Packard MA, Mustard JF: Platelet adhesion, *Prog Hemost Thromb* 7:211-288, 1984.

Packham MA: Role of platelets in thrombosis and hemostasis, *Can J Physiol Pharmacol* 72:278-284, 1994.

Page CP: The involvement of platelets in nonthrombotic processes, *Trends Pharmacol Sci* 9:66-71, 1988.

Palmer BF: Nephrotic edema: pathogenesis and treatment, *Am J Med Sci* 306:53-67, 1993.

Palmer BF, Alpern RJ: Pathogenesis of edema formation in the nephrotic syndrome, *Kindey Int* 59(suppl):S21-S27, 1997.

Phillips DR, Charo IF, Parise LV, Fitzgerald LA: The platelet membrane glycoprotein IIb-IIIa complex, *Blood* 71:831-843, 1988.

Pietra GG: Biology of disease: new insights into mechanisms of pulmonary edema, *Lab Invest* 51:489-494, 1984.

Ploysongsang Y, Michel RP, Rossi A, Zocchi L, Milic-Emili J, Staub MC: Early detection of pulmonary congestion and edema in dogs by using lung sounds, *J Appl Physiol* 66:2061-2070, 1989.

Robbins KC, Barlow GH, Nguyen G, Samara MM: Comparison of plasminogen activators, *Semin Thromb Hemost* 13:131-138, 1987.

Rosenberg RD: The biochemistry and pathophysiology of the prethrombotic state, *Annu Rev Med* 38:493-508, 1987.

Rosenberg RD, Aird WC: Vascular-bed-specific hemostasis and hypercoagulable states, *N Engl J Med* 340:1555-1564, 1999.

Rosenberg RD, Rosenberg JS: Natural anticoagulant mechanisms, *J Clin Invest* 76:1-5, 1984.

Rosendaal FR: Risk factors for venous thrombosis: prevalence, risk and interaction, *Semin Hematol* 34(3):171-187, 1997.

Ruf W, TS Edgington: Structural biology of tissue factor, the initiator of thrombogenesis in vivo, *FASEB J* 8:385-391, 1994.

Ruggeri ZM, Ware J: Von Willebrand factor, *FASEB J* 7:308-316, 1993.

Ruggeri ZM: New insights into the mechanisms of platelet adhesion and aggregation, *Semin Hematol* 31:229-239, 1994.

Ryan U: The endothelial surface and responses to injury, *Fed Proc* 45:101-108, 1986.

Sadler JE: Biochemistry and genetics of von Willebrand factor, *Annu Rev Biochem* 67:395-424, 1998.

Sahhah S: Inhibitors to clotting factors, *Ann Hematol* 75:1-7, 1997.

Saito H: Contact factors in health and disease, *Semin Thromb Hemost* 13:36-49, 1987.

Saksela O: Plasminogen activation and regulation of pericellular proteolysis, *Biochim Biophys Acta* 823:35-65, 1985.

Saksela O, Rifkin DB: Cell-associated plasminogen activation: regulation, and physiological functions, *Annu Rev Cell Biol* 4:93-126, 1988.

Scarborough RM, Kleiman NS, Phillips DR: Platelet glycoprotein IIb/IIIa antagonists: what are the relevant issues concerning their pharmacology and clinical use? *Circulation* 27:437-444, 1999.

Schafer AI: Focussing of the clot: normal and pathologic mechanisms, *Annu Rev Med* 38:211-220, 1987.

Schaub RG, Simmons CA, Koets MH, Romano PJ II, Stewart GJ: Early events in the formation of a venous thrombus following local trauma and stasis, *Lab Invest* 51:218-224, 1984.

Simeonescu M, Simionescu N: Functions of the endothelial cell surface, *Annu Rev Physiol* 48:279-293, 1986.

Sixma HJJ, Van Zanten H, Danga J-D, Niewenhus HK, deGroot PG: Platelet adhesion, *Semin Hematol* 32(2):89-98, 1995.

Slauson DO, Gribble DH: Thrombosis complicating renal amyloidosis in dogs, *Vet Pathol* 8:352-363, 1971.

Staub NC, Taylor AE: *Edema,* New York, 1984, Raven Press.

Steen VM, Holmsen H: Current aspects on human platelet activation and responses, *Eur J Haematol* 38:383-399, 1987.

Stemerman MB, Colton CK, Morell EM: Perturbations of the endothelium, *Prog Hemost Thromb* 7:289-324, 1984.

Stern DM, Carpenter B, Nawroth PP: Endothelium and the regulation of coagulation, *Pathol Immunopathol Res* 5:29-36, 1986.

Thomas DP: Venous thrombogenesis, *Annu Rev Med* 36:39-50, 1985.

Thomas JS, Green RA: Clotting times and antithrombin III activity in cats with naturally developing diseases: 85 cases (1984-1994), *J Am Vet Med Assoc* 213:1290-1295, 1998.

Thomas JS: Von Willebrand's disease in the dog and cat, *Vet Clin North Am Small Anim Pract* 26:1089-1110, 1996.

Wachtfogel YT, DeLa Cardena RA, Colman RW: Structural biology, cellular interactions and pathophysiology of the contact system, *Thromb Res* 72:1-21, 1993.

Wallis WJ, Harlan JM: Effector functions of endothelium in inflammatory and immunologic reactions, *Pathol Immunopathol Res* 5:73-103, 1986.

Welles EG: Antithrombotic and fibrinolytic factors, *Vet Clin North Am Small Anim Pract* 26:1111-1127, 1996.

Welles EG, Prasse KW, Moore JN: Use of newly developed assays for protein C and plasminogen in horses with signs of colic, *Am J Vet Res* 52:345-351, 1991.

White JG: The secretory pathway of bovine platelets, *Blood* 69:878-885, 1987.

Wickremasinghe RG, Hoffbrand AV: Biochemical and genetic control of apoptosis: relevance to normal hemostasis and hematological malignancies, *Blood* 93(11):3587-3600, 1999.

Willerson JT, Zoldhelyi P: Future directions in thrombolysis, *Clin Cardiol* 22(suppl 8):44-53, 1998.

Wu KK, Thiagarajan P: Role of endothelium in thrombosis and hemostasis, *Annu Rev Med* 47:315-332, 1996.

Wu KK: Genetic markers: genes involved in thrombosis, *J Cardiovasc Risk* 4:347-352, 1997.

Zucker-Franklin D, Benson KA, Myers KM: Absence of a surface-connected canalicular system in bovine platelets, *Blood* 65:241-249, 1985.

CHAPTER 4

Inflammation and Repair of Tissue

Philip N. Bochsler
David O. Slauson

OUTLINE

Inflammation is one of the most important and most useful of our host defense mechanisms, and without an adequate inflammatory response none of us or our patients would be living. Ironically it is also one of the most common means whereby our own tissues are injured. Inflammation is among the oldest of recognized pathophysiological phenomena, and the history of medicine itself is closely paralleled by the history of inflammation. As in many other fields, knowledge of inflammation grew through the careful observations of curious individuals, and what we will discuss in this chapter is a synopsis of the combined efforts and intellect of many dedicated scientists who have made discoveries in this field; the last chapter of discoveries in this area has by no means yet been written (Table 4-1).

The inflammatory process is closely interdigitated with the responses that constitute *healing* and *repair*. Inflammation fundamentally acts as a host defense mechanism, but there is no distinct line between where inflammation leaves off and repair begins. It is best to view *inflammation* and *repair* as a continuum, and much evidence has accumulated to indicate that repair processes begin during the earliest phases of inflammation. The *vascular* and *cellular* events that highlight *acute inflammation* are aimed at mobilization of host defenses to neutralize whatever the offending agent might be, and these events overlap and are shared by the early events of the healing and repair process.

The word *inflammation* itself takes us back a long way in the history of medicine, and it literally means a "burning." Inflammation was studied for hundreds of years before any true insight was obtained with respect to the mechanisms by which it occurred. In the first century of our era, observations of patients had allowed the Roman *Cornelius Celsus* to formulate his famous "cardinal signs" of inflammation: *calor, rubor, tumor,* and *dolor.* These are still true today: "Now the characteristics of inflammation are four; heat and redness with swelling and pain" (Table 4-2). To this classic list of four

signs must be added *functio laesa,* or 'injured or impaired function' (or loss of function). This fifth sign is often attributed to *Galen* (AD 130-200), but it really originated with *Rudolf Virchow* (1821-1902), the father of modern pathology. It is now clear that most of these clinical signs relate to the early vascular events of the inflammatory response. By the middle of the nineteenth century, one of Virchow's students, *Julius Cohnheim* (1839-1884), had described in considerable detail the vascular changes in inflammation. He observed injured blood vessels in thin membranes such as frog mesentery and detailed the vasodilatation, augmented blood flow, and increased vascular permeability that occurred.

Despite their obvious importance, these vascular changes are not the sum total of inflammation. It remained for the Russian zoologist *Elie Metchnikoff* (1845-1916), in his interesting book on the comparative pathology of inflammation, to draw our attention to the central theme of inflammation as the activities of the "wandering mesodermal cells" (leukocytes) against an irritant. Metchnikoff discovered the process of phagocytosis by observing the ingestion of rose thorns by amebocytes of starfish larvae and concluded that the purpose of inflammation was to bring phagocytic cells to the injured area such that they could engulf invaders. It was at about this same time that sweeping changes in medicine were taking place related to the discoveries of *Louis Pasteur* (1822-1895) and *Robert Koch* (1843-1910), in that microorganisms like bacteria were important in the cause of disease. Thus the phenomenology of inflammation was fairly well described almost a century ago; it had become clear that the vascular phenomenon detailed by Cohnheim set the stage for the cellular events of Metchnikoff.

Although both the vascular and cellular aspects of the inflammatory response are closely interdigitated, a substantial argument regarding which part was more important occupied early investigators

TABLE 4-1 Giants in the Early History of Inflammation

NAME	TIME	CONTRIBUTION
Cornelius Celsus	1st century AD	*Calor, rubor, tumor, dolor*
Rudolf Virchow	1821-1902	Father of modern pathology, *functio laesa*
Julius Cohnheim	1839-1884	Vascular phenomena
Elie Metchnikoff	1845-1916	Importance of leukocytes, phagocytosis
Louis Pasteur	1822-1895	Microbial causation
Robert Koch	1843-1910	Koch's postulates
Paul Ehrlich	1854-1915	Humoral theory of host defense

for some time. The same type of argument followed the discovery that blood serum could have a protective effect against microorganisms that was equal to or even greater than phagocytosis. It was somehow fitting, then, that *Paul Ehrlich (1854-1915)*, who developed the "humoral theory" of host defense (antibodies), and Metchnikoff shared the Nobel Prize in 1908. For the first time, both cellular (phagocytosis) and serum factors (antibodies) were jointly recognized for their importance to host defense.

Neither Cohnheim, Metchnikoff, nor Ehrlich considered the role of biochemical mediators in inflammation, however. That was left for *Sir Thomas Lewis*, who, in a series of beautifully simple experiments with skin reactions published in 1927, established that locally produced chemical substances mediate the vascular changes in inflammation. The "triple response" described by Lewis can be elicited when one firmly rubs one's own forearm with a blunt instrument like a pencil or the edge of a ruler. Within seconds, a dull red line forms along the line of the stroke, followed by a bright red halo around the stroke mark. The third feature, swelling of the stroke mark accompanied by its blanching, follows soon thereafter. Lewis postulated that these vascular phenomena were attributable to a chemical he called "H-substance" (histamine), and thus was ushered in the modern era of biochemical and molecular approaches to the study of inflammation.

The history of inflammation and healing and repair is a fascinating one, but it is not our purpose to provide a detailed account. Interested readers would greatly profit from Guido Majno's excellent book cited in the reference list. Henry Movat's book also provides a variety of interesting historical information on the subject.

INFLAMMATION IN GENERAL

What is inflammation? Inflammation has long been considered simply as the reaction of tissues to an irritant. More specifically, it is the *reaction of vascu-*

larized living tissues to local injury which comprises a series of changes in the terminal vascular bed, in the blood, and in the connective tissues that are designed to eliminate the offending irritant and to repair the damaged tissue. Because it is such a complex series of events and because it is difficult to usefully define, some generalities about inflammation may help to place it in perspective (Box 4-1).

Ten Generalities About Inflammation

1. *Inflammation is a process involving many components.* An understanding of the complexity of the inflammatory response can be facilitated by first noting that it is a process involving multiple cellular, humoral and tissue participants. It comprises a complex series of events, some sequential, others virtually simultaneous but overlapping and many of which are interdependent. Inflammation begins with or is preceded by cell or tissue injury, which leads to the hemodynamic and permeability adjustments that follow. Affected vessels readily exude fluids, plasma proteins, and white blood cells. The machinery activating such events includes a cluster of biochemical mediators. Once gathered into a focus of injury the various types of white blood cells contribute to the defense reaction by virtue of their ability to migrate, release enzymes and often inflammatory mediators, and phagocytose particulate matter.

In inflammatory reactions that evoke systemic responses, there is often an increase in circulating leukocytes in the bloodstream *(leukocytosis)*, and the leukocytes that are already in

| TABLE 4-2 | Classical Clinical Signs of Inflammation |

SIGN	ORIGINATOR	TRANSLATION
Calor	Celsus	Heat
Rubor	Celsus	Redness
Tumor	Celsus	Swelling
Dolor	Celsus	Pain
Functio laesa	Virchow	Loss of function

| BOX 4-1 | Ten Generalities about the Inflammatory Response |

1. It is a process involving multiple participants.
2. It occurs only in living tissue.
3. It is a series of events overlapping into a continuum.
4. It is an evoked response that requires initiation by a stimulus.
5. It can be more harmful than the initiating stimulus.
6. It is fundamentally a defense reaction.
7. It is fairly stereotyped irrespective of the initiating stimulus.
8. It has most of its reactive components in the blood.
9. It is highly redundant with many promoters and regulators.
10. It is largely a surface-oriented phenomenon.

tissues and other types of cells throughout the body usually become involved. Although most inflammatory responses tend to be alike in their early phases, many factors relating to both the inciting agent and to the host modify the evolving reaction.

2. *Inflammation occurs only in living tissue.* Cells can die in the living organism (necrosis), or they can die after the entire organism has ceased living (postmortem autolysis). Intravascular blood clots can form in the living animal (thrombosis), or they can form in the dead animal (postmortem clots). In both of these situations, some experience may be necessary before one can discern whether the events took place before or after death. In contrast, *postmortem inflammation does not occur.* The inflammatory process, with its many vascular and cellular subsets, depends wholly on viable tissue. If one were examining a histological section of kidney in which thrombi filled the vessels, the tubular epithelium was dead, and numerous neutrophils were present in the interstitium, one might wonder about the authenticity of the thrombi (ante or post mortem?) and about the dead tubular epithelial cells (necrosis or autolysis?), but one would not have to worry about the inflammatory aspects of the lesion. The neutrophils present in this example migrated into the inflamed kidney while the animal was still alive. This is *always* the case. Inflammation cannot occur in a dead organism.

3. *Inflammation is an overlapping series of events that form a continuum.* The terms "acute," "subacute," and "chronic" as applied to disease in general and to inflammation in particular have survived over the years because they are practical. We can assume they are here to stay. It is easy to use such terms but more difficult to define their significance in the light of the modern biology of inflammation. Although such terms are useful to pathologists and clinicians, it is more correct to envision inflammation as a single continuum that cannot truly be split on the basis of its course in time. It is a well-planned mechanism of defense, with multiple overlapping pathways leading to similar effects, no matter what the cause. The inflammatory response has two themes, inflammation and repair, but the two processes are so closely interdigitated that they really represent different parts of a single continuing process. Inflammation begins with injury to tissue and ends with permanent destruction of tissue or with healing.

4. *Inflammation is a response to an initiating event.* Inflammation does not occur without a cause; it is always an *evoked* response set into motion by some kind of a stimulus, usually one that injures tissue. It is therefore appropriate to think of inflammation in terms of a cause-and-effect relationship. Bacteria, viruses, mycoplasmas, fungi, protozoa, chemicals, physical injury, immunological injury, and a variety of other kinds of stimuli can evoke an inflammatory response. In addition, the products of injured tissue (such as dead cells) can themselves serve as an inflammatory stimulus. Thus the inflammatory response, once set into motion by a variety of stimuli, can become self-perpetuating by virtue of its ability for cyclic self-stimulation. It is important to conceptualize inflammation as an evoked response that *always* requires an initiating stimulus. If the stimulus can be identified and removed, inflammation should cease.

5. *Inflammation can be harmful.* Although engineered as a part of host defense, in many situations the host may suffer more tissue damage as a result of an inflammatory reaction than would have been caused by the initiating stimulus had there been no inflammatory response at all. Some of the best examples of this paradox come from immunopathology (see Chapter 5). Horse serum, for example, is by itself nonpathogenic when injected into an animal for the first time, but repeat injections can lead to the production of a violent, destructive, and sometimes fatal localized or generalized inflammatory response (Arthus reaction, anaphylaxis, or serum sickness) in which the reaction of the host is considerably more damaging than the horse serum itself. Thus, within certain limits, the inflammatory reaction cannot distinguish readily between those instances in which it is called into play to protect the host and those instances in which the host is unnecessarily harmed. Indeed, it is probably true that *all* inflammatory reactions, no matter how useful to host survival, produce some damage to host tissue. Another example is seen in sick calves: if neutrophil depletion is accomplished by experimental means in calves with experimentally induced pneumonic pasteurellosis, the calves are partially protected against the development of severe pneumonia and the resultant hypoxia. These changes are therefore, in large part, *neutrophil mediated* rather than being attributable to the direct effects of the causative agent, *Mannheimia* (formerly *Pasteurella*) *haemolytica*.

The problem is that an intense inflammatory reaction occurs in the lung in which the tissue-damaging contributions of the inflammatory host-defense mechanisms (leukocytes, fibrin, and so forth) are worse than the tissue-damaging contributions of the original infectious agents (Fig. 4-1). An inappropriately excessive level of host inflammatory reaction develops and becomes a major contributor to the ongoing disease process rather than fulfilling its function as a defensive maneuver. A thorough understanding of the inflammatory process will assist in providing the necessary tools for a greater appreciation of what is actually occurring in the tissues of patients with such inflammatory lesions.

Inflammation is therefore like certain other vital life processes that may become harmful. For example, hemostasis is a vital process in the arrest of bleeding, yet the same coagulation pathways can produce fatal thrombosis, that is, infarcts. Insulin is necessary for life, but its excessive production by a neoplasm of the pancreatic islet cells can result in death. Many diseases such as rheumatoid arthritis, asthma, and glomerulonephritis are associated with inflammatory reactions that provide the host no obvious benefit but rather inflict considerable harm. These are clinical problems that must be dealt with on a regular basis. It is for this reason that our pharmacies are loaded with a wide variety of antiinflammatory drugs that we employ in attempts to limit, control, or otherwise modify inflammation. The inflammatory response is a crucial host defense mechanism, but it has a potentially harmful, destructive side as well.

6. *Inflammation is fundamentally a defensive reaction.* Our ability to recover from various infectious and noninfectious injuries is related to the fact that the inflammatory response is a survival-oriented process. It is one of the most fundamentally important host defense systems in virtually all living things; mammals, birds, reptiles and amphibians, fish, invertebrates, and plants have their own responses to local injury. Without effective inflammatory responses, bacterial infections are difficult to contain, wounds do not heal well, and damaged tissues are not repaired.

The result of inflammatory activity usually includes *repair,* which begins during the active phases of inflammation but reaches completion only after the initiating stimulus has been removed or walled off. The damaged cells and

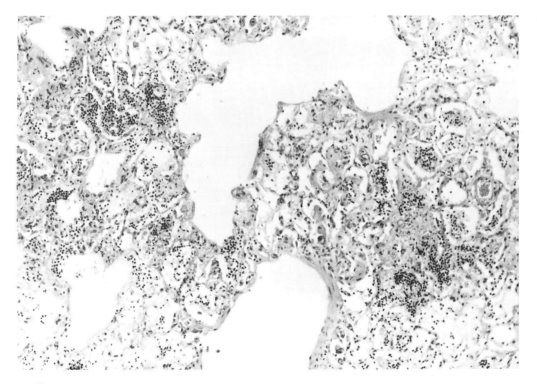

Fig. 4-1 Acute inflammation. There are many neutrophils as well as fibrin deposition in this acutely inflamed dog lung. These typical hallmarks of inflammation are host-derived contributors to the inflammatory process.

tissues are either replaced by vital cells *(repair by regeneration)* or by replacement with less specialized fibroblasts (repair by connective tissue replacement, or *scarring*). A prompt and effective response destroys or neutralizes most injurious agents before much cell and tissue destruction takes place, and the need for repair is minimized with little or no scarring. If, on the other hand, the injury is severe and repair by regeneration cannot occur, scarring will result. The inflammatory process itself is aimed at maximizing normalcy as an end point. Ideally this can be accomplished by removal of the initiating stimulus and regenerative repair of the injured tissue.

Perhaps some of the best examples of the importance of inflammation as a survival-oriented defense mechanism come from patients in which the inflammatory response is defective because of disorders of phagocyte function. A syndrome in humans of severe recurrent infections is known as *chronic granulomatous disease* because of the persistent infections of skin, lymph nodes, lung, liver, gastrointestinal tract, genitourinary tract, and bones. Such patients have a profound impairment in leukocyte oxidative metabolism, that is, generation of oxygen radicals, leading to defective microbicidal function. The *Chediak-Higashi syndrome* (CHS) has been described in humans, Aleutian mink, beige mice, partial albino Hereford cattle, albino whales, and cats. CHS is a genetically determined autosomal-recessive disease characterized by neutropenia and recurrent pyogenic infections associated with abnormal, giant phagocyte lysosomal granules and defective microbicidal activity. *Leukocyte adhesion deficiency* (LAD) is a rare disease described in humans, cattle (BLAD, bovine LAD), and dogs in which leukocytes lack a related group of functional adhesion molecules on their surface, the CD11/CD18 integrins. The disease was at one time *not* rare in Holstein cattle in the United States because the defective gene was spread widely through the use of artificial insemination; it has since been reduced in prevalence. In LAD some leukocytes, most notably neutrophils, are unable to efficiently leave the bloodstream and enter the tissues. These patients are thus predisposed to serious bacterial infections and may die relatively early in life. Another adhesion-molecule deficiency has also been described in humans, LAD2. These examples represent naturally occurring illustrations of situations in which a defective cellular in-

flammatory response exists and underscore the importance of inflammation as a vital defense mechanism.

7. *Inflammation is fairly stereotyped.* The long list of potential causes of tissue injury is *not* paralleled by an equally long list of types of inflammatory responses. Indeed, the basic character and progression of events in the inflammatory response has many common events, despite the variability of initiating stimuli. There are some variations in the inflammatory reaction, however, and these are determined by both the nature and severity of the injurious stimulus, the ability of the host to respond with an inflammatory response, and some species variation in response. The intensity and duration of inflammatory reactions may be viewed as a delicate balance between attacker and host. Depending on the severity of the injury and the adequacy of the defense, inflammation may remain localized to its site of origin and evoke no systemic reactions or may involve dramatic systemic responses.

Despite these variables, the early phases of the inflammatory response are often similar in many cases, almost irrespective of the nature of the initiating stimulus. Local increases in blood flow *(hyperemia)* develop. Increased vascular permeability occurs. Leukocytes leave the bloodstream and enter the inflamed tissues. The reactions usually differ only in timing and magnitude during the early phase. In these cases, the nature of the leukocytic infiltrate may differ over time; for example, lymphocytes and plasma cells may predominate. When the irritant is difficult to degrade, such as a lipid or an insoluble foreign body, macrophages may predominate.

8. *Many of the components of inflammation are in the blood.* Many of the components of an inflammatory response are normally found in the blood, whereas injury is almost always in the "solid" tissues. (Some anatomists also consider blood to be a tissue.) When we look microscopically at the inflamed tissue, protein-rich edema fluid, fibrin, leukocytes, and injured tissue are visible. Except for the injured tissue itself, all these typical components of the acute reaction are blood derived, largely white blood cells and serum proteins (Fig. 4-2). You will see as we further dissect the inflammatory process in this chapter that many other participants in this vital host defense mechanism are also blood derived: the platelets, the coagulation factors, the fibrinolytic enzymes, the complement system,

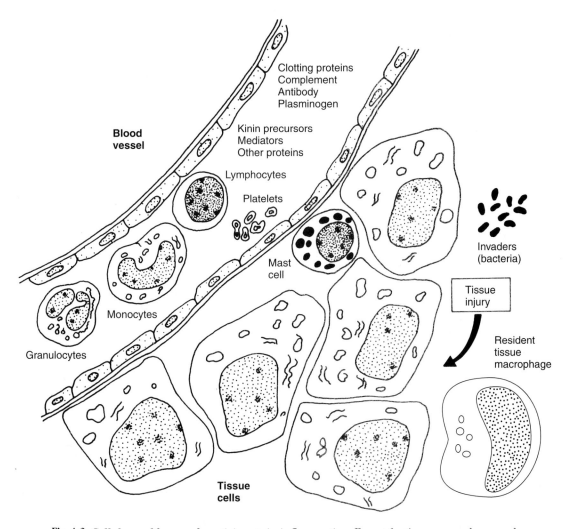

Fig. 4-2 Cellular and humoral participants in inflammation. Except for tissue macrophages and mast cells, most of the host defenses that are involved in inflammation are blood borne. Therefore the blood vessel walls become critical barriers across which the defenders must pass.

antibody, the kinins, and so on. This makes practical sense in that it is a mobile reservoir that can be quickly delivered to almost any body location.

It should also be clear that a very important barrier exists between the *tissue*, where injury takes place, and the *blood*, where the defenses are marshaled. The barrier is the wall of the vascular bed across which the blood-borne defenses must move to gain access to the injured tissue itself. This places the *vascular endothelium* in a unique position as the only continuous cellular layer between the leukocytes and plasma proteins and the tissue sites of injury. It is not surprising, then, that the microvascular bed and endothelial cells play a vitally important role in the development of inflammatory reactions.

9. *There are multiple overlapping pathways in the inflammatory response.* The inflammatory response is a beautifully orchestrated defense mechanism essential to life. Because of its importance, it makes sense that there are usually multiple ways to get any one aspect of it initiated (in case an individual has a defect) as well as complicated feedback loops and control mechanisms. It would make no biological sense for neutrophils to exhibit directed migration *(chemotaxis)* toward only one specific chemical signal; indeed, they will respond to many such chemotactic stimuli. This is in keeping with the importance to the inflammatory response and the survival dependence of their successful employment. There are two major pathways for initiating blood coagulation, each with interconnecting loops, and several routes by which

fibrin removal can be achieved. The list of stimuli that will cause lysosomal enzyme release from leukocytes is a long one. Collagen, thrombin, epinephrine, and ADP, among other stimuli, will cause platelets to aggregate at inflammatory foci. The more refined and detailed our ability to look at inflammatory mechanisms becomes, the more we discover the incredible orchestration and complicity of molecular and cellular interactions and the redundancy of initiation and control signals. This will become a recurrent theme in our discussion of inflammation.

If all the interlacing activation and control pathways involved in inflammation could be drawn on a single piece of paper (not possible, we think), it would make those giant intermediary metabolism charts and signal-transduction charts that hang in research laboratories look tame. The cascades of closely interdigitated events that constitute the reaction of tissues to injury over a variable time scale involves a large cast of cellular participants, each with numerous functions that are mediated, modulated, and orchestrated by a multiplicity of biochemical messengers that influence and determine the vascular, extravascular, and cellular sequelae of inflammation. It is easy to get lost in the labyrinthine interlacing of the inflammatory pathways and to lose sight of the forest for the trees: to forget that inflammation is a vital host defense mechanism and a healing response.

10. *Much of the inflammatory response is a "surface phenomenon."* It is interesting to understand how much of inflammation is "surface oriented." Bacteria become opsonized to make them more readily available (by surface receptors) for phagocytosis. Leukocytes crawl on surfaces; they do not swim in fluids; their locomotor activities involve reversible adherence of receptors on the leukocyte exterior to the surface over which they move. Mast cell activation and degranulation involves stimulation by surface-related membrane events. Platelets adhere to subendothelial collagen by surface receptors for von Willebrand factor, which is bound to the collagen. The Hageman factor–dependent pathways are initiated by contact activation on negatively charged surfaces. The leukocytes basically respond to membrane events related to perturbation of surface membrane receptors, and so on.

These surface-related phenomena, particularly as they relate to cells, are manifestations of the basic "irritation level" of the responding cells. Since inflammatory cells can neither hear nor see as we do, their membranes act as their eyes and ears. By perceiving various signals in the immediate microenvironment, the leukocytes "read" the messages and act accordingly. The stimulus, whether it be a phagocytic stimulus, chemotactic attraction, movement along a surface, interaction with immune reagents, or whatever, involves specific surface membrane receptor interaction, which can then subsequently activate the signals necessary for the intracellular events necessary for specific cellular functions. The messages responsible for this intense cellular activity are received at the cell surface for translation into functional activity by the events of intracellular biochemistry and molecular biology. Viewed as such, inflammation is certainly a special subset of the larger field of cell biology.

Inflammation: Are These Things Real?

In the pages that follow, we will dissect the inflammatory response into its component parts and explain how the various vascular, cellular, and humoral ingredients function and relate to each other. In so doing, there is a decided risk that one can lose sight of the "big picture," a risk that, for example, the molecular events in leukocyte activation and the biochemistry of phagocytosis somehow become more important than knowing what *pus* is. Knowledge about inflammation is a wonderful thing, for it allows us to begin to understand how and why things happen in a certain way. The greater our level of understanding, the more likely we are to be able to *interpret* clinical signs and to approach inflammatory lesions with rational, specific therapy. We must remember, however, that all the world's molecular information is not worth the paper or Internet pages it is printed on if it seduces us into forgetting the overall clinical nature of inflammation as it occurs in living animals.

TYPES OF INFLAMMATION

Although many types of inflammatory responses have similar mechanistic backgrounds as far as the cells participating, the vascular phenomena, and the biochemical mediators are involved, the result in tissue does not always look the same. Many factors relating to both the inciting agent and the host modify the evolution and appearance of the reaction, the nature of the local exudate, the distribution in tissue, the time course of the reaction, and its severity. It would be impossible to discuss all these variables in great detail or enumerate each particular disease. Rather, we will focus on features of inflammation that are useful to clinicians and pathologists in the interpretation of inflammatory lesions in disease settings. We will direct our attention to the various appearances of inflamed tissues that reflect differences in severity, time frame, distribution, and types of exudate as fundamental manifestations of inflammation in tissue. In later sections, we will explore the fascinating *biology* of the cells involved and the *mechanisms* by which inflammatory reactions develop.

Understanding the Nomenclature of Inflammatory Reactions

In the naming and classification of inflammatory reactions, what winds up on the bottom line often reflects a general rather than a specific designation. A lengthy and detailed examination of an inflamed lung deserves a better diagnosis than just the general term "pneumonia." Why? Because the details of the *type* of pneumonia often point toward the cause. What was the distribution of the lesion? How severe was the process? How long had the process been underway? What type of exudate or injury pattern characterized this particular inflammatory response? Did the pneumonia largely involve airways and contiguous parenchyma or was it predominately interstitial? This type of information possibly can be extracted from a pathologist's description of the lesion, but it is far preferable that it is included as part of a succinct *morphological diagnosis* that describes the process and lesions. (This is part of the "bottom line" of pathology reports.) It also forces one to think in terms of the process rather than the end point and provides a language

that both clinicians and pathologists can understand (Tables 4-3 and 4-4). Thorough designation of the character of inflammatory lesions as they are reflected in tissue reactions allows a far better understanding of the processes that underlie the lesion. In addition, there is also a thing called the *etiological diagnosis*. This is a short, two- or three-word diagnosis that indicates the *cause* and the *organ location* of the lesion. It is a useful, quick way to describe a lesion when talking to colleagues or clients. It does not, however, include all the information that a morphological diagnosis does. Examples of etiological diagnoses are "coliform mastitis," "viral pneumonia," and "flea-bite dermatitis."

Severity: How Bad Is It?

Inflammation can be minimal or mild, as in the reaction to a tiny wood splinter in one's finger, or it can be severe and life threatening, as in a severe bronchopneumonia. In between lies a gray zone in which other degrees of inflammation occur. Much of this reflects a value judgment on the part of the individual making the assessment as to mild, moderate, or severe, but certain guidelines are useful. *Mild* reactions usually include little or no tissue destruction, slight evidence for vascular involvement (hyperemia and edema), and little in the way of exudation. *Minimal* reactions are even more minimal than just described and may be visible only histologically. *Moderate* reactions usually contain some damage to host tissue and an easily visible clinical or histological host reaction to the injury manifest by leukocytic accumulation and vascular phenomena. *Severe* reactions are an extension of moderate

TABLE 4-3 Classification of Inflammatory Lesions—The Morphologic Diagnosis

SEVERITY	DURATION	DISTRIBUTION	EXUDATE	ANATOMIC MODIFIERS	ORGAN
Minimal	Peracute	Focal	Serous	Interstitial	Nephritis
Mild	Acute	Multifocal	Catarrhal	Broncho-	Hepatitis
Moderate	Subacute	Locally extensive	Suppurative/purulent	Glomerulo-	Enteritis etc.
Severe or marked	Chronic	Diffuse	Fibrinous	Submandibular	
	Chronic-active		Serofibrinous	Bilateral etc.	
			Fibrinopurulent		
			Necrotizing		
			Granulomatous		
			Nonsuppurative		
			Caseous etc.		

Examples

Severe chronic focal caseous submandibular lymphadenitis
Severe acute locally extensive fibrinopurulent bronchopneumonia

TABLE 4-4   Some of the Anatomic Prefixes Used for Classification of Inflammatory Lesions (add "-itis")

WORD ROOT	ORGAN/TISSUE
Arter-	artery
Oste-	bone
Osteomyel-	bone marrow, or bone and bone marrow
Encephal-	brain
Encephalomyel-	brain and spinal cord
Bronch-	bronchi
Burs-	bursa(e)
Typhl-	cecum
Typhlocol-	cecum and colon
Col-	colon
Conjunctiv-	conjunctiva(e)
Cellul-	connective tissue (usually under the skin)
Duoden-	duodenum
Ot-	ear
Endocard-	endocardium
Esophag-	esophagus
Ophthalm-	eye (does not specify area[s] of the eye)
Panophthalm-	eye, the entire eye
Kerat-	eye, just the cornea
Keratoconjunctiv-	eye, cornea, and conjunctivae
Uve-	eye, just the uveal tract (iris, ciliary body, choroid)
Blephar-	eyelid
Cholecyst-	gallbladder
Aden-	gland (generic)
Balan-	glans penis
Gingiv-	gum
Valvul-	heart valve
Lamin-	hoof
Enter-	intestine
Arthr-	joint
Nephr-	kidney
Laryng-	larynx
Laryngotrache-	larnyx and trachea
Cheil-	lip
Hepat-	liver
Pleuropneumon-	lung and pleura
Pneumon-	lung Note: inflammation of the lung is usually, by common convention, referred to as "pneumonia," not "pneumonitis." Likewise, inflammation of the pleura and lungs is called "pleuropneumonia," not "pleuropneumonitis."
Lymphaden-	lymph node
Mast-	mammary gland(s)
Mening-	meninges
Meningoencephal-	meninges and brain
Stomat-	mouth
Myocard-	myocardium

WORD ROOT	ORGAN/TISSUE
Myos- (my-)	muscle
Neur-	nerve
Rhin-	nose
Salping-	oviduct
Pericard-	pericardium
Periost-	periosteum
Periton-	peritoneum/abdominal cavity
Pharyng-	pharynx
Pleur-	pleura
Posth-	prepuce
Prostat-	prostate
Proct-	rectum or anus, or both
Dermat-	skin
Pododermat-	skin (and often deeper structures) of the foot
Funicul-	spermatic cord
Myel-	spinal cord
Splen-	spleen
Gastr-	stomach
Synov-	synovium
Tendin-	tendon
Orch(id)-	testicle
Gloss-	tongue
Tonsil-	tonsil
Odont-	tooth
Trache-	trachea
Omphal-	umbilicus
Ureter-	ureter
Cyst-	urinary bladder
Metr-	uterus
Vagin-	vagina
Phleb-	vein

As seen in the list, by common convention some of the anatomic word roots may be linked together to indicate inflammation in two tissues or organs, such as gastroenteritis, tracheobronchitis, encephalomyelitis. These word roots may also be used, when appropriate, in combination with the suffixes "-osis" and "-opathy."

"-osis" indicates a noninflammatory insult that results in damage to a tissue or organ and is often used when necrosis is a prominent feature. Example: renal damage as a result of ethylene glycol toxicity is referred to as "nephrosis."

"-opathy" is used to indicate that there is a problem or lesion in an organ or tissue, but the cause/pathogenesis/nature of the lesion is not entirely clear. Examples: hepatopathy, nephropathy, encephalopathy.

reactions, in which considerable tissue damage is present, usually with abundant exudation. Such designations are useful and helpful in communicating value judgments and opinions about patients between clinicians, pathologists, and clients.

Duration

All inflammatory reactions have a beginning, and most have an end. In between lies a variable span of

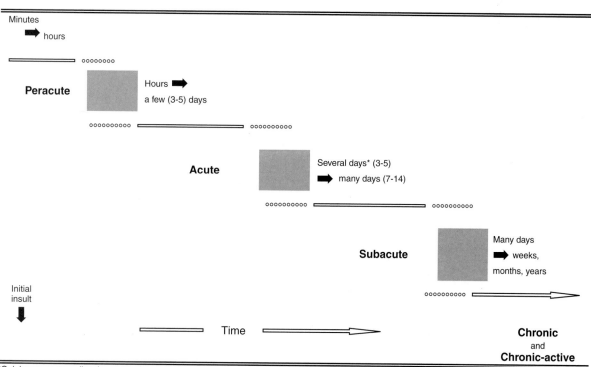

Minutes
→ hours

Peracute
Hours →
a few (3-5) days

Acute
Several days* (3-5)
→ many days (7-14)

Subacute
Many days
→ weeks,
months, years

Initial
insult

Time →

Chronic
and
Chronic-active

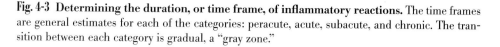

*Opinions vary regarding the appropriate transition times when the term "subacute" is used.

Fig. 4-3 Determining the duration, or time frame, of inflammatory reactions. The time frames are general estimates for each of the categories: peracute, acute, subacute, and chronic. The transition between each category is gradual, a "gray zone."

time in which the character of the evolving reaction can change (Fig. 4-3). *Peracute* inflammation is manifest very soon after its initiation, perhaps only a few hours, and usually is caused by a potent stimulus. A good example is a bee sting. There may be little evidence at this point in time of host contributions in terms of exudation. Rather, tissue reaction with some of the vascular events of inflammation are often all that is visible. Hence, edema, hyperemia, perhaps hemorrhage, and a few leukocytes beginning to infiltrate the damaged tissue may be the only visible markers.

Acute inflammation usually begins within 4 to 6 hours, and the evidence of vascular involvement is readily visible. Vessels are dilated and engorged with blood and occasionally even contain thrombi. Local hemorrhage and edema may be present. Fibrin is often visible. Clinically the involved tissues are warm and reddened (increased blood flow), swollen (edema), and painful (biochemical mediators of inflammation). These cardinal signs of inflammation were originally described in Latin as *calor, rubor, tumor,* and *dolor.* The leukocytic contribution in acute inflammation is variable and may be sparse early but usually is well developed within a day or two. Neutrophils are often predominant, though in some cases mononuclear cells can be

present in large numbers in acute inflammation. Edema and hyperemia are prominent in acute inflammation. This is the picture we usually think of when imagining what an inflammatory reaction looks like (see Fig. 4-2). The lymphatics play a major role in transporting away the fluid and cells of an acute inflammatory reaction. This function of the lymphatic system begins early in an acute inflammatory reaction, and the transportation of the inflammatory flotsam may lead to an acute regional *lymphadenitis* as the lymphatics carry away inflammatory mediators and cells. It is useful to look "upstream" for a primary lesion when an enlarged lymph node is encountered.

The distinction between acute inflammation and subacute inflammation is not an abrupt one, but rather there is a gradual change in character. *Subacute* inflammation usually is characterized by a decline in the magnitude of the vascular contribution (edema and hyperemia) and often by a change in the character of the infiltrating leukocytes. The declining evidence of edema and hyperemia can be explained both by gradually moderating vascular contributions and by the lymphatic drainage that occurred during the more acute phases. Although subacute inflammation still may be predominately neutrophilic, the infiltrate usually becomes mixed,

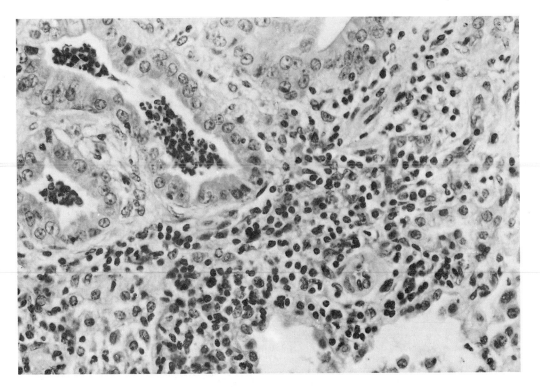

Fig. 4-4 Subacute inflammation. Mixed populations of inflammatory cells are present here, including many mononuclear cells (lymphocytes and macrophages), though the glandular lumens still contain acute phase debris and neutrophils. No hyperemia is visible.

with mononuclear cells (lymphocytes, macrophages, and maybe a few plasma cells) visible along with the neutrophils (Fig. 4-4). Subacute inflammation occupies the time span between truly acute reactions and those in which evidence of chronicity is apparent. It is an intermediate time frame that can vary from a few days to a few weeks, depending on the nature of the inciting stimulus. The designation of subacute often is used for inflammatory reactions up until evidence of host tissue reparative responses (angiogenesis, fibroplasia, and so on) are clearly manifest, at which time the lesions begin to grade into what is called "chronic inflammation."

Chronic inflammation is a clinical and pathological concept pertaining to prolonged duration of an inflammatory lesion, and it has some sufficiently unusual characteristics to warrant our special attention. It is really more than just a time frame. It represents an entity in which ongoing inflammation is often accompanied by evidence of host tissue reparative responses (Fig. 4-5). Although the transition from acute to subacute to chronic is hard to precisely pinpoint in every case, we can nonetheless define certain key features of chronicity: (1) it is caused by persistent inflammatory stimuli, and the host has been unable to rid itself of it (microbes,

foreign bodies, immune reactions, and so on); (2) the inflammatory response (innate immunity) may be accompanied by an immune response (acquired immunity) attributable in part to the duration of the insult and in part to the persistence of the invader; (3) it is usually accompanied by evidence of host tissue reparative responses. This may be by parenchymal regeneration, but *fibrosis* (scarring) remains the most reliable criterion of chronicity, and (4) it is characterized histologically by both mononuclear cell infiltrates (such as macrophages) and by connective tissue cells such as fibroblasts. Proliferation of small blood vessels (angiogenesis, neovascularization) is also often present.

Chronic inflammation usually presents clinically in one of two forms; it may follow an obvious acute inflammatory phase, or it may develop as an insidious, low-grade, subclinical process in which there is no history of a prior acute episode. The latter is particularly true in veterinary medicine, since we may not see our patients until they are sick enough to get the attention of their human owners, and acute lesions have already evolved into chronic ones.

Remember that the terms "acute," "subacute," and "chronic inflammation" may have somewhat different meanings and time frames in different spe-

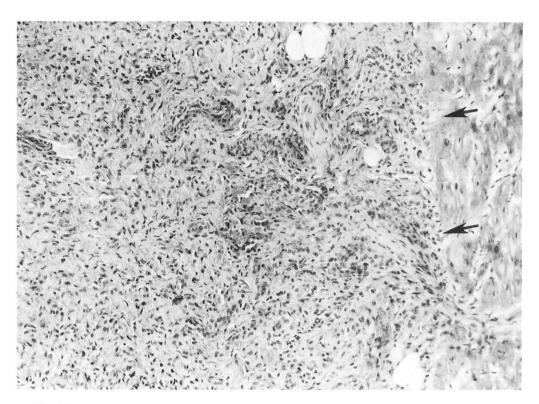

Fig. 4-5 Chronic inflammation. On the epicardial surface, *arrows*, of this bovine heart, there is active fibrovascular connective tissue (scarring) as well as scattered numbers of inflammatory cells. Fibrosis is the single best indicator of chronicity.

cialty areas of medicine, but the generalities are the same.

Macrophages at sites of subacute or chronic inflammation and wound repair consist of two populations, both having their origin in the bone marrow. The first are the "resident" tissue macrophages. They and their macrophage-derived counterparts are present in most types of tissue at all times, and under suitable stimuli are capable of entering the mitotic cycle and undergoing cell division. The other major numerical component of macrophages at most sites of chronic inflammation is directly recruited from hematogenous precursor cells, the monocytes, which themselves are derived from a rapidly dividing pool of stem cells in the bone marrow. In fact, most macrophages at sites of inflammation are derived from the monocytes in the blood, with the name change to "macrophage" occurring when the cells leave the blood and enter the tissue. Macrophages are the cells principally responsible for phagocytosis and tissue débridement in a chronic lesion.

As already mentioned, the ultimate causes of chronicity are related to a failure to eliminate an irritant or stimulus. The use of a wide variety of ra-diolabeled irritants has failed to reveal any instance where a chronic reaction is not accompanied by tissue persistence of the irritant, or where disappearance of the irritant is not accompanied by disappearance of the reaction. Clinical situations of this sort include diseases such as tuberculosis or foreign-body reactions. In contrast, there are some cases where no irritant can be seen or recovered. However, since a small amount of irritant, especially microbiological, can provoke a chronic response, the persistent stimulus may nevertheless be present, even though we cannot easily detect it.

Persistence of an irritant within cells or tissues may be caused by survival of living organisms but also may follow failure of macrophages to degrade dead organisms to diffusible products, that is, persistence of inflammatory stimuli. This has been demonstrated by quantitative analysis of the degradation by macrophages of various kinds of bacteria. Breakdown of bacteria is initially rapid, proceeding to completion for simple organisms but ceasing at 48 to 72 hours in the case of bacteria that induce chronicity. The reason for this cessation of degradation by macrophages is not entirely clear, but it appears to be attributable in part to the protective chemical nature of the cell coat on certain microorganisms as well as to more complicated intracellular dysfunctions in leukocytes such as inhibition of phagosome-lysosome fusion and failure of degranulation mechanisms.

Macrophages usually play an essential role in the pathogenesis of chronic inflammatory lesions. Macrophages are phagocytic cells, and ingested materials are degraded by enzymes within the large number of lysosomes present in the cells. Enzymes may also be released from macrophages into the local tissue environment, in much the same way as enzyme release occurs from neutrophils, and this can contribute to chronic inflammation. Macrophages also secrete numerous other biologically active products, including an array of cytokines and chemokines, which play significant roles in the inflammatory process. We explore the biology of the all-important macrophage in greater detail later.

Chronic inflammation may be accompanied by acute exacerbations in which the tissues exhibit all the usual features of chronicity upon which are superimposed features of acuteness. That is, it is not unusual to find acute suppurative inflammation side by side with fibrosis and tissue regeneration. Such lesions are often designated as *chronic-active* inflammation, and this implies that repeated episodes of inflammation have occurred and overlapped in their evolutionary cycles; that is, failure of host defenses to adequately contain the invaders has led to episodes of local reappearance to elicit new acute responses. Such lesions are not at all uncommon.

Before leaving the subject of chronic inflammation, we should note that the line between chronic inflammation and repair of injured tissues is often a blurred one. Many of the features of chronicity also are found in healing wounds, as we discuss later.

Distribution of Inflammatory Lesions

It often is useful to evaluate the inflammatory response on the basis of its distribution within the involved tissue, and this distribution is part of the morphological diagnosis. Such designations generally are used for both gross and microscopic description of lesions. Lesions may be focal, multifocal, locally extensive (or "focally extensive," as some tend to say), or diffuse (Fig. 4-6). *Focal* lesions are usually a single abnormality or inflamed area within the tissue. Such an area is called a *focus* of inflammation. These can be very small lesions of a few millimeters or less, or they can be up to several centimeters or more in diameter. They are surrounded by relatively normal tissue. *Multifocal* lesions represent several or many scattered *foci* of in-

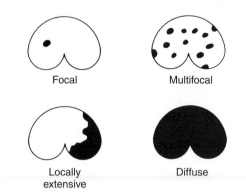

Fig. 4-6 Distribution of lesions. Lesions usually are described as either local, multifocal, locally extensive, or diffuse.

flammation within the tissue. Again, the size can be variable, but each focus of inflammation is separated from other inflamed foci by an intervening zone of relatively normal tissue. An example of these lesions is a shower of septic emboli into kidneys from an infected and inflamed heart valve.

Locally extensive lesions involve all of a considerable zone of tissue within the inflamed organ. They may arise from severe local reactions that spread into adjacent normal tissue or may evolve by the coalescence of foci in a multifocal reaction. A good example of inflammation having this type of distribution would be the pulmonary lesions of pneumonic pasteurellosis in cattle in which the cranioventral aspect of the lungs are involved whereas the dorsal portions usually are spared. Such lesions often have a bacterial or a combined viral and bacterial cause. *Diffuse* lesions involve all the tissue or organ in which they are found. There may be variations in severity within the diffusely inflamed tissue, but all the tissue exhibits inflammation. An example to contrast with the locally extensive distribution of pneumonic pasteurellosis would be the diffuse distribution of many of the interstitial pneumonias. Lesions of such distribution are often viral in cause, but toxicants can produce a similar pattern.

Types of Inflammatory Exudates

Just as the severity and distribution of inflammation can be variable, so can the nature of the exudate that characterizes inflammation. The variations in fluid, plasma protein content, and cellular composition are generally reflections of the duration and severity of the inflammatory process though variations related to the causative agent are also notable. There are certain common, repetitive patterns that warrant our attention.

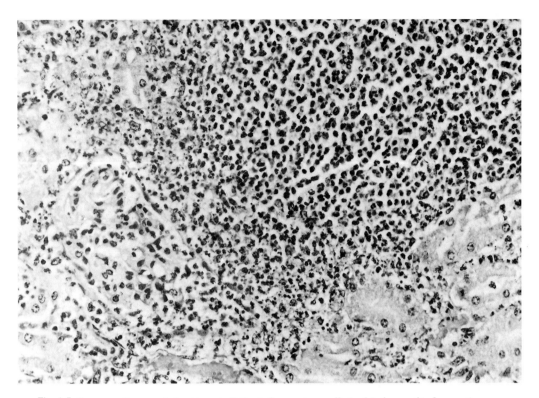

Fig. 4-7 Suppurative exudate. Almost all the inflammatory cells in this focus of inflammation are neutrophils. This makes the lesion suppurative, or purulent, and the exudate is called "pus."

SUPPURATIVE EXUDATION

Suppurative exudates are composed largely of neutrophils along with dead cells including both dead host-tissue cells and dead inflammatory cells (Fig. 4-7). A synonym for "suppurative" is *purulent*, which means that the predominant feature of the exudate is the formation of *pus*. The process by which pus is formed is called *suppuration* and, in general, implies that neutrophils and their proteolytic enzymes are present and that necrosis of host tissue cells has occurred. Pus itself is composed largely of accumulated dead cells, both tissue cells and inflammatory cells, and usually also contains a variable number of viable leukocytes as well as fluids added by the inflammatory edema-forming process. *Abscesses* are a localized form of suppurative inflammation that frequently are surrounded by a connective tissue capsule, a reaction of the host to "wall off" the lesion. Suppurative lesions are often bacterial in origin.

FIBRINOUS EXUDATION

The increased vascular permeability accompanying acute inflammation permits leakage of large amounts of plasma proteins including fibrinogen into tissues. The fibrinogen may then polymerize into fibrin coagula in the inflamed tissue or body cavities. Fibrin formation is an acute phenomenon, and it takes only seconds for fibrin to form under normal circumstances. This is characteristic of some kinds of inflammation that, not surprisingly, are termed *fibrinous* (Fig. 4-8). An example would be the "shipping-fever" types of pneumonia in beef cattle, which often are decidedly fibrinous in character (Fig. 4-9). Fibrinous pericarditis occurs in cattle in which foreign bodies penetrate the pericardial sac from the reticulum (traumatic reticulopericarditis). One must be careful not to mentally or visually confuse *fibrin* with *fibrosis*, the latter being a chronic event composed of fibroblasts and tough collagen, a "scar." Fibrin, on the other hand, can be identified by the ease with which it can be broken down; that is, if you pull on it, it breaks. Histologically, fibrin is a chaotic, fibrillar meshwork. Fibrin provides a microscopic scaffold for the ingrowth of fibroblasts and neocapillaries, which can eventually transform the fibrinous exudate of an early inflammatory response into the well-vascularized connective tissue seen later, a process known as *organization* of the fibrinous exudate. This can be a harmful sequel, as obliterative scarring may be the result.

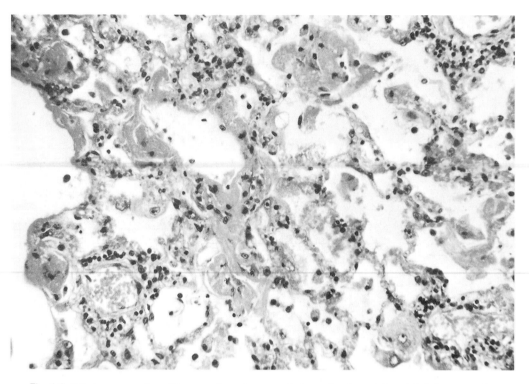

Fig. 4-8 Fibrinous exudate. The strands and accumulations of pale-staining debris here consist largely of fibrin deposits in this acutely inflamed bovine lung.

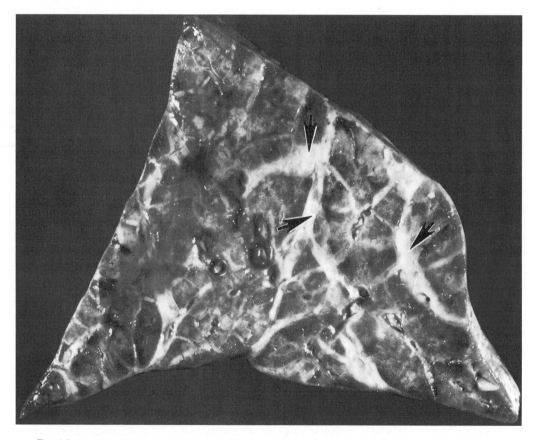

Fig. 4-9 Bovine fibrinous pneumonia. The interlobular deposition of fibrin, *arrows*, is a typical finding in the acute infectious "shipping-fever" pneumonias of cattle.

Much fibrin in acute exudates is, however, dissolved by enzymatic fibrinolysis or by phagocytosis by macrophages before organization can occur. When many neutrophils are present along with fibrin, the exudate is properly termed *fibrinopurulent* or *fibrinosuppurative*.

SEROUS EXUDATION

When inflammatory lesions are characterized by accumulation of fluid relatively rich in protein on body surfaces, especially serous surfaces, the lesion is said to represent serous inflammation. The oozing of clear fluid that results from first- or second-degree burns is a good example of serous inflammation. Blisters are another example. Within the blister is a volume of fluid derived partly from the bloodstream and partly from the locally injured cells. This type of exudate can be characteristic of the very early aspects of some kinds of evolving inflammatory responses.

OTHER TYPES OF EXUDATES

Necrotizing inflammation is characterized largely by necrosis, obviously, and may also have evidence of vascular or leukocytic contributions. When this occurs on an epithelial surface (such as the trachea, intestine, nasal passages) that is well vascularized, serum often oozes out to produce fibrin, and *fibrinonecrotic exudation* results. Such exudates sometimes form thin layers of adhesive debris over their damaged surfaces, which are termed *pseudomembranes*. The term *diphtheritic membranes* was coined to refer to pseudomembranes formed during the human disease of diphtheria. Infectious bovine rhinotracheitis (IBR) often is characterized by a fibrinonecrotic or diphtheritic tracheitis (Fig. 4-10). If hemorrhage is the predominant feature of an inflammatory lesion, the designation *hemorrhagic* inflammation is used. Such lesions are usually acute or peracute and often include necrosis of blood vessels. *Mucoid* exudate obviously consists largely of mucus but often is mixed with neutrophil infiltrates, in which case the lesion is called *mucopurulent*. Such lesions can occur only on mucous membranes where the appropriate secretory cells are present, and a good example of this is inflammation and infection of the nasal cavity. A semisynonym for mucopurulent or mucoid is *catarrhal*, which refers to inflammation of mucous membranes. If the lesion in question is composed largely of eosinophils, as can occur with many kinds of parasitic lesions and some kinds of allergic diseases, then *eosinophilic* inflammation is present. Flea-bite der-

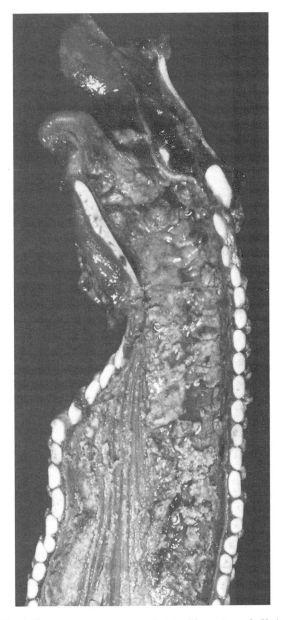

Fig. 4-10 Fibrinonecrotic tracheitis. Necrosis and fibrin deposition on the damaged tracheal mucosa occurs quite commonly in infectious bovine rhinotracheitis. Such lesions also are called "pseudomembranous," or "diphtheritic," tracheitis.

matitis in dogs and cats often has an eosinophilic component.

Lesions in which mononuclear cells, such as macrophages or lymphocytes and plasma cells, predominate are sometimes lumped together with the general term *nonsuppurative*, which is rather nonspecific and merely differentiates these inflammatory reactions from the suppurative lesions in which neutrophils predominate. The virus of canine distemper, for example, produces a nonsuppurative encephalitis. If one type of cell predominates such as the lymphocyte, we usually choose to call it a *lymphocytic* exudate, rather than using the term "nonsuppurative." The viral disease lymphocytic chorio-meningitis is named for its characteristic lymphoid infiltrate, as is lymphocytic thyroiditis.

Granulomatous inflammation is a category that warrants our special attention. Granulomatous inflammation is always chronic and may have variations in histological appearance, but central to the definition of granulomatous inflammation is the presence of *macrophages*. The related term *granuloma* refers to one or more isolated foci or nodules of granulomatous inflammation, which are surrounded by or separated by normal host tissue. A granuloma is merely a subset of the larger category of granulomatous inflammation. The term *granuloma* originally defined the tiny, pale, granular foci that could be seen with the naked eye in tissues as a result of systemic, hematogenous spread of the tuberculosis organism. This was before the invention of the microscope, and the lesions looked "grainy" to early physicians and healers. The term was later redefined according to certain microscopic criteria. At present, granulomatous inflammation refers to an inflammatory response characterized by the presence of numerous macrophages, with a variable number of lymphocytes and with or without plasma cells; the predominant cell is the macrophage. A few other types of leukocytes in smaller numbers, such as neutrophils or eosinophils, may be scattered among the other cells. If numerous neutrophils are present along with the macrophages, we refer to the exudate as *pyogranulomatous*. Macrophages are often clustered in a characteristic semispherical formation around the causative agent or around a central necrotic area (Fig. 4-11). Large cells, larger than the usual macrophages but still with a single nucleus, may appear. These macrophages with abundant cytoplasm are referred to as *epithelioid cells*, or *epithelioid macrophages*, and they are derived from macrophages that have been stimulated at the site of inflammation. Epithelioid macrophages were apparently named by an imaginative microscopist because of their vaguely similar appearance to cells in the lower and middle layers of the epidermis. It also is common to see multinucleated *giant cells* associated with granulomas; these cells are derived from fusion of macrophages. In addition, fibroplasia often is seen around granulomas and within granulomatous inflammation; this is a result of the chronicity of the reaction. The relative amounts of these

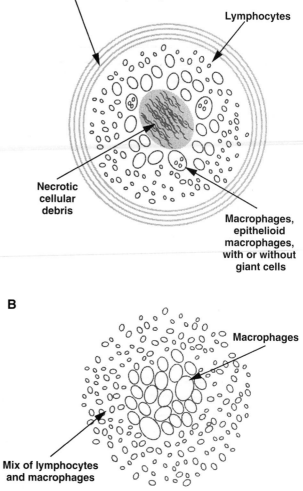

Fig. 4-11 Granulomas. A, Granulomas often contain a central necrotic area surrounded by a variable mixture of macrophages of different morphologic types: regular, epithelioid, and multinucleated giant cells. Lymphocytes appear together with the macrophages, sometimes in greater concentration at the periphery. If the granuloma has been present for a sufficient period of time, the body will usually react with surrounding fibrosis. **B,** Very small or new granulomas may not have a necrotic center or peripheral fibrosis. *(Copyright © The University of Tennessee College of Veterinary Medicine, 2000.)*

various components can vary considerably in different lesions; hence granulomatous inflammation can have a wide range of histological forms and still qualify as granulomatous (Fig. 4-12). Central to this form of inflammation is the presence of some indigestible organism or particle that serves as a chronic inflammatory stimulus. Delayed-type hypersensitivity reactions are the driving immunological mechanism of some granulomas. This is true

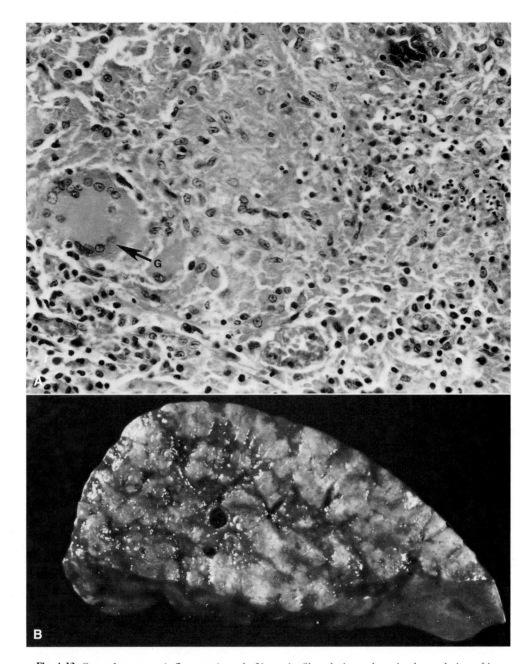

Fig. 4-12 Granulomatous inflammation. A, Necrosis, fibroplasia, and a mixed population of inflammatory cells, including lymphocytes and many macrophages are seen in this section of lung from a tuberculous monkey. Giant cells, *G*, are commonly seen in granulomatous inflammation. **B,** This lung from a case of canine blastomycosis shows numerous irregular pale zones, which represent areas of granulomatous inflammation. The unitized nature of the lesions here and their separation from each other by relatively normal tissue are typical, and each inflamed focus represents a discrete granuloma.

for some of the infectious granulomas, as in tuberculosis, and for granulomas that occasionally form at vaccination sites. This type of inflammation also characterizes the tissue response to certain kinds of microorganisms that tend to be persistent in tissue, including *Mycobacterium, Leishmania,* and some fungal infections, to name just a few.

Generalizations about the various types of inflammatory exudates, and the interpretation of their presence are summarized in Table 4-5.

TABLE 4-5 Types and Significance of Various Inflammatory Exudates

TYPE	COMMENTS/SIGNIFICANCE
PRIMARILY ACUTE REACTIONS	
Suppurative	Often a response to microbes, especially bacteria. Synonym: Purulent.
Purulent	See Suppurative.
Fibrinous	Often seen in combination with purulent lesions.
Fibrinopurulent	Often a response to microbes, especially certain bacteria.
Serous	Usually peracute. The protein-rich and cell-poor fluid is often a result of burns, blisters, etc.
Mucinous/mucoid	Associated with irritation of the respiratory and gastrointestinal tracts, often by microbes. Synonym: Catarrhal.
Mucopurulent	Mucoid/catarrhal and purulent. Usually caused by microbes on respiratory and intestinal surfaces.
Hemorrhagic	Synonym: Sanguineous. Serosanguineous refers to a dilute serum-blood mix.
Necrotizing	Often used in combination with suppurative, hemorrhagic. Toxins from certain microbes can cause this.
ACUTE OR CHRONIC	
Eosinophilic	May be acute, subacute, or chronic. Often a response to allergic or hypersensitivity diseases or to parasites.
USUALLY SUBACUTE, CHRONIC, OR CHRONIC-ACTIVE REACTION	
Granulomatous	Frequently a response to persistent microbes or foreign bodies.
Pyogranulomatous	Similar to granulomatous but may be a slightly "younger" lesion or a chronic-active lesion. Suggestive of certain microbes, including *Blastomyces* species and other fungi.
Lymphocytic, plasmacytic, or lymphoplasmacytic	Can be caused by persistent, nonpyogenic microbes (such as *Mycoplasma*) or other chronic immune stimuli.
Nonsuppurative	Refers to lymphoplasmacytic, granulomatous, or a combination of both.

MANIFESTATIONS OF ACUTE INFLAMMATION

Acute inflammation may produce clinical signs localized to the site of injury or may be accompanied by profound systemic changes. For example, an infected cut on the digit usually causes only local signs, whereas bronchopneumonia may produce not only local signs but also a significant systemic reaction, including leukocytosis and fever. The local clinical signs of inflammation have been mentioned previously and classically have been characterized as heat, redness, swelling, pain, and loss of function (see Table 4-2). The local heat and redness are the result of dilatation of the microcirculation in the local environment of the injury. The swelling is largely produced by the escape of fluid ("inflammatory edema") containing plasma proteins and other solutes from the blood to the perivascular tissues. Leukocytes also escape, and the high protein content of the fluid with the presence of leukocytes is known as *exudation*. The origin of the pain is multifactorial but can be attributed to irritation of local nerves by biochemical mediators. Function is usually a result of physiological and anatomic normalcy of the various cells and tissues, and it is reasonable to conclude that damaged and inflamed tissues should exhibit some degree of loss of function if the problem is severe enough.

We mentioned previously the terms "exudate" and "transudate" (Table 4-6). An *exudate* is an extravascular fluid with a high content of proteins, cellular debris, and leukocytes; it is usually a result of inflammation. The white blood cells and cellular debris within it impart the yellow-white appearance of pus; the medical term is a "purulent" or "suppurative exudate." In contrast, a *transudate* is a low-protein fluid that is essentially an ultrafiltrate of the blood plasma consisting primarily of water, small proteins, and dissolved electrolytes. A *modified transudate* occupies the middle ground between these parameters. The origin and role of transudates and exudates in inflammation will become more clear as our discussion progresses.

With regard to inflammation, there is some correlation between the severity of the injury and the

TABLE 4-6 Exudates and Transudates

CHARACTERISTIC	EXUDATE	PURE TRANSUDATE
Appearance	Turbid to opaque; variable color	Clear or lightly colored
Etiology	Inflammation, occasionally neoplasia	Hemodynamic imbalances
Protein content	>3 g/dL	<3 g/dL
Clottable	Sometimes	Rarely
Nucleated cells/μL	>1500*	<1500
Bacteria	Sometimes	Almost never

*>5000 cells/μL are present before an exudate is suspected in horses.

TABLE 4-7 Sequence of Events in Acute Inflammation

EVENT	MECHANISM
Transient vasoconstriction (usually lasts a few seconds)	Neurogenic
Vasodilatation (begins in a few minutes and lasts minutes, hours, or longer)	Release of histamine from mast cells and generation of nitric oxide and prostaglandins (PGD_2, PGE_2).
Increased volume of blood flow in the area	A result of vasodilatation.
Increased vascular permeability	Histamine, leukotrienes C_4, D_4, E_4, bradykinin, and platelet activating factor (PAF) cause "contraction" of endothelial cells resulting in gaps in the small vessels. C5a and C3a indirectly participate by inducing release of histamine by mast cells.
Rate/speed of flow decreases	Caused by vasodilatation in the area.
Margination of leukocytes along vessel walls	The decreased rate of flow results in decreased shear force on WBC as they contact the vessel wall. As a result, adhesion molecules on WBC and endothelial cells are able to remain engaged. Adhesion molecules also are upregulated in numbers or avidity in many cases. When vascular permeability is significantly increased, more protein leaks into tissue.
Exudation	WBCs migrate out into the tissue.

composition of the inflammatory fluid. Even very mild injuries can produce a protein-poor watery transudate. With progressively more potent injurious stimuli, the inflammatory fluid will acquire higher and higher concentrations of plasma proteins, red blood cells, and white blood cells and will become an exudate. This local manifestation of acute inflammation highlights *three major parts of the inflammatory response:* (1) hemodynamic changes, (2) permeability changes, and (3) events involving leukocytes. Each of these is discussed separately, but we must emphasize that such a separation is arbitrary. The hemodynamic changes that first signal the inflammatory response are followed very soon thereafter by alterations in the permeability of the affected vessels and by reactions involving white blood cells. Overlap in these three aspects of the reaction results in a continuum of events.

Vascular Events in Inflammation

HEMODYNAMIC CHANGES

Most of the local signs of inflammation arise from changes in the microcirculatory bed in the area of the injury. The hemodynamic alterations are an integrated chain of events activated by biochemical mediators but in some cases are transiently initiated by neurogenic mechanisms. These vascular events are usually manifested in the following order (Table 4-7):

1. Arteriolar dilatation, sometimes preceded by transient vasoconstriction.
2. Increased volume of blood flow through the arterioles.
3. Opening of additional capillary and venular beds in the area to accommodate the increased flow.

4. Congestion of the veins.
5. Increased permeability of the microvasculature with the outpouring of fluid into the extravascular tissues.
6. This results in a modest concentration of red blood cells in the capillaries and venules.
7. If the concentration progresses, this can result in slowing or stasis of blood flow in these small vessels.
8. Meanwhile, peripheral margination of white blood cells in the capillaries and venules increases.
9. This results in a sequence of subsequent white blood cell events (adhesion, chemotaxis, phagocytosis, and so on) if the inflammation is severe enough to warrant these leukocyte events.

Many of these changes begin at the same time but develop at varying rates depending on the severity of the injury. In virtually all inflammatory reactions, dilatation of arterioles associated with increased blood flow through the capillaries and venules occurs (Fig. 4-13). This is the *acute local active hyperemia of inflammation* associated with the opening of precapillary sphincters and the active perfusion of additional capillaries and venules; it also results from the dilatation of these small vessels. Overload of the venous drainage can lead to congestion of these vessels, which contributes to the vasodilatation. By this time, the permeability of the microcirculation usually has been altered, and fluid begins to leak out of the vessels. This leakage may at first be strictly a watery transudate, but, in significant inflammatory responses, the progressive increase in permeability—as a result of endothelial cell contraction and creation of microgaps in the venules—permits the escape of larger macromolecules, forming a protein-rich exudate. The magnitude of this event follows a simple rule: "The greater the extent of acute inflammation, the greater the leakage." In severe cases, the loss of plasma fluid from the bloodstream in the small vessels causes local hemoconcentration, and the small vessels contain crowded erythrocytes, which move at a decreased rate of speed. The slowing of blood flow facilitates the adhesive interactions between activated leukocytes and endothelial cells, and an increased number of white cells assume a peripheral orientation along the endothelial surfaces of the affected vessels. We discuss the mechanisms of this event soon. The *venules* are the principal participants in the early phases of this evolving acute inflammatory drama; capillaries play a larger role in the latter phases, particularly in more severe injuries.

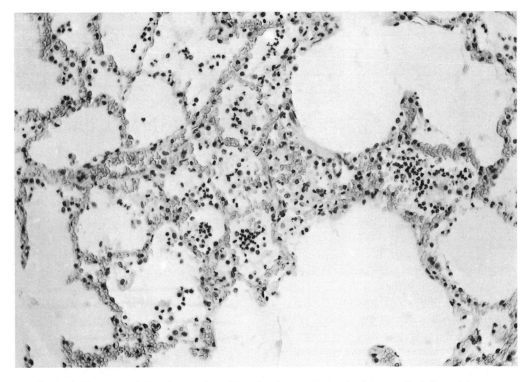

Fig. 4-13 Hyperemia of inflammation. The alveolar capillaries in this acutely inflamed bovine lung are engorged with blood. This is the acute, local, active hyperemia typical of inflammation.

PERMEABILITY CHANGES

The leakage of fluid that occurs as a consequence of changes in the permeability of the microvasculature is a major characteristic of virtually all acute inflammatory reactions. The fluid is at first a watery transudate or plasma ultrafiltrate when the endothelial gaps are small (edema), but the permeability changes within the venules and capillaries soon permit the escape of more and larger plasma proteins, leukocytes, and sometimes red blood cells. This protein-rich, cell-containing exudate appears in all but the most trivial of inflammatory responses. Transudation often attends noninflammatory congestion of vessels, as in the edema accompanying congestive heart failure, but exudation *often* indicates inflammation. (Note: Some kinds of cancer, such as lymphosarcoma, can also result in accumulation of an exudate; for example, protein-rich fluid and exfoliated neoplastic cells can accumulate in body cavities.)

Understanding the pathogenesis of inflammatory exudation requires an understanding of the normal permeability of the microcirculation. Adjacent endothelial cells have cell junctions with a potential space existing between contiguous cells (Fig. 4-14). This varies depending on the type of endothelium. Using particles of known molecular size visible in electron micrographs, investigators have been able to demonstrate filtration of small proteins through the normal intercellular junctions whereas larger molecules are withheld.

Passage of fluid between the endothelial cells implies a passive role for the endothelium in the exchange of fluids. This is not entirely true. Endothelial cells have, on their luminal surfaces, small invaginations (caveolae) that become pinched off to create small endocytotic *vesicles* containing plasma. Transport of these vesicles across the endothelial cell with discharge of the contents on the other side constitutes an active-transport mechanism. It is likely that this contributes to the limited passage of the large protein macromolecules characteristic of normal interstitial fluid.

Two major mechanisms are operative in the development of edema at sites of acute inflammation. The first is purely hydrostatic, and the second involves alterations in vascular permeability effected by the biochemical mediators of inflammation. Remember that arteriolar dilatation leads to an increased volume of blood flow in inflamed tissues. Accompanied by congestion of the venous drainage and increased hydrostatic pressures, this forces fluid, essentially an ultrafiltrate of plasma relatively free of protein, out of the vessels. Some protein may

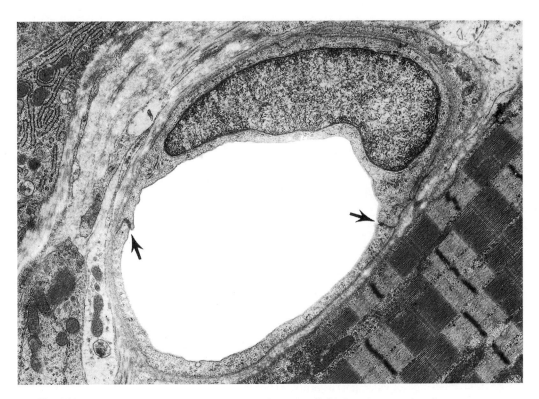

Fig. 4-14 Capillary endothelium. It is through the intercellular junctions, *arrows*, that serum proteins and leukocytes pass to gain entry to inflamed tissue.

escape but not enough to produce a characteristic exudate. Exudation soon follows transudation, however, as the permeability of the microcirculation increases. Using experimental techniques with intravascular tracers, investigators have demonstrated varying patterns in the rise and ebb of increased permeability. These responses have been classified into different phases of altered permeability (Fig. 4-15).

Histamine secreted by mast cells is an important mediator of the first phase of increased vascular permeability as well as leukotrienes C_4, D_4, E_4, serotonin (only in rodent mast cells), and platelet-activating factor (PAF). All these mediators are either preformed and stored in cells for rapid release, such as histamine in mast cells, or can be synthesized very rapidly. The early phase of vascular permeability can be responsive to treatment with antihistamines, underscoring the importance of this mediator. The histamine-dependent phase can be transient. If the inflammation is severe enough, within 2 to 4 hours a prolonged and quite different phase occurs. In contrast to the histamine-dependent phase, the secondary phase is prolonged, lasting over the next 3 to 4 hours or more. It is during this period that leukocytes begin to migrate out of blood vessels. No single mediator is responsible for this second, more prolonged phase of permeability increases. A large number of different chemical mediators of inflammation can evoke increased vascular permeability in this phase (Table 4-8) as we discuss in greater detail later (see Other Biochemical Mediators of Inflamma-

TABLE 4-8 Mediators of Vascular Permeability

TYPE OF MEDIATOR	COMMENTS AND CHARACTERISTICS
Vasoactive amines	Histamine, serotonin; stored in granules of mast cells, basophils, and platelets.
Plasma kinins	Generated from plasma precursors by enzymatic cleavage. The principal vasoactive kinin is bradykinin. Activated by plasma proteinases, including Hageman factor (XIIa).
Complement fragments (anaphylatoxins C5a and C3a)	They work indirectly by inducing mediator release from leukocytes, e.g., mast cells.
Leukotrienes	Some work independent of PMN (LTC$_4$, LTD$_4$, LTE$_4$), but LTB$_4$ can provoke PMN-dependent permeability changes.
Prostaglandins	PGE$_2$ and PGI$_2$ cause vasodilatation and potentiate vascular leakage. Thromboxane A$_2$ causes vascular leakage.
Some cytokines (IL-1, TNF-α)	Induce the "second phase" of vascular leakage; derived from leukocytes.
Platelet-activating factor	Has actions on endothelium and on leukocytes.

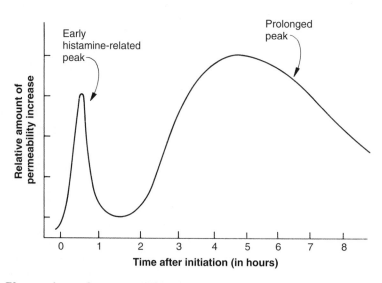

Fig. 4-15 Phases of vascular permeability. Antihistamines can eliminate or diminish the first peak of increased permeability but have little effect on the second, more prolonged, phase of vascular leakage in which cytokines and other mediators play a role.

tion, p. 206). The *leukocytes* also participate to a lesser extent in the mediation of vascular permeability by virtue of their activity of secreting mediators upon the endothelial cells and perhaps to a very minor extent by physically leaving the small blood vessels by opening and squeezing through inter–endothelial cell gaps and the basement membrane.

These phases of increased vascular permeability are associated with the loss of fluids from the blood, not through endothelial cells but *between* endothelial cells. Electron microscopic studies with tracer molecules have elegantly documented how proteins, electrolytes, and water percolate through the junctional zones between endothelial cells, through the basement membrane of the vessel, and into the area around the blood vessel. As just mentioned, the same is true for leukocytes. They normally migrate between endothelial cells, not through them.

In summary, vascular leakage after local injury can occur by two distinct mechanisms: (1) *directly,* as an effect of any kind of structural injury to the microvasculature, or (2) *indirectly,* as an effect of biochemical substances that appear in and around the site and affect the walls of small vessels (Fig. 4-16). Vascular labeling techniques show that direct injury

can affect all types of vessels (arterioles, capillaries, and venules), a statement that seems obvious, whereas indirect, biochemically mediated vascular leakage shows a high degree of specificity for the venules. Since much of the inflammatory response is dependent on biochemical mediators, the venules are the primary anatomic site for inflammation-related leakage. An example of this is that bacteria in the tissue produce and release substances that activate resident tissue macrophages; a good example is endotoxin (LPS, lipopolysaccharide) released from the cell wall of gram-negative bacteria. This results in activation of the tissue macrophages and synthesis and secretion of vasoactive mediators, such as cytokines, and vascular leakage from venules ensues. Last, some of the leakage induced in the venules can be neutrophil mediated because these cells leave the small blood vessels en route to the offending bacteria.

Thus, chemical mediators of vascular permeability in acute inflammation can exert their effects either by direct effects on the microvasculature (such as histamine and the leukotrienes C_4, D_4, and E_4) or by use of the leukocytes as an intermediary (such as cytokines) (Figs. 4-16 and 4-17). The redundancy of

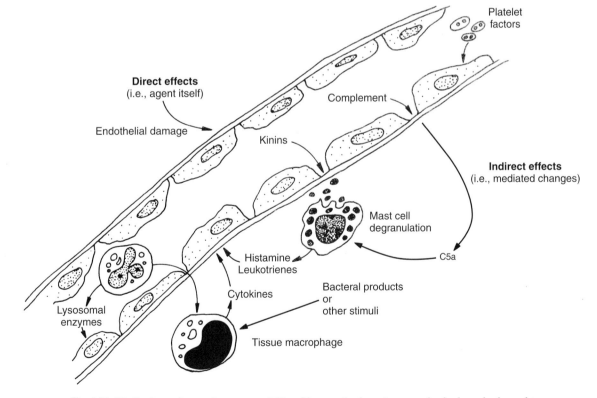

Fig. 4-16 Mediation of vascular permeability. Changes in the microvascular bed can be brought about directly by injury to the endothelium or indirectly by means of mediators generated from both cellular and plasma sources. Some mediators work directly on the endothelium, whereas others employ neutrophils as a cellular intermediary.

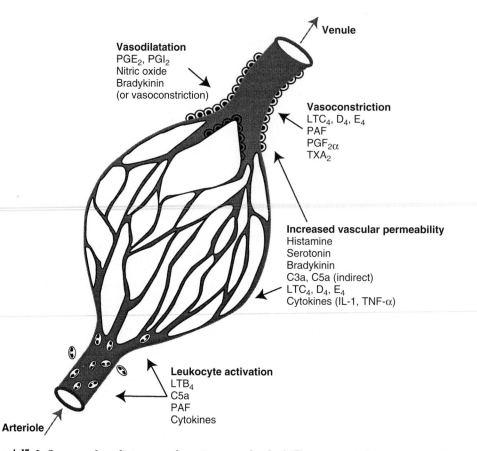

Fig. 4-17 Influence of mediators on the microvascular bed. The various inflammatory mediators work at different levels to influence both vascular dilatation and constriction as well as permeability and may function by means of different mechanisms. PGE_2 can potentiate vascular leakage by causing vasodilatation. The vasoactive amines and others can cause increased permeability directly, whereas some mediators (LTB_4, C5a) promote leukocyte-dependent increased permeability. *(Copyright © The University of Tennessee College of Veterinary Medicine, 2000.)*

ways to increase vascular permeability ensures its presence in an evolving inflammatory reaction.

CELLS OF THE INFLAMMATORY EXUDATE

The basic groups of leukocytes that take part in inflammatory reactions are neutrophils, eosinophils, basophils, and granulocytes, mast cells, monocytes and macrophages, and lymphocytes and plasma cells. All these leukocytes, save the plasma cells and mast cells, are normal inhabitants of the circulating blood, and the relative proportions of the different white blood cells may be greatly modified in systemic responses to inflammation. Each cell type plays a fairly distinctive role and enters into the inflammatory response in response to specific stimuli as we have indicated previously. The discussion that follows will be concerned principally with the

major characteristics of these different types of leukocytes.

Granulocytes: Red, White, and Blue

The term "granulocyte" derives from the fact that these cells have recognizable granules in their cytoplasm. The *eosinophil* has eosinophilic (red) granules as a result of a chemical affinity for the red eosin stain. The *basophil* has (blue) basophilic granules as a result of its liking for basic dyes such as hematoxylin. The *neutrophil* has granules that take neither type of dye very well and hence are "neutral." Notice that this is true for human neutrophils, from which the name was coined, but some of our veterinary species have neutrophils that take up some of the red eosin stain, albeit less avidly than eosinophils. Nevertheless, we have followed and also adopted the name "neutrophil." These cells also are sometimes referred to as *polymorphonuclear* leukocytes because their nuclei are multilobed, in contrast to the mononuclear lymphocytes, monocytes, and plasma cells. In practical usage, however, the terms "polymorphonuclear leukocyte"—a real mouthful—or simply "polymorph," "poly," or "PMN," refer to neutrophils.

NEUTROPHILS

These cells are usually the first leukocytes to gather at sites of acute inflammation, and their specialty is killing microbes. Like all the granulocytes, neutrophils develop in the bone marrow, arising from a population of hematopoietic stem cells. Maturation proceeds through stages, beginning with myeloblasts and proceeding to promyelocyte, myelocyte, metamyelocyte, juvenile or band forms, and eventually mature neutrophils called "segs" (those with a segmented nucleus). This maturation process usually takes about 2 weeks but can be speeded up when the demand for circulating neutrophils is high. When demand is high, as in severe stress situations, even immature neutrophils such as bands can be released to the peripheral blood. Once released from the bone marrow, mature neutrophils remain in the circulation for only a short time (less than a day, on average) and then migrate into tissues where they may survive for up to 1 to 2 days. Radiolabeling studies have shown that this is a one-way ticket; once neutrophils leave the vasculature to enter tissue, they do not return to the circulation. Neutrophils do not have the ability to divide and give rise to new cells once they have been released from the bone marrow. There are normally two functional pools of neutrophils in the blood, a *marginated* (or marginal) pool, consisting of cells within the lumen of blood vessels but closely apposed to the walls, and a *circulating* pool, which is the free-flowing one we sample when drawing blood. Margination along vessel walls, primarily in the microcirculation and especially in the postcapillary venules, is a dynamic event. Some of the leukocytes transiently slow down and roll along the endothelial surface, an interaction largely controlled by adhesion molecules (discussed in detail later). They may then go on to migrate into tissues (if inflammation is present) or quickly release and return to the mainstream blood flow. Any pharmacological or biochemical mediator that affects the level of leukocyte or endothelial cell function can affect the balance between the marginated and circulating pool. Highly stimulated leukocytes and endothelial cells (as by cytokines) will bear activated adhesion molecules on their surface, and the balance will shift to the marginal pool in a localized area of inflamed tissue. Drugs that suppress leukocyte function (such as corticosteroids) promote systemic loss of adhesiveness, release of leukocytes, and their return to the central pool (Fig. 4-18).

Neutrophils range from about 10 to 12 μm in diameter, have polymorphonuclear characteristics, and contain abundant cytoplasmic granules, which are membrane-bound small bags of enzymes and other proteins. This last morphological feature of neutrophils is suggestive of some of their major functions. When the granules fuse with the membrane surrounding phagocytized particles, the membranes of the granules and the membrane surrounding the particle also fuse. The *phagolysosome* therefore not only contains the newly delivered granule contents such as proteinases and antibacterial substances, but it also expresses the membrane contents of the granule. The same is true of shared membrane content when granules fuse with the plasma membrane of the leukocytes, as when the leukocyte is discharging its granule contents outside of the cells; that is, granule membrane content is now expressed in the cell membrane. This is important because some of the granules contain receptors that can be moved and therefore "upregulated" on the surface of the leukocyte.

Ultrastructurally, neutrophils are characterized by a scarcity of organelles, except for the granules. The mature neutrophil contains little endoplasmic reticulum, a small Golgi apparatus, and a few small mitochondria; glycogen is present in the cytoplasm as an energy source (Fig. 4-19). Their synthetic ability is relatively small, consistent with their short lives and their provision of preformed granule content. Two, three, four, or five classes or subclasses of granules (or compartments) have been identified in neutrophils of various species, depending on the amount of research that has been done, species differences, and perhaps the willingness of scientists to subdivide. We consider and briefly discuss the five-compartment/granule model, since it seems possible that neutrophils of many other species may also have this many types and some just await discovery. (The species currently identified with five or so is humans.) Each of the major granule types has a different profile of enzymes (Table 4-9), and the enzyme profile can also vary with species; Table 4-9 lists generalities of three of the granule types. Also notice that the different granules appear at different stages of neutrophil development in the bone marrow, and the azurophil, or primary, granules are the first to appear.

Normal conditions in microcirculation

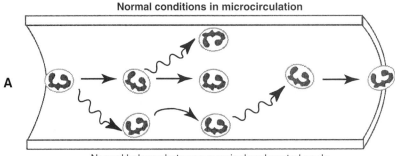

Normal balance between marginal and central pools

Local inflammation

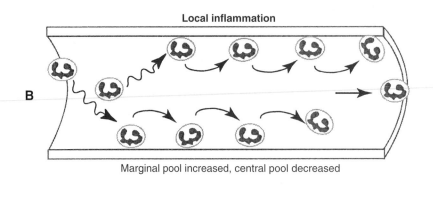

Marginal pool increased, central pool decreased

Corticosteroids

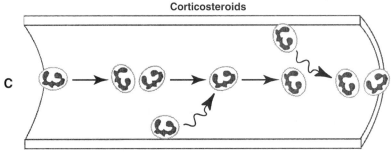

Central pool increased, marginal pool decreased

Fig. 4-18 The marginated and circulating pools of neutrophils in the peripheral vasculature. **A, B,** and **C,** Local conditions in the tissue or systemic administration of some drugs may affect the balance between the marginated and circulating pools. (Copyright © The University of Tennessee College of Veterinary Medicine, 2000.)

The *azurophil*, or primary, granules are large, oval, and electron dense. The *specific*, or secondary, granules are smaller, less dense, and more numerous. Study of the granules used to be simpler, since only these two types were known. Now, the azurophil granules may be divided into two groups; one group contains large quantities of the antibacterial peptides called "defensins," or "beta-defensins" (in cattle), and the other group does not, but their enzyme profile does not otherwise vary much. The defining characteristic of the azurophil granules is the presence of myeloperoxidase, an important component of one of the oxygen-dependent micro-

bicidal systems (discussed later). The specific/secondary granules do not contain myeloperoxidase but, as seen in Table 4-9, contain plenty of other things. One of their components, cytochrome *b*, is essential for production of microbicidal oxygen radicals in the phagolysosome (also discussed later, in the section on oxygen- and non–oxygen dependent microbicidal mechanisms.) Another type of granule has been identified in neutrophils from many species, and they have been referred to as "tertiary granules," or "gelatinase granules"; they were discovered third, after azurophil and specific granules. Gelatinase, a extracellular matrix-

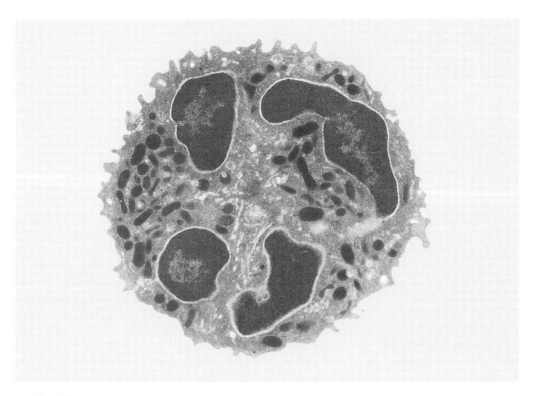

Fig. 4-19 Neutrophil. The segmented nucleus and numerous lysosomal granules in the cytoplasm of this sheep neutrophil are typical of this kind of granulocyte.

TABLE 4-9 Some of the Neutrophil Granule Constituents

AZUROPHIL GRANULES†	SPECIFIC GRANULES	TERTIARY (GELATINASE) GRANULES
Myeloperoxidase*	Collagenase (MMP-8)	
Elastase	Gelatinase (MMP-9)	Gelatinase (MMP-9)
Lysozyme*	Lysozyme*	Lysozyme*
Cathepsin G and several other cathepsins	Histaminase	
	Heparinase	
Proteinase-3	Cytochrome *b**	Cytochrome *b**
β-Glucuronidase	Lactoferrin	
α-Mannosidase	Vitamin B_{12}—binding protein*	
Defensins*	TNF-α receptor	
Bactericidal/permeability-increasing protein (BPI)*	CD11b/CD18 β_2-integrin (adhesion molecules)	CD11b/CD18 β_2-integrin (adhesion molecules)
	Urokinase plasminogen activator (uPA)	
	uPA receptor	uPA receptor

This table is not intended to be a specific or complete listing of granule content applicable to all species.
*These constituents have a function more specifically directed to microbicidal activity.
†Azurophil granules can also be subdivided into two types in some species, based on the finding that some are rich in defensins and some contain little or no defensins.
Abbreviations: *MMP*, matrix metalloproteinase; *TNF*, tumor necrosis factor.

dissolving enzyme, is quantitatively their greatest component, though they also contain cytochrome *b*–like specific granules. A last type may not technically be a granule; it does not contain enzymes. This compartment is called a "secretory vesicle." The se-cretory vesicles are rich in receptors and also contain some plasma, alkaline phosphatase, urokinase plasminogen activator (uPA), and a few other chemicals. Receptors in the secretory vesicles include complement receptor-1 (CR1), CD11b/CD18 (a type of adhesion molecule), CD14 (an endotoxin receptor), and others. The secretory vesicles are considered to be the most easily and quickly mobilized of the granules, and when swiftly fused with the plasma membrane of the neutrophil, the cell has increased amounts of complement receptors and adhesion molecules (CD11b/CD18), to name just two, presumably becoming a more highly responsive cell to surface stimuli. The relative ease or speed with which the various granules or compartments can be mobilized in neutrophils is believed to be: (fastest) secretory vesicles > gelatinase granules > specific granules > azurophilic granules. Other novel granule constituents in granules have been and are still being identified, and Table 4-9 should be viewed as a primer.

Proteinases

This is a good place to digress and discuss proteinases in leukocyte granules. The array of proteinases and other enzymes present in leukocytes varies depending on the type of leukocyte, such as a neutrophil, macrophage, or mast cell. Because of this complexity, we initially focus much of this discussion on the enzymes in the neutrophil. But keep in mind that many or most of the enzymes, such as collagenase, are present in more than just one type of leukocyte. Also keep in mind that the type of enzyme, the quantity of the enzyme, and probably the granule location of the particular enzyme in leukocytes can vary somewhat depending on the species of animal. Hence the following information discusses generalities that do not hold true for every kind of creature; bear this in mind when looking at Table 4-9 or other sources.

The proteinases can be classified in several different ways, the biochemical nature of their active site, the substrate or substrates they prefer, or the pH at which they work most efficiently, such as "acid hydrolases." Although the literature seems to use a mixture of these schemes, it is worth mentioning the classification according to the biochemical nature of their active sites. These four classes of leukocyte proteinases are serine, metallo-, cysteine, and aspartic proteinases. The serine proteinases have a catalytically essential serine residue at their active site, hence the name. Overall, they constitute the largest class of mammalian proteinases. These and also the metalloproteinases are most active at a near-neutral pH (7-9) and serve well to degrade extracellular matrix proteins. The pH at which activity occurs is important because it varies tremendously between the inside of a phagolysosome (acid environment) versus the extracellular matrix tissue.

Serine proteinases in neutrophils include leukocyte elastase (also in macrophages, eosinophils, and mast cells), cathepsin G (also in macrophages), proteinase-3 (also in macrophages and mast cells), and urokinase-type plasminogen activator (uPA, also in macrophages). As you can see, many of the proteinases are in more than just one type of leukocyte, which is a general truism. Elastase, cathepsin G, and proteinase-3 are stored in *active* form in granules, or lysosomes, and do not require limited cleavage for activation, but most of the other enzymes do.

By the way, the names for some of these enzymes are a little misleading. Leukocyte elastase implies that the substrate for this enzyme is elastin, of course. That's true, but it can work on many substrates other than elastin including several types of collagen, fibronectin, laminin, various plasma proteins, and other substrates. The same tenet of multiplicity of substrates and action is true of most of the other leukocyte proteinases.

The matrix metalloproteinases (MMPs) rely upon Zn^{++} and Ca^{++} for full activity, thus the latter part of their name. The first part of their name, "matrix," refers to the fact that this group of enzymes is specialized for degrading extracellular matrix (ECM) proteins, the structural proteins between the cells. There are many enzymes in the MMP family, and taken as a group, they can degrade just about any structural protein in the ECM. They include neutrophil collagenase (MMP-8), which is also present in eosinophils, and a gelatinase (MMP-9) present in neutrophils and macrophages. Gelatinases not only degrade many different types of collagen, elastin, and other substrates but also further degrade "gelatins," which are defined as already partially degraded collagens ("Jell-O"). Macrophages but not neutrophils also contain another collagenase (MMP-1, also in eosinophils), another gelatinase (MMP-2), several stromelysins (MMP-3, -10, -11), matrilysin (MMP-7), and another type of elastase (metalloelastase, MMP-12). All MMPs are secreted from the leukocytes as proenzymes (zymogens) and require extracellular activation by enzymes such as plasmin, cathepsin G, or bacterial proteinases to achieve activity. Besides their activity in inflammation *per se,* they are important in degrading and the subsequent remodeling of tissue, as occurs during wound repair.

The cysteine proteinases and aspartic proteinases are most active at acid pH (pH 3-6 and 2-5 respectively) as in phagolysosomes and in localized tissue sites loaded with inflammation-associated acidity. They are named because of the requirement for a particular amino acid for their catalytic activity.

They include cathepsins B, D, H, L, and S, which are contained in the lysosomes of most leukocytes.

The proteinases in leukocytes participate in many different activities, including degradation of phagocytized particles, degradation of extracellular matrix proteins (important in wound repair, as mentioned), and enzymatic activation of other proteins, such as complement components. If all this happens according to plan, these enzymes behave as useful and helpful components of our immune system. But what keeps these proteinases under control; what keeps them from spreading to other sites and damaging our tissues? Antiproteinases. Our bodies and those of our patients are replete with a range of antiproteinases, which are designed to contain and confine the actions of the proteinases to a given locale. The most universal of the antiproteinases is alpha$_2$-macroglobulin; it is produced in the liver, circulates in the plasma, and inhibits all four classes of leukocyte proteinases. Serine proteinase inhibitors, or serpins, are abundant in plasma and include alpha$_1$-proteinase inhibitor, plasminogen-activator inhibitors, antithrombin III, and others. The MMPs are inhibited by the tissue inhibitors of metalloproteinases (TIMPs), which are synthesized by leukocytes and other cells of the connective tissues.

Back to our discussion of neutrophils. Neutrophils constitute a major cellular defense system of all higher organisms against bacteria and are a big part of the "innate" immune system, which does not rely on prior exposure and sensitization to a microbe for activity. They are well equipped for their job by virtue of their motility, responsiveness to chemotactic stimuli, phagocytic abilities, and bactericidal activities. A major function of neutrophils in the inflammatory response involves their participation in phagocytosis, the release of their lytic lysosomal enzymes, and the formation of chemotactic factors. Certain complement components can be activated by neutrophil enzymes, yielding chemoattractants for more neutrophils (such as C5a), and neutrophils produce leukotriene B$_4$ (see the discussion of arachidonic acid cascade, p. 212) providing for a cyclic reaction of neutrophil attraction and activation.

The purpose of phagocytosis is to ingest, neutralize, and, whenever possible, destroy the ingested particle; in essence, the neutrophils are well-designed little killers. This function is accomplished with the aid of intracellular substances located within the granules of the neutrophil. The enzymes and other substances in neutrophil granules (known as "lysosomes") are numerous (Table 4-9 and Box 4-2), and many of the enzymes in the granules are proteolytic and digestive in nature. When neu-

BOX 4-2 Partial List of the Array of Enzymes and Other Substances in Lysosomes of Various Leukocytes

ENZYMES ACTING ON PROTEINS

Cathepsins (B, D, G, H, L, S)
Collagenases (matrix metalloproteinases (MMP-1, -8)
Gelatinases (MMP-2, -9)
Leukocyte elastase
Metalloelastase (MMP-12)
Urokinase plasminogen activator
Tryptase
Chymase
Matrilysin (MMP-7)
Stromelysins (MMP-3, -10, -11)
Granzymes (NK cells and cytotoxic T lymphocytes)

ENZYMES ACTING ON CARBOHYDRATES

β-Acetylgalactosaminidase
α-Acetylglucosaminidase
α-Galactosidase
β-Galactosidase
α-Glucosidase
β-Glucosidase
β-Glucuronidase
α-L-Fucosidase
β-D-Fucosidase
Hyaluronidase
Lysozyme
α-Mannosidase
Neuraminidase

ENZYMES ACTING ON LIPIDS

Acid lipase
Cholesterol esterase
Glucocerebrosidase
Galactocerebrosidase
Phospholipase A$_1$
Phospholipase A$_2$

ENZYMES ACTING ON NUCLEIC ACIDS

Acid deoxyribonuclease
Acid ribonuclease

MISCELLANY

Acid phosphatase
Anticoagulants
Arylsulfatase
Myeloperoxidase
Peroxidase
Phosphodiesterase
Phosphoprotein phosphatase
Antimicrobial peptides and proteins (bactericidal permeability–increasing protein [BPI], defensins)
Some cytokines

trophils ingest bacteria or other particulate material, a cell membrane wraps around the particle forming *phagosomes*. These fuse with the lysosomes to form *phagolysosomes*, and in this process the particle is subject to attack and subsequent digestion. Videomicroscopy has allowed demonstration of fusion of the lysosomes with the phagosomes and discharge of the granule contents into the phagolysosome, and this is similar in appearance to fusion of small soap bubbles with a larger one. As mentioned, many of the lysosomal enzymes do not actually participate in bacterial killing but rather serve as digestive enzymes to degrade bacteria that have already been phagocytized and killed by means of both oxygen-dependent and oxygen-independent mechanisms. We discuss phagocytosis and the mechanisms of bacterial killing soon.

EOSINOPHILS

Eosinophils are particularly abundant at sites of allergic, parasitic, or certain types of fungal inflammatory disease, but they can be part of any exudate. Their significance in such tissue reactions is related to their unique function as effector cells for damaging or killing helminths and other pathogens and their propensity for both causing and assisting in the regulation of hypersensitivity diseases, particularly type I hypersensitivity reactions. The eosinophils are phagocytic but are less active phagocytes than neutrophils, and they are distinguished from the neutrophils in routine stains by the great affinity of their large cytoplasmic granules for the red dye eosin. Eosinophils have a shape and nuclear morphology similar to those of neutrophils. The eosinophil granules vary considerably in size from species to species, with the equine granules being the largest. The eosinophil leukocytes of the horse contain 25 to 50 granules, each approximately 1 μm in diameter, whereas those of the rat have up to 400 granules, measuring only about 0.2 μm. The eosinophil granules of virtually all species have the commonality of containing crystalloid structures (Fig. 4-20).

Eosinophils make up a variable percentage (1%-5%) of the total circulating leukocytes. They are produced in the bone marrow, and their differentiation and maturation are particularly dependent on three cytokines, IL-3, IL-5, and GM-CSF. IL-5 is particularly important ("eosinophil differentiation factor") and stimulates release of eosinophils from

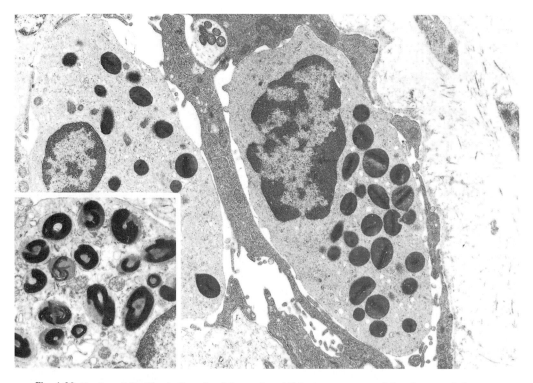

Fig. 4-20 Eosinophils. The hallmark of the eosinophil is the structure of the characteristic cytoplasmic granules, which have a dense central core. This dense core is the source of "major basic protein," an important eosinophil constituent. These eosinophils are from a rhesus monkey. To show the variation in granules between species, feline eosinophil granules are shown in the inset. *(Courtesy Drs. W.L. Castleman, Gainesville, Fla., and J.M. Ward, Bethesda, Md.)*

the bone marrow. In tissues, they are found mainly in contact areas within the external environment, such as the intestinal wall, lungs, skin, and mucous membranes, though other sites are also possible. This makes sense, since these are frequent anatomic locations for parasitic disease (such as intestine) and Type I hypersensitivity reactions (such as skin or lung). Eosinophils are influenced by glucocorticosteroids, and increased secretion of them or therapeutic administration can result in eosinopenia, attributable in part to transient inhibition of the release of eosinophils from the bone marrow.

Some of the enzymes demonstrable in neutrophils and macrophages are also found in eosinophils, including collagenases (MMP-1, -8) and leukocyte elastase. Hence eosinophils have the capability of degrading extracellular matrix proteins. When gathered in large numbers, eosinophils can degrade masses of collagen in the dermis, as seen in the eosinophilic granulomas of domestic species, including horses, dogs, and cats. Importantly, eosinophil granules also contain several granule proteins that are not components or not significant components of neutrophils. These include *major basic protein* and *eosinophil cationic protein,* which are antiparasitic

in function. Eosinophils can adhere to helminths and degranulate against them, thus bringing the helminthotoxic proteins into play (Fig. 4-21). As already mentioned, eosinophils have a remarkable ultrastructural feature, in that large cytoplasmic granules, as a class, are composed of a crystalloid core surrounded by a less-dense matrix. The predominant protein of the core is major basic protein, which constitutes about 50% of the granule protein content and is strongly cationic, meaning that it interacts with negatively charged surfaces of its targets by virtue of its strong positive charge. Major basic protein has several functions: it binds to parasites and is toxic to them as well as some other kinds of cells, it can cause histamine release from mast cells and basophils, and it can neutralize heparin. The other helminthotoxic eosinophil granule protein, eosinophil cationic protein, also reacts with the negative surface charge of some parasites. In addition, it also has other functions, including shortening coagulation time and altering fibrinolysis (Table 4-10).

We discuss mast cells soon, but it is germane to also mention them here in this section on eosinophils. Activation of mast cells in allergic or parasitic disease leads to the elaboration of a wide

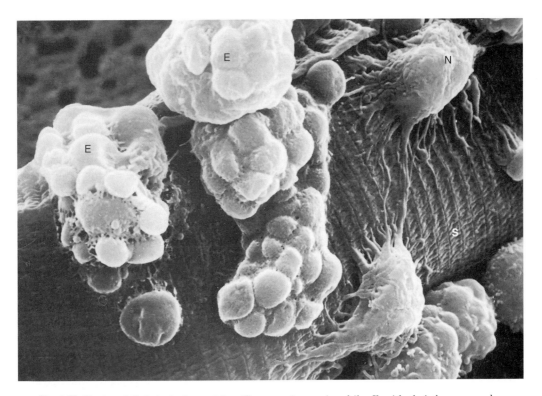

Fig. 4-21 Eosinophil helminthotoxicity. These equine eosinophils, *E,* with their large granules are degranulating against the surface of a strongyle, *S.* Such activity releases major basic protein and other toxic agents against the parasite. A few neutrophils, *N,* are also adherent to the parasite. *(Courtesy Dr. Thomas R. Klei, Baton Rouge, La.)*

TABLE 4-10 **Distinctive Contents of Eosinophils**

CONSTITUENT OR PRODUCT	FUNCTION
Major basic protein*	Parasite killing
	Induces histamine release from mast cells
	Neutralizes heparin from mast cells
Eosinophil cationic protein	Parasite killing
	Shortens coagulation time
	Alters fibrinolysis
Arylsulfatase B*	Inactivates leukotrienes (LTC$_4$, LTD$_4$, LTE$_4$)
Histaminase*	Inactivates histamine
Phospholipase D*	Inactivates PAF

LT, Leukotriene; *PAF*, platelet-activating factor.
*These may neutralize some mediators released from mast cells.

array of chemical mediators including both those released from preformed stores, such as histamine, heparin, and peptides, and those generated *de novo*, such as the lipid-derived platelet-activating factor (PAF) and prostaglandins and leukotrienes. Release of large amounts of these potent mediators from mast cells can result in excessive inflammation unless they are kept under control. It seems more than just coincidence that eosinophils are usually attracted to sites of mast cell degranulation, since eosinophils have the biochemical potential to help neutralize some of these mast cell–derived mediators. (A reason for their attraction to sites of mast cell degranulation is generation of a specific eosinophil chemotaxin, appropriately named "eotaxin," which is discussed a bit more later.) As already mentioned, the major basic protein can neutralize heparin presumably by virtue of a charge interaction. Eosinophil *histaminase*, like that of the neutrophil, can inactivate mast cell–derived histamine (see Table 4-10). Eosinophil *arylsulfatase B* can inactivate leukotrienes LTC$_4$, LTD$_4$, and LTE$_4$, which are potent arachidonic acid metabolites released from activated mast cells. *Phospholipase D* can inactivate PAF. Both arylsulfatase B and phospholipase D are found in greater quantities in eosinophils than in other leukocytes. It thus appears that the eosinophil has also evolved as a "regulator cell" while maintaining its role as an effector cell that can damage or kill some parasites and other pathogens.

Eosinophils respond to some of the same stimuli and chemotaxins as the neutrophils, such as soluble bacterial factors and activated components of com-

plement. However, eosinophil-specific chemotaxins ("eotaxins"), which are members of the chemokine family of chemoattractant and activators of leukocytes, have been recently discovered in some species (see Table 4-15). The small eotaxin proteins are apparently synthesized at tissue sites by several cell types, including fibroblasts and some epithelial cells, at least in part as a response to release of contents from stimulated mast cells, such as histamine. So it appears that the mast cells, in response to activation by IgE and antigen (Type I hypersensitivity/allergy) or other stimuli are therefore indirectly responsible for the subsequent accumulation of eosinophils in tissue. If the system works the way it should, upon arrival the eosinophils play a role in helping to destroy offending antigens or pathogens and may help to neutralize excess mast cell mediators, which might otherwise cause excessive inflammation. Unfortunately, if the antigenic or inflammatory stimulus is persistent or the host's immune system is too sensitive to it, *too many* eosinophils arrive in tissue over *too long* of a period of time and can contribute to adverse tissue reactions and tissue damage.

MAST CELLS AND BASOPHILS

These two cell types have been of interest to biomedical scientists for over a century since they were first described by Paul Ehrlich. Mast cells are found principally in perivascular sites in tissues, whereas basophils are rare circulating granulocytes. Basophils and mast cells are very closely related functionally and have many similarities, such as a cytoplasm that is literally loaded with coarse granules, which appear dark blue with the usual blood stains. The granules are also metachromatic, meaning they have a "color shift" and stain violet-purple, rather than blue, with special histological stains such as toluidine blue. This is related to their rich content of sulfated mucopolysaccharides, principally heparin, as well as histamine, several proteinases, and other potent biologically active mediators, and you will occasionally see reference to "metachromasia" when reading surgical biopsy reports of mast cell tumors. Both mast cells and basophils also have receptors that bind the Fc portion of IgE antibody with high affinity. An explosive degranulation with release of histamine and many other potent inflammatory mediators occurs when basophils and mast cells are appropriately stimulated, as when specific antigen binds to cell-bound IgE molecules. Mast cells are major cellular sources of histamine, which is so important to the vascular phenomenon of acute inflammation, and they also generate some cytokines depending on the species being studied;

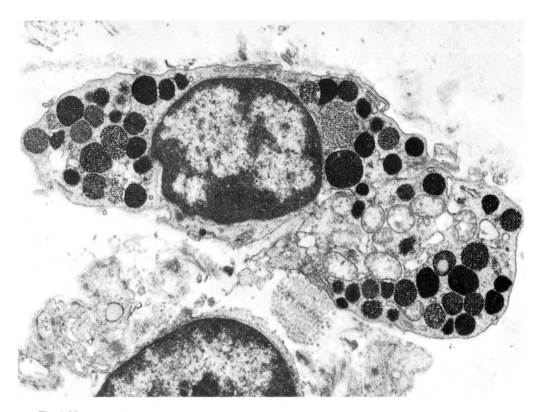

Fig. 4-22 Mast cell. Equine subcutis. The mononuclear mast cell is strikingly similar ultrastructurally to the basophil. Notice that the variation in granule morphology is similar to that of the basophil. These granules also contain potent mediators of inflammation. *(Courtesy Dr. John F. Cummings, Ithaca, N.Y.)*

the much-studied rodent mast cells make TNF-α, IL-1, -3, -4, -5, -6, -8, IFN-γ, and a few others. A few of the cytokines are preformed and stored for rapid release from granules when cells are activated, whereas others must be synthesized upon mast cell stimulation.

Mast cells are found throughout the tissues in virtually every organ of the body (Fig. 4-22). They are "born" in the bone marrow, circulate in the blood as undifferentiated and unrecognizable cells, and then migrate into tissues where they differentiate and are histologically identifiable. It is widely recognized that there is heterogeneity in populations of mast cells, as between the *mucosal* mast cells found principally in the gastrointestinal and respiratory tracts and the *connective tissue* mast cells found in the skin and stroma of other tissues and organs, as well as other specialized types. There are apparent species differences in the distribution of the mast cell subtypes. The reasons for the heterogeneity are debatable and perhaps multifactorial but could be attributable to the fact that they complete their differentiation at different tissue sites and are influenced by the local microenvironments.

Although we may tend to think of mast cells as a relatively minor cell population and as being present in only modest numbers in tissue, this is apparently not the case. It has been estimated that if all the mast cells in the body were grouped together in one mass their bulk might equal that of the spleen. They are most numerous at sites of "contact" with the external environment such as skin, respiratory tract, and gastrointestinal tract. Mast cells are most numerous around small blood vessels, which fits well with their function as inducers of vascular permeability. They are slightly larger and have mononuclear nuclei and somewhat more abundant cytoplasm than the basophil has. Immunological, inflammatory, and allergic stimuli activate the cells and produce degranulation with mediator release. After secreting their products, such as heparin and histamine, cytokines, and proteinases, the cells can gradually regenerate their supply of granules and mediators; that is, degranulation is not linked to cell death. In fact, mast cells have not only regenerative capability but can proliferate in tissue as well. In some rodents, some subtypes of mast cells are rich in serotonin, which is not the case in most species.

These cells are intimately involved in the pathogenesis of acute inflammation because it is their release of histamine that triggers many of the immediate clinical manifestations arising from smooth muscle contraction (such as bronchoconstriction) and increased vascular permeability (such as accumulation of edema fluid). As already mentioned in the section on eosinophils, mast cells play a major role in recruitment of eosinophils to tissue sites. There may be numerous reasons for this, but premier in this regard is mast cell–mediated generation of eosinophil-specific chemotaxins ("eotaxins"), which are members of the chemokine family of chemoattractants and activators of leukocytes (to be discussed). The small eotaxin proteins may be synthesized at tissue sites by several cell types in part as a response to release of contents from stimulated mast cells. So it appears that the activated mast cells can also promote the participation of eosinophils in tissue reactions, such as allergic disease.

The basophil (Fig. 4-23) is a granulocyte of bone marrow origin and is a rare member of the white cell population of the blood where they usually constitute less than 1% of the circulating leukocytes. In the size and shape of their nuclei they closely resemble neutrophils. Bone marrow–derived blood basophils are recruited into the tissues by immune mechanisms in some hypersensitivity responses, and as already mentioned, their mediators and function are similar to those of mast cells. Thus one consequence of the arrival and accumulation of basophils at hypersensitivity reactions would be to augment the anaphylactic potential of a given tissue site. In reactions to parasites, release of mediators by tissue basophils seems to aid in the expulsion of these organisms. Thus basophils and mast cells and their mediators, such as vasoactive amines, are involved in the onset, development, and function of various tissue inflammatory responses.

Macrophages

Most of the macrophages that are prominent in tissue inflammatory reactions have migrated there and are derived from circulating blood monocytes of bone marrow origin. A smaller proportion originates from resident macrophages in the tissues (called "histiocytes"), which can undergo cell division, but these cells are ultimately of bone marrow origin as well. Macrophage-derived or macrophage-related cells are present in many or most of the tis-

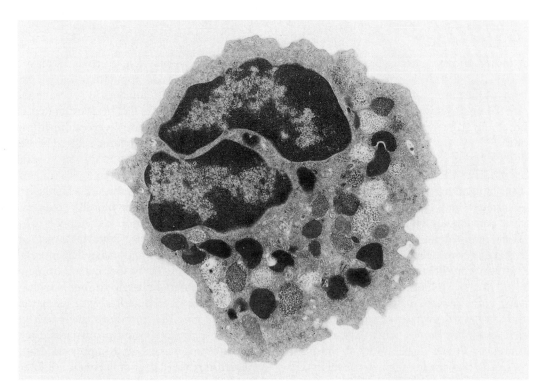

Fig. 4-23 Basophil. Sheep blood. The granules of the basophil vary from dense structures to more loosely associated aggregates of smaller, electron-dense granules sometimes organized into tubular or chainlike arrays. The granules contain potent inflammatory mediators.

sues of the body (Table 4-11). The macrophages are larger than neutrophils and, in routine blood stains, possess a gray-blue cytoplasm that has very fine granules. Their nuclei are large, usually central, and may be folded or kidney shaped, that is, "reniform." The macrophage contains many lysosomes and has cytoplasmic extensions called "pseudopodia" (Fig. 4-24).

Macrophages are the most dynamic and gifted of the leukocytes. They have some of the same basic functions of neutrophils, such as phagocytosis and killing of microbes, but this is just the surface of their abilities and activities. They arrive in numbers at inflammatory sites after the first wave of neutrophils and are key players in marshaling and controlling the inflammatory reaction from that point on (Box 4-3). They also have a longer life span (weeks) than neutrophils have and may actually proliferate at sites of protracted inflammation. Macrophages are capable of synthesizing a huge array of immunoinflammatory mediators, including proteins (cytokines, chemokines, complement fragments, proteinases, and so on), oxygen radicals and nitric oxide, and lipid mediators of inflammation (PAF, prostaglandins, and leukotrienes). These mediators recruit and influence the activities of other leukocytes and also stromal cells such as fibroblasts in the area (Table 4-12).

The macrophages at inflammatory sites have other functions too. One is in the mundane role of garbage collection and disposal; macrophages phagocytize cellular debris and literally help keep the tissue clean. Another function is related to production of cytokines. Cytokines such as IL-1, TNF-α, and IL-6 have local autocrine- and paracrine-stimulating effects but also have far-reaching systemic effects. These include induction of an "acute-phase response" (which we discuss later), which includes fever and malaise, signs that are ob-

vious indicators of infection, inflammation, or other disease. Stimulated macrophages also synthesize and secrete many growth factors, which stimulate the regeneration and reparative response in the damaged tissue. Both neutrophils and monocytes can emigrate simultaneously into tissue, but neu-

---

BOX 4-3 **Multifunctional Macrophages**

1. **ANTIMICROBIAL AND PHAGOCYTIC**
   - Oxygen radicals
   - Reactive nitrogen intermediates
   - Antimicrobial granule contents, including antimicrobial peptides (such as defensins)

2. **RECRUIT OTHER LEUKOCYTES TO TISSUE**
   - Chemokine synthesis
   - Synthesis of other mediators that upregulate leukocyte and endothelial adhesion molecules, such as cytokines

3. **STIMULATE OR MODULATE OTHER CELL ACTIVITY IN THE TISSUE**
   - Antimicrobial, antiviral, antitumor activity
   - Stimulate lymphocytic immune responses (cytokines)
   - Vascular effects (prostaglandins, leukotrienes, etc.)
   - Healing and repair (growth factors)

4. **CLEAN UP DEBRIS IN THE TISSUE**
   - Phagocytosis
   - Breakdown of fibrin (plasminogen activators)

5. **INDUCE SYSTEMIC EFFECTS, "ACUTE-PHASE REACTION"**
   - Paracrine and endocrine responses to macrophage-synthesized cytokines (IL-1, TNF-α, etc.)

TABLE 4-11 **Cells Closely Related to Macrophages**

Monocytes	In blood
Histiocytes/macrophages	Resident in connective tissue
Alveolar macrophages	Resident in the air space of the lung
Pulmonary intravascular macrophages	Resident in the capillaries of the lung
Kupffer cells	Resident in the sinusoids of the liver
Microglia	Resident in the CNS ("gitter cells" refer to large, active cells with phagocytized debris, and many of these probably are newly emigrated from the blood, not microglia)
Osteoclasts	Resident in bone
Epithelioid cells	At some sites of chronic inflammation
Multinucleated giant cells	At some sites of chronic inflammation

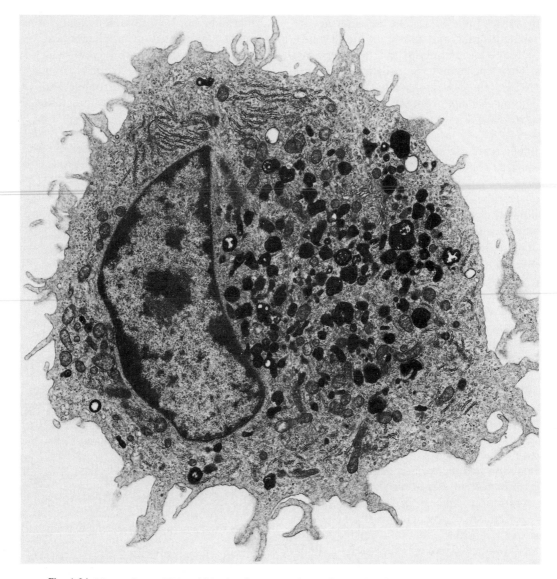

Fig. 4-24 Macrophage. This rabbit alveolar macrophage shows abundant cytoplasmic granules, many of which represent phagocytosed debris. Notice the numerous cytoplasmic processes at the cell surface. *(Courtesy Jan Henson and Dr. Peter Henson, Denver.)*

TABLE 4-12 **Some of the Cytokines and Other Mediators Synthesized and Secreted by Stimulated Macrophages or Monocytes**

SOURCE	TYPE OF MEDIATOR	EXAMPLES
Macrophages or monocytes	Interleukins and TNF:	IL-1α, -1β, IL-1ra, IL-4, -6, -8, -10, -12, -15, -18, TNF-α
	Chemokines:	IL-8, GRO-α/MGSA, MCP-1/MCAF, MIP-1α, MIP-1β, interferon-inducible protein-10 (IP-10)
	Interferons:	IFN-α, IFN-β (not IFN-γ)
	Hematopoietic growth factors:	G-CSF, GM-CSF, M-CSF
	Other growth factors and miscellaneous:	TGF-β, TGF-α, PDGF, leukemia inhibitory factor (LIF), hepatocyte growth factor (HGF), oncostatin M (OSM)
	Others:	Some complement components, prostaglandins and leukotrienes, nitric oxide (NO), platelet-activating factor (PAF)

See also Tables 4-14 and 4-15 for chemokine information.

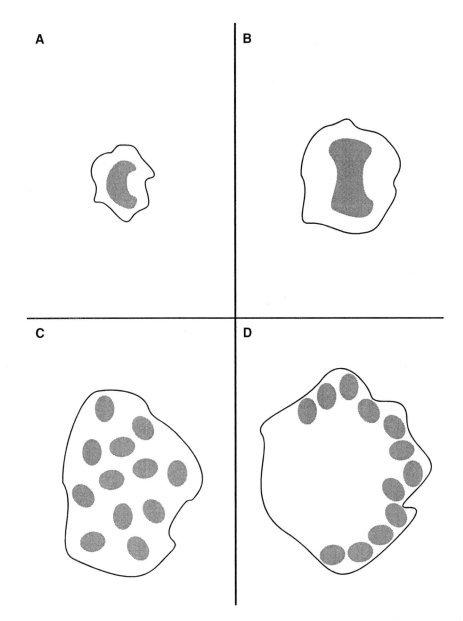

Fig. 4-25 Various morphological forms of macrophages at tissue sites of inflammation. A, Regular macrophage, also called a histiocyte. **B,** Epithelioid macrophage; larger with ample cytoplasm. **C,** Multinucleated giant cell, with scattered nuclei throughout. **D,** Langhans' type of giant cell, with numerous peripheral nuclei. *(Copyright © The University of Tennessee College of Veterinary Medicine, 2000.)*

trophils are "faster cells" when on the move and are in greater numbers, and so macrophages tend to appear as a group later in the tissue reaction. As mentioned, macrophages have a longer life span than neutrophils have and may actually proliferate at sites of protracted inflammation, accounting for their larger numbers in long-standing reactions.

Macrophages are the sources of the multinucleated *giant cells* present in some chronic inflammatory reactions (see Fig. 4-12) in which the stimulus for giant cell formation is usually some rather frustrating, indigestible object; such as foreign bodies or

certain kinds of microorganisms such as mycobacteria. Giant cells are formed by the coalescence of macrophages, and this coalescence may be a result of macrophages attempting to engulf the same objects, highly stimulated and coexisting in the same area, bumping together, and fusing under the influence of cytokines. Two types of macrophage-derived giant cells are commonly seen: Langhans' type and the foreign-body type, depending on the location of the nuclei; there does not seem to be any particular functional distinction between the two types of cells (Fig. 4-25). A third type, the Touton giant cell, is similar to the Langhans' type except that the peripheral cytoplasm is foamy, rather than eosinophilic. Another type of macrophage seen in some kinds of chronic inflammatory reactions is the *epithelioid cell*. These are large, pale-staining macrophages that have an ovoid nucleus and an angular shape vaguely resembling epithelial cells. They often result when macrophages are chronically stimulated by hard-to-kill microbes, such as those in the submucosa of the ileum in Johne's disease of cattle (caused by *Mycobacterium paratuberculosis*).

Unlike the neutrophils, the monocytes do not have a large reserve pool in the bone marrow but remain longer in the circulation, with a half-life of about 24 to 72 hours. Like circulating neutrophils, the blood monocytes require further "activation" under the influence of various chemical mediators before they can achieve their maximal functional competence as macrophages. Thus one major difference between a *monocyte* and a *macrophage* relates to the state of activation. More importantly, perhaps, it has been traditional to divide these cells into two camps based on a territorial separation; once monocytes have migrated into tissues they are referred to as "macrophages." This definition of a macrophage also includes the hepatic Kupffer cells, which are technically still in contact with the bloodstream yet are specialized liver macrophages (see Table 4-11).

The interesting *pulmonary intravascular macrophages* (PIMs) are a unique category of mononuclear phagocytes. They are found in ruminants (cattle, goats, sheep), cats, and pigs but apparently not in dogs, most laboratory animals, or humans. Located adherent to the capillary endothelium of the lung, they are morphologically similar to hepatic Kupffer cells and apparently serve similar functions in those species that have them, possibly being as important as Kupffer cells in the removal of blood-borne particulates. These cells are highly responsive to bacterial endotoxins and other stimuli, which induce release of a host of cytokines and other mediators from the macrophages. This creates a situation where the fixed-tissue macrophages can induce organ-specific immunoinflammatory responses.

As mentioned, one of the functions of the macrophage, like that of the neutrophils, is to phagocytize and degrade ingested material. In addition to bacteria and other pathogens, the organ- or tissue-specific macrophages can act as collectors of tissue debris and even participate in recycling of substances the body prefers to conserve, such as iron from heme products. Examples are alveolar macrophages and inhaled particles, Kupffer cells and particles or material absorbed by the intestine, and dermal and subcutaneous macrophages and injected material. Macrophages contain granule contents that are similar in many ways to those of neutrophils, which have already been discussed.

Lymphocytes and Plasma Cells

Both lymphocytes and plasma cells as cell types are principally involved in immune reactions. If you need a brief review of the various types of lymphocytes and their participation in the immune system, you may wish to consult the appropriate section of this book in Chapter 5 or a textbook devoted in its entirety to immunology. In a conventional blood smear, lymphocytes are heterogeneous in both size and morphology but are generally smaller than neutrophils and have a densely staining nucleus and a scant amount of cytoplasm (Figs. 4-26 and 4-27). These cells usually appear somewhat later than neutrophils in most inflammatory reactions and may be prominent cellular features of the exudate in the subacute and chronic phase of many types of inflammatory lesions. There are exceptions to this, however. A few infectious agents seem to provoke a lymphocytic response almost from the beginning. The renal lesions of acute leptospirosis in dogs, for example, are often lymphocytic as *Mycoplasma* infections in many species are. At one time, it was believed that the presence of plasma cells in lesions always indicated infection. We now know that this is an oversimplification, but the principle that lymphocyte and plasma cell infiltrates usually indicate a local immune reaction in response to some kind of an agent or antigen is still valid.

Lymphocytes are less motile than neutrophils in an active "crawling from here to there" sense, yet they have their own sophisticated methods of traversing the tissues of the body. Lymphocytes are produced by the primary lymphoid organs and migrate through the circulation to secondary lymphoid tissues such as the spleen and lymph nodes. Unlike neutrophils, lymphocytes have relatively long lives and recirculate among and between various lymphoid tissues through the blood and lymphatics. Some lymphocytes leave the bloodstream through nonspecific venules at sites of inflammation, similar to neutrophils, using various adhesion molecules to accomplish this (Table 4-13). In addition to this, however, lymphocytes "home" to noninflamed tissue sites on a regular basis and leave through specialized portions of the postcapillary venules; some of these venules are known as *high endothelial venules* (HEV) (Fig. 4-28). The HEV were named because these endothelial cells appear "plump" or "high," rather than the usual flattened

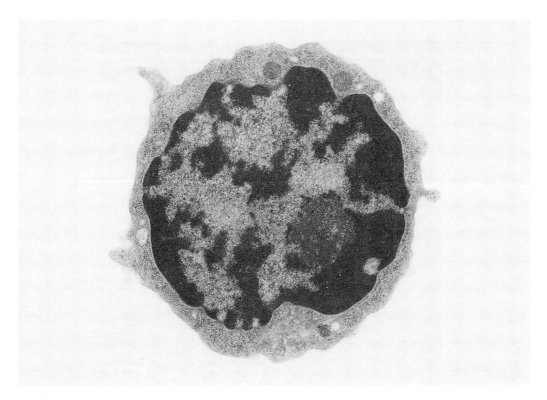

Fig. 4-26 Lymphocyte. This typical sheep lymphocyte has only scant amounts of cytoplasm containing abundant polyribosomes, a few profiles of endoplasmic reticulum, mitochondria, and a Golgi zone. The nucleus has the usual pattern of peripheral heterochromatin.

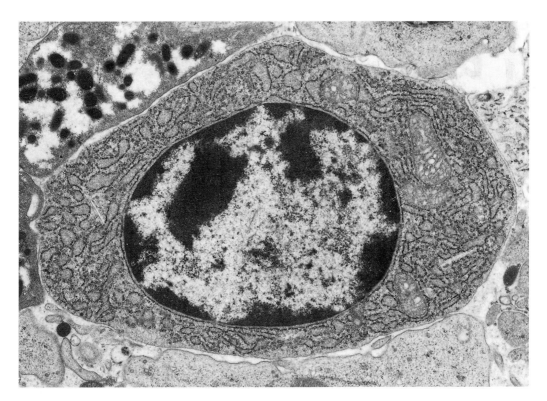

Fig. 4-27 Plasma cell. This sheep plasma cell shows the abundant, rough-surfaced endoplasmic reticulum (RER) that fills the cytoplasm of most plasma cells. It is on these profiles of RER that immunoglobulins are synthesized and assembled.

TABLE 4-13 Adhesion Molecules Present on Leukocytes and Corresponding Receptors or Adhesion Molecules They Recognize on the Surface of Endothelial Cells

ADHESION MOLECULE (WBC)	PRESENT ON THESE WBC	ADHESION MOLECULE (COUNTERRECEPTOR ON EC)
β₂-INTEGRINS		
CD11a/CD18 (LFA-1)	L, M, N, E, B (all WBC) (enriched on L)	ICAM 1, 2, 3 (immunoglobulin superfamily)
CD11b/CD18 (Mac-1)	N, M, E, B, some L (enriched on myeloid cells)	ICAM 1 (CD54), binds a region different from that of CD11a; also binds C3bi (CR3) and fibrinogen
CD11c/CD18	M, N, some L (enriched on M)	ICAM-1(?), also fibrinogen and C3bi
CD11d/CD18	Primarily M	ICAM-3
NON-β₂ INTEGRINS		
VLA-4 (CD49d) (a β1 integrin)	M, E, L (*not* N)	VCAM-1 (CD106); also binds fibronectin
α4β7 integrin	L	MadCAM-1 (immunoglobulin superfamily) and VCAM-1
SELECTINS		
L-Selectin (CD62L)	L	CD34, GlyCAM-1, and MadCAM-1 (mucosa)
	N	Mucin-like molecules
	E	?
IMMUNOGLOBULIN SUPERFAMILY		
CD31 (PECAM-1)	N, M, L, platelets	CD31 (PECAM-1)
MUCIN-LIKE (CARBOHYDRATE LIGANDS; "STICKY SUGARS")		
SialyLeˣ, Lewisˣ (Leˣ)	N, L, M, E (E recognizes only P-selectin)	E- and P-selectin (CD62E and -P), glycosaminoglycans

B, Basophils; *E*, eosinophils; *EC*, endothelial cells; *GlyCAM-1*, glycosylation-dependent cell adhesion molecule-1; *ICAM*, intercellular adhesion molecule; *L*, lymphocytes; *LFA-1*, lymphocyte function-associated antigen-1; *M*, monocytes; *MadCAM-1*, mucosal addressin cell adhesion molecule-1; *N*, neutrophils; *PECAM-1*, platelet–endothelial cell adhesion molecule-1; *VCAM-1*, vascular cell adhesion molecule-1; *VLA-4*, very late antigen-4; *WBC*, white blood cells.
•Many of the ICAM molecules are also present on leukocytes, not just on endothelial cells.
•MadCAM-1 is typically found on mucosal high endothelial venular endothelium (HEV) in the gastrointestinal tract, such as Peyer's patches, and in mesenteric lymph nodes. It is a vascular addressin for lymphocytes homing to the gut; it is not found in peripheral lymph nodes. MadCAM-1 is also constitutively expressed on flattened endothelial cells in the lamina propria of the small and large intestine. Other molecules regulate specific homing of lymphocytes to HEV in peripheral lymph nodes, including CD34, and GlyCAM-1.
•SialyLeˣ, Lewis-X (Leˣ) are sialylated and fucosylated structures related to the sialylated Lewis-X blood group antigen of humans, hence their name. They also appear as CD15 or PSGL-1 (P-selectin glycoprotein ligand-1 in some lists).
•L-, E-, and P-selectins are three of a family of "lectin cell adhesion molecules."

morphology when seen microscopically. It seems likely that not all endothelia that serve this function are microscopically recognizable as plump cells, however. It is this group of specialized endothelial cells that not only express an array of the common leukocyte-attracting adhesion molecules, but also express specific ones that enable capture of subsets of tissue-specific lymphocytes from the blood and permit their return to lymph nodes and other lymphoid tissue, that is, "homing." There is evidence that specialized tissue or organ sites that regularly contain recirculating lymphocytes have their own special combination of adhesion molecules on endothelial cells in that area, such as gut-associated

Peyer's patches (MadCAM-1), peripheral lymph nodes (GlyCAM-1, or "peripheral lymph node addressin"), and other mucosal sites in the genitourinary tissue, respiratory tissue, and skin. The adhesion molecules that identify different tissues and organs for circulating leukocytes have been collectively and aptly referred to as "addressins." A group of lymphocytes that preferentially home to one tissue site are not all strictly limited to a return to that site, however. For example, some lymphocytes from the intestinal mucosa may eventually circulate through other tissue sites such as lymph nodes and also different mucosal sites. This allows their antigenic experience and antigenic awareness

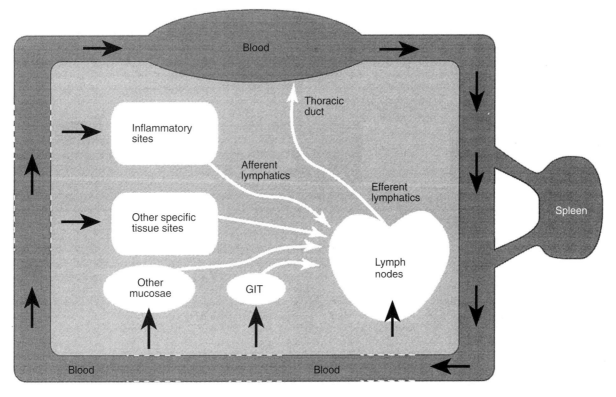

Fig. 4-28 Emigration of lymphocytes to tissue and specific mucosal sites. *Dashed lines* represent endothelial cells that express adhesion molecules to retain lymphocytes at that vascular site. *GIT,* Gastrointestinal tract. See text for details. *(Copyright © The University of Tennessee College of Veterinary Medicine, 2000.)*

to be on board at other tissue sites in the body, that is, a shared mucosal awareness of pathogens. Hence an oral vaccine may provide mucosal immunity at other organ and tissue sites. We further discuss leukocyte adhesion and migration later, in the section on cellular events during inflammation.

In addition to the traditional division of lymphocytes into T-cells and B-cells, studies have shown tremendous functional heterogeneity among different lymphocyte subclasses in several species, resulting in the TH1 and TH2 paradigm. The roles of the various functional lymphocyte types in immunological reactions are discussed at greater length in Chapter 5. Beyond their obvious importance in the generation of immune responses, lymphocytes are also consequential to the inflammatory response in several specific ways. B-Lymphocytes and their progeny, plasma cells, are of importance in the production of antibody. Antibody constitutes one of the major *opsonins* and thus interfaces directly with the cellular, phagocytic arm of the host defense mechanism. In addition, TH1 lymphocytes represent the cellular sources of the potent *lymphokines,* IFN-γ, TNF-α, and IL-2, which can modulate and expand local inflammatory reactions, like certain

kinds of granulomas (see Chapter 5 and Type IV hypersensitivity reactions).

Platelets as Inflammatory Cells

The blood platelets tend to be ignored by pathologists because they are too small to be readily seen in routine histological slides of inflamed tissue. When we think of platelets, we do not usually associate them with inflammatory processes other than to acknowledge that they play a role in coagulation. However, in a local inflammatory reaction, platelets are almost always involved because damaged vessels leave subendothelial structures exposed to the circulating blood cells, and platelets bind at these sites.

One of the earliest steps in the primary hemostatic defense mechanism involves the adhesion of circulating platelets to subendothelial collagen and basement membrane in the vicinity of a damaged endothelial surface. Adhesion relies on binding of surface adhesion molecules on platelets (glycoprotein Ib, or gpIb) to von Willibrand factor (vWF), which is also known as "factor VIII–related antigen." vWF is synthesized in endothelial cells and in

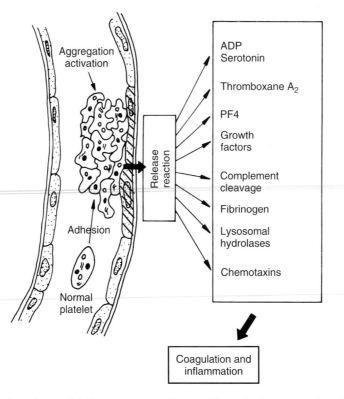

Fig. 4-29 Platelet release of inflammatory mediators. When platelets are activated and aggregated, the ensuing platelet release reaction causes the secretion of many chemical mediators of importance to inflammation and coagulation. *ADP,* Adenosine triphosphate; *PF,* platelet factor.

megakaryocytes, stored in cytoplasmic granules called Weibel-Palade bodies (in endothelial cells), and secreted from endothelial cells both into the plasma and toward the subendothelial basement membrane and collagen; it sticks to the latter. When vessels and endothelial cells are damaged, the exposed vWF is ready to act as an anchor for the platelet gpIb receptor, and the platelet phase of coagulation begins.

Once the first few platelets are stuck they release intracellular granule constituents from their two types of granules, alpha and dense bodies (Figs. 4-29 and 4-30 and Box 4-4). Granule contents include adenosine diphosphate (ADP), serotonin, platelet factor 4 (PF4), platelet-activating factor (PAF), fibrinogen, fibronectin, products of the arachidonic acid pathway, especially thromboxane A_2 (TXA$_2$), and many other factors. In addition, they contain and release growth factors, including platelet-derived growth factor (PDGF), fibroblast growth factors (FGF), and transforming growth factors (TGF), which participate in and stimulate the ensuing healing process (Fig. 4-29). The released ADP, thromboxane A_2, and other stimuli activate additional platelets, and such activation leads to the formation of a large platelet aggregate, which even-

BOX 4-4 **Some of the Products of Platelets Related to Coagulation, Inflammation, and Healing**

Platelet factor 4
Fibrinogen
Fibronectin
Coagulation factors VIII and V
Serotonin
Histamine
ADP, ATP
Ca^{++} cations
The arachidonic acid product TXA$_2$
Complement-cleaving protease (resulting in C5a)
Platelet-activating factor
Growth factors: PDGF, TGF-β, FGF
P-selectin (CD62P, adhesion molecule)

ADP, Adenosine diphosphate; *ATP,* adenosine triphosphate; *FGF,* fibroblast growth factor(s); *PDGF,* platelet-derived growth factor(s); *TGF-β,* transforming growth factor–beta; *TXA$_2$,* thromboxane A$_2$.

tually plugs and seals off the disrupted vessel. Formation of the aggregate requires platelet-platelet adhesion. This adhesion occurs as a result of expression of adhesion molecules (gpIIb-IIIa, a member of the integrin adhesion molecules) on the sur-

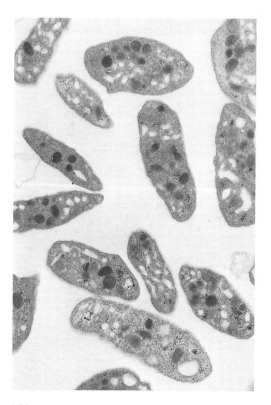

Fig. 4-30 Platelets. Rabbit blood. These typically anucleate platelets show the cytoplasmic granules and dense bodies as well as the open cytocavitary network typical of most platelets and through which granule constituents are secreted to the exterior. *(Courtesy Jan Henson and Dr. Peter Henson, Denver, Colo.)*

face of activated platelets, which bind fibrinogen; fibrinogen more or less forms the "glue" that holds the platelet aggregate together. Platelets also apparently contribute to subsequent neutrophil accumulation at sites of vascular damage. Platelets store an adhesion molecule (P-selectin, CD62P) in their granules, and that molecule is moved to the surface of activated platelets during the process of degranulation. P-selectin adhesion molecules exposed on the surface of platelets, which are now stuck to the damaged vessel wall and collagen, recognize a receptor on neutrophils that are flowing by. Some of the neutrophils stick to the platelets and are thus encouraged to remain at the site of vascular damage and tissue damage.

Endothelial Cells and Fibroblasts

For completeness, it is necessary that we include the endothelial cells and fibroblasts as part of the cast of cellular participants in inflammation. To leave the bloodstream and enter tissue sites of inflammation, the leukocytes must first adhere to and then migrate through the microvasculature, and the endothelium is an active participant in these leukocyte–endothelial cell interactions. In addition, the endothelial cells have high proliferative potential and play a critical role in healing and repair responses (see discussion of Healing and Repair, p. 225). Fibroblasts are important cells by virtue of the fact that they can synthesize an array of cytokines, which influence leukocytes. Fibroblasts are obviously important in the healing and repair of injured tissues by virtue of their ability to synthesize and lay down collagen. In addition, many of the important extracellular matrix proteins (see Chapter 3) are fibro-blast products, and many of these are important to leukocyte activation and locomotion. Thus, although the endothelial cells and fibroblasts are not leukocytes, they are vital tissue participants in inflammation. Their role in healing and repair responses is discussed in greater detail later in this chapter.

CELLULAR EVENTS IN INFLAMMATION

Leukocytes and their products constitute the third leg (along with the hemodynamic and permeability changes) of the tripod on which the inflammatory process stands. An important question is: How do these cells get to the precise focus of injury, and what do they do once they arrive? The sequence of leukocytic events can be divided into (1) margination, (2) pavementing, (3) emigration, (4) chemotaxis, and (5) phagocytosis and synthesis of biochemical mediators (Fig. 4-31). Many of these events involve complicated biochemical and functional changes in the leukocytes themselves as they become converted from resting cells into *activated* cells.

Adhesion of Leukocytes to Blood Vessels and Emigration to Tissue

Adhesion to and migration through the vascular endothelium is, of course, a prerequisite for the extravasation of leukocytes from the blood to tissue sites of inflammation. The endothelium and leukocyte–endothelial cell interaction is therefore of central importance to the entire inflammatory drama. We already have briefly mentioned margination or peripheral orientation of leukocytes from the moving bloodstream in our discussion of the hemodynamic changes in inflammation. Many red and white cells in the normal blood flow within the microvessels are in the "central" area of fast-moving blood, and other leukocytes are in relatively close

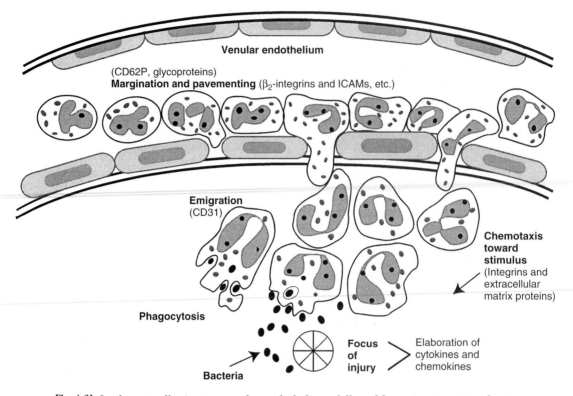

Venular endothelium

(CD62P, glycoproteins)
Margination and pavementing (β₂-integrins and ICAMs, etc.)

Emigration
(CD31)

**Chemotaxis
toward
stimulus**
(Integrins and
extracellular
matrix proteins)

Phagocytosis

Bacteria

**Focus
of
injury**

Elaboration of
cytokines and
chemokines

Fig. 4-31 Leukocyte adhesion to vascular endothelium, followed by emigration into the tissue. At the focus of injury or inflammation, cells such as resident tissue macrophages are stimulated to synthesize and secrete chemoattractants and activators of cells, such as cytokines and chemokines. These diffuse from the site, contact small blood vessels, and stimulate leukocyte–endothelial cell adhesion in local venules, resulting in attraction of leukocytes to the tissue. *(Copyright © The University of Tennessee College of Veterinary Medicine, 2000.)*

contact with the endothelial lining of the vessel wall. With the onset of inflammation, the small venules in that area are seen to have more and more leukocytes that are in contact with them. This may be attributable in some part to slowing of the blood flow, some of which can result from the hemodynamic changes of inflammation. More of the leukocytes move out of the central column of blood flow and are seen toward the edges of the moving stream of blood and are now in position to more readily contact the endothelium. The cells roll relatively slowly along the walls of the capillaries and venules and may momentarily stop; this phenomenon is known as *margination* (see Fig. 4-31). Although margination is, in part, accomplished by vasodilatation and a decrease in the speed of blood flow, much of it is attributable to adhesion molecules on the surface of leukocytes and endothelial cells. There are numerous adhesion molecules that have been discovered, and it is not possible to discuss them all, but a general outline for leukocyte–endothelial cell adhesion is presented here, and Table 4-13 (p. 182) describes many of them. When endothelial cells are

stimulated (inflammation, infection, trauma), they rapidly move the preformed adhesion molecules, such as P-selectin (CD62P) stored in cytoplasmic granules to the surface. This takes only a few minutes. Endothelial P-selectin recognizes its counter-receptors on the surface of neutrophils (such as glycoproteins), and the neutrophils slow down, roll, or transiently stop (see Fig. 4-31). P-selectin expression on endothelial cells is preferentially dense at the margins or edges of individual endothelial cells, and this denseness helps to conveniently localize the neutrophils at the inter–endothelial cell junctions where they can eventually force their way out of the bloodstream and into the tissues. The P-selectin–glycoprotein link is not a strong bond, however, and has only the weak staying power of a Post-it Note. If the inflammatory stimulus is weak and no other adhesion molecules become involved to strengthen the bond, the neutrophils will break away after a few seconds or minutes and return to the regular blood flow.

If the inflammatory stimulus is stronger, however, other adhesion molecules come into play. On the leukocytes, the β_2 integrins are an important, archetypal group. These heterodimeric molecules are always present on the surface of the leukocytes but are quickly upregulated in adhesiveness when the leukocytes are stimulated. This occurs either by a conformational change of the integrins (as with CD11a/CD18, also known as LFA-1) or by a combination of conformational change and increased surface expression (as with CD11b/CD18, also known as Mac-1) as a result of movement of adhesion molecules—stored in granules/lysosomes—to the surface when the cells are stimulated. If the developing inflammation near the blood vessels is sufficiently intense, biochemical mediators diffusing throughout the tissue in that area, often cytokines like IL-1 and TNF-α, contact the endothelial cells. This causes the endothelium to produce still other mediators like PAF and IL-8. The endothelial cells can directly expose the adhered or rolling leukocytes to PAF and IL-8, and such exposure stimulates the neutrophils and other leukocytes. Some tissue-derived mediators may also diffuse from the tissue into the vessels, onto the endothelial cells, and directly contact the leukocytes. Chemokines fit into this category; they bind to the surface of endothelial cells, probably to heparin molecules. The various chemokines demonstrate some *selectivity* for attracting and activating subsets of leukocytes, and this is a major way in which groups of leukocytes such as neutrophils, eosinophils, or lymphocytes are specifically attracted. The upregulated, sticky β_2 integrins on stimulated leukocytes then recognize their counterreceptors on endothelial cells, which include the intercellular adhesion molecules (ICAM-1, -2, -3). ICAM-1, -2, and -3 are constitutively expressed, but ICAM-1 is normally expressed only at a modest level until endothelial cells are stimulated, and then it is upregulated. E-selectin (CD62E) and VCAM-1 (CD106) are other adhesion molecules on the endothelium that take part in leukocyte adhesion, and these require cell stimulation, that is, developing inflammation, for expression to occur (see Table 4-13). Their expression is induced by various cytokines (IL-1, TNF-α, and so on) and also by bacterial endotoxin. This second phase of leukocyte–endothelial cell bonding is much stronger than the initial bond between P-selectin (on endothelium) and leukocytes, and leukocytes can be firmly arrested at the site. The visual image of rows or layers of leukocytes stuck to and hugging vessel walls resulted in the term "pavementing."

Stimulated and now having a firm grip on the surface of the endothelial cells, the leukocytes can crawl around a bit in response to the mediators they

sense. The term *chemotaxis* refers to directed movement of cells toward a chemical attractant, and the term *chemokinesis* refers to random, excited movement. The cells likely do some of both at this stage of the process. Neutrophils soon contact inter–endothelial cell junctions, and another adhesion molecule is present on endothelial cells at that site, CD31. Neutrophils also have these same adhesion molecules (CD31), and these recognize and bind to their twins on the endothelial cell junctions. This is, more or less, an exit signal for the neutrophils. They squeeze through the inter–endothelial cell junction, secrete proteinases to get through the basement membrane, and crawl into the perivascular tissue.

The term *emigration* refers to the process by which leukocytes escape from their location in the blood to reach the perivascular tissues. Neutrophils, eosinophils, basophils, monocytes, and lymphocytes use similar routes, crawling *between* the endothelial cell junctions in moving from the bloodstream into tissue. It is interesting to notice how correct Cohnheim's early descriptions of the morphodynamics of the emigration process were; we know much more now about mechanisms, but little has been added to his descriptions. The motile leukocytes force their pseudopodia (large cytoplasmic extensions) into gaps between adjacent endothelial cells. These gaps can be created through the actions of histamine and other chemical mediators on endothelium and also can apparently be created by the leukocytes themselves. Once the pseudopod has passed, the entire cell slips through the widened inter–endothelial cell junctions. The leukocyte may then pass through the basement membrane and between cells of the vessel wall into the perivascular connective tissues and beyond (see Fig. 4-31). Electron microscopic observations have shown the incredible plasticity of the white cells as they crawl through the narrow pathways opened between endothelial cells (Figs. 4-32 and 4-33). It is remarkable to observe that the whole migrating cell changes its shape and even the nucleus elongates itself to an extreme. When circulating, neutrophils have a diameter of approximately 10 μm but are capable of reducing their width to an amazing 1 μm when migrating. Monocytes seem no less flexible.

Segmental differences in the vasculature with regard to the number and types of inter–endothelial cell junctions and receptors may be of considerable importance to sites of leukocyte emigration. The small venules, which are so important to inflammation, have a combination of open and loose junctional complexes, which renders them uniquely susceptible to the development of interendothelial gaps

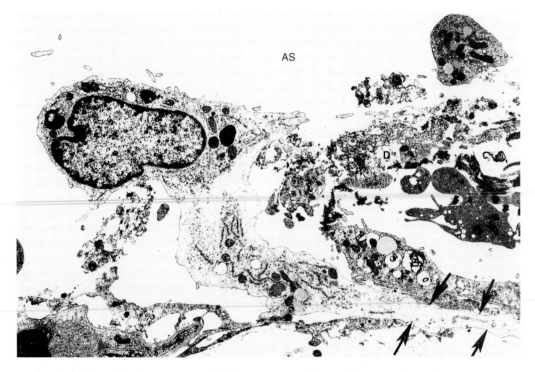

Fig. 4-32 Macrophage penetrating the basement membrane. This macrophage has inserted a long pseudopod, *arrows*, through the basement membrane in this inflamed lung. Debris, *D*, consisting of red blood cells, fibrin, and cell fragments is in the alveolar space, *AS*. *(Courtesy Dr. W.L. Castleman, Gainesville, Fla.)*

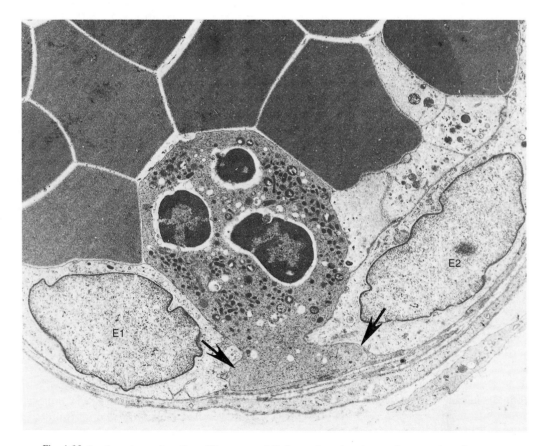

Fig. 4-33 Leukocyte emigration. The neutrophil shown here has inserted a pseudopod, *arrows*, into the interendothelial space between two adjacent endothelial cells, *E1* and *E2*.

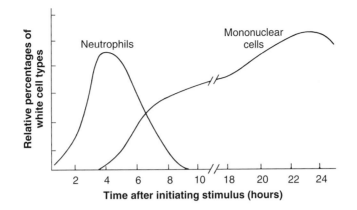

Fig. 4-34 Leukocyte accumulation. In many typical inflammatory reactions, the neutrophils arrive first and are followed by a more prolonged phase of mononuclear cell accumulation.

under the influence of histamine. It is also apparent that venular endothelium contains more specific histamine receptors on the luminal endothelial cell surface than other types of endothelia have. This greater amount may also help to promote endothelial cell contractility in this region. In the postcapillary venules, where most of the leukocyte emigration important to inflammation takes place, tight junctions, or desmosomes, which might otherwise hinder the formation of endothelial gaps and easy egress of leukocytes, are normally absent or rare.

When leukocytes reach the basement membrane, the membrane may be opened by the collagenase type of enzymes. The "lysed" segment of the basement membrane rarely exceeds 1 μm in length, permitting only the passage of the elongated migrating cell. However, massive migration of neutrophils during intense inflammation can result in extensive penetration of the basement membrane, allowing the *passive* extravasation of red blood cells; these resulting microhemorrhages are often observed in acute inflammation.

The number of cells migrating into inflammatory exudates can be measured after the injection of inflammatory agents into the peritoneal cavity, into the pleural cavity, or into small chambers placed over minor skin abrasions. The findings show that, with relatively mild irritants, neutrophil accumulation reaches a peak at about 4 to 6 hours and then declines rapidly, whereas the total number of mononuclear cells begins to rise only after 4 hours and reaches a sustained peak at 18 to 24 hours (Fig. 4-34). The height of the peak shows great variation with different stimuli. When living microorganisms are injected intrapleurally, massive numbers of neutrophils accumulate progressively throughout the 24 hours of observation; no mononuclear response can be detected in this period. It previously was sug-

gested that neutrophils and mononuclear phagocytes migrate simultaneously into inflammatory exudates and that the neutrophils rapidly disappear, thus exposing the less-numerous but more long-lived mononuclear cells at the later stages. This was supported, at the time, by the belief that neutrophils and monocytes showed no differences in chemotactic reactivity to various stimuli. Evidence is suggestive, however, that the entry of monocytes into the exudates usually starts as neutrophil emigration declines and continues for a considerably longer period.

It is important to remember that adhesion molecules other than those mentioned here are involved in this process, depending on the type of leukocyte, the duration of the inflammation, and, in some cases, the location of the endothelial cells, such as "regular" endothelium, or HEV. As a reminder, a list of many of the adhesion molecules is presented in Table 4-13. It is true, of course, that most of these adhesion molecules were first discovered in humans or in animal models of human disease, such as mice, and fewer have been identified in domestic animals. This is a result of the large funding base for human research, of course. Nevertheless, receptors have also been identified in some domestic animal species, such as the β₂-integrins and selectins, and others await discovery at the time of this writing. The workings of adhesion molecules in leukocyte–endothelial and leukocyte–extracellular matrix adhesion that are discussed in this chapter are also largely based on discoveries made with human or human-animal model cells. Although some species variation in the details undoubtedly occurs, it is reasonable from what we know thus far to accept a similar paradigm for leukocyte–endothelial cell interactions of domestic and wild vertebrates. It is also worth emphasizing that, despite the variation concerning which particular adhesion molecules are involved, all significant leukocyte–endothelial cell adhesive interactions and all leukocyte–extracellular matrix interactions rely on functioning adhesion molecules.

Chemotaxis

The leukocytes are now outside of the vessel and in the tissue. Neutrophils and other leukocytes can sense minute directional differences in the concentration of chemotactic mediators ("chemotaxins"). The probable reason is that more of their receptors for chemotaxins become occupied on one side of the cell, the side nearest the largest site of inflammation with the greatest concentration of inflammatory mediators and chemotaxins.

It has been clear since the time of Metchnikoff that activated leukocytes are highly motile and seem

---

BOX 4-5 **Some Factors That are Chemotactic for Leukocytes**

PLASMA-DERIVED

C5a, C5a des-Arg
Fibrinopeptides (fibrin degradation products)

INFLAMMATORY CELL-DERIVED

LTB$_4$ ⎫
HETEs ⎬ Arachidonic acid derivatives
Platelet-activing factor
Chemokines (see separate Tables 4-14 and 4-15)

OTHER ORIGINS

Bacterial chemotaxins, including fMLP-like peptides
Dead cells (necrotaxis)

des-Arg, Terminal arginine residue enzymatically cleaved away; *fMLP*, N-Formyl-Met-Leu-Phe; *HETE*, hydroxyeicosatetraenoic acid; *LTB$_4$*, leukotriene B$_4$.

---

to possess direction sense; that is, their wanderings in tissue are not random but directed. The phenomenon of *chemotaxis,* or directional migration in response to a gradient of chemoattractant, explains this phenomenon. Leukocytes are not the only cells that display chemotaxis. Bacteria, cellular slime molds, tumor cells, fibroblasts, endothelial cells, and other cells also exhibit varying degrees of chemotactic responsiveness.

Neutrophilic granulocytes respond to chemotactic signals quickly, a response that is reminiscent of their behavior *in vivo*. These cells require only about 90 minutes to complete their response in an *in vitro* experimental chemotactic chamber. This is in sharp contrast with the course of response for mononuclear cells, which may take several hours. Eosinophils are somewhat intermediate in chemotactic responsiveness.

At the site of a well-developed acute inflammatory reaction, there is a veritable chemical soup of potential chemoattractants, and a large number of these different chemotactic factors have been studied (Box 4-5). An important plasma-derived chemotaxin is the complement fragment *C5a*. *Fibrinogen* is another likely source of chemotactic activity, since both fibrinopeptide B and the plasmin-generated degradation products of fibrinogen and fibrin are chemotactic. Many of the other chemotaxins, such as the arachidonic acid metabolite *LTB$_4$* and *platelet-activating factor,* are cell-derived.

CHEMOKINES

The largest single group or family of chemotactic mediators is also the most recently discovered, and this is arguably the most important group; these are the chemokines (Tables 4-14 and 4-15). Their importance as a group is attributable to their potency in attracting and activating an array of virtually every

---

TABLE 4-14 **Families of Chemokines and their General Selectivity for Leukocytes**

FAMILY	SOME EXAMPLES	SELECTIVITY (WBC)
α-Chemokines with ELR (C-X-C)	IL-8, NAP-2, GRO-α, -β, -γ, ENA-78, etc.	Potent attractant and activators of neutrophils
α-Chemokines without ELR (C-X-C)	IP-IO, SDF-1, PF4, MIG, etc.	Attract various leukocytes but not neutrophils
β-Chemokines (C-C)	MIP-1α, -β, MCP-1, -2, -3, RANTES, Eotaxin-1, -2, -3, etc.	Attract various leukocytes but not neutrophils
"C" chemokine	Lymphotactin	"Resting" T lymphocytes
C-XXX-C chemokine	Fractalkine	NK cells

ELR, Glutamic acid, leucine, and arginine; *ENA-78*, Epithelial cell–derived neutrophil-activating factor; *GRO*, growth-regulated oncogene; *IL-8*, interleukin-8; *IP-10*, interferon-inducible protein-10; *MCP*, monocyte chemoattractant protein; *MIG*, monokine induced by interferon-γ; *MIP*, macrophage inflammatory protein; *NAP-2*, neutrophil-activating peptide 2; *PF4*, platelet factor 4; *RANTES*, regulated upon activation normal T-cell expressed and secreted; *SDF-1*, stromal cell–derived factor-1.

kind of leukocyte and on the fact that their great variety, receptor diversity, and preferential action on certain types of leukocytes helps to create, along with other factors, a degree of *selectivity* in leukocyte recruitment and activation (Fig. 4-35). The selectivity afforded by chemokines constitutes much of the explanation why some leukocyte infiltrates at inflammatory sites are primarily eosinophilic, or lymphocytic, or other types, or a mixture of various proportions of leukocytes. The generation of chemokines at sites of inflammation is central to the evolution of an inflammatory or immune response.

The chemokines are a group of small proteins (usually 8 to10 kD) that are further subdivided into families based upon the placement and presence of conserved cysteine residues near the amino terminus. This is the sort of thing that many of us might regard as only of interest to biochemists and molecular biologists, but in the case of chemokines it translates into interesting and important functional differences among the chemokine families, which are worth discussing. The number and placement of the conserved cysteine (C) residues results in differences in conformation of the molecules, creating differences in receptor binding. Different groups and combinations of chemokine receptors are expressed on different types of leukocytes, that is, neutrophils versus T lymphocytes versus macrophages and so forth. The result is a complex but logical method for attracting some types of leukocytes to an inflammatory site but not to others.

The families of chemokines have been grouped as follows. The alpha (α) chemokine group is designated "C-X-C" because one amino acid separates the first two conserved cysteines near the amino terminus. The α-chemokines have two branches of the family depending on whether a characteristic three–amino acid sequence precedes the C-X-C motif; this is glutamic acid, leucine, and arginine, or ELR. This has functional significance, as we shall see in a moment. The β-chemokines have a "C-C" configuration, without the intervening amino acid. There are two other known configurations at the present time: "C" and "C-X-X-X-C," each with only one known member, but like most newly discovered things in biology this may change. Table 4-14 shows the general selectivity of these groups. Notice that our discussion has focused on leukocytes, but chemokines and their receptors have diverse and important roles in many other processes such as angiogenesis and in the

TABLE 4-15   Some of the Chemokines and their Receptors on Several Common Types of Leukocytes Involved in the Inflammatory Response

PRINCIPAL LEUKOCYTES ATTRACTED OR ACTIVATED	CHEMOKINES	CHEMOKINE RECEPTOR
Neutrophils	IL-8, GCP-2	CXCR1
	IL-8, GRO-α, -β, -γ; NAP-2, ENA-78	CXCR2
Monocytes and macrophages	MIP-1α, MCP-3, RANTES	CCR1
	MCP-1, -2, -3, -4, -5	CCR2
	MIP-1α, -1β, RANTES	CCR5
	others	
Eosinophils	MIP-1α, MCP-3, RANTES	CCR1
	Eotaxin-1, -2, -3, MCP-3, RANTES	CCR3
T-cells	MIP-1α, MCP-3, RANTES	CCR1
	MCP-1, -2, -3, -4, -5	CCR2
	IP-10, MIG	CXCR3
	TARC	CCR4
	MIP-1α, -1β, RANTES	CCR5
	Fractalkine	CX₃CR1
	Lymphotactin (resting T cells)	XCR1(?)
Erythrocytes*	IL-8, GRO-α, RANTES, MCP-1, TARC	DARC "Duffy antigen"

DARC, Duffy antigen receptor complex; *ENA-78*, epithelial cell–derived neutrophil-activating factor; *GCP*, granulocyte chemotactic protein; *GRO*, growth-regulated oncogene; *IL-8*, Interleukin-8; *IP-10*, interferon-inducible protein-10; *MCP*, monocyte chemoattractant protein; *MIP*, macrophage inflammatory protein; *NAP-2*, neutrophil-activating peptide 2; *RANTES*, regulated upon activation normal T-cell expressed and secreted; *TARC*, thymus and activation-regulation chemokines.
•The chemokines generated at inflammatory sites provide some chemotactic selectivity for certain types of leukocytes, though it is apparent that a great deal of overlap or redundancy is built into the system.
•This is a much-simplified and only partial list of a large and growing family of chemokines.
*The DARC receptor on erythrocytes does not stimulate or chemoattract erythrocytes. It probably functions to bind and neutralize excess chemokines that have leaked into the circulatory system and apparently provides a measure of safety against a circulating excess of chemokines.

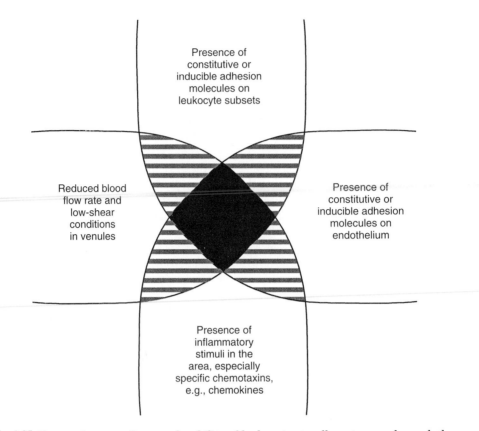

Fig. 4-35 Factors that contribute to the ability of leukocytes to adhere to vascular endothelial cells. If all these factors are present *(area of shaded overlap)*, the chances are good that leukocytes will adhere and be in position to migrate out of the vasculature and into the tissues. *(Copyright © The University of Tennessee College of Veterinary Medicine, 2000.)*

pathogenesis of many diseases. For example, α-chemokines with ELR are generally angiogenic, whereas α-chemokines without ELR are angiostatic and inhibit the activity of the ELR(+) group. This has implications for the inflammatory and healing and repair responses, tumorigenesis, and other processes and diseases.

Interactions between some chemokine receptors and pathogens have also been shown to occur, at least with human cells. For example, chemokine receptors CXCR4 or CCR5 can be subverted and used by HIV as coreceptors to bind to and gain entry to T-cells and macrophages. Another chemokine receptor on erythrocytes called DARC (Duffy antigen) is targeted and serves as a binding site for *Plasmodium vivax*, the agent of malaria. Interactions such as these may be discovered in animals.

At a focus of tissue injury caused by inflammation or infection, resident cells in the tissue, including fibroblasts, macrophages and many others, are stimulated to secrete an array of cytokines, chemokines, and other mediators (Fig. 4-31). The concentration of mediators is highest at the focus of injury. These mediators diffuse out from the primary focus like ripples in a pond, interacting with other cells and creating a concentration gradient of mediators and chemotaxins. Chemokines bind to extracellular matrix proteins as they diffuse, with their concentrations decreasing as they get further from the inflammatory focus; they also bind to the luminal surface of endothelial cells as they seep into small vessels. These mediators activate endothelial cell adhesion molecules, leukocytes and their adhesion molecules, and the chemokines in particular provide a chemotactic stimulus, or "scent," for the leukocytes to follow into the tissue. As the leukocytes get closer and closer to the focus of injury, the concentration of mediators increases, such that they arrive at the focus highly stimulated and ready for action. The leukocytes presumably "know" they have arrived at the proper site (and so stay there) when there is no longer an increasing chemotactic gradient to follow; that is, the stimuli are maximal in the focus of tissue damage or inflammation. Perhaps there are also other signals to stop. The growing length of the list of chemoattractants for leukocytes illustrates once again the enormous complexity and redundancy built into the inflammatory response.

Before we leave the topic of chemotaxins, it is important to mention bacterial products. Many kinds of bacteria produce chemoattractants, but these are of no apparent advantage to most bacteria because, by calling leukocytes into play, they invite their own demise. (An important exception to this would be those bacteria or other intracellular pathogens that prefer to survive and grow *within* the leukocytes, such as *Mycobacterium* species within macrophages). Biochemical studies of different bacterial chemoattractants led to the development of the structurally similar synthetic *N-formylated oligopeptides*, of which N-formyl-methionyl-leucyl-phenylalanine (N-formyl-Met-Leu-Phe, fMet-Leu-Phe, or simply *fMLP*) has been the most widely studied. Neutrophils of some species, notably humans, have receptors that bind fMLP, and much of our present knowledge of the cell biology of leukocyte chemotaxis is based on observations made with synthetic oligopeptides like fMLP. Bovine neutrophils, however, fail to respond to fMLP.

ENDOTOXIN

Another potent bacterial product is endotoxin, also known as "bacterial lipopolysaccharide" (LPS), which is a structural component of the wall of gram-negative bacteria, and some of it is shed as bacteria when they multiply and die. This discussion is included here because endotoxin can *indirectly* cause inflammation; it induces the synthesis and release of other proinflammatory agents. LPS is not a potent chemotaxin for leukocytes, either, but it induces synthesis of potent chemotaxins by cells in the tissues, such as chemokines, as already discussed. Some experiments have demonstrated that LPS alone actually decreases chemotactic responsiveness of PMN and may decrease PMN migration, though the biological relevance of this *in vitro* finding should be reconsidered in light of the other chemotactic agents, which it can induce. The ability of PMNs to generate oxygen radicals, either for use in killing bacteria or perhaps resulting in inadvertent tissue damage in the host, is also increased by exposure to endotoxin. If released into the bloodstream in large amounts, endotoxin can cause the condition in patients variably referred to as "endotoxemia," "sepsis," or, if severe, "septic shock." There are technical differences in the definitions of these terms, but they can be pathophysiologically grouped together.

Endotoxin, or LPS, is a potent activator of many different types of leukocytes but has much of its effect on the immune system by activation of macrophages. LPS is important in medicine because it and some other bacterial products initiate the conditions of sepsis and septic shock, as just mentioned. Interestingly, LPS does not directly activate macrophages but instead combines with body proteins to do so. When LPS is released from gram-negative bacteria, it is recognized and bound by a protein synthesized in the mammalian liver, LPS-binding protein (LBP). LBP normally circulates in the plasma; its concentration is increased during inflammatory disease (LBP is one of the acute-phase proteins, which are discussed later in this chapter); and it will leak into various tissues. LBP greatly enhances the efficiency (100- to 1000-fold) of transfer and presentation of LPS to the CD14 receptor on the macrophage's (or neutrophil's) surface (Fig. 4-36). The LPS molecule is composed of a "lipid A" portion at one end of the molecule with the rest of it being polysaccharide or oligosaccharide. The lipid A portion is responsible for inducing the immunoinflammatory reaction, and both LBP and the CD14 receptor recognize and bind to LPS at the lipid A site. When LPS binds to it, the CD14 receptor on the cell surface is unable to transmit a cellular signal on its own and cooperates with other receptors (in the "toll-like" receptor family) to cause signal transduction and upregulation of NF-κB and AP-1 transcription factors. This results in leukocyte activation, cytokine/mediator synthesis and secretion, and general immune stimulation.

What's the purpose; why would we be designed to be hypersensitive to LPS at the risk of perhaps succumbing to septic shock? The increased efficiency in recognizing LPS, provided by LBP and CD14, constitutes an "early warning system" for the body's immune system to "gear up." Without it, bacteria would be able to proliferate much more before the macrophages/monocytes recognize the presence and threat of gram-negative bacterial invaders. This early alert of the immune system results in increased synthesis of numerous cytokines (IL-1, TNF-α, IL-6, and others), leukocyte-activating chemokines (IL-8 and others), lipid-derived molecules (arachidonic acid metabolites, platelet-activating factor), and other mediators. The desired net effect should be to suppress or eliminate the threatening gram-negative bacteria. The system is in delicate balance, however. Overstimulation of the immune system and excessive production of mediators can cause life-threatening reactions that are mechanistically part of the pathogenesis of sepsis and septic shock. Self-destructive elements of the latter often include fever (or if death is approaching, a low temperature), hypotension, disseminated intravascular coagula-

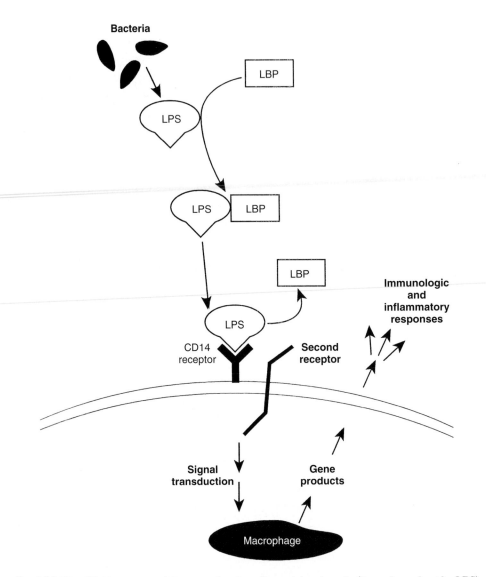

Fig. 4-36 The CD14 receptor-driven mechanism. Bacterial endotoxin (lipopolysaccharide, LPS) stimulates macrophages to synthesize and secrete products that are important to the immunoinflammatory response and host defense. *(Copyright © The University of Tennessee College of Veterinary Medicine, 2000.)*

tion, perfusion abnormalities and acidosis, and cellular and multiorgan ischemia, which may result in organ failure and death. The sensitivity of different species of vertebrates to LPS derived from gram-negative bacteria varies greatly, but a full explanation for this is lacking. Humans and horses are among the most sensitive.

The CD14 receptor for LPS also has a soluble, free-floating version of itself in plasma and other protein-rich body fluids. This is not unusual for receptors associated with the immune system; for example, many of the cytokine receptors exist in soluble form, in addition to their cell-bound form. Soluble CD14 will also bind LPS, and the LBP molecule can catalyze this transfer, but the results are different. Soluble CD14 will efficiently transfer the

bound LPS to cells that do not normally express the membrane-bound CD14 and activate these cells. An example is endothelial cells, which become stimulated upon contact with soluble CD14-LPS complexes and express adhesion molecules and generate other types of inflammatory activity (Fig. 4-37). The other main route for soluble LPS-CD14 complexes is efficient transfer of LPS to lipoproteins in plasma. This results in neutralization of the biological activity of LPS, which is transferred to the liver and degraded.

The CD14 receptor has other functions too. It can participate in phagocytosis of microorganisms; that is, its surface expression on macrophages enhances phagocytosis of microbes by those cells. CD14 can also recognize and bind microbial com-

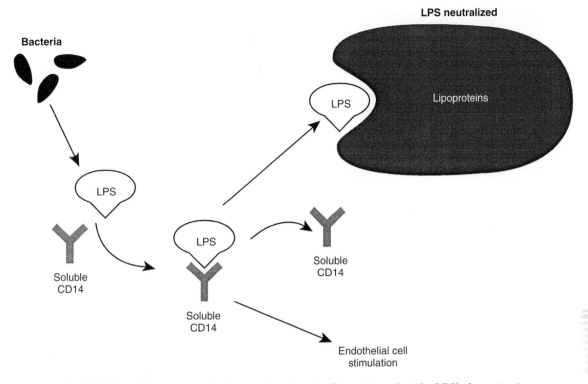

Fig. 4-37 The CD14 receptor for bacterial endotoxin (lipopolysaccharide, LPS) also exists in a soluble form in plasma. This receptor can bind LPS and activate some kinds of cells, such as endothelial cells, or can transfer LPS to plasma lipoproteins, neutralizing LPS. *(Copyright © The University of Tennessee College of Veterinary Medicine, 2000.)*

ponents other than LPS and thus participate in macrophage activation by bacteria other than those of the gram-negative variety. Lastly, CD14 is perhaps the best known receptor for LPS, but it is not the only one. The leukocyte integrins CD11$_x$/CD18, best known for their active roles in leukocyte adhesion (see Table 4-13), also have been reported to recognize and bind LPS and may induce signal transduction in the cell. The macrophage scavenger receptor also binds LPS, but meaningful signaling does not occur, and this may be a prelude to disposal of LPS by the cell.

MECHANISMS OF CHEMOTAXIS

It is not difficult to imagine the assorted chemical attractants oozing out of inflammatory foci to serve as "come hither" signals for the various leukocytes. Let's look at the phenomenon morphologically. Based on a large number of careful ultrastructural and cinemicrographic studies, several conclusions have been reached.

1. Leukocytes crawl. Unlike some microbes, they do not swim. Proper locomotion requires reversible adhesiveness to a surface.
2. The cells undergo characteristic morphological changes that begin with increased surface mem-

brane ruffling within 30 seconds of stimulation (Fig. 4-38).
3. Transient dose-dependent leukocyte aggregation may occur within the first few minutes of stimulation.
4. Responding leukocytes assume a characteristic polarized orientation during locomotion with broad-spreading lamellipodia at the leading edge, which, when assessed by phase microscopy, are fairly free of organelles. A narrow, blunt tail (uropod) is at the rear of the cell.
5. In a gradient of chemoattractant, the population of cells migrate toward the source of the chemotactic factor.
6. Leukocytes easily become deformed as they migrate through narrow places.

These morphological observations contribute important correlative data to what is known about molecular mechanisms of chemotaxis. The best models for understanding the mechanisms of chemotaxis are based on the idea that chemotaxis requires careful integration of adherence, secretion, and locomotion. The first component of the model, increased adhesiveness, is attributable to upregulation of adhesion molecules, as already discussed, usually as a result of stimuli binding to chemoattractant receptors.

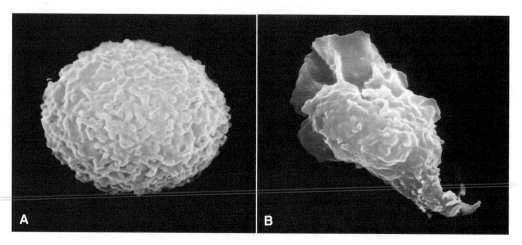

Fig. 4-38 Bovine neutrophil response to chemoattractant C5a. The resting cells, **A,** shown by scanning electron microscopy exhibit only normal small surface membrane projections; 30 seconds after exposure to C5a the stimulated cells, **B,** exhibit pronounced ruffled membrane activity with the formation of large surface lamellipodia.

The initiating event in chemotaxis is binding of the chemoattractant to the cell surface; this is a receptor-mediated event. What happens next in terms of cell physiology occurs very rapidly (Fig. 4-39). There have been described several biochemical processes that develop within 5 seconds or so after ligand-receptor interaction; many stages occur almost simultaneously. One of the early consequences of chemoattractant binding to the cell is release of calcium from intracellular stores and membrane translocation of calcium. This leads to a measurable rise in cytosolic Ca^{++}, which is necessary for triggering both degranulation and changes in membrane polarity. An initial membrane depolarization is followed by a hyperpolarization within 1 minute of stimulation.

Increased intracellular Ca^{++} also influences the submembranous actin-myosin network, the "muscles" of the leukocyte used in cell movement. After the initial increase in intracellular calcium, cell recovery before the next wave of Ca^{++}-mediated movement involves the sequestration of calcium intracellularly. Chemotaxis is optimal in the presence not only of Ca^{++} but also Na^+, K^+, and Mg^{++}. Cells exposed to chemotaxins undergo rapid changes in monovalent cation fluxes, and activation of a membrane-bound Na^+, K^+-ATPase may function as a cation pump.

Alterations in the intracellular levels of cyclic nucleotides also contribute to the regulation of chemotactic responses. A rise in cyclic AMP (cAMP) occurs within 5 to 15 seconds after ligand-receptor interaction and probably follows the rise in cytosolic Ca^{++}. Cyclic nucleotides play important roles as "second messengers"; agents that stimulate cAMP

formation inhibit chemotaxis, whereas agents stimulating increases in cyclic GMP (cGMP) enhance the chemotactic response.

Several important reactions that involve changes in membrane phospholipids occur. After receptor-ligand interaction (with fMLP, C5a, or numerous other chemotaxins), activation of membrane *phospholipase A_2* occurs and correlates well with the release of arachidonic acid from its esterified position in membrane phospholipids such as phosphatidylcholine. Arachidonate liberated from stimulated cells triggers the energy-producing hexose monophosphate shunt, and its subsequent metabolism generates several other powerful mediators such as LTB_4, which is also a potent chemoattractant (see Arachidonic Acid Metabolites, p. 209). The discovery of this phospholipase A_2 pathway has helped to explain one of the mechanisms of the well-known antiinflammatory effects of *glucocorticoids*, since they induce the synthesis in many cells of an inhibitor of phospholipase A_2 known as *lipocortin* or *lipomodulin*, thus inhibiting the synthesis of prostaglandins and leukotrienes, which are part of the inflammatory response.

In a gradient of chemoattractant, orientation of leukocytes seems to occur before movement; that is, the cells initially become polarized like tiny football players lined up on the scrimmage line before they start to move, with their leading edge in the direction of the highest concentration of chemoattractant. Indeed, it has been shown that if the gradient is suddenly reversed neutrophils will stop and reorient themselves in the correct direction before they again start to move. The ability of cells to properly orient in a chemotactic gradient is a func-

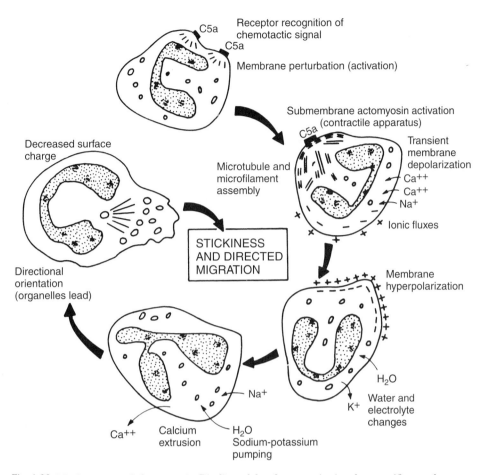

Fig. 4-39 Mechanisms of chemotaxis. Binding of the chemotactic signal to specific membrane receptors causes membrane perturbation and activation of the cellular contractile apparatus. Microtubule and microfilament assembly allows cell motility and directed migration. A series of ionic fluxes and membrane electrical changes is also involved, and the result is an actively motile cell that exhibits specifically directional movement.

tion of the *microtubules,* whereas locomotion itself is tied to the *microfilaments.* Agents such as *cytochalasin B,* which disrupts microfilaments, prevent locomotion even though the cells remain oriented in the gradient. *Colchicine,* on the other hand, disrupts microtubules and produces disorientation though not interfering with locomotion. In a properly responding cell, coordinated microtubule and microfilament activity permits both direction sense and movement.

The biological basis for this activity involves the interaction of actin and myosin with several other important regulatory and modulating proteins. Orientation and sustained locomotion require that these events not be diffuse but occur in a restricted location within the cell. Degranulation at the leading edge of the cell provides new membrane with chemoattractant receptors and integrin adhesion molecules, some of which are known to be present on the granule membranes. There are many differ-

ent integrins that bind different extracellular matrix proteins. Once attached, the leukocyte's tiny "muscles," that is, actin-myosin filaments, contract and pull the leukocytes forward. Then they relax, and the adhesion molecules are downregulated at that spot, releasing the matrix proteins to which they were clinging. Many of these receptors are internalized, recycled, and used again. As the process repeats itself at multiple areas on the leading edges of the leukocyte, the result is a smoothly flowing (or crawling) cell.

To summarize, the phases in the chemotactic response (see Fig. 4-39) are (1) recognition of the chemoattractant followed by (2) transduction of the recognition of the chemoattractant signal into locomotion, which implies (3) an activation of the cellular locomotor apparatus, which is not so very different from the contractile apparatus of muscle cells, (4) ionic fluxes to maintain membrane and submembrane organelles, (5) changes in membrane charge and polarity, and (6) sustained locomotion with its implicit reversible adhesion and renewable facility for gradient detection. Since the highest concentrations of chemoattractant are presumably at the center of the site where injury and inflammation is underway, arriving cells might be expected to follow the chemical gradient until they reach this high concentration of chemoattractant and then become deactivated for further movement. Having "arrived," they need go no farther; downregulation of surface chemotaxin receptors may be involved.

Phagocytosis

Cellular endocytic activity traditionally has been divided into two categories: *phagocytosis*, or "eating," and *pinocytosis*, or "drinking" (see also Chapter 2). Most cell biologists use the term "phagocytosis" to describe the active cellular uptake of larger particulate matter, such as bacteria, whereas "pinocytosis" is used to describe the vesicular uptake of virtually everything else, particularly soluble material, but also very small particles. We focus our attention here on phagocytosis, which is the more important of the two events in terms of inflammation and host defense.

This fascinating biological phenomenon has interested scientists for a long time. Nearly a century ago Metchnikoff stated that phagocytic cells were responsible for protecting the host from invasion by the innumerable microorganisms in the internal and external environment and was among the first to propose that phagocytosis was a basis for survival against infection. Time has proved Metchnikoff to have been partly right. We now know that phagocytic cells cooperate with a variety of humoral factors, collectively called *opsonins,* in improving the efficiency of the process. George Bernard Shaw focused scientists and nonscientists alike on this concept in *The Doctor's Dilemma:*

> *The phagocytes won't eat the microbes unless the microbes are nicely buttered for them. Well, the patient manufactures the butter for himself all right; but my discovery is that the manufacture of that butter, which I call opsonin, goes on in the system by ups and downs; there is at the bottom only one genuinely scientific treatment for all diseases, and that is to stimulate the phagocytes.*

Phagocytosis and the subsequent or concomitant release of enzymes by neutrophils and macrophages are two of the major functions associated with the accumulation of leukocytes at a focus of inflamma-

tion. The lysosomal granules of neutrophils and macrophages are rich in a wide variety of enzymes that can participate in the degradation of foreign materials (see Table 4-9 and Box 4-2). These enzymes and antibacterial products are central to the effectiveness of the phagocytic capacity of these cells.

The phagocytic process involves specific membrane-recognition events, surface attachment of the leukocyte to the particle, engulfment, formation of a phagocytic vacuole, and fusion of that vacuole with lysosomes, exposing the imprisoned object to the action of the lysosomal contents (Fig. 4-40). This sequence is particularly important in the defense against bacterial invasion. In the course of this action, the neutrophils and the monocytes become progressively degranulated; that is, they use their granule contents to try to kill or degrade the particle. Many events increase the vulnerability of bacteria to engulfment. Perhaps the most important is the phenomenon of *opsonization. Opsonins* are naturally occurring and acquired substances that coat bacteria and render them more susceptible to phagocytosis. Although several different potentially useful opsonins have been characterized, by far the most important ones are antibody (which interacts with the Fc receptor on phagocytic cells) and the complement fragment C3b, for which phagocytes also possess receptors. *Fibronectin* is a large dimeric glycoprotein that can bind to many surfaces and may influence phagocytosis both as an opsonin and by increasing cell adhesiveness. Phagocytosis is favored by higher body temperatures, which commonly occur during infection, and febrile reactions in inflammation thus favor this phenomenon.

Engulfment begins with a recognition event at the cell surface. This is obviously favored if the stimulus has been opsonized but may also proceed anyway through nonspecific receptor systems. Upon contact, the cell extends small cytoplasmic extensions, or pseudopods, which become closely applied to the surface of the attached particle; these flow around the particle until it is engulfed. The cytoplasmic processes pinch together, meet, and fuse around the particle, and the resulting phagosome is drawn into the cell. This is accompanied by the movement of the lysosomal granules toward the developing phagosome. By means of cinemicrography and electron microscopy it has been demonstrated that the lysosomal granules converge on the forming phagosome, fuse with it to form the *phagolysosome,* and discharge their contents into the vacuolar lumen around the particle. This process is called phagocyte *degranulation.* In neutrophils, it appears that the specific granules fuse with the phagosome slightly

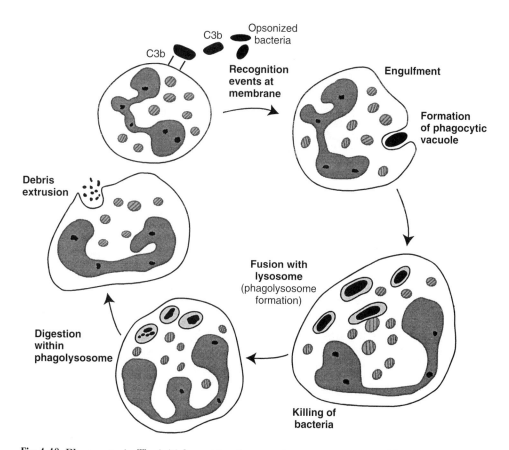

Fig. 4-40 Phagocytosis. The initial event involves membrane receptor-recognition events that trigger the formation of the phagocytic vacuole. Phagolysosome formation exposes the imprisoned object to the hydrolytic enzymes in the lysosome. After digestion, the residual debris often is extruded.

before the azurophil granules. This sequential fusion may relate to pH changes inside the vacuole.

The cellular mechanisms by which phagocytosis occurs seem to involve many of the same processes that are central to chemotaxis. Activation of the engulfment sequence is a response to receptor-ligand interaction, and the factors involved in propagation of the pseudopods rest in activation of the leukocyte "motor" by the interaction of actin with other actin-modulating proteins in a Ca^{++}-dependent way. The proteins that control actin filament length are the same as those involved in chemotaxis: actin, actin-binding proteins, and myosin. These assembled cytoskeletal networks control the shape and development of the pseudopods and are apparently of importance in the distribution of organelles and the consistency of the cytoplasm. Ca^{++} acts as a second messenger here to help convert the recognition events at the membrane into ingestion. It has been well documented that actin-rich microfilaments are numerous in submembrane locations in the portions of the pseudopods that are in contact with phagocytosable particles. The movement of

the lysosomes toward the developing phagosomes is also believed to be under microtubular control.

MICROBICIDAL MECHANISMS

The ultimate purpose of bacterial phagocytosis is to kill and degrade bacteria. Two somewhat different oxygen-dependent killing systems, an *oxygen radical system* and the *H_2O_2-myeloperoxidase-halide system*, as well as oxygen-independent bactericidal mechanisms have been identified.

Oxygen-Dependent Killing Mechanisms

During phagocytosis, neutrophils show a burst of metabolic activity, characterized by a two- to threefold increase in oxygen consumption, an increase in superoxide anion (O_2^-) generation and hydrogen peroxide (H_2O_2) formation, and an increase in the amount of glucose metabolized by means of the hexose monophosphate shunt (HMPS). This collectively has been called the *respiratory burst of phagocytosis* (Box 4-6). Much of this biochemical activity in

BOX 4-6 **Major Features of the "Respiratory Burst" of Phagocytosis**

Increased oxygen utilization by the cell
Increased glucose oxidation by the hexose monophase shunt (HMPS)
Generation of reactive oxygen species, including superoxide anion (O_2^-), hydrogen peroxide (H_2O_2), and hydroxyl radical (HO·)
Generation of hypochlorous acid (HOCl)

phagocytes is attributable to a membrane-bound *NADPH oxidase*; cytochrome *b* is also part of this system and is present in specific and tertiary (gelatinase) granules of neutrophils. These granules fuse with the engulfed particle (such as one containing bacteria), which is also membrane bound, making cytochrome *b* and also numerous other granule constituents available for microbicidal activity. The activated NADPH oxidase reduces molecular oxygen by electron transfer from NADPH and in so doing forms the oxygen radical O_2^- and NADP; the latter is required for operation of the HMPS. Most of the superoxide generated reacts rapidly and spontaneously dismutates to produce oxygen and H_2O_2. The NADP-activated HMPS metabolizes glucose to provide the energy that is needed to regenerate NADPH, which was consumed in the initial reaction involving NADPH oxidase, and the system can then cycle again and again.

The production of superoxide anion (O_2^-) and hydrogen peroxide (H_2O_2) during the respiratory burst is important because they provide a direct link to the oxygen radical and myeloperoxidase-based systems of phagocyte microbicidal and cytotoxic activities. Neither superoxide anion nor hydrogen peroxide are hugely potent microbicidal molecules themselves. Superoxide anion, however, contributes to formation of the very toxic hydroxyl radical (HO·), which is very reactive and damaging to biological molecules. Bacterial killing by these radicals is a result of oxidant damage and peroxidation of membrane lipids. It is also worth noting that much of the superoxide generated occurs on the surface of the phagolysosome. Without this mechanism, these reactions could occur internally—in the cytosol of the cell—and could damage the phagocyte. The chemistry of the steps in the four-electron reduction of oxygen is as follows:

One electron accepted: $O_2 + e^- \rightarrow O_2^-$ (superoxide anion)

Two electrons accepted: $O_2^- + e^- + 2H^+ \rightarrow H_2O_2$ (hydrogen peroxide, just like that in the bottle from the pharmacy)

Three electrons accepted: $H_2O_2 + e^- \rightarrow HO· + OH^-$
(The Fenton reaction)   (hydroxyl radical, HO·, a very potent, damaging oxidant)

Four electrons accepted: $HO· + e^- + H^+ \rightarrow H_2O$

Another antimicrobial reaction results from combination of superoxide anion with hydrogen peroxide, both produced and available from the reduction of oxygen. This also results in production of the extremely reactive oxidant, hydroxyl radical, and is called the Haber-Weiss reaction:

$$O_2^- + H_2O_2 \rightarrow HO· + OH^- + O_2$$

The Haber-Weiss reaction is catalyzed by iron. The iron for these reactions can come from many sources, including iron within the leukocytes and iron outside of the leukocyte; the latter is available in the form of heme proteins and iron-transport proteins like transferrin.

The hydrogen peroxide produced in these reactions can also combine with the azurophil granule enzyme *myeloperoxidase* within the phagolysosome and, along with a *halide ion,* such as iodide, bromide, or chloride (the last being the usual physiologically relevant halide), forms a potent bactericidal blend known as the *H_2O_2-myeloperoxidase-halide system.* The molecular combination of these components produces bactericidal activity many times stronger than the effect that might be produced by any one of the molecules acting singly. The "killer" molecule produced in this reaction,

$$H_2O_2 + Cl^- \rightarrow HOCl + H_2O$$

is hypochlorous acid (HOCl), a powerful oxidant and antimicrobial agent that is similar to bleach sold in supermarkets (sodium hypochlorite). Again, this activity takes place within the phagolysosome so as not to kill the phagocyte itself.

Potent oxidizing agents such as these can damage membrane lipids, proteins, and DNA. The intent is to wreak havoc on microbes, but when produced or released outside of a leukocyte's phagolysosome, they can commit damage to our own tissues. Such damage can occur when excessive oxidative reactions occur during inflammation and also in other traumatic disease. As an added risk, the oxygen radicals can inactive antiproteinases (such as α_1-antiproteinase) in the extracellular environment. This increases the risk of excessive tissue destruction as a result of the unavailability of antiproteinases to control the powerful proteinases released from leukocytes and other cells. As always, a way to balance this potential risk exists. Cytosolic and plasma molecular "scavengers" of oxyradicals are present and are designed to limit damage to cells and tissue. For example, superoxide dismutases

(SODs) convert or dismutate O_2^- to H_2O_2, and catalase or the substrate glutathione (GSH) and its enzyme glutathione peroxidase, both in cells, convert H_2O_2 to H_2O and O_2.

$$2O_2^- + 2H^+ + SOD \rightarrow H_2O_2 + O_2$$
$$2H_2O_2 + Catalase \rightarrow O_2 + 2H_2O$$

and

$$H_2O_2 + 2GSH + Glutathione\ peroxidase$$
$$\rightarrow GSSG + 2H_2O$$

We need to pause for a moment and put oxygen radical production by leukocytes in perspective: leukocytes are not the only sources of oxygen radicals produced in the body. Oxygen radicals are produced daily in our body by normal oxidative metabolism, as in the electron-transport chain in mitochondria, as a by-product of arachidonic acid metabolism, by exposure of our cells to ionizing radiation, by air pollution (ozone), and by exposure to some types of drugs, herbicides, or pesticides. The same protective antioxidant enzymes mentioned above also help to provide a measure of safety for us against these other sources of oxygen radicals.

Another important pathological process when oxygen radicals come into play is during *reperfusion injury*. Reperfusion injury occurs when normal blood flow is transiently interrupted to tissues, as in thromboembolism or in torsion of the bowel, when aerobic metabolism is interrupted. If medical intervention or just plain luck results in restoration of blood flow, aerobic metabolism resumes, but oxygen radicals may then be produced in excess as a result of metabolic changes in the tissues and sudden reperfusion with oxygen-rich blood. If the antioxidant systems are overwhelmed, tissue injury can result in the area that is being reperfused; this is double jeopardy for the area of tissue that was ischemic. Reperfusion injury is an important pathological process that is covered in greater detail in diseases of the circulatory system.

Lastly, another reactive molecule that can be produced by some cells, particularly macrophages, is nitric oxide (NO). NO and its reactive intermediates have some antimicrobial activity too, and NO can combine with superoxide anion to form another highly reactive molecule, peroxynitrite. NO also has other important functions and is discussed later in this chapter in the section on mediators of inflammation.

Oxygen-Independent Killing Mechanisms

Bactericidal mechanisms not dependent on oxygen metabolic events are also very important, and the components are found in the leukocyte granules (lysosomes). The cationic enzyme *lysozyme* attacks bacterial cell walls, especially gram-positive cocci, and hydrolyzes the muramic acid–N-acetylglucosamine bond found in the glycopeptide coat of many bacteria. *Lactoferrin* is an iron-binding glycoprotein found in the specific granules that may be detrimental to some microbes that need iron to grow. *Cathepsin G* is a proteinase of azurophil granules that has antimicrobial properties for both gram-positive and gram-negative bacteria, as well as some fungi.

A group of related arginine- and cysteine-rich peptides known as *defensins* are very important constituents of leukocyte granules and have broad-spectrum antimicrobial properties, including both gram-negative and gram-positive bacteria, fungi, and even some enveloped viruses. The defensins and defensin-like peptides are just one group of a much larger collection of *antimicrobial peptides* that occur throughout nature. Various members of this group exist in everything from plants and insects to mammals. The antimicrobial peptides occur in numerous kinds of cells but, in general, are concentrated in locations and cells that are likely to contact microbes, that is, epithelial surfaces (skin, respiratory tract, gastrointestinal tract) and phagocytic leukocytes. The antimicrobial activity of these peptides and small proteins varies in its biochemistry but is sometimes related to insertion of the peptides into the microbial membrane and the creation of "holes," much like the activity of the terminal components of complement. An example of the group of mammalian antimicrobial peptides and proteins is bactericidal permeability–increasing protein (BPI; see Table 4-9). BPI has particular affinity for LPS on the external surface of gram-negative bacteria. BPI is present in high concentration in neutrophil granules and, when released into phagolysosomes, not only punches holes in the bacteria but also neutralizes LPS. Others that have been identified in veterinary species include the β-defensins in bovine neutrophils, and the cathelicidins PR-39 and protegrin in porcine neutrophils; cathelicidins have also been identified in other animals, including cattle, horses, sheep, and goats, and antimicrobial peptides have also been discovered in poultry. Interestingly it seems that some antimicrobial peptides and the other oxygen-independent mechanisms are specialized for certain groups of bacteria or other microbes, whereas the oxygen-dependent systems attack all microbial cell walls nonspecifically. Fortunately, in a properly functioning phagocyte both systems are operational, and the most effective microbicidal activity rests on this combined action.

Antimicrobial peptides are relatively newly discovered compared to many other aspects of host defense, and their importance is huge, whether discussing their presence in leukocytes or in other cells. Consider for a moment the bovine respiratory mucosa, constantly exposed to inhaled particulates including microbes. In addition to the day-to-day protective effects of mucociliary clearance and phagocytic activity of alveolar macrophages, defensins can be produced by respiratory epithelial cells to help keep bacteria at bay; defensins are also part of the armament of alveolar macrophages. Consider the small intestinal tract, where bacterial overgrowth can result in enteritis. Antimicrobial peptides have been demonstrated to be produced in the intestinal crypt cells, helping to keep microbes in check. Frogs have antimicrobial peptides that are produced in their skin, helping them to resist waterborne bacteria. There are many other examples. The concept of epithelial barriers such as skin or gastrointestinal mucosa as a first line of defense against microbes is an established idea and is made even stronger in light of the fact that antimicrobial peptides are produced and present at these sites.

There is another recently discovered protein that is very important in the antimicrobial armament, *Nramp1*, which is the acronym for "natural resistance–associated macrophage protein one." *Nramp1* may be the prototypical representative of a family of similar proteins that have transporter function. *Nramp1* supports increased cytoplasmic flux of iron, and its activity apparently is sensitive to and increased by some of the cytokines associated with the inflammatory response. After phagocytosis of bacterial pathogens, *Nramp1* appears in the membrane of the phagolysosome of cells of macrophage lineage. Evidence argues in support of the hypothesis that *Nramp1* is an iron pump that depletes the phagolysosome of this nutrient and therefore helps starve the engulfed bacteria of this essential nutrient needed for their survival and growth. *Nramp1* has also been shown to affect intracellular phagosomal pH and negatively affect the ability of bacteria such as mycobacteria to grow. Other important antimicrobial properties and activities of the *Nramp* family of proteins will doubtless be discovered.

What then of all those other enzymes in the leukocyte lysosomes; are they antimicrobial too? (See Table 4-9 and Box 4-2.) Many of the lysosomal enzymes do not have direct bactericidal activity but are *digestive*. That is, after killing, the acid hydrolases and other lysosomal enzymes degrade and digest the bacteria within the phagolysosomes before either subsequent extrusion of the debris from the cell, or death of the cell. After phagocytosis and with the help of proton pumps, the pH of the phagolysosome drops to a range of about 4 to 5, which is the optimum pH for the action of such enzymes. Thus, many of the enzymes serve only a terminal degradatory role after the killing systems have completed their task.

These systems are formidable and might seem unbeatable, but despite the fact that these phagocytic and bactericidal systems are usually successful, they are not always so. There are various examples of diseases in which the primary problem is failure of the phagocyte killing systems. The significance of phagocytosis in the body's defense against bacterial infections is perhaps best illustrated by the vulnerability of patients who suffer from defects in the phagocytes; infections often cause the death of these predisposed individuals. Other strategies used by pathogens are exemplified by those organisms that are sufficiently virulent to destroy the phagocytes. Others, like the tubercle bacillus, seem to happily survive within the phagocytes that have engulfed them, whereas still other organisms seem to be able to escape from the phagosome and replicate in the cytoplasm or to somehow interfere with phagosome-lysosome fusion. Various "escape mechanisms" are discussed in greater detail elsewhere. Another risk that occurs when phagocytic cells like macrophages fail to kill microorganisms is that the organisms may take up residence inside the macrophages, and the macrophages may then migrate through lymphatic or vascular channels, spreading the infectious agent.

RELEASE OF LYSOSOMAL ENZYMES AND TISSUE INJURY

Three basic mechanisms whereby phagocytic cells can release their potent chemicals into the tissues at sites of inflammation and thus contribute to tissue injury have been recognized. These have been variously referred to by the colorful designations of (1) "lysosomal suicide," (2) "regurgitation during feeding," and (3) "frustrated phagocytosis." We briefly consider each of these.

Lysosomal Suicide

When a phagocyte internalizes pathogenic bacteria, sometimes the bacteria overwhelm the leukocyte rather than vice versa. When this occurs, the phagolysosome may rupture into the cell cytoplasm, spilling out potent lysosomal enzymes, which can then kill the leukocyte (Fig. 4-41). Also, when leukocytes die at sites of inflammation, stores of lysosomal enzymes are released into the local environment after lysis or rupture of the limiting cell membranes.

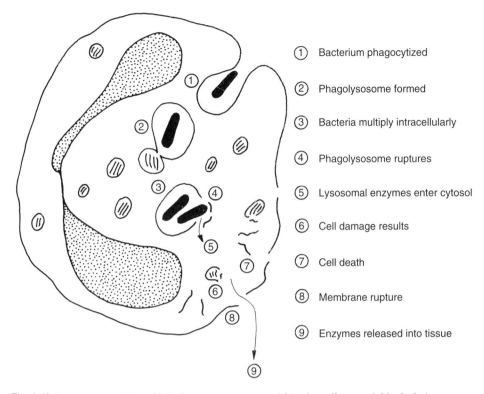

① Bacterium phagocytized

② Phagolysosome formed

③ Bacteria multiply intracellularly

④ Phagolysosome ruptures

⑤ Lysosomal enzymes enter cytosol

⑥ Cell damage results

⑦ Cell death

⑧ Membrane rupture

⑨ Enzymes released into tissue

Fig. 4-41 Lysosomal suicide. If the lysosome ruptures within the cell, powerful hydrolytic enzymes are released and can ultimately cause death of the cell itself. Rupture of the cell membrane releases lysosomal contents into tissue sites.

The resulting cellular debris is what we clinically recognize as "pus." Fortunately, a minimal amount of this occurs in the noninflammatory, daily turnover of short-lived neutrophils. Many senescent and apoptotic neutrophils and other leukocytes are phagocytized and digested by macrophages in places like the spleen, disappearing without a ripple, and thus tissue damage is avoided.

Regurgitation During Feeding

In the face of large numbers of bacteria (or some other phagocytic stimulus), the leukocytes sometimes make critical errors of timing, which no doubt have their basis in the membrane and microtubule-microfilament events associated with internalization of the phagocytic stimulus and lysosomal granule movement. During a serious phagocytic feeding orgy in which large numbers of bacteria are present, fusion of the lysosome with the developing phagosome may occur before the complete internalization of the bacterium. That is, fusion of lysosome to phagosome takes place before the plasma membrane has completely surrounded the bacterium (Fig. 4-42). In such an event, it is not difficult to imagine that the lytic enzymes present in the lysosome have direct access to

the extracellular environment. The result is enzymatic damage to host tissues.

Frustrated Phagocytosis

Sometimes phagocytes encounter phagocytic stimuli that are simply too large to be internalized. Examples might be bacteria immobilized against a fibrin meshwork or complexes of antigen and antibody fixed against a basement membrane or joint surface. Here, the cell responds appropriately to the phagocytic stimulus by attempting to internalize it, but because the stimulus is too large, formation of a phagosome does not take place. Rather, the membrane events associated with phagosome formation occur and set into play the intracellular mechanisms responsible for fusion of the lysosome with the developing phagosome (Fig. 4-43). Since the phagosome never really develops because of the size of the nonphagocytosable stimulus, union of the lysosome with the membrane results in discharge of the lysosomal contents against the nonphagocytosable stimulus, almost as though the leukocyte were frustrated at its inability to internalize the bulky stimulus. If this occurs where the stimulus is adjacent to or integrated into host tissue, the enzymes released can

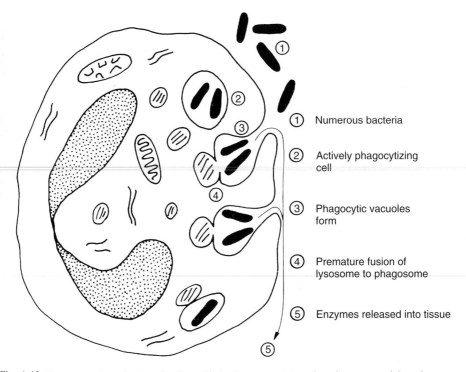

① Numerous bacteria

② Actively phagocytizing cell

③ Phagocytic vacuoles form

④ Premature fusion of lysosome to phagosome

⑤ Enzymes released into tissue

Fig. 4-42 Regurgitation during feeding. If the lysosome joins the phagosome (phagolysosome formation) before the complete closure of the cell membrane around the phagocytic stimulus, enzymes escape into the surrounding tissues.

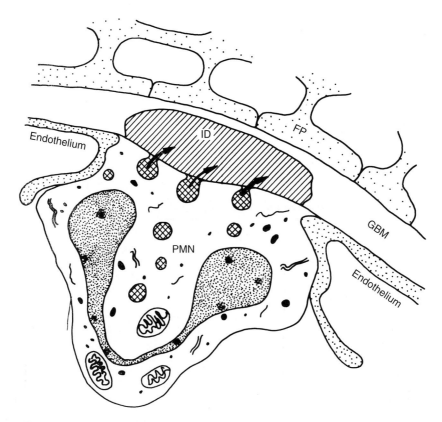

Fig. 4-43 Frustrated phagocytosis. The neutrophil, *PMN*, here has encountered a phagocytic stimulus (immune deposit, *ID*) too large to internalize because it is fixed against the glomerular basement membrane, *GBM*. Fusion of the lysosome to the surface occurs, and enzymes are discharged. *FP*, Foot processes of epithelial cells.

damage that tissue substrate, adding to the injury process. Such a mechanism is believed to be operative in some cases of immune-mediated diseases such as glomerulonephritis and rheumatoid arthritis.

We have already discussed mechanisms in place for limiting damage of host tissue by leukocyte enzymes, but it is a good idea to reemphasize it here while we are discussing the release of leukocyte enzymes. These enzymes can, of course, behave as useful and helpful components of our immune system, but the antiproteinases are needed to keep them under control. We have a range of antiproteinases that are designed to contain and confine the actions of the proteinases to a given locale. The most universal of the antiproteinases is α_2-macroglobulin, which is produced in the liver, circulates in the plasma, and inhibits all four classes of leukocyte proteinases. Serine proteinase inhibitors, or serpins, are abundant in plasma and include α_1- proteinase inhibitor, plasminogen-activator inhibitors, anti–thrombin III, and others. The matrix metalloproteinases (MMPs) are inhibited by the tissue inhibitors of metalloproteinases (TIMPs), which are synthesized by leukocytes and other cells of the connective tissues. Mechanisms are in place to limit the damage if the potent proteinase enzymes are spilled into our tissues.

LEUKOCYTE ACTIVATION: STIMULUS-RESPONSE COUPLING

As we have stated, much of the leukocytic activity associated with inflammation occurs after these cells are stimulated by means of membrane receptor-ligand interactions. This linking of a stimulus at the cell membrane with some functional response has been known as *stimulus-response coupling*. Normal leukocytes in the peripheral blood are at a low level of activity, and leukocyte functions such as oxidative burst activity, exocytosis, and phagocytosis are absent or minimal. In short, all these functions of leukocytes are induced responses and require leukocyte *activation*. Huge progress has been made in recent years in our understanding of the intracellular machinery responsible for signal transduction within cells, including leukocytes. Fig. 4-44 presents

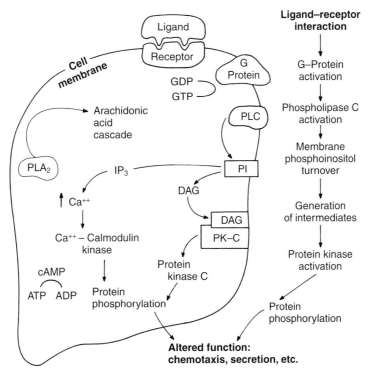

Fig. 4-44 Leukocyte activation and stimulus-response coupling. The sequence of events by which membrane-ligand interaction at the surface is translated into functional activity involves several important intermediate steps and the generation of second messengers. Receptor occupancy alters receptor affinity for the ligand and changes its conformation to activate G-proteins, which in turn excite the membrane phospholipase, *PLC*. Activated PLC acts on membrane phosphoinositol, *PI*, to generate the intermediates inositol triphosphate, *IP₃*, and diacyl glycerol, *DAG*. IP₃ acts to increase intracellular calcium for activation of Ca^{++}-dependent protein kinases, whereas DAG directly activates protein kinase C, *PK-C*. Both kinases phosphorylate different substrates, and altered functional activity results. *PLA₂*, Phospholipase A₂.

a venerable and still valid schema showing a wee part of the receptor-initiated biochemical activity that results in activities such as upregulation of adhesion molecules, chemotaxis, and the oxidative burst. Fig. 4-44 legend tells the basic story.

But what about more complex receptor-driven events and signal transduction, some of which eventually result in activity in the nuclei of leukocytes including transcriptional regulation and synthesis of cytokines, chemokines, and other molecules involved in the inflammatory process? Ten years ago it was possible to present a concise overview of this, but it is not possible today. Receptor-ligand binding still is the usual event that occurs at the surface of the leukocyte or other cell to start the process, but the following events depend on what kind of stimulus was present, what kind of receptor was activated, and what kind of cell we are talking about. There are numerous different ligands (stimuli), there are several different receptor families, and there are many different possible intermediate steps and second messengers in cells that may cross-talk with yet other pathways. Multimembered families of signal-transducing messengers have been discovered, including the Janus kinases (JAKs), signal transducers and activators of transcription (STATs), mitogen-activated kinases (MAP kinases) and related kinases, and many others. Some kinds of receptors have tyrosine kinase activity as a result of autophosphorylation after ligand-receptor binding, resulting in activation of *ras* and then phosphorylation and activation of MAP kinases. Thousands of manuscripts have been written on this topic, and it is beyond the scope and possibility of this textbook to incorporate it into this chapter; you can find some references on this at the end of this chapter and many more by doing a literature search.

But why study this at all unless you just happen to find it interesting? Much of the currently employed therapy for various inflammatory diseases uses pharmacological agents that are not yet highly refined or effective in taking aim at specific chemical mediators involved in inflammatory diseases. In terms of controlling leukocyte activity to reduce inflammation, many of the currently available drugs cause only rather general and nonspecific depression of leukocyte or other cellular function. Useful cell functions as well as damaging ones can be altered. This situation will likely change within the professional lifetimes of most of the readers of this book, as ways to manipulate specific signaling pathways in specific groups of cells and leukocytes are developed. We will hopefully reach for drugs and recombinant products aimed at specific mediators, selected secretory products, and precise cell functions. It should be very interesting.

OTHER BIOCHEMICAL MEDIATORS OF INFLAMMATION
General Features of Mediators

A simple definition of a biochemical mediator of inflammation might be any messenger that acts on blood vessels, inflammatory cells, or other cells to contribute to an inflammatory response. A large number of agents fulfill this definition, and we have already had occasion to mention or discuss some of these in this chapter; we will take a closer look at more of them now. Since the *vascular* and *cellular* aspects of inflammation remain its central features, it stands to reason that many of the important mediator molecules are those that enhance blood flow, increase vascular permeability, or induce the emigration of leukocytes from the bloodstream to the site of injury. Because of the importance of these functions in host defense, a large number of chemical mediators can induce these changes. This reiterates the theme of redundancy of pathways within the inflammatory response.

Where do the mediators of inflammation come from and what are they like? Chemical mediators can be *exogenous* ('coming from outside the body'), such as endotoxin (bacterial lipopolysaccharide, LPS), or they can be *endogenous* ('coming from within the body'), such as histamine. In keeping with the view that inflammation is a host defense system, most of the useful chemical mediators are endogenous. The endogenous mediators can be derived from plasma sources such as bradykinin, from leukocyte sources such as LTB_4 and IL-1, or from the other cells of the host tissues, such as endothelial cells and fibroblasts. Virtually all these mediators interact with their targets by means of specific receptor-ligand interactions at the cell surface.

Some mediators are *preformed* and require only release from their cellular stores, such as histamine, whereas others are newly *synthesized* by stimulated cells, such as prostaglandins or platelet-activating factor. Others are generated as a consequence of multiple enzymatic steps involving sequential activation of different molecules by limited proteolysis, such as the complement and coagulation systems. Some mediators are very small, such as histamine (MW 200) or bradykinin (only 9 amino acids); some are intermediate in size, such as tumor necrosis factor, 17 kD; and some are much larger. Some are amines like histamine and serotonin, some are lipids like the leukotrienes and platelet-activating factor, some are glycoproteins like interferon, and many are polypeptides like C5a.

The biochemical mediators of inflammation have generated intense interest among biochemists, physiologists, cell biologists, pathologists, pharmacologists, and clinicians. Since our focus here is on understanding the biology of the inflammatory response, we emphasize the function of the various mediators in terms of their relationship to the vascular and cellular events of inflammation, some of their unique biochemical features, and the means by which they are generated.

Injury precipitates the inflammatory response largely by stimulating the release of biochemical mediators. Their existence was long suspected because whatever the nature of the injury, the ensuing inflammatory changes compose a fairly uniform, almost stereotyped reaction. The relative significance of different mediators to a developing inflammatory reaction varies somewhat depending on the animal species, the location in the body, and the nature of the injurious agent. A well-developed inflammatory reaction involves many mediators acting simultaneously. Although differing widely in chemical structure and in mechanisms of release or activation, the mediators have one general characteristic in common: they are readily available wherever needed. They are either distributed widely throughout the body or can be synthesized at most locations, so that release or activation can occur locally at almost any inflammatory focus. To protect ourselves from the potentially negative effects of "too many mediators" some of the molecules of inflammation have rather short tissue half-lives and can be quickly inactivated. Many of them do not circulate systemically in high concentration except in unusual circumstances; the presence in the systemic circulation of significant concentrations of these potent agents would pose a difficult problem in regulating and limiting the response and might well prove disastrous in many instances. Lastly, natural inhibitors of most mediators are found in normal plasma, a condition that helps to limit the extent of inflammatory responses.

The mediation of inflammation involves an extensive network of interacting biochemicals that provide the system with a high degree of redundancy. This guarantees that both amplification and preservation of the response can be maintained even if one component or another of the system is deficient. There are virtually no parts of the inflammatory response that are dependent on a single mediator; indeed, most functions can be elicited by multiple mediators, and most mediators serve multiple functions. The potent and important complement fragment C5a, for example, can stimulate neutrophil adhesiveness and aggregation, chemotaxis, and lysosomal enzyme release as well as several other functions and is an important initiator of acute inflammation, yet genetic deficiency of C5 is not a major impairment to inflammatory respon-

siveness. This demonstrates the value of compensatory collateral mediation systems.

Before we look at a few more of the mediators involved in the inflammatory response, we need to acknowledge the chemokines and cytokines. Chemokines have previously been covered in this chapter. Many of the cytokines have also already been mentioned in this chapter in context of their involvement in events and progression of the inflammatory response. As we all know, there are literally dozens of cytokines and chemokines, and to discuss them all in adequate detail would require volumes, not just a few pages in this chapter. For those who would like more detailed information on the cytokines refer to Chapter 5 in this book, other books devoted exclusively to immunology, and good reviews in the literature. Table 4-16 is included here with a warning that it is a vast oversimplification in terms of actions and functions of these cytokines. As a group, the cytokines are incredibly pleiotropic, and the table serves only as the briefest of primers. The previous Tables 4-14 and 4-15 show the chemokines and their actions.

Vasoactive Amines: Histamine and Serotonin

Histamine is a *preformed* mediator that is largely from the granules of tissue mast cells and peripheral blood basophils and, in some species, the platelets. It is formed by the decarboxylation of the amino acid L-histidine. Histamine has long been known to play an important part in the initiation of the vascular aspects of a wide variety of inflammatory states. It is undoubtedly important in mediating the immediate active phase of increased vascular permeability. Histamine produces not only increased vascular permeability but has profound effects on vascular and bronchial smooth muscle as well. Histamine is unquestionably of major importance in the pathogenesis of systemic anaphylaxis.

In mast cells and basophils, histamine is stored within granules in the cytoplasm and is bound within the granules by electrostatic forces to heparin. When these granules are extruded from the cell, histamine is released. Histamine promotes the contraction of extravascular smooth muscle in the bronchus yet dilates arterioles. It also elicits an increase in vascular permeability by causing the endothelial cells of venules to contract and round up, and so gaps appear between the margins of adjacent cells. Soon after release it is inactivated by histaminase or by oxidative deamination.

Serotonin (5-hydroxytryptamine, 5-HT) is an important mediator of inflammation in some animal species and is formed from dietary tryptophan. It is

TABLE 4-16 Brief Overview of Some of the Cytokines Involved in Inflammatory and Immunological Responses

CYTOKINE	QUICK SYNOPSIS OF FUNCTION(S)
IL-1α, -1β	Stimulates a vast number of types of cells. Involved in producing the acute-phase response. IL-1 is truly a pluripotent "master cytokine."
TNF-α, -β	Similar to IL-1 in many of its actions. Also can induce apoptosis of some cells. Another "master cytokine."
IL-2	A very potent stimulus for most lymphocytes, especially related to cell-mediated immunity (CMI).
IL-3	A pluripotent colony-stimulating factor ("multi-CSF") that synergizes with other factors to stimulate progenitor cells of the bone marrow.
IL-4	Important for humoral immunity. Stimulates proliferation and differentiation of B cells and T_H2 cells. Has some inhibitory and antiinflammatory actions in some circumstances. Important in allergic diseases.
IL-5	An eosinophil growth and differentiation factor. Also a stimulant for B-cell proliferation. Important in allergic diseases.
IL-6	Another pluripotent "master cytokine" with some of the same actions as IL-1 and TNF-α. Can stimulate both B-cell and T-cell proliferation.
IL-7	A lymphocyte growth factor.
IL-8	The first chemokine discovered and was named as an interleukin. Chemotaxis and activation of neutrophils and some other cell types.
IL-9	Stimulates proliferation and enhances survival of some T lymphocytes; also stimulates mast cells.
IL-10	Can act as a potent downregulator of cytokine synthesis by some cells; can dampen the immunoinflammatory response.
IL-11	Stimulates platelet development and generation in the bone marrow; promotes osteolysis; other actions.
IL-12	A strong stimulus for T_H1 lymphocytes and NK cells; dampens the T_H2 lymphocyte response; a potent factor in CMI.
IL-13	A B lymphocyte growth and stimulatory factor. May be important in allergic diseases.
IL-14	Another B lymphocyte growth and stimulatory factor.
IL-15	Stimulates multiple types of lymphocytes to proliferate or differentiate, especially T cells; overlaps with IL-2.
IL-16	Is actually a chemokine ("lymphotactin") that is a specific chemotaxin for T cells.
IL-17	Extremely diverse actions; generally proinflammatory.
IL-18	Also known as "interferon-gamma inducing factor"; activates T_H1 and NK cells to synthesize IFN-γ. Has many more actions than just this.
IFN-α	Broad stimulatory action on many cells; has antiviral activity.
IFN-β	Similar to IFN-α
IFN-γ	Plays a key role in activation of cells involved with host defense, especially macrophages. Numerous other activities.
MIF	"Macrophage migration inhibitory factor." First described as a lymphokine that induces macrophages to stay in a localized tissue area. A probable counterregulator of corticosteroid suppression of cytokine synthesis; that is, generally enhances cytokine secretion, which would otherwise be suppressed by corticosteroids.
G-CSF	"Granulocyte colony–stimulating factor." A stimulant for neutrophil granulocyte development in the bone marrow and also a stimulant for mature neutrophils.
M-CSF	"Macrophage colony–stimulating factor." Similar to G-CSF but directed toward monocytes/macrophages. Also called CSF-1.
GM-CSF	"Granulocyte-macrophage colony–stimulating factor." Has overlapping activity with G-CSF and M-CSF.

In this list of cytokines, their actions are by necessity vastly understated and oversimplified. Most or all of these cytokines have numerous, diverse activities that are addressed in other sources, such as chapters and texts devoted to immunology. We do not mean to imply that these are the only actions of these cytokines. This simple table is presented as a primer for students new to the field.

found in certain cells of the gastrointestinal tract, the brain, the lung, and the platelets. In rodents it is also found in mast cells and basophils, but this is not the case for most species. Serotonin has a variety of effects on smooth muscle, blood vessels, and nerves in different regions of the body and can produce pain. It is inactivated by monoamine oxidases.

Release of vasoactive amines, that is, histamine or serotonin, from mast cells occurs in response to a wide variety of stimuli such as physical injury, mechanical trauma, irradiation, heat, various chemical agents, snake venoms, melittin from bee venom, toxins, trypsin, bile salts, ATP, immunological processes, antigenic challenge of IgE antibody–sensitized cells, and exposure to complement components C3a and C5a. Release of serotonin from platelets occurs during the platelet-release reaction triggered by stimuli such as thrombin, trypsin, collagen, antigen-antibody complexes, globulin-coated surfaces, snake venoms, epinephrine, and ADP. In addition, vasoactive amines can be secreted from platelets after interaction with platelet-activating factor.

The mechanisms involved in the release of amines and other mediators from mast cells, basophils, and platelets have been intensively studied. Of particular interest is the role of IgE antibody in mediator release and how this can explain the pathogenesis and manifestations of some anaphylactic reactions (see Chapter 5). Both histamine and serotonin induce contraction of smooth muscle and increased vascular permeability. Recently it has been reported that histamine probably stimulates stromal cells to synthesize and release eotaxins, which are chemokines with potency for chemotaxis of eosinophils. This helps to explain the influx and localization of eosinophils in some allergic hypersensitivity reactions.

Kinins

The kinins are a group of related polypeptides that are split from protein precursors in plasma (kininogens) by enzymes termed "kallikreins." The prototype kinin is *bradykinin* and its biologically active metabolite des-Arg bradykinin (meaning that a terminal arginine residue has been enzymatically cleaved away). The term *"brady-"* indicates that it is *slow* to produce a full contraction of smooth muscle in comparison to histamine. Bradykinin is a polypeptide consisting of nine amino acids and is derived from a circulating high-molecular-weight kininogen (HMW kininogen). The related peptides lysyl-bradykinin and methionyl-lysyl-bradykinin are also produced but are not so important as bradykinin. Other kinins are derived from tissue kininogens by the action of tissue kallikreins. *Leukokinins* are kinins derived from leukocytes. An additional kinin *(C-kinin)* is derived from one of the early-acting complement components. After generation, kinins are quickly inactivated (in minutes) by kininases, enzymes that split amino acids from the carboxy terminus of these polypeptides.

Bradykinin results from activation of the enzyme *kallikrein* (from its precursor, prekallikrein), which cleaves it from the substrate high-molecular-weight

kininogen *(HMW kininogen)* as just mentioned. Activation of this pathway occurs in a "contact reaction" also involving coagulation factors XII (Hageman factor) and XI (plasma thromboplastin antecedent, PTA), prekallikrein, and plasminogen. This is the same plasma "contact system" responsible for intrinsic coagulation and fibrinolysis (Fig. 4-45). This means that whenever blood clots, kinins are generated, especially bradykinin. Proteinases released from neutrophils and other leukocytes at sites of inflammation will also activate this pathway; hence the kinins are present whenever inflammation and plasma are present.

Bradykinin and des-Arg bradykinin are potent mediators that have a variety of effects on blood vessels and various cell types. Bradykinin and des-Arg bradykinin bind to their respective receptors B_2 and B_1, which are constitutively expressed (B_2) or upregulated during inflammation (B_1). The kinins act on peripheral vessels to cause either vasodilatation or vasoconstriction, depending on local conditions, and they cause bronchoconstriction. They can reduce arterial smooth muscle tone and can increase vascular permeability by the same mechanism as histamine, namely, contraction and separation of endothelial cells. Kinins can also stimulate the release of histamine from mast cells and activate the arachidonic acid cascade for prostaglandin and leukotriene production. Along with the prostaglandins, bradykinin is believed to be a major mediator of the *pain* of acute inflammation by virtue of its effects on afferent nerve fibers. Through either direct or indirect mechanisms, kinins are able to increase peripheral blood flow, affect vascular permeability, and produce pain. They can thus induce *rubor, calor, tumor,* and *dolor,* four of the cardinal signs of inflammation.

Arachidonic Acid Metabolites

Our understanding of the importance of arachidonic acid and its metabolites in inflammation dates from the 1970s when it was discovered that drugs like aspirin work, at least in part, by interfering with arachidonic acid metabolism. This was a major breakthrough, since aspirin had been used medically for many years without knowledge of its mechanism, and it opened the door to an arena of modern research into antiinflammatory drugs and pain control. Many of the over-the-counter and prescription antiinflammatory drugs available today stem from this research, and Dr. John Vane was later awarded a Nobel prize for his early work in this field.

The metabolites of arachidonic acid function in a variety of biological processes, of which inflamma-

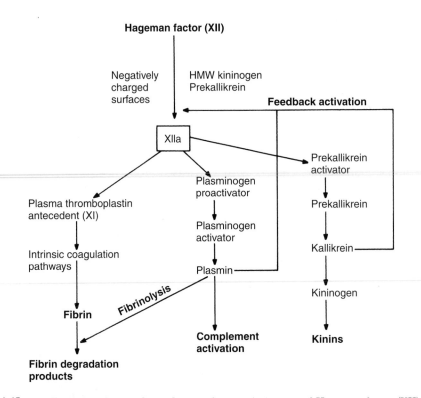

Fig. 4-45 The Hageman factor–dependent pathways. Activation of Hageman factor (XII) provides a means of access to four systems of importance to inflammation: intrinsic coagulation, fibrinolysis, kinin generation, and complement activation. Cyclical activation can occur by means of plasmin and kallikrein. *HMW,* High molecular weight.

tion is an important one. These metabolites are sometimes referred to as *autocoids,* which are rapidly formed short-range hormones that decay spontaneously or are quickly destroyed enzymatically. Arachidonic acid metabolites are important in a variety of situations, including vasodilatation and vascular leakage, coagulation and thrombosis, and pain, and in the pathophysiology of the cardiopulmonary, renal, endocrine, and other systems.

Arachidonic acid is a 20-carbon polyunsaturated fatty acid (5,8,11,14-eicosatetraenoic acid) derived directly from dietary sources or by conversion from essential fatty acids like linoleic acid. It is esterified into membrane phospholipids such as phosphatidylcholine in many types of cells in the body, including inflammatory cells (Fig. 4-46). For the cellular metabolism of arachidonic acid to proceed, it must first be freed from its esterified position in these membrane phospholipids to "feed" the arachidonic acid cascade. Cleaving arachidonic acid from the membrane is accomplished through the activity of various cellular phospholipases, principally isoforms of phospholipase A_2 (PLA$_2$), which have activity on several of the membrane phospholipid substrates, but also phospholipases C and D, which have more limited substrate specificity. (Keep in mind that various isoforms of PLA$_2$ are implicated in the pathogenesis of many other body functions and diseases, and their importance is not just limited to the arachidonic acid cascade.) The phospholipases can be activated when appropriate membrane receptors on the cell surface bind proinflammatory stimuli such as cytokines, growth factors, chemotactic peptides, or any of a variety of signaling molecules relevant to a particular cell. These phospholipases are the enzymatic axes that cut the membrane-bound arachidonic acid loose to feed the flow of the cascade. This is a rate-limiting step in the production of prostaglandins and leukotrienes and is one of the points at which antiinflammatory drugs may work, as we discuss soon in more detail. The freed arachidonic acid can then be metabolized by one of two major pathways (Fig. 4-47).

The *cyclooxygenase* pathway is named for the enzymes responsible for the conversion of arachidonic acid into the unstable prostaglandin endoperoxide PGG_2, which is subsequently reduced to a second endoperoxide, PGH_2, which can then be used as a substrate to synthesize several different prostaglandins: prostaglandin E$_2$ *(PGE$_2$),*

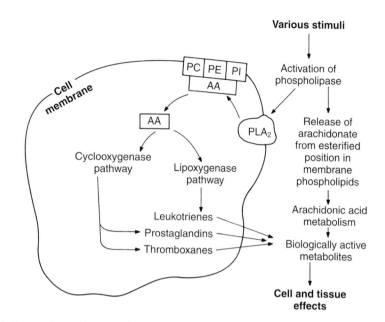

Fig. 4-46 Generation of biologically active arachidonic acid metabolites. The various potent prostaglandins, thromboxanes, and leukotrienes so important to the inflammatory process have their origin in arachidonic acid, *AA*, esterified into membrane phospholipids such as phosphatidylcholine, *PC*; phosphatidylethanolamine, *PE*; and phosphatidylinositol, *PI*. Arachidonic acid is freed from these cell membrane phospholipids by means of phospholipases such as phospholipase A_2, *PLA_2*, and metabolized by one of two major pathways.

TABLE 4-17   **Common Arachidonic Acid Metabolites and Some of Their General Actions**

METABOLITE	PHYSIOLOGICAL ACTIONS
PGI_2	Vasodilatation; inhibits platelet function. Endothelial cells are a major source.
TXA_2	Vasoconstriction; promotes platelet function. Platelets are a major source.
PGD_2	Vasodilatation.
PGE_2	Vasodilatation, potentiates accumulation of edema, pain (sensory nerve stimulation).
$PGF_{2\alpha}$	Vasoconstriction; bronchoconstriction.
LTB_4	Leukocyte chemotaxis and activation, especially neutrophils.
LTC_4, LTD_4, LTE_4	Vasoconstriction; increased vascular permeability; bronchoconstriction.

LTB_4, LTC_4, LTD_4, LTE_4, Leukotrienes B_4, -C_4, -D_4, and E_4; PGD_2, PGE_2, $PGF_{2\alpha}$, prostaglandins D_2, E_2, and $F_{2\alpha}$; PGI_2, prostacyclin; TXA_2, thromboxane A_2.

prostaglandin D_2 (*PGD_2*), and prostaglandin $F_{2\alpha}$ (*$PGF_{2\alpha}$*). These prostaglandins, which are sometimes referred to as "prostanoids," are collectively associated with the pain associated with inflammation, can cause vasodilatation, and can assist with other mediators in producing increased vascular permeability and edema (Table 4-17). PGH_2 may also be converted either by prostaglandin I_2 synthase to produce *prostacyclin (PGI_2)*, primarily in endothelial cells, or by thromboxane A_2 synthase to produce *thromboxane (TXA_2)*, primarily in

platelets. PGI_2 and TXA_2 are unstable, short-lived molecules with important biological properties in inflammation and blood coagulation (see also Chapter 3). PGI_2 is a potent vasodilator and inhibitor of platelet aggregation, and TXA_2 is an important vasoconstrictor and potent platelet aggregator; they form a rival duo positioned in a delicate balancing act. Whichever is in greater concentration in a locale has an edge in exerting its own effects and influencing local vascular conditions.

For many years only one cyclooxygenase enzyme

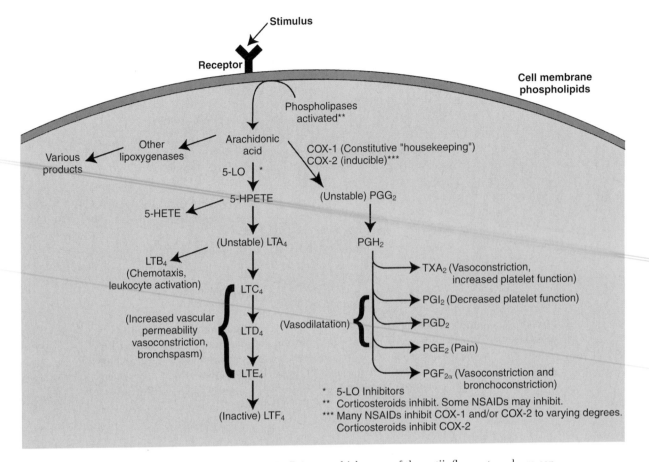

Fig. 4-47 The arachidonic acid cascade. Points at which some of the antiinflammatory drugs can inhibit the cascade are indicated with asterisks (*). Abbreviations: *COX*, cyclooxygenase; *HETE*, hydroxyeicosatetranoic acid; *HPETE*, 5-hydroperoxyeicosatetraenoic acid; *LTB₄*, *LTC₄*, *LTD₄*, *LTE₄*, *LTF₄*, leukotrienes; *LO*, lipoxygenase; *NSAID*, nonsteroidal antiinflammatory drug; *PGD₂*, *PGE₂*, *PGF₂α*, *PGG₂*, prostaglandins; *PGI₂*, prostacyclin; *TXA₂*, thromboxane A₂. (*Copyright © The University of Tennessee College of Veterinary Medicine, 2000.*)

was known to exist, but a second enzyme was recently discovered. The two are now referred to as cyclooxygenase-1 (COX-1) and cyclooxygenase-2 (COX-2), or alternatively as PGH synthase-1 and PGH synthase-2. This discovery was a major research and medical breakthrough, and the reasons for this accolade will be evident as you read on. COX-1, the previously known enzyme, is responsible for promoting production of constitutive, day-to-day needs of cells for arachidonic acid metabolites. These include the need for prostaglandins to help regulate blood flow in tissues by inducing moderate, normal physiological variations in vasodilatation, for normal stimulation of cells of the gastric mucosa to produce mucus (to protect from ulcers), and other functions. COX-1 is, more or less, an enzyme that needs to be available and functional for everyday activities, that is, "housekeeping" activities.

COX-2 is different. It is fed by the same flow of arachidonic acid from the cell membrane that COX-1 is, but COX-2 is transcriptionally regulated and becomes present in "unusual" circumstances, as during inflammation. (Exception: some cells in the body normally have a little COX-2 around on a day-to-day basis because they are routinely exposed to noxious stimuli; such are the Kupffer cells of the liver. Note also that COX-2 expression is an important topic in cancer research, not discussed in this chapter.) The presence of COX-2 presumably allows generation of greater quantities of prostaglandins and thromboxane than what would normally be produced at a particular tissue or organ site, and this of course contributes to the inflammatory process. Because of this, COX-2 is an obvious medicopharmacological target for inhibition. The commonly available nonsteroidal antiinflammatory drugs (NSAIDs), including aspirin, ibuprofen, phenylbutazone, flunixin, and others, are known to or assumed to inhibit (or partially inhibit) either COX-1 only or both COX-1 and COX-2 to varying degrees, depending on the particular drug and dose employed. As we all know, these drugs usually ameliorate some of the adverse effects of inflammation. However, because they are linked to some disruption of the normal "housekeeping" functions of the COX-1 products, this results in a risk for undesirable side effects such as gastric ulcers, among other things. Although some animals and humans can tolerate the COX-1 only, or COX-1 + COX-2 inhibitory drugs, other individuals cannot, especially when the drugs are used long term for chronic diseases. Newer COX-2 selective (or predominantly COX-2 selective) NSAIDs are now available and provide some selective control over this pathway of inflammation, with the intent of preserving some or all of the housekeeping activity of COX-1 and thus avoiding classic side effects such as ulcers. The implications and advantages of the mechanism of action of these new drugs are significant.

Glucocorticosteroids, those medically important and powerful inhibitors of inflammation, also inhibit expression or activity of the COX-2 enzyme. In addition, they inhibit PLA_2 enzymes, which results in inadequate cleavage of arachidonic acid from the cell membrane.* (Corticosteroids do this by inducing a protein inhibitor of PLA_2 enzymes called "lipocortin.") Without adequate arachidonic acid available, the result is that the COX-1 enzyme is starved of its substrate, arachidonic acid (see Fig. 4-46). This means that corticosteroids can inhibit the arachidonic acid cascade at two points; that is, at least two known so far. Again, these effects are dose dependent. Both COX-1 (starved for arachidonic acid) and COX-2 (inhibited) are suppressed by corticosteroids. In light of this, one can understand the basis for the powerful antiinflammatory activity of the corticosteroids.† The body needs to maintain some COX-1 activity for housekeeping activity, of course, and if used at high doses or for long periods of time the corticosteroids therefore also have the risk of side effects, as we have just discussed with the NSAIDs. In light of this, the med-

ical rationale for using the lowest possible daily dose of shorter-acting corticosteroids for certain medical problems in individuals prone to side effects, when appropriate and allowable, may be the most logical way to try to preserve some of the COX-1 function, rather than using long-acting formulations of corticosteroids.

The alternative chief branch of the arachidonic acid cascade, other than that of the COX enzymes, leads to the lipoxygenase (LO) enzymes, 5-LO, 12-LO, and 15-LO (which yields lipoxins). The 5-LO enzyme and its products are the best characterized and are very important in the inflammatory response. The first step in metabolism of arachidonic acid by this pathway involves activation of the 5-LO enzyme by a 5-lipoxygenase-activating protein, called FLAP, resulting in synthesis of *5-hydroperoxyeicosatetraenoic acid (5-HPETE)*, which is the precursor of the potent *leukotrienes* (see Fig. 4-47). They are named "leukotrienes" because of their triene chain structure and the fact that they were first isolated from leukocytes. One branch metabolite of 5-HPETE is 5-HETE, which is chemotactic for leukocytes, but most of the 5-HPETE is usually converted to the intermediate leukotriene A_4 *(LTA₄)*. LTA_4 is subsequently metabolized to give rise to the rest of the leukotrienes. Leukotriene B_4 *(LTB₄)* is a potent inflammatory mediator and induces leukocyte (especially neutrophil) chemotaxis, aggregation, increased adhesiveness, lysosomal enzyme release, and superoxide anion generation. Alternatively, LTA_4 can be processed to produce leukotriene C_4 *(LTC₄)*, which is subsequently converted to leukotriene D_4 and leukotriene E_4 *(LTD₄ and LTE₄)*; at the end of this pathway is LTF_4, which is an inactive degradation product. The combination of LTC_4, LTD_4, and LTE_4 account for the biological activity formerly known as the *slow-reacting substance of anaphylaxis*. In sufficient concentration, leukotrienes C_4, D_4, and E_4 can produce intense vasoconstriction and are more potent than histamine in producing increased vascular permeability. The leukotrienes are therefore logical targets for antiinflammatory drugs. Research in this area is very active and will doubtless result in new insights into the mechanisms of action of antiinflammatory drugs on the LO, COX, and PLA_2 enzymes and, one would hope, yield new and even better antiinflammatory drugs for our use.

With all these potential products of the arachidonic acid, what determines which ones will be made by the cells, or are they all made by every cell? Most cell types predominantly make one, or just a few products of the arachidonic acid cascade, and this is dependent on which of the active enzymes or

---

*It is also suggested that some of the NSAIDs may inhibit transcription of PLA_2 enzymes and thus may control arachidonic acid metabolism at this point too.

†This is just one way in which corticosteroids can suppress inflammation. They suppress transcription of some proinflammatory cytokine genes and therefore suppress the concentrations of some cytokines as well as the inducible nitric oxide synthase (iNOS). Corticosteroids also inhibit the function of some of the cells in the immune system.

synthases that particular type of cell possesses and can put to work. For instance, a major arachidonic acid product made by endothelial cells is PGI_2 because they have abundant prostacyclin synthase; PGI_2 is a vasodilator and inhibits platelet function. Platelets have abundant thromboxane synthase and therefore produce TXA_2 as a major product; TXA_2 promotes platelet function and vasoconstricts. One of the products from neutrophils is LTB_4 as a result of their supply of the 5-LO enzyme; LTB_4 serves to activate neutrophils and chemoattract others to the area. Mast cells make abundant PGD_2, which promotes vasodilatation, a common sequela of mast cell activation, and so on.

Finally, some food for thought. Arachidonic acid metabolism is a basic, important cellular function in day-to-day life but can obviously play a significant role in the inflammatory response. Some foods contain arachidonic acid *per se*, and many foods contain common fatty acids such as linoleic, which will yield arachidonic acid upon metabolism, and it can then be incorporated into our cell membrane phospholipids for later use in the arachidonic acid cascade. We all have heard of the much-advertised benefits of a diet rich in fish or fish oils. Many fish oils contain eicosapentaenoic (EPA) and docosahexaenoic (DHA) fatty acids (ω-3 fatty acids), and when present in sufficient amounts in the diet, they will become incorporated into cell membrane phospholipids, displacing some of the arachidonic acid. When the arachidonic acid cascade is activated, EPA and DHA will compete with arachidonic acid for entry into the cascade, that is, compete for binding sites on the COX and 5-LO enzymes. The apparent result is that less arachidonic acid is metabolized and less of the proinflammatory prostaglandins and leukotrienes are generated, and the fatty acids in fish oils that trickle through the arachidonic acid cascade also do not yield the usual inflammatory prostaglandins and leukotrienes either; the variant products of EPA and DHA metabolism are not so biologically active as the arachidonic acid metabolites. In summary, what this basically means is that the phospholipids in fish do not contain as much of the usual substrate for the arachidonic acid cascade, and so if these become incorporated into *our* cell membranes, this theoretically decreases the amount of arachidonic acid–related inflammation that can develop in *us*. This is not the only potential medical benefit of having fish for dinner, of course, but the general message is clear: we are what we eat.

Hageman Factor–Dependent Pathways

Hageman factor, which is factor XII of the intrinsic clotting cascade, also sets in motion other enzymatic cascades as a result of its serine protease activity. Activation of Hageman factor caused by contact with collagen, activated platelets, or various negatively charged surfaces (including glass) results in (1) *blood clotting*, (2) nearly simultaneous activation of the *fibrinolytic system*, (3) generation of *kinins*, and (4) *activation of the complement cascade* (see Fig. 4-45). The latter two play significant parts in the inflammatory response. Activation of Hageman factor can set all these pathways in motion, and it is worth noting that Hageman factor can also be activated and these cascades set in motion by neutrophil/leukocyte proteinases, which are invariably present whenever there is significant inflammation. In addition, both plasmin and kallikrein are produced in these cascades, and they can feed back into the system to cleave or activate additional Hageman factor, thus providing a mechanism for cyclic activation.

Complement System and Inflammation

The complement system really is a multicomponent system, even though it is often referred to as a single entity, "complement." It was discovered in the late 1800s as a heat-labile principle in fresh guinea pig serum that was required for bactericidal activity. Complement thus *complements* the action of antibody in the killing of bacteria. It is an important means by which antibodies function in host defense against most bacterial infections, and many complement components also participate in other functions important to host defense and the inflammatory reaction. Complement is a complex series of interacting protein components designated as C1, C2, C3, C4, C5, C6, C7, C8, and C9 for the *classical pathway* as well as factor B, factor D, factor H, factor I, and properdin (P) for the *alternative pathway* of activation and a variety of regulatory protein molecules (see Table 4-15).

Like the coagulation system, the complement proteins circulate as precursor soluble proteins (zymogens) that are inactive or hypoactive unless triggered. The activated complement components, however, are *enzymes*, and they interact sequentially in an ordered and well-understood fashion in the classical pathway of antibody-directed cell lysis. Complement components can also be activated by pathways not requiring antibody, as in the *alternative pathway*, which is induced by bacterial cell wall components. A variety of enzymes from other sources—not intrinsic to the classic complement sequence—such as plasmin, kallikrein, and the lysosomal enzymes of leukocytes, can activate some of the complement components. Consequently, complement has the potential to be activated in any situation in which leukocytes have accumulated, since lysosomal enzymes are released from leukocytes during the course of phagocytosis or after their degeneration or death.

Upon activation, the various components of the complement sequence (see Table 4-15) interact sequentially in a self-assembling cascade fashion reminiscent of the coagulation cascades. The primary target of most complement-mediated reactions is biological membranes, and the ultimate result is perforation of the membranes with holes, thus leading to cytolysis. In addition, the by-products of the cascade, such as C5a and C3a, can cause activation of cellular functions resulting in enhanced vascular permeability, smooth muscle contraction, chemotactic attraction of leukocytes, release of mediators from mast cells, immune adherence, degranulation and release of lysosomal enzymes from neutrophils, and enhanced phagocytosis. It is in these diverse biological activities of the cells affected by complement that the system participates in inflammatory reactions.

Complement Activation

Two major pathways for activating the complement sequence are the *classical* pathway and the *alternative* pathway. In a nutshell, the so called "classical" pathway is activated when complement compo-

nents bind to antibody; by corollary, if antibody is not bound, the classical pathway cannot be activated. The so called "alternate" pathway does not use or need antibody to become activated; it can do so by coming in contact with microbial products, such as endotoxin. It has been theorized that the alternate pathways is the more ancient, evolving and existing before immune systems of primitive organisms had developed antibodies. The classical system presumably evolved later, along with the advent of sophisticated immune systems that produce antibodies. The function of both systems is the same, however, regardless of how they are activated: enhancing the body's ability to disable and kill microbes.

The sequence of biochemical events involved in the classical activation of complement is a well documented, although somewhat complicated, story. In the presence of two or more molecules of IgG or at least one molecule of IgM bound to a cell wall (bacterium), the three subunits of C1, named *C1q, C1r,* and *C1s,* are associated in equimolar amounts as a precursor macromolecular complex (Fig. 4-48). C1q is a unique globular protein with six protruding appendages capable of interacting with a site on the Fc portion of certain complexed or aggregated immunoglobulins. This interaction leads to a conformational change in C1q that is transmitted to C1r, and the C1r subunit becomes a proteolytic enzyme (a serine protease) that cleaves C1s to yield

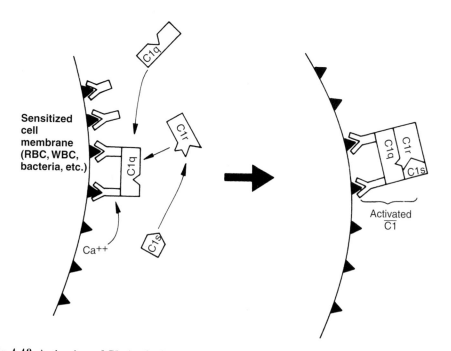

Fig. 4-48 Activation of C1. Antibody binds to antigen on the cell surface. Serum C1q binds to the Fc portion of immunoglobulin, and the C1r and C1s attach to bound C1q in the presence of calcium ions. The binding and activation of C1s completes the activation of C1.

activated C1s. The natural substrates of activated C1s are C4 and C2 (Fig. 4-49). C4 is cleaved by activated C1s, and the major fragment, C4b, is bound to the complex, markedly enhancing the subsequent cleavage of C2 by activated C1s. The major fragment of C2, C2a, binds to C4b to form a new enzymatically active bimolecular complex, C4b2a, or *C3 convertase*. This complex is unstable and rapidly decays, releasing C2d into the fluid phase, but the active C42 site may be regenerated with native C2. In the course of activation of C2, a kinin-like activity, *C-kinin*, which is distinct from bradykinin, is generated.

In the next stage of the complement sequence, the newly formed enzyme C3 convertase splits C3 into two fragments (Fig. 4-50). The smaller fragment, *C3a*, is a potent inflammatory mediator. The larger fragment is either bound to the complex as the important opsonin *C3b* or is released into the fluid phase as the decay fragment *C3bi*. Even though it has decayed a bit, C3bi can serve as an opsonin. When bound to the complex, C3b confers the property of *immune adherence*, the ability of the complex to bind to erythrocytes, neutrophils, platelets, and bone marrow–derived lymphocytes. In fact, C3b can bind independently of C4 and C2.

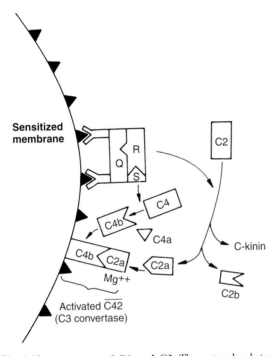

Fig. 4-49 Activation of C4 and C2. The natural substrates for activated C1 are C4 and C2. The cleavage fragments C4b and C2a become bound in a molecular complex in the presence of magnesium ions, and the activated C4b2a enzyme is known as C3 convertase, which can act upon native C3 to produce cleavage.

Fixation of C3b to the complex modifies the activated C4b2a enzyme so that it develops new enzymatic specificity termed *C5 convertase* (activated C4b2a3b), which is able to split C5 into two fragments (Fig. 4-51). The smaller fragment, *C5a*, is released into the fluid phase and is both an activator and a chemotactic factor for polymorphonuclear leukocytes and monocytes; it and its cousin, C3a, are referred to by some as anaphylatoxins. The larger fragment, *C5b*, becomes complex bound but is unstable and rapidly decays.

This nascent C5b fragment becomes the focal point for the eventual assembly of C6, C7, C8, and C9 into the *C5b-C9* cytolytic complex capable of behaving as the *"membrane attack complex"* (MAC) in complement-mediated cell lysis. When C5 is cleaved by C5 convertase and C5b is produced, self-assembly of the MAC is initiated. C5b and C6 form a stable bimolecular complex that binds to C7, causing C7 to express a site through which the C5b-7 complex can bind to the target cell's membrane. This C5b-7 complex bound to the cell membrane becomes the receptor for C8 binding, and the subsequent C5b-8 complex can finally bind and polymerize C9. In this regard, it should be noted that C8 has no detectable affinity for membranes by itself and is therefore entirely dependent on the mediating function of C5b-7, which determines not only the site of membrane attack but also serves as the C8 receptor. The fully assembled complex is a unique molecular creature containing a single molecule each of C5b, C6, C7, and C8 and multiple molecules of C9. It is basically a large complex made up of the tetramolecular C5b-8 complex and tubular poly-C9. The big MAC becomes inserted into the cell membrane and is so large that it is actually visible in electron micrographs as "holes" in the cell membrane that have a 10 nm–wide central circular pore surrounded by a 5 nm–wide rim. These characteristic and well known images of the MAC and the membrane lesions produced by complement are by and large attributable to the tubular poly-C9 contained in the MAC. The tubular poly-C9 inserted into the cell membrane represents the major complement transmembrane channel.

Actual membrane leakiness can be detected before complete assembly of the MAC. In the absence of C9, the C5b-8 complex tends to aggregate in the cell membrane, and these large protein aggregates produce structural and functional membrane damage evidenced by moderate leakiness. With the binding of C9, an accelerated influx of water and sodium ions into the cell occurs, and intracellular potassium is lost to the extracellular fluid. These water and electrolyte fluxes across the transmembrane channel create severe ionic disequilibrium, which eventually leads to osmotic rupture of the cell. The cell becomes an empty sac and is removed by the phagocytic systems.

The *"alternate pathway"* (properdin system) can be activated by bacterial cell wall components; it is a more nonspecific mechanism of host defense. The alternate pathway is independent of and does not rely on immunoglobulin and the "early components" C1, C4, and C2. The properdin system consists of at least three active factors, factor B, factor D, and C3, as well as the regulatory molecules factor H, factor I, and properdin (P). Activation of the alternate pathway may be initiated by microorganisms or their products, such as certain polysaccharides like endotoxin. It can also be activated by *aggregated* immunoglobulins of certain classes, but the site on rabbit and guinea pig immunoglobulins responsible for the activation of the alternate pathway is distinct from the C1q fixing site used by the classical pathway and resides in a part of the heavy chain near the hinge region on both the Fc fragment and the F(ab)$_2$ fragment.

The initial reactions of the alternate pathway occur when factors B, D, and certain microbial products interact with C3 to produce cleavage of C3. The major cleavage product of C3 is C3b (as in classical cleavage), which then interacts with alternate pathway components B and D to form a C3 convertase (activated C3bBb), which can activate more C3, thus forming the so-called C3 amplification loop. The larger fragment (Bb) remains bound to the activated complex of C3bBb, which can cleave native C3, thus gaining access to the terminal classical complement sequence beyond C3. Properdin binds to the alternate pathway C3 convertase, C3bBb, and increases the stability of the complex. Factor H also binds to C3b and modulates its functions; it is believed to restrict the formation of the C3bBb convertase by competing with factor B for its binding site on C3b. Factor I is also a regulatory molecule that cleaves and inactivates C3b as well as other components. Functions and actions of the multitude of complement fragments are summarized in Tables 4-18 and 4-19.

Amidst all these hieroglyphics, two major facts emerge. *First*, the key complement component around which both the classical and alternate pathways revolve is C3. *Second*, after C3 cleavage either

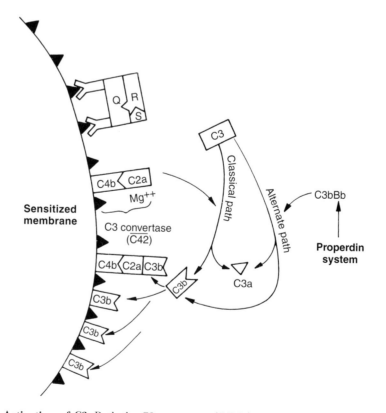

Fig. 4-50 Activation of C3. Both the C3 convertase (C4b2a) generated by the classical pathway and the C3 convertase (C3bBb) generated by the alternate pathway can cleave native C3 into two major fragments. The C3a fragment is an anaphylatoxin, whereas the C3b fragment becomes bound to the complex, where it modifies the activated C4b2a enzyme so that C5 convertase activity (C4b2a3b) is generated.

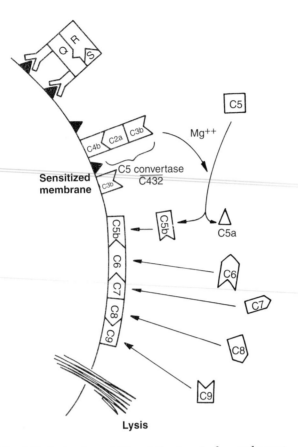

Fig. 4-51 Activation of C5 and the terminal complement sequence. The C5 convertase (C4b2a3b) generated cleaves native C5 into two major fragments. The C5a fragment is a potent anaphylatoxin and chemotactic agent, whereas C5b becomes membrane bound. The binding of C6 stabilizes the bound C5b, and the subsequent binding of C7, C8, and C9 produces lysis by forming transmembrane channels in the lipid bilayer of the membrane.

by C3 convertase (activated C4a2b) in the classical pathway or by C3 convertase (activated C3bBb) in the alternate pathway, activation of the terminal complement components proceeds in a similar fashion, regardless of which pathway started the cascade, and the biological activities that result are identical. Thus, although two activation schemes provide flexibility in host defense, the ultimate functional consequences of complement activation are the same.

Complement Functions in Inflammation and Host Defense

In discussing the complement activation sequence earlier, we have talked largely in terms of membrane events leading to lysis of a target cell or bacteria. Equally important to inflammation is the elaboration of soluble fluid-phase products and cell-bound

fragments that act as important mediators of the inflammatory and other biological response. Some of these biological functions merit our special attention.

Virus neutralization by antibody can be enhanced in the presence of C1 and C4 and, in the case where antibody concentrations are low, by fixation of C3b. It seems likely, then, that complement may be extremely helpful in the early stages of some viral infections when antibody titers are low.

Hereditary angioedema (HAE) is a disease of humans mediated by a low-molecular-weight fragment derived from C2 cleavage that has kinin-like activity (C-kinin). The action of C1 is normally regulated by a plasma glycoprotein called C1-inhibitor (C1-INH). This inhibitor binds stoichiometrically with C1r and C1s in the C1qrs complex to inhibit their activities thus preventing C1 activation and the further assembly of the C3 convertase (activated C4b2a). A deficiency of this control protein has been defined in human HAE patients. In the absence of C1-INH, uncontrolled production of the C2 kinin occurs and is apparently responsible for producing the episodic attacks of cutaneous, respiratory, and gastrointestinal edema characteristic of HAE. There are no well-defined HAE-like syndromes in animals.

Immune adherence is the phenomenon by which cells or particles bind to specific receptor sites on neutrophils, monocytes, macrophages, and platelets thus enhancing phagocytosis (opsonization). This important biological phenomenon is attributable to C3b binding to the surface of the cells or particles. The binding of C3b to lymphocytes also may facilitate antibody production by B cells and enhance antibody-dependent cellular cytotoxicity.

Anaphylatoxin generation refers to the biological activities of the complement cleavage peptides C3a and C5a (Table 4-20). The C3 convertase generated from either classical or alternate pathway complement activation along with other noncomplement proteolytic enzymes like plasmin, trypsin, lysosomal enzymes from leukocytes, and certain bacterial proteinases can release C3a by cleavage of native C3. This fragment obeys the definition of an anaphylatoxin in that it can cause increased vascular permeability, smooth muscle contraction, and release of mediators such as histamine from mast cells. Similar activity can be generated by C5a, which is cleaved from native C5 by C5 convertase as well as a similar group of noncomplement proteolytic enzymes that can function to cleave C5.

As mentioned, the biological functions of C5a are similar to those described above for C3a. Although these peptides have similar biological activities, they

TABLE 4-18 Principal Components of the Classical and Alternate Complement Pathways

COMPONENT	FUNCTION
CLASSICAL	
C1q	Binds to antibody; reveals active site on C1r
C1r	Cleaves C1s to reveal active subunit
C1s	Cleaves C4 and C2 to form the C3 convertase
C2	Converted by C1s to C2a and C2b
C4	Converted by C1s to C4a and C4b
C4b2a	Classical C3 convertase
C3	Most abundant component; cleaved by classical C3 convertase
C3a	Cleavage product of C3; anaphylatoxin
C3b	Cleavage product of C3; opsonin; part of C5 convertase
C4b2a3b	Classical C5 convertase
C5	Substrate for C5 convertase
C5a	Cleavage product of C5; anaphylatoxin
C5b	Binds C3b on membrane; initiates membrane attack sequence
C6	Binds to C5b as bimolecular complex
C7	Binds to C5bC3b; inserts into lipid bilayer
C8	Binds to C5b-7 and inserts in membrane; initiates leakage
C9	Bound to and polymerized by C5b-8; insertion of poly C9 into membrane produces lesion leading to lysis
C1-INH	Control molecule; inhibits C1 activation as well other enzymes
ALTERNATE	
C3	Source of C3b for alternate pathway C3 convertase activity
Factor B	Cleaved by Factor D to form Bb for C3 convertase
Factor D	Active serine protease; cleaves factor B bound to C3b
C3bBb	Alternate C3 convertase; can bind additional C3b
C3bBbC3b	Alternate pathway C5 convertase
Factor H	Control molecule; restricts alternate C3 convertase formation
Factor I	Control molecule; cleaves C3b to inactive form C3bi
Properdin	Positive regulator; binds to and stabilizes C3bBb convertase

TABLE 4-19 Selected Biologic Activities of Complement-derived Mediators

COMPONENT OR FRAGMENT	BIOLOGIC FUNCTION
C1q	Binds to IgG and IgM
C14, C1423	Viral neutralization
C4a	Weak anaphylatoxin
C4b	Immune adherence and enhancement of phagocytosis; antibody-formation
C2 fragment	C2 kinin; (increase vascular permeability, edema)
C3a	Histamine release, smooth muscle contraction, increased capillary permeability, lysosomal enzyme release
C3e	Induction of leukopenia and leukocytosis
C3b	Activation of the alternative complement pathway, immune adherence, enhanced opsonization, enhanced induction of antibody formation, enhancement of antibody-dependent cellular cytotoxicity, stimulation of B cell lymphokine production, etc.
C3d	Immune adherence via receptors on lymphocytes and macrophages
C5a	Histamine release, smooth muscle contraction, increased capillary permeability, chemotaxis of leukocytes, leukocyte secretion, increased adhesiveness and aggregation, etc.
C5b	Opsonization of fungi; initiates membrane damage
C6	Promotion of blood coagulation
C5b-9	Membrane attack sequence

TABLE 4-20 Biological Activities of the Anaphylatoxins

FUNCTION	C3a	C5a
Leukocyte chemotaxis	no	yes
Smooth muscle contraction	yes	yes
Increased vascular permeability	yes	yes
Neutrophil membrane-ruffling	no	yes
Increased leukocyte stickiness	no	yes
Neutrophil aggregation	no	yes
Superoxide anion generation	no	yes
Neutrophil secretion	no	yes
Mast cell degranulation	yes	yes
Stimulate respiratory burst	no	yes

differ in potency and receptor specificity. C3a is less potent than C5a, and each peptide seems to react with different membrane receptors. It is of further interest that C5a can promote chemotaxis and mediate the release of lysosomal enzymes from neutrophil leukocytes. This gives the system a self-amplification loop in that initial complement activation will generate C3a and C5a, which, by their effects on neutrophils, causes release of enzymes capable of cleaving additional native C3 and C5 to generate more C3a and C5a.

In our discussion, we have stressed the phlogistic (proinflammatory) properties of the complement system with little attention paid to control mechanisms. It should be obvious that to avoid total complement consumption by any single complement-fixing reaction, numerous inhibitors and built-in control mechanisms must be operational. It also should be recalled that many of the active components (cleavage products) are unstable and decay rapidly. The extrinsic factors (inhibitors or inactivators of complement peptides) combine with or destroy the activated components and thus prevent the progression of the reaction sequence or destroy the pathobiological activity of the activated product. This limits uncontrolled or poorly controlled spontaneous activation of the complement system.

Nitric Oxide

Nitric oxide (NO) is a tiny, uncharged molecule composed of only two atoms and is one of the smallest mediators known. It is produced in a wide variety of mammalian cells and tissues and has multifunctional and widespread actions in a variety of pathophysiological settings. These include effects induced within the vascular system, lung, nervous system, gastrointestinal tract, liver, reproductive system, and immune system. The best known roles of nitric oxide are threefold: (1) in the cardiovascular system, as a potent physiological mediator of vascular tone, specifically of vasodilatation; (2) as an effector of host defense against certain pathogens; and (3) as a signaling molecule, particularly in the nervous system. Its roles in vascular and immunoinflammatory responses are significant and warrant some discussion here.

The amino acid L-arginine is the substrate for NO synthesis (Fig. 4-52). In the presence of oxygen, a nitrogen of L-arginine undergoes oxidation, and the result is nitric oxide and L-citrulline as a by-product. The ability of any given cell to synthesize NO is dependent on the presence and activity of nitric oxide synthase (NOS) and its cofactors (NADPH, FAD, FMN, BH_4), which are needed to catalyze the reaction. There are three distinct isoforms of the NOS enzyme, and these are differentially expressed and regulated in various tissues and cells; this allows for selective control and specific, site-directed activity of NO when it is generated. Modulation of NOS isoenzyme activities is regulated by transcriptional, translational, or posttranslational mechanisms depending on the particular isoform, and variations in this can influence both normal and pathological processes. Like many of the other mediators of cellular function in the body, there is some interest in the possibility of pharmacological manipulation of NO levels for medical purposes.

The three basic isoforms of the NOS enzymes can be separated into two functional categories: (1) *constitutive* forms of NOS, which are continuously present in certain cells, and (2) *inducible* NOS (iNOS), which is transcriptionally regulated and not normally present in significant amounts in the absence of inflammation (Table 4-21). Cells with constitutive NOS intermittently turn the enzyme on and off, producing small quantities of NO in response to stimuli, which then acts as an autocrine and paracrine signaling molecule. This is, more or less, a normal physiological "housekeeping" type of activity. Cells that use NO as a signaling agent for normal physiological processes include vascular endothelial cells (*e*NOS isoform, also called "NOS3") and neurons (*n*NOS, or NOS1), but many other types of cells also rely on the constitutive function of NOS.

The endothelial cell–related function of NO is not only important in normal physiology but also in pathological processes. Stimulated endothelial cells use constitutive NOS to generate NO in a calcium-dependent fashion; the NO diffuses out of the endothelial cells a short distance (before rapid inactivation) and induces soluble guanylyl cyclase in smooth muscle cells of the vascular wall (Fig. 4-53). The result is protein kinase–dependent relaxation of vascular smooth muscle and *net vasodilatation*. Before

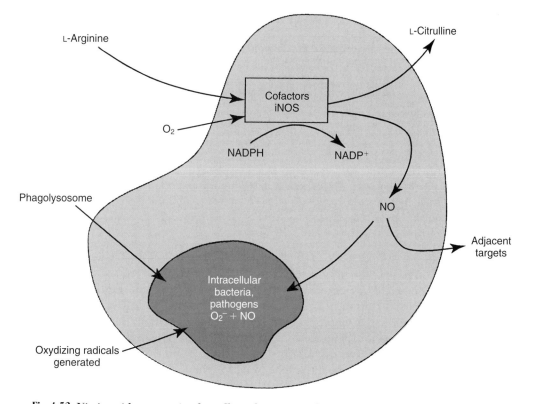

Fig. 4-52 Nitric oxide generation by cells such as macrophages. *NADPH,* Nicotinamide adenine dinucleotide phosphate, reduced; *NO,* nitric oxide; *iNOS,* inducible nitric oxide synthase; O_2^-, superoxide anion. *(Copyright © The University of Tennessee College of Veterinary Medicine, 2000.)*

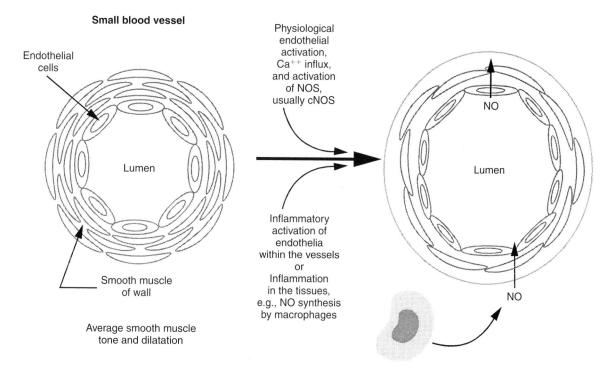

Fig. 4-53 Nitric oxide can induce smooth muscle relaxation in the walls of small blood vessels, resulting in vascular dilatation. *NO,* Nitric oxide; *cNOS,* constitutive nitric oxide synthase. *(Copyright © The University of Tennessee College of Veterinary Medicine, 2000.)*

TABLE 4-21   **The Nitric Oxide Synthase (NOS) Enzymes**

The nitric oxide synthase enzymes are essential for generation of nitric oxide (NO). Enzymatic activity differs between the inducible (iNOS) and the constitutive (cNOS) isoforms.

iNOS	cNOS (eNOS, nNOS)
Long-lasting release of NO (hours)	Short-lasting release of NO
Regulated by transcription	Ca^{++}/calmodulin-dependent regulation
Is a high-output NO pathway (nmoles NO/min·mg protein)	Is a low-output NO pathway (pmoles NO/min·mg of protein)
Is inhibited by corticosteroids	Not affected by corticosteroids

Other: These cofactors are necessary for NOS activity: BH$_4$ (tetrahydrobiopterin), FAD, FMN, NADPH, heme, and calmodulin; but note that calcium and calmodulin are required for cNOS but not iNOS activity.

eNOS, Endothelial nitric oxide synthase; *nNOS*, neuronal nitric oxide synthase.

NO was discovered, an elusive "mystery factor" termed "endothelial cell-dependent (or -derived) relaxing factor" was recognized, and this turned out to be NO. In terms of medicine and pathology, if conditions in the patient result in excess synthesis of NO, severe hypotension caused by massive vasodilatation can result. A well-known situation where this can occur is sepsis or septic shock. In septic shock, eNOS is highly stimulated in endothelial cells. Compounding this is that iNOS is likewise highly induced in monocytes and macrophages as a result of bacterial toxin–induced generation of cytokines. Making matters worse, iNOS can also be induced in the highly agitated endothelial cells. The result is that the peripheral vasculature becomes highly vasodilated, peripheral pooling of blood occurs, and the patient becomes hypotensive.

Many cell types are capable of expressing inducible NOS (iNOS), including endothelial cells, but macrophages and monocytes are the most significant producers in most species. (Curiously, the ability of human macrophages to generate NO is nominal under the same conditions that stimulate macrophages of many other species.) Transcriptional induction of iNOS occurs, and NO is synthesized after macrophages are stimulated with combinations of bacterial toxins such as endotoxin and various cytokines such as interferon-γ, interleukin-1, and tumor necrosis factor-α. Various interacting features of the immunoinflammatory system must exist in a balance to maintain life, of course, and transcriptional regulation of iNOS can be suppressed by glucocorticosteroids, transforming growth factor-β, IL-4, IL-10, and the exogenous cyclosporin A.

Macrophages use the iNOS isoform to sustain synthesis of relatively *large* amounts of NO over a longer period of time than that for cNOS. For example, after induction in macrophages, iNOS results in synthesis of about a hundredfold more NO than the diminutive cNOS isoforms are capable of.

The larger quantity and sustained synthesis of NO is enough to have an effect on immunoinflammatory events, as in sepsis and hypotension, as we have just discussed. In addition to the vascular events, however, high concentrations of NO is inhibitory or destructive to many but not all pathogens. These include bacteria, such as *Mycobacterium* spp. and *Staphylococcus aureus;* fungi, such as *Cryptococcus neoformans;* protozoa, such as *Leishmania major, Trypanosoma brucei* and *T. cruzi,* and *Plasmodium* spp.; and metazoa, such as *Schistosoma mansoni.*

How does NO cause these deleterious effects? NO reacts with superoxide anion (O$_2^-$), which is commonly and conveniently produced at sites of inflammation, to produce a very reactive hybrid intermediate molecule, peroxynitrite (ONOO·); this molecule also breaks down into other reactive nitrogen intermediates. These are free radicals with unpaired electrons, oxidizing agents similar in this respect to the oxygen radicals that we have already discussed, and interaction with biological molecules often damages them. The molecular targets of NO are varied but commonly consist of iron-sulfur–containing proteins, where the reactive NO-derived intermediates result in formation of nitrosyl–iron-sulfur complexes. Examples of enzymatic targets in cells include cis-aconitase in the TCA cycle, Fe-S proteins in the electron-transport chain, and ribonucleotide reductase. The result is that important synthetic and metabolic pathways can be damaged or ruined in targets, which hopefully belong to pathogens, not our own cells. Damage to our cells is normally limited because NO and the reactive intermediates are usually short lived and therefore can diffuse only a small distance before decaying. NO is also inactivated by heme groups, and so whenever it comes into contact with blood, it is inactivated.

A few final thoughts about NO. Although we have concentrated the discussion on NO produced

TABLE 4-22 Some of the Pathophysiologic Responses and Results of Acute-phase Reactions

RESPONSES	EXPLANATION OR POSSIBLE RATIONALE FOR THIS RESPONSE
Fever	Increased resistance to some pathogens.
Malaise and somnolence	Decreased need for caloric intake.
Anorexia	?
Neutrophilic leukocytosis	Increased leukocytes for host defense.
Increased cortisol secretion	Increases synthesis of acute-phase proteins. Also can suppress transcription of some cytokines and other proteins associated with the inflammatory response.
Anemia of chronic disease	Caused (at least in part) by sequestration of iron by iron-binding acute-phase proteins and macrophages.
Loss of muscle mass	Muscle is catabolized and provides amino acids needed for synthesis of proteins during a time of anorexia, a time of negative nitrogen balance.
Loss of adipose stores	Lipolysis to provide energy substrate.
Osteoporosis	?
Cachexia	The term refers to a "wasted" or emaciated body condition as a result of a very chronic, disease-related acute-phase reaction (loss of muscle mass, adipose, tissue, or bone) or other conditions such as cancer.

during inflammation, NO is also a normal physiological mediator in the body, and many other cells besides macrophages and endothelial cells can synthesize it. The difference is related to the amount of NO synthesized. During inflammation a lot can be made using the high-output iNOS isoform, but during healthy, normal physiological processes only tiny amounts are needed and synthesized, usually by the cNOS isoforms. It is also worth noting that a place exists for NO in pharmacology and therapeutics. For instance, NO and its reactive intermediates can react with proteins to form *S*-nitrosothiols. The *S*-nitrosothiols have longer half-lives than NO has and act as a "reservoir" for the bioavailability and bioactivity of NO in the body. *S*-Nitrosothiols are believed to be key intermediates in the action of important nitrovasodilators, such as nitroglycerin and sodium nitroprusside.

OTHER ASPECTS OF THE INFLAMMATORY RESPONSE
Acute-Phase Response and Acute-Phase Proteins

The acute-phase response (APR), or, alternatively, acute-phase reaction, is a medical expression that can be used to indicate either (1) the pathophysiological and behavioral changes that may result from a significant round of either acute or chronic inflammation or (2) may refer to the actual plasma *proteins* whose concentrations vary during inflammation. In either case, it is an adaptive response of the host, the theoretical purpose of which is to better position the host animal for survival and healing. Keep in mind

that, even though the name of this response includes the word "acute," many chronic conditions are also accompanied by this response.

Some of the behavioral changes of an APR are well known to us, since most of us have experienced them during intermittent bouts of sickness such as the "flu." They include malaise, increased sleep, and anorexia. Logical speculation would indicate to us that some of these symptoms may be of some survival value when we or our patients are faced with a significant inflammatory or infectious challenge. Both malaise and somnolence would decrease physical activity and therefore also decrease the energy needs during this time period, allowing for the decreased caloric intake as a result of anorexia and also allowing needed substrates for synthesis of proteins to be shunted and used for the inflammatory response. A survival-oriented rationale for anorexia, on the other hand, is an enigma. In terms of other physiological responses of the APR, fever may have value in terms of enhancing immunity against some pathogens.

A term that frequently arises when discussing patients with chronic diseases and poor health is "cachexia." This describes a state of ill health resulting in a severely wasted body condition. This term and the condition it refers to may be included in the list of potential findings in a long-standing acute-phase reaction, but, in fact, cachexia can result, and the term can be applied to many different causes, including cancer. There are other medical or pathophysiological events that can be observed or measured during an APR. Some of these events are summarized in Table 4-22, and an explanation or rationale is suggested. Taken as a group, the overall purpose seems to be centered around host defense and survival-oriented adaptive responses.

The definition of an acute-phase *protein* is that it is one whose plasma concentration either increases or decreases by a minimum of 25% as a result of an inflammatory reaction. The acute-phase proteins are numerous. Most of them increase and are called "positive," though the individual proteins can vary a great deal in the amount of increase, such as a halffold to thousandfold increases, depending on the protein. The positive acute-phase proteins are subgrouped as either major or minor based on their fold induction. Some proteins decrease in plasma concentration and are therefore referred to as "negative" acute-phase proteins. The label of "negative" does not refer to a class of proteins with adverse consequences, just ones whose concentration decreases. The host-adaptive rationale for decreased concentration of negative acute-phase proteins such as albumin may be that synthetic activity is redirected toward more essential proteins during the in-

flammatory event. Some of the acute-phase proteins are listed in Table 4-23. Note that not all these proteins have been identified in all species, and not surprisingly the species with the most identified is *Homo sapiens*. Also note that there is species variation of which proteins may be produced during an acute-phase reaction and to what degree they increase or decrease; that is, the presence and importance of many of the acute-phase proteins is species variable.

How does the APR evolve? Cytokines that are synthesized in increased quantity during the inflammatory response are the major drivers for synthesis of acute-phase proteins and for inducing many of the signs and symptoms of the APR. Some of the principal cytokines involved are interleukin-6, interleukin-1, and tumor necrosis factor-α, though others can also be involved. Remember that synthesis of cytokines often results in synthesis of other cytokines; that is, a networked cascade results. Synthesis of IL-1 or tumor necrosis factor-α can induce

TABLE 4-23 Some of the Acute-phase Proteins and their Known or Suspected Functions

PROTEINS	FUNCTIONS
SOME "POSITIVE" ACUTE-PHASE PROTEINS (CONCENTRATION INCREASES)	
Complement components (C3, -4, -9, C1 inhibitor, others)	Host defense: microbial killing, leukocyte activation.
C-reactive protein (CRP)	Host defense: can activate the complement system, bind to microbes. Other roles likely.
Antiproteases (α_1-protease inhibitor, α_1-antichymotrypsin, others)	Limits "bystander" proteolysis or damage of host tissues during inflammation.
Iron or other metal-binding proteins (haptoglobin, hemopexin, ceruloplasmin)	Transport proteins that can bind and "sequester" metals when in increased concentration. The iron binders may decrease availability of iron for microbial growth and other reactions.
Coagulation-related proteins	Provide increased substrate or catalytic enzymes for regulation of clotting, inflammation-associated fibrin formation, or dissolution of fibrin
These include:	*Fibrinogen:* substrate for clot formation
	Plasminogen: degrades fibrin/clots, cleaves other protein substrates
	Plasminogen activators (tissue and urokinase forms)
	Plasminogen activator inhibitors
	Protein S: anticoagulant
Lipopolysaccharide-binding protein (LBP)	*Host defense:* increases the ability of macrophages and other cells to detect and respond to gram-negative bacteria.
Serum amyloid A (SAA) family	Various members of the acute-phase SAAs are known or suspected of being involved in lipid metabolism and transport, chemotaxis of leukocytes, and induction of extracellular matrix-degrading enzymes. Can be deleterious if in high concentration for extended periods as a result of deposition of amyloid in tissues.
Serum amyloid P (SAP) family	Biological functions not clear yet, but binds many ligands, including endotoxin.
SOME "NEGATIVE" ACUTE-PHASE PROTEINS (CONCENTRATION DECREASES)	
Albumin	
Transferrin	
Factor XII	
Insulin-like growth factor I	

synthesis of IL-6, and so on. (TNF-α was originally named "cachectin," by the way, since it was present in association with cases of cachexia.) Many of the acute-phase proteins are synthesized in the liver, and the cytokine signals transcriptionally regulate their synthesis. Cytokines and the molecules they induce also act in other tissues such as the brain to induce some of the typical pathophysiological responses, such as fever.

In summary, some of the biological relevance of the APR remains to be determined, but it is worth remembering that the evolutionary intent of it seems to be host defense and survival, though some aspects of it could potentially be detrimental for us and our patients.

Perspective

It should now be clear to readers that our assertion that the inflammatory response is complex is perhaps an understatement. The basic hemodynamic and permeability changes and the infiltration of leukocytes represent its common themes, but different time courses, different initiating stimuli and tissue sites, different combinations of mediators, and dissimilar outcomes complicate predictions of the clinical manifestations of the inflammatory response. The underlying cellular and biochemical processes encompass complicated and interlacing networks of signals and responses to stimulation. It would be good at this point to reiterate or summarize the key features of these complicated host defense mechanisms to ensure that the intricacies of the response do not wind up masking an appreciation for the overall nature of the reaction.

Two major aspects of the inflammatory response are paramount: (1) the vascular phenomena of hemodynamic and permeability changes and (2) the biochemical and cellular events that permit blood-borne proteins and leukocytes to enter inflamed tissues. The latter includes synthesis and release of biochemical mediators of the inflammatory response. Throughout the response, we continually encounter two important arms of the defense reaction, humoral and cellular, which dominate discussions of inflammation much as they do immunology. Clearly, they are both vital and closely interactive parts of the whole, so carefully interdigitated and interdependent as to be inseparable.

The relatively uncomplicated past in the fields of inflammation, immunology, and host defense is gone. We must continue to probe disease mechanisms with new ideas and new tools. As clinicians and pathologists, we are used to dealing with lesions in our patients but not necessarily with their molecules. We often function as visually oriented medical scientists, trained to recognize the abnormal and to interpret its significance. It can be difficult for us to think of injury to molecules when viewing a swollen joint or a focus of coagulation necrosis, but we must learn to speak the language of the cell and of the molecule while not losing sight of what it all means to the tissues, the organs, and the entire organism. We must remember that although the underlying basis may be molecular only the entire animal can develop clinical signs and present them for our questioning. Our ability to answer those questions at the highest possible level of resolution will continue to be the challenge of modern medicine.

> "Our own wronged flesh
> May work undisturbed, restoring
> The order we try to destroy, the rhythm
> We spoil out of spite: valves close
> And open exactly, glands secrete,
> Vessels contract and expand
> At the right moment, essential fluids
> Flow to renew exhausted cells,
> Not knowing quite what has happened."
> W.H. AUDEN

HEALING AND REPAIR

Healing and repair of injured tissue is undoubtedly the final, desired end point of the inflammatory response. Remember that from the outset, *inflammation* and *repair* are intimately linked. Events aimed at healing actually begin almost as soon as injury has taken place, and features of inflammation usually occur throughout the repair phases. As such, it is highly appropriate to view healing and repair as part of a continuum of loosely timed events stretched between the moment of initial injury and the final result of healing.

The repair of injury is a phylogenetically important process that occurs throughout the animal kingdom and, indeed, also occurs in plants and most or all living things. It seems that the "lower" one goes on the phylogenetic tree, the more complete is *tissue regeneration* as a type of healing response. If an earthworm is decapitated, it may simply form a new head, and this process can be repeated several times. An additional example comes from the ocean starfish, where they can grow new "arms" if they are cut off. In some vertebrates such as amphibians, whole limbs and tails can also sometimes be regenerated. Such durable responses are not, however, the luck of most of the animals with which one deals in veterinary medicine, and the acquisition of mammalian status has apparently been accompanied by certain evolutionary exchanges. We have lost the capacity for wholesale organ and limb regeneration, and some tissues do not regenerate much at all. Instead, mammals often rely upon their phenomenal capacity for the repair or replacement of damaged cells and tissues with less specialized connective tissue. Because of this, even mild injuries can result in some scar tissue formation.

Healing and repair are among the more remarkable of biological phenomena. If even the most sedate and quiescent of tissues are incised or otherwise damaged, within 24 hours intense cellular activity is underway to try to heal the defect created by the wounding process. This commonplace activity is deceptively simple; under its seemingly quiet surface the complex waters of cell biological processes run deep.

The healing and repair processes in any tissue are dependent not only on the cellular composition of that tissue but also on the nature of the injury process itself and its effect on the integrity of tissue architecture. Using the kidney as an example, a toxic injury that destroys renal tubular epithelium in the nephron without injuring the underlying connective tissues may be repaired by *regeneration,* whereas a kidney abscess that destroys the connective tissue framework as well as the epithelium will be repaired by *scarring.* In real life, the healing responses to many types of injury often involve combinations of repair by regeneration as well as scarring, but it will enhance our understanding of the underlying biology to categorize the major healing processes. We therefore divide the repair process into two subcategories that have clinical and biological significance: (1) healing by *parenchymal regeneration* and (2) healing by *connective tissue replacement.*

Healing by Parenchymal Regeneration

At a simplistic level, repair is in the replacement of dead or damaged cells by new, healthy cells derived from either the parenchymal or connective tissue elements in the damaged tissue. If the repair is accomplished largely by the regeneration of parenchymal cells, almost perfect reconstitution of the original tissue can result. (Parenchymal cells are defined as the essential cells or parts of an organ that are concerned with its function, not its supporting framework.) A good example can be drawn from clinical medicine. People use antifreeze in their vehicles to keep the engine cooling system from freezing in cold weather. Unfortunately, the sweet taste of the ethylene glycol in antifreeze has lured many dogs and some cats into drinking it, and many of these animals presented to veterinarians have acute

renal failure. This is attributable to necrosis of the renal tubular epithelial cells caused by the toxicity of ethylene glycol metabolites as well as other metabolic disturbances. If these patients can be kept alive by dialysis, both structural and functional recovery of the kidneys is theoretically possible. The reasons for this are in the *repair by parenchymal regeneration* that is possible in the patient's kidneys. While the *function* of those kidneys is being replaced by dialysis in a hospital, the *structure* can be restored by the regeneration of tubular epithelial cells (Fig. 4-54).

This type of clinical example can be used to illustrate two important points about parenchymal regeneration (Box 4-7). First, it can obviously occur only in tissues that have the cellular capability for regeneration. We discuss this in more detail later on. Second, it can occur only if the connective tissue framework of the tissue is maintained so that the regenerating cells have an architectural framework upon which to rebuild. In the example above, the metabolic products of the antifreeze kill the tubular epithelial cells but do not destroy the underlying tubular basement membranes or the connective-tissue supporting network for the tubules, and hence the framework of the kidney is maintained. To better understand parenchymal regeneration we must understand something about the regenerative capabilities of various tissues and cells.

CELLULAR REGENERATIVE CAPABILITY

The various cells of the body can be divided arbitrarily into three major groups based on their regenerative capability: *labile, stable,* and *permanent* cells. As we will see, such a classification scheme is only a generalization, but it is nonetheless a useful one for our purposes. Labile and stable cells usually are in constant turnover or in a resting phase, respectively, and as a group they retain the ability for regeneration. On the other hand, permanent cells cannot reproduce themselves, or regeneration is limited. The latter are differentiated end-stage cells and have little or no regenerative capability. From this background, it is immediately clear that any serious attempts at regeneration as a means of tissue reconstitution after

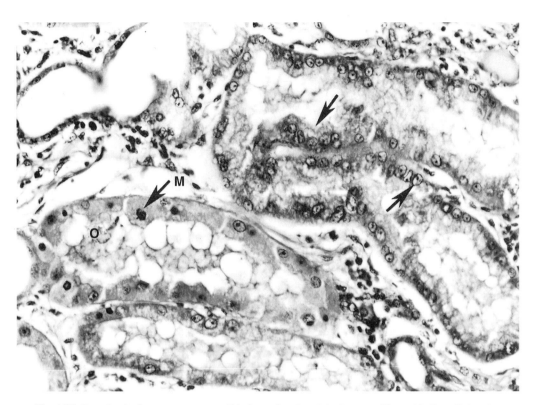

Fig. 4-54 Renal tubular regeneration. Ethylene glycol toxicity in a cat. The epithelium lining the tubules has proliferated, *arrows*, along the intact basement membrane, and a mitotic figure is seen, *M*. There are oxalate crystals, *O*, in the tubules.

injury normally occurs only in tissues composed of labile or stable cell populations. In general, if cells of the permanent type become injured and die as a result of that injury, repair will occur by proliferation and replacement by less specialized connective tissue cells. An additional point is worthy of emphasis: even when regeneration occurs (as in labile and stable cell populations) and the cellular mass of the injured tissue is replaced, the original architecture of the tissue may not be perfectly imitated. In this regard art and science are similar: numerous copies of the works of Van Gogh and Rembrandt have been made, but they always lack the value of the original masterpiece.

Labile Cells

Those cells of the various tissues and organs that under normal physiological conditions continually multiply at a fairly rapid rate throughout life are referred to as "labile cells." Their replication is a means of replacing cells that are continually being lost as a matter of day-to-day life processes. Such cells exist as part of the lymphoid and hematopoietic elements and the surface-oriented epithelia. *Bone marrow* cells are in a constant state of proliferation throughout life to maintain the normal cellular composition of the circulating blood. In short, the rapid turnover of blood cells is continually being compensated for by the formation of new, mature cellular elements in the labile cell populations of the bone marrow. Only when the precursor stem cells in the marrow itself are destroyed is the proliferative capability of this system altered. When this happens, proliferation of fibroblasts and connective tissue replacement follows, as it might in any other tissue, and scarring (in this case called "myelofibrosis") results. With respect to the *lymphoid organs* including the spleen, renewal of cell populations can occur from the surviving lymphoblastic cells in those tissues or from the primitive mesenchymal stem cells of the splenic and lymphoid sinuses. In a sense, what happens in the lymphoid tissues is somewhat analogous to what happens in the bone marrow.

The situation with respect to the *epithelia* is somewhat different and of interest to our study of repair by regeneration. Note that the labile epithelia do not include all forms of epithelium in the body but are limited to the epithelia that make up the cellular content of surfaces throughout the body. This includes the stratified squamous epithelia of the skin and of mucosal surfaces such as the oral cavity and some portions of the reproductive tract; the columnar epithelia of the respiratory and gastrointestinal mucosae; the epithelial cells of most excretory ducts such as the biliary tract and ducts of glands like the salivary glands and pancreas; the columnar epithelium of the fallopian tubes and uterus; and the transitional epithelium of the urinary tract. At these various anatomical locations, there occurs a continuum of maturation and sloughing that is normally compensated for by the proliferative capability of more primitive and less well-differentiated reserve or stem cells located deep to the surface, the basal cells of the epithelia. The continual turnover of the gastrointestinal epithelium forms an additional good example. Here, superficial cellular elements are continually being sloughed into the intestinal contents to be replaced by the proliferative activity within the deeper crypts. Maturation proceeds as the cells move from the crypts to the surface of the villi. Indeed, it is common to see mitotic figures in the intestinal crypts of normal animals.

After injury, almost perfect reconstitution of tissues composed of labile cell populations can occur by proliferation of remaining cells at the margins of the wound or area of injury. It must be stressed again, however, that this can occur only with an intact connective tissue framework or scaffolding upon which the regenerating epithelium can grow. Epithelia on surfaces also try to regenerate over large, cavitated defects in tissue such as ulcers, but here the process is delayed until the large tissue defect becomes filled with less specialized fibrovascular granulation tissue, which forms a foundation for the epithelium. In such injuries, a combination of repair by connective tissue replacement and repair by regeneration occurs; the bulk of the defect is eventually filled by connective tissue replacement, whereas the surface is healed by regeneration of the epithelium.

Stable Cells

Cells that are generally classified as stable differ from the labile cell populations discussed previously in that they normally have a rather low rate of turnover during adult life. Instead, they retain the *capacity* for rapid division and cell proliferation in response to a variety of stimuli or insults. These cells are also capable of reconstitution of the injured tissue to almost perfectly normal architecture. Cells that fit into this category are the parenchymal cells of most of the glandular tissues of the body such as the pancreatic acinar cells and salivary glands, the renal tubular epithelium, hepatocytes, and a wide range of mesenchyme-derived cells such as fibroblasts, vascular endothelial cells, osteoblasts, chondroblasts, and smooth muscle cells. A good illustration of the regenerative capability of stable cells already has been presented in the example of ethylene glycol (antifreeze) toxicity and renal tubular epithelial regeneration. An additional example can be found in the regenerative capacity of the liver. The liver is sometimes a target for toxic injury, and it is fortunate in this regard that it has such an enormous functional reserve. It has been shown that up to 70% or to 80% of the liver can be removed by surgical excision and that regeneration of the original mass or weight of the liver occurs quite rapidly. Such regenerative capability allows the liver to repair some of the injuries caused by toxic, viral, or chemical injury.

It must be noted that although stable cells are entirely capable of regeneration such repair does not necessarily occur in every situation. The additional necessary ingredient is that the underlying framework or supporting connective tissue stroma be preserved (see Box 4-7). With respect to most parenchymal tissues, the critical structural component in this regard is the integrity of the basement membrane or, more properly, the retention of an appropriate arrangement of the basement membranes such that *tissue architecture* is maintained. Many types of epithelia as well as endothelial cells are capable of synthesizing basement membrane components upon which to grow, but, in the absence of proper architectural arrangement, chaotic regrowth results. Thus the stimuli for cell proliferation may be operative even in the absence of an appropriate connective tissue framework, but the result is a haphazard proliferation of cells into disorganized clusters and masses that have little structural or functional resemblance to the original tissue. Cell proliferation by itself is inadequate to ensure regeneration, and the result must include restoration of structure-function relationships that are dependent on the architectural arrangement of the connective tissue framework if regeneration is to be successful.

An additional hindrance to proper regeneration is excessive exudation at the sites of tissue injury, such as accumulation of pus. Where there has been sufficient exudation that the exudate cannot be quickly resolved or removed by enzymatic and phagocytic degradation and reabsorption, the exudate will delay healing and provoke a connective tissue response that leads to scarring. For example, a badly infected skin wound that contains pus and does not receive prompt medical attention will take much longer to heal, and the resulting scar will be larger because of the increased amount of tissue damage and connective tissue at the site.

The proliferative capability of mesenchymal cells is well known. The intense proliferation of fibroblasts that accompanies or precedes scarring is a good example of a stable mesenchymal cell population being called into action. In the repair of a bone fracture, osteoblast proliferation is essential to the ultimate formation of a solid bony union. Vascular endothelium normally has a rather slow rate of turnover. If, however, a segment of a vessel becomes denuded of endothelium, cells from the margin of the wound quickly migrate into the injured area and proliferate to fill the defect. Endothelial proliferation also is a prominent component of granulation tissue formation in which the proliferation of endothelium in small venules, arterioles, and capillaries results in the formation of a new vascular bed for the injured tissue, a process referred to as "neovascularization." These newly formed capillary beds become the sites of egress for phagocytic cells that infiltrate the wound to perform their defensive functions as well as providing a nutrient supply for the proliferating cells in the healing wound.

In a fashion somewhat analogous to endothelial cells, the smooth muscle cells making up the walls of hollow viscera and blood vessels also have a very low turnover rate in the normal adult. The smooth muscle cells do, however, have considerable proliferative capability. Although not a wound, possibly the best example of this can be drawn from the rapid smooth muscle proliferation that occurs under hormonal influence in the pregnant uterus. Smooth muscle also can proliferate in the walls of blood vessels in response to various kinds of injury. It is particularly responsive to lowered oxygen tension (hypoxia) and to increases in blood pressure (hypertension). In both of these settings, smooth muscle proliferation occurs in the walls of medium-sized and larger muscular arteries. When a vessel is severed or otherwise injured, local smooth muscle proliferation occurs. Smooth muscle proliferation in response to injury is also involved in the pathogenesis of degenerative vascular diseases such as atherosclerosis.

Permanent Cells

Cells that are classified as permanent are those in which regenerative attempts are generally absent or limited. To this group would belong cells such as neuron and cardiac muscle cells, for which tissue repair by regeneration is, at best, of little practical importance. The dogma has long been that when neurons in the central nervous system (CNS) are lost they are gone forever. The space they vacate can be filled in by the proliferation of the supportive cellular elements of the CNS, the glial cells, but these cells cannot do what neurons do. Restoration of structure-function relationships does not occur, and for most practical purposes a neuron lost is indeed a neuron gone forever. Perhaps on-going stem cell research will some day reveal new information and hope for replacement of permanent cells.

The situation in the peripheral nervous system (PNS) is a little different and more complicated. Here, the sequelae to injury depend on where within the peripheral neuron injury takes place. If the injury spares the cell body, damaging only the peripheral axon, regeneration can occur from the intact proximal axonal segment. On the other hand, if the cell body is damaged and lost, the entire neuron, including the peripheral axon, dies, and regeneration does not occur. Therefore regeneration within the PNS depends largely on the anatomic location of the damage. As mentioned, cell body damage means total neuronal loss without regeneration. However, if an axon is severely injured, the portion of the axon distal to the injury usually degenerates completely, whereas the axonal segment proximal to the injury degenerates only to the level of the nearest node of Ranvier; this is referred to as "wallerian degeneration." Regeneration of the damaged distal axon can proceed from the node of Ranvier, provided that the axonal tube or membrane is intact and the axon has a structural framework to follow. Regeneration can be quite rapid, and regenerating proximal segments have been clocked at the biologically blazing speed of up to 5 mm per day.

There is a familiar theme here. In a fashion analogous to the need for an intact connective tissue stromal architecture if parenchymal regeneration is to succeed in other organs, the regrowth of the damaged axon also has similar needs. The regenerating proximal segment must contact and have or gain continuity with the old channel of the original nerve fiber if successful regeneration of the distal axon is to succeed. If, on the other hand, the axonal tube is cut and displaced, the regenerating proximal segment becomes separated from the distal segment, and there results a disorganized sprout of axonal fibers that fail to restore the continuity of the original fiber. This is basically what takes place in the formation of the *amputation* or *traumatic neuroma*, which is basically a mass of regenerating axonal fibers lacking orientation and a reason to be. Such growths do nothing for the patient but cause pain.

Skeletal and cardiac muscle provide an interesting biological contrast. Skeletal muscle is able to regenerate fairly well if injured. Again, restoration of structural and functional integrity depends on the preservation of the arrangement of basement membrane and other connective tissue elements. When the basement membrane is intact, regeneration of skeletal muscle is good. When the basement membrane is disrupted, regeneration of muscle fibers is less effective. If the edges of a wound in skeletal muscle are separated, as by a blood clot, muscle cells will proliferate but cannot effectively bridge the gap, which becomes filled by scar tissue. The muscle then loses a portion of its contractile or mechanical ability and with it some of its functional strength. Unfortunately, cardiac muscle has little ability to regenerate. For this reason, injuries to the myocardium, such as infarcts, are healed by replacement with scar tissue.

Thus the situation with respect to permanent cells and their regenerative capability is not a happy one. Even in the face of an intact connective tissue framework, regeneration is not much of an option. Fig. 4-59 should help to place the relative value of cellular regenerative capability into perspective with other features of the healing and repair process.

Healing by Connective Tissue Replacement

In many situations in which injury to tissue occurs, the amount of tissue destruction is such that not only are host parenchymal cells destroyed and lost but also the framework of supporting connective tissue elements is also destroyed. Healing by regeneration of the tissue then cannot occur. In these situations, the defect ultimately becomes filled with less specialized fibroblastic cells that effect a "gluing and bonding together" type of repair of the damaged tissue by replacing the injured portion with collagen-rich scar tissue. For obvious reasons, this is a less desirable result than parenchymal regeneration is.

These sorts of defects and injuries are initially characterized by the formation of *granulation tissue*. This term is derived from the appearance of the soft, developing fibrovascular scar. Grossly it has a red, slightly rough, granular appearance that reflects its characteristic histological features: the proliferation of fibroblasts and newly formed small blood vessels. This is what you see at the base of a large healing ulcer and is mostly what gives it a red appearance. Thus, granulation tissue is best defined as *fibrovascular connective tissue*. By the way, it is important not to confuse the somewhat similar-sounding terms *granulation tissue, granuloma,* and *granulomatous*. "Granuloma" is a term used to describe a particular form of chronic inflammation in which macrophages predominate and the lesion is discrete, that is, surrounded by other tissue. "Gran-

ulomatous" is a term used to define a similar morphological type of chronic inflammation in which the character of the lesion is more extensive, not discrete. Thus it is important to make a clear distinction between "granuloma" and "granulomatous" as types of inflammation and "granulation tissue" as a form of healing response.

FORMATION OF GRANULATION TISSUE

The development of granulation tissue in a large ulcerated lesion proceeds to form a mass of red tissue ("healing by second intention"), but the healing of a simple surgical incision ("healing by first intention") also includes formation of granulation tissue, just less of it and difficult to see. In the case of a mature granulating wound, it often is possible to recognize several different zones as one proceeds from either the margins or the deep edge to the surface (Fig. 4-55). At the deep edge of a mature granulating wound, there is a *zone of mature connective tissue* that represents the oldest portion of the healing process. Here, the entire healing process has virtually run its course, and mature collagenous scar tissue has resulted. Because of the nature of the overlying defect, however, this mature connective tissue is still well vascularized. It is these vessels in the zone of mature connective tissue that are the source for the growth of neocapillaries seen in the *zone of capillary proliferation*, which lies superficially to the zone of vascularized mature connective tissue. Here, budding young vessels grow from the more mature vessels in the deeper zone up into the "granulating wound." These vessels often have a somewhat parallel arrangement as they grow perpendicularly to the surface of the defect (Fig. 4-56). Anastomotic branches of these neovascular structures ensure a substantial collateral circulatory supply. This can give the appearance of a fine gridwork of plump young vessels in the area.

Between the growing young vessels there are proliferating fibroblasts laying down extracellular matrix components and scattered inflammatory cells. Superficial to this morphological region is a *zone of capillary sprouts and arches* where migration and mitosis of the endothelial cells occur at the leading edge. These newly formed capillaries form by budding from existing neocapillaries in the zone of capillary proliferation. At first the buds and sprouts are not perfused with blood because they are solid buds of endothelium. Differentiation soon proceeds, however, and the buds develop lumens to allow blood to move through them. As these sprouts advance into the inflamed area toward the surface of the wound, they form anastomotic arches with each other. The walls of these delicate young vessels have

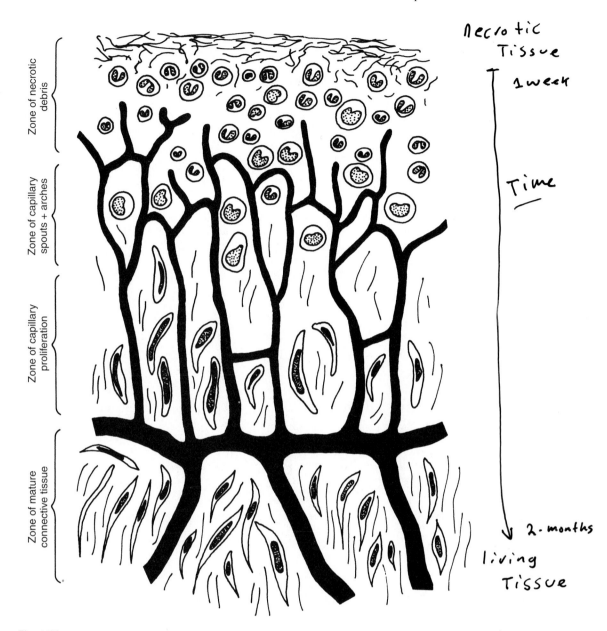

Fig. 4-55 Zones in granulation tissue. Schema of the four major zones in a granulating wound. The lesion is oldest at the base where the mature connective tissue is found.

enhanced vascular permeability and easily permit the movement of fluids, plasma proteins, and red and white cells from the bloodstream into the healing lesion. For this reason, newly formed granulation tissue is often edematous, and this yields the shiny, wet appearance of healing ulcers (if the "scab" is removed). These developing capillary sprouts and anastomotic arches are basically growing into an inflamed area that is filled with clotted blood, fibrin, and necrotic debris; the desiccated appearance of the latter is referred to as a "scab," or a "serocellular crust."

Scattered between these neocapillaries are numerous phagocytic cells performing their cleaning-up functions. Large numbers of *macrophages* are pres-

ent, but closer to the ulcerated surface there are usually many *neutrophils* as well. On the surface and extending down to the level of neovascular sprouts and arches is a *zone of necrotic debris,* which may be covered with a scab, depending on the level of medical care and also whether the patient has "picked it off." Here are many dead cells, coagulation products, and usually a fair number of dying neutrophils. If there is substantial contamination of the surface by bacteria, the numbers of leukocytes and the percentage of them that are neutrophils will be increased.

At the epithelial edges of the wound is abundant evidence of attempts at epithelial restitution (Fig. 4-57). Much proliferation of the basal layer is seen,

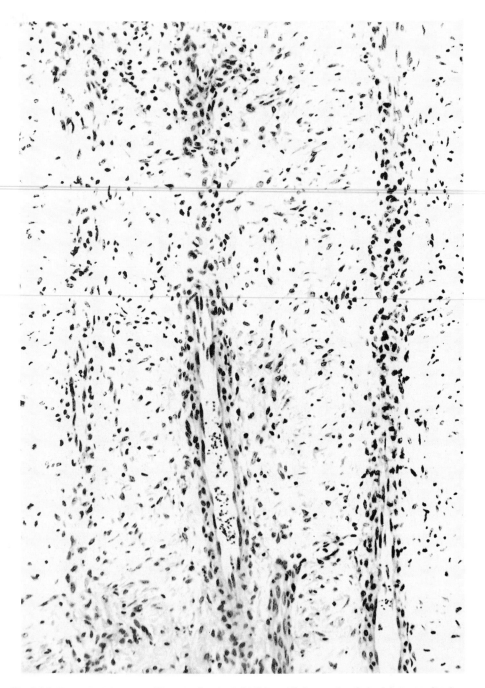

Fig. 4-56 Granulation tissue. The vessels are typically parallel to each other and perpendicular to the surface. Between the vessels is active fibroplasia along with a few scattered macrophages.

and there is usually a considerably thickened epithelium that sends pegs and fronds of proliferating cells down along the margins. Such epithelium is attempting to restore surface continuity by growing down *under* the moist coverlet provided by the dried surface scab. Because the edges in a large wound may be far apart, successful reepithelialization usually cannot take place until wound contraction and the granulation process have proceeded to a point where closer apposition is possible. These

proliferating edges of epithelium invade the edges of the granulating defect and sometimes, because of a slight morphological resemblance to neoplastic change, have been referred to as *pseudoepitheliomatous hyperplasia*. Such changes are not cancerous, of course, and can be seen at the margins of many granulating wounds on epithelial surfaces.

These typical morphological characteristics of granulation tissue provide a useful map for what is happening. The healing process is most advanced at

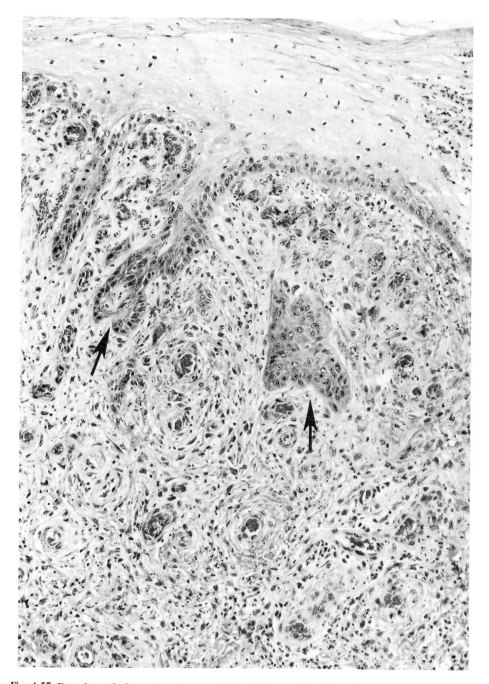

Fig. 4-57 Pseudoepitheliomatous hyperplasia. Active proliferation of squamous epithelium at the edge of a granulating wound. There are pegs and islands of proliferating epithelium, *arrows*, which appear to "invade" the underlying fibrovascular connective tissue.

the base and proceeds from there toward the surface, laying down connective tissue components as it goes. Because the surface remains exposed, a reaction continues, one that basically can be resolved only by restitution of the physical barrier provided by an intact epithelial surface.

The cellular features of granulation tissue warrant a little more of our attention. There are basically three cell types that always are found in a heal-

ing or granulating wound: the *macrophage*, the *fibroblast*, and the *endothelial cell*. Their activities are central to the healing process.

MACROPHAGES

We have already discussed the arrival of macrophages at sites of inflammation and have noted their importance and prominence in the later, more chronic stages of an evolving inflammatory reaction. It is during these more chronic phases in the evolution of a successful inflammatory response that the distinction between "inflammation" as a host defense mechanism and "healing" as a reparative effort becomes blurred. The highly important macrophages play a pivotal role in the transition between inflammation and wound healing and are essential cells for the phagocytic removal of necrotic debris and exudate that have accumulated within the damaged tissue as well as synthesis of growth factors important to the wound-healing process.

The inflammatory response resulting from tissue injury is characterized by a relatively rapid accumulation of numerous neutrophils and macrophages at the site of injury. Although both of these cell types may begin to emigrate from blood vessels adjacent to the injured tissue at about the same time, the neutrophils quickly reach a maximum level in the wound and then decline in number, provided that the wound is not infected. Macrophages reach maximal levels somewhat later and usually become the principle phagocytic cell in chronic injuries and are of prominent importance in granulation tissue.

The role of the macrophage in wound repair has been exemplified in venerable experiments in which attempts were made to eliminate macrophages from healing wounds and to inhibit phagocytosis by those remaining cells. Such experiments were attempted using antimacrophage serum (AMS), but AMS alone seems to have variable effects on the macrophages in healing wounds. Because the effects of AMS alone seemed to be inconclusive, attempts were made to eliminate the circulating sources of replacement cells. Since tissue macrophages are largely derived from blood monocytes, hydrocortisone was used to produce monocytopenia. Using this system, the number of macrophages in wounds was reduced to approximately one third. This reduction in macrophage levels was accompanied by inhibition of wound débridement, as evidenced by increased levels of fibrin deposition and a decreased rate of disappearance of both fibrin and neutrophils. When AMS was used together with hydrocortisone in such studies, the effects were dramatic, and the result was virtually complete disappearance of macrophages from the wounds.

What do these studies of wound healing when the macrophages were diminished tell us? Macrophage-depleted animals have defective wound repair, and hence the macrophages are key elements of the process. There are many reasons for this, and one of the most important is that they provide a rich source of growth factors, which we discuss soon.

FIBROBLASTS

For many kinds of open wounds and tissue defects, the morphological expression of those reparative phenomena is the formation of *granulation tissue,* as we have discussed previously. As such, granulation tissue can be regarded as a sort of "temporary tissue" present as long as it is useful and then disappearing, to ultimately be replaced by a collagenous scar. It is an interim solution to a temporary problem, the filling of space where tissue has been damaged and lost. Along with the macrophages (and, as we shall see, endothelial cells), the fibroblasts are of critical importance to wound healing; without them, healing of most types of wounds would never proceed.

The fibroblasts are ubiquitous connective tissue cells and the most widespread of the mesenchymal cells, present in substantial numbers in virtually every organ and tissue. They are classified as "stable cells retaining proliferative capability," and they certainly maintain the capacity for rapid growth. Fibroblasts are essential to wound repair by virtue of their ability to proliferate locally and to synthesize and lay down extracellular matrix components such as collagen to restore functional and structural integrity to the damaged tissue and to provide the wound with tensile strength. Fibroblasts are also potent producers of growth factors. When an effective cellular defense has been mounted within the damaged tissue, the reparative phenomena that follow almost always involve at least some fibroblast proliferation; some scarring almost inevitably accompanies virtually all injuries.

EXTRACELLULAR MATRIX COMPONENTS

The importance of extracellular matrix components like collagen in wound healing has been appreciated for a very long time for the simple reason that the ultimate result of many repair processes is the formation of some amount of collagenous scars. However, since the complex processes of cell proliferation, cell migration, cell differentiation, and cellular interaction are involved in wound healing and repair, we must take a broader look at the extracellular matrix as more than merely the source of the end-stage product, collagen.

Wound repair can be arbitrarily divided into inflammatory, proliferative, and reorganization or remodeling stages; the fibroblast is involved during all three stages. *Healing begins at the moment of injury.* The fibroblast product collagen is even important in the early hemostatic events that occur in the damaged tissue. The escape of blood from damaged vessels coagulates to form the blood clot. A primary step here is the adhesion of platelets to molecules on the exposed collagen. Collagen also can provide a negatively charged surface, which can activate Hageman factor to initiate the intrinsic coagulation cascade. Thus, by virtue of its initial interaction with platelets and Hageman factor, collagen occupies a key position in wound healing from the very beginning of the process. The provisional, or temporary, matrix in the wound, which will serve as a scaffold upon which fibroblasts and other cells can ultimately rebuild and heal the wound, contains structural components including fibrin (from the blood clot), fibronectin, and hyaluronic acid.

During the inflammatory phase, the leukocytes that invade the tissue also play a role in the wound matrix. Proteolytic enzymes in neutrophils, macrophages, and other cells facilitate the movement of cells in the wound by enzymatic degradation of some of the tissue matrix in which they are seated. We have already discussed many of these enzymes previously in this chapter when discussing the enzymes contained in leukocytes, and they include familiar names such as leukocyte elastase, collagenase (matrix metalloproteinase-8, or MMP-8), and gelatinase (MMP-9). The MMPs are important in various phases of the process of wound healing, and many of them are also synthesized by cells other than leukocytes, such as fibroblasts. As a group, the MMPs can degrade—and help remodel—virtually any kind of extracellular matrix. Thus the collagenolytic and matrix-dissolving activity assists in allowing wound healing to enter the proliferative phase by freeing cells for migration and proliferation. This in turn can be shown to be associated with a burst in collagen synthetic activity by the proliferating fibroblasts. The final stages of healing involve the production, maturation, and remodeling of collagen and other matrix synthesized during the proliferation phase. The newly synthesized collagen fibrils bridge the gap between the edges of the damaged tissue to form a scar of appreciable tensile strength (Fig. 4-58).

Collagen is a term that encompasses a family of at least 11 types of molecules, all of which consist largely of the unique collagen triple helical structure. The primary types of collagen deposited during fibroplasia and granulation tissue formation are *type I* and *type III* collagen; the percentages of other types of collagen participating in wound repair are lower. Both type I and type III collagen are fibrillar types of collagen that have uninterrupted triple helices. It is the deposition of these rigid helical collagen macromolecules that gradually provides the healing tissue with increased tensile strength. This process takes time, but scar tissue never really does fully regain the tensile strength of the original, intact tissue. It has been estimated that most skin wounds have regained only about 20% of their final strength after 3 weeks, and at maximum strength a scar is only about 70% as strong as intact skin. The increase in tensile strength that wounds develop after collagen deposition is not only related to the amount of collagen being deposited but also to the eventual *remodeling* of the collagen with reorganization of collagen bundles to better resist tensile forces, which can take weeks and months to complete.

Depending on the nature of the wounding process and the involved tissue, formation of new *basement membrane* can also occur. This has been best documented in the process of reepithelialization in skin wounds. Epithelial cells initially migrate over a provisional matrix, and a true basement membrane is formed when migration has ceased and epithelial continuity has been restored. Basement membrane reformation appears to occur in sequential stages, with the deposition of *laminin* and *type IV collagen* proceeding from the original margin of the wound toward the center.

The extracellular matrix components thus accumulate in wound healing in a fairly predictable fashion, with the initial hyaluronic acid and fibronectin deposits being replaced in older wounds by types I and III collagen for greater tensile strength. This sequence of events allows extracellular matrix components to exert their own special influences on the evolving cellular and biochemical activity central to wound repair.

WOUND CONTRACTION AND THE MYOFIBROBLAST

During the development and maturation of granulation tissue, some of the fibroblasts acquire ultrastructural, chemical, immunological, and functional characteristics that distinguish them from fibroblasts of normal tissues. A fibrillar system develops within the cytoplasm, with the appearance of bundles of parallel fibrils resembling those of smooth muscle cells. Strips of active granulation tissue tested *in vitro* behave like smooth muscle in that they are contracted and relaxed by agents that contract or relax smooth muscle, including serotonin, angiotensin, bradykinin, epinephrine, and some of the prostaglandins. When granulation tissue regresses after the healing of a wound, these various phenomena can no longer be demonstrated. Thus it is accepted that the forces producing wound contraction reside in the modified fibroblasts typical of granulation tissue. Because of their functional and

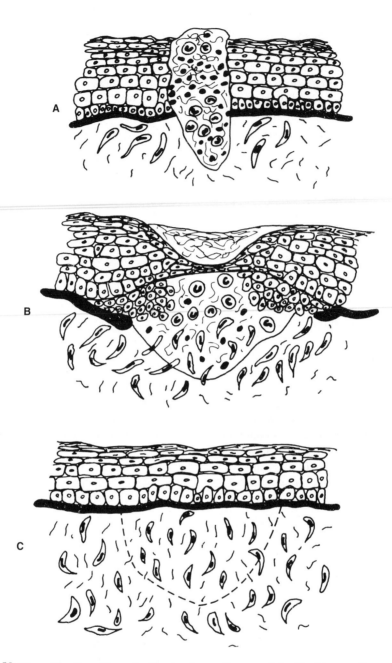

Fig. 4-58 Wound healing. Tissue healing involves collagen and the fibroblast at all stages. **A,** The initial lesion exposes collagen to bring about coagulation and platelet aggregation for hemostasis. **B,** The infiltrating leukocytes remodel the wound using granulocyte collagenase while fibroblasts begin to proliferate and synthesize collagen at the base. **C,** The wound has been repaired and the defect filled by mature collagenous connective tissue synthesized and elaborated by the fibroblasts.

morphological similarity to smooth muscle cells, these modified fibroblasts are known as *myofibroblasts*. These cells seem to progressively develop intracytoplasmic "muscles" as well as cell-to-cell and cell-to-stroma connections. They are functionally active cells that can contract and apparently can do so at the same time that collagen is being laid down. This provides a unique sort of "lock-step" arrange-ment so that the tightening and shrinkage of the scar tissue occurs simultaneously with its acquisition of additional tensile strength. When healing is completely finished, these cells disappear. The myofibroblasts provide an explanation for the age-old observations regarding wound contraction.

Although wound contraction is usually a useful phenomenon in the healing of open wounds, it also can occur where it is not cosmetically or functionally wanted. It can result in serious disfigurement of the head and face and can also cause serious functional problems such as luminal strictures in organs such as the intestine.

ENDOTHELIAL CELLS

The endothelial cell is critically important in wound repair because of its function as the cell lining the new blood vessels, which are conduits of nutrients and other cells into the wound. Endothelial cells also produce platelet-derived growth factor (PDGF), which stimulates healing; PDGF is also produced and secreted by other types of cells. As we have mentioned previously, vascular endothelium normally has a fairly low turnover rate, but endothelial cells in the microvasculature start proliferating relatively early in the course of an inflammatory injury in response to growth factors such as vascular endothelial growth factor (VEGF), and low oxygen tension in the disordered, wounded area may also provide a trigger for angiogenesis. Buds of endothelial cells grow out from existing blood vessels at the wound margins, undergo canalization, and form a series of vascular arcades by joining with their neighbors. These newly formed vessels are extremely permeable and leak protein readily so that the fluid bathing the injured area consists of dilute plasma. It forms an excellent nutrient medium for the various proliferative activities of the fibroblasts and also for the phagocytic activities of the leukocytes because it contains antibodies and complement components; the bacteria that can also thrive in plasma are likely hindered by the latter. This highlights one of the major functions of endothelium in the healing process in granulation tissue (and elsewhere): to proliferate and provide a permeable microvasculature to provide nutrients and support the activities of the various cellular members of the healing drama. The same newly formed vessels that are so permeable to protein also readily exude leukocytes and thus form a conduit for the movement of phagocytic cells from the vascular compartment to the injured area.

ROLE OF GROWTH FACTORS IN HEALING AND REPAIR

The entire preceding discussion has an underlying theme: in order for healing and repair to take place, *cell proliferation* must occur. Not only must parenchymal cells proliferate if repair by regeneration is to take place, but also the critical processes of reepithelialization, neovascularization, and fibroblast proliferation central to granulation tissue formation depend on enhanced mitotic activity within the involved cell populations.

What causes these cells to proliferate? Much of the cellular activity central to healing and wound repair is under the influence of *growth factors* derived from a variety of sources. Growth factors involved in wound healing are proteins that have the ability to stimulate cell proliferation and cell differentiation and stimulate synthesis of structural matrix proteins by cells; some are also chemotactic, attracting additional cells to the area. Growth factors can push quiet, stable, drowsing cells back into the growth cycle from the G_0 (resting) phase or may stimulate cells to undergo mitosis while in the growth cycle. These factors work by binding to cells that express their receptors and initiate signal transduction, DNA synthesis, and eventually mitosis. In general, growth factors can have endocrine, paracrine, or autocrine activity on cells, but in terms of wound healing most are produced or secreted locally at the site of wounds by many cell types, including platelets, macrophages, fibroblasts, and epithelial cells. Some of the most well-known and important growth factors involved in wound healing are presented in Table 4-24, along with some of their actions and characteristics.

There are growth factors, other than just those listed in Table 4-24, of course, that are variably involved in growth and development, differentiation of cells, and other stimulatory activity upon cells. Some of the others (not mentioned in Table 4-24) are known or suspected of being involved with repair of tissues and organs, that is, wound healing, at least in some circumstances. These include growth hormone (somatotropin); insulin-like growth factor-II (IGF-II); bone morphogenetic proteins (BMPs), which are involved with bone and cartilage; colony-stimulating factors (CSFs), important in growth and differentiation of hematopoietic cells of the bone marrow, including monocyte CSF (M-CSF), granulocyte CSF (G-CSF), granulocyte-macrophage CSF (GM-CSF), interleukin-3 (IL-3), which collaborates with the other CSFs in stimulatory activity, and erythropoietin, which stimulates erythrocyte growth and development. Others include nerve growth factor, melanocyte growth factor, and hepatocyte growth factor. Even the cytokines TNF-α and IL-1 can be considered growth factors in some situations, since they stimulate fibroblast activity and can chemoattract cells to the area of the wound. Some of the growth factors have been used experimentally to spur or speed healing, albeit with variable success, and this is an interesting area that will probably continue to evolve and find important medical applications.

TABLE 4-24 Some of the Growth Factors and their Sources and Actions in the Process of Wound Healing

GROWTH FACTORS	SYNTHESIZED BY	SOME OF THEIR ACTIONS, AND COMMENTS
Platelet-derived growth factors (PDGF)	P, Mac, EC, SMC	Mitogenic for mesenchymal cells, like fibroblasts, but not EC. Chemoattracts and stimulates fibroblasts, macrophages, and neutrophils. Stimulates angiogenesis indirectly by chemoattracting and stimulating macrophages. An initial "trigger" for wound healing since platelets secrete PDGF (and other growth factors) during bleeding. There are three dimeric forms.
Fibroblast growth factors (FGF)	Mac, SMC, Ep	Stimulates new growth of blood vessels (angiogenesis). Chemotactic for macrophages, and chemotactic and stimulatory for EC, F. Two forms, acidic (aFGF) and basic (bFGF) exist and have similar actions.
Keratinocyte growth factor	F	Is in the FGF family. Stimulates epidermis.
Epidermal growth factor (EGF)	P (also produced by the kidney and salivary and lacrimal glands)	Potent stimulator of epithelial cell proliferation. Also stimulates endothelial cells and fibroblasts. Angiogenesis.
Transforming growth factor–α (TGF-α)	P, Mac, Ep	Similar actions as EGF and uses the same receptor. More potent for angiogenesis than EGF.
Transforming growth factor–β (TGF-β)	P, Mac, L	Truly pleiotropic effects. Chemotactic for Mac and F. Stimulates Mac to secrete other growth factors; stimulates F to divide. Angiogenesis. May have (+) or (−) effects on cell stimulation related to the stage of healing. Several isoforms; a superfamily. TGF-β receptors are found on most mammalian cells. No homology to TGF-α.
Vascular endothelial growth factors (VEGF)	Mac, Ep	Hallmark is promotion of angiogenesis. Receptors for VEGF are found only on EC, and VEGF is a potent mitogen. Also promotes vascular permeability, which enhances release of important plasma factors into the wound. There are several isoforms of VEGF.
Insulin-like growth factor–1 (IGF-1)	Liver, F, muscle	Increased levels are present in regenerating skeletal muscle and peripheral nerve. Has homology to proinsulin. Also called somatomedin-c.

Many other growth factors exist and are important in growth, differentiation, and repair of tissue.

EC, Endothelial cells; *Ep,* epidermis; *F,* fibroblasts; *L,* lymphocytes; *Mac,* macrophages; *P,* platelets; *SMC,* vascular smooth muscle cells.

WOUND HEALING: OTHER CONSIDERATIONS

There can be confusion with the interchangeable use of the terms "healing," "repair," and "regeneration." As we have discussed previously, *regeneration* refers to the replacement of lost tissue by tissue of the same type. *Repair* is a somewhat more general term that encompasses both regeneration and connective tissue replacement. There is really no precise definition of *healing*, but it generally includes all means (including connective-tissue replacement and regeneration) by which restoration of tissue continuity is achieved. It can be difficult to pinpoint an exact end point for healing. For example, a skin wound may appear "healed" when epithelial regrowth over the surface has occurred, but below the surface, remodeling of the connective tissue may continue for weeks or months depending on the magnitude of the initial defect. Healing is an amazing phenomenon, the ultimate value of which is determined by its effectiveness in restoring the tissue to complete normalcy of structure and function.

Several important concepts in cell biology are central to the healing process. First, the *movement* of cells is essential. Second, the ability of cells to *proliferate* is vital, for without cell proliferation, neither parenchymal regeneration nor scarring can take place. Third, the cells must *differentiate* and *mature* for the restitution of normalcy. Importantly, *cell death* and the removal of dead cells plays a large part in the inflammatory and maturational phases of healing. Exudates must be resolved, and dead cells must be removed before tissue continuity can be restored. But what turns the system off? Why, for example, do proliferating endothelial cells and fibroblasts in a healing wound eventually stop proliferating; what (usually) stops them from continuing until there is a huge, cumbersome mass of fibrovascular tissue as is sometimes the case when "exuberant granulation tissue" or "proud flesh" forms on the limbs of horses? It appears that a combination of negative signals and events are involved when the system works right. The cessation of cell proliferation that occurs when epithelia from opposite sides of a wound meet infers the existence of a mechanism that recognizes that coverage is complete; otherwise there would be a piling up of epithelium. The cellular events involved in this *contact inhibition* may involve cell-to-cell communication by changes in membrane permeability or surface electrical charge. The equivalent of "anti-"growth factors also contributes to a large extent, such as the antiangiogenic factor called "angiostatin"; there are others. In addition to the cessation of cell proliferation, apoptosis comes into play, resulting in a reduction of cells such as endothelial cells and fibroblasts when they are no longer needed in great numbers to heal the wound.

HEALING AND REPAIR IN PERSPECTIVE AND REVIEW

In review, several well-defined stages can be reconstructed in the progression of a simple healing skin wound with scar formation. First, there is formation of the *blood clot* within the disrupted tissue and the subsequent development of a scab. Second, *epithelial continuity* is restored, often as quickly as the first 48 to 72 hours if edge apposition is good. Third, an *inflammatory reaction* develops in the incised dermis with neutrophil infiltration followed by macrophage infiltration. Fourth, *neovascularization* occurs with the ingrowth of new capillary buds to bridge the wound. Fifth, *fibroblast proliferation* occurs to provide a sufficient cellular base for the manufacture and laying down of *collagen*. However, there is often not a clear distinction between these early stages and the timing of these events in early wound healing; they are ongoing, and they overlap. Thereafter, the process is one of progressive accumulation of collagen and other structural matrix components within the wound. The sixth event, gradual *devascularization* of the wound, results from "negative" factors. In the absence of a nutrient vasculature, the seventh stage of *departure of inflammatory cells* occurs, and, as the wound becomes progressively avascular, *fibroblast regression* takes place as an eighth step. This leaves us with the final stage of a pale, collagenous *scar* as an end product of wound healing. It must be emphasized that although it is possible to arbitrarily divide the process into these sorts of staged events there is overlap between stages of this dynamic process, which forms a continuum from initiation of the wound to the terminal scar.

The clinical relevance of an increased understanding of the biology of healing is readily apparent. An enlightened approach to understanding the healing process at the cellular and molecular levels gives us as clinicians a better understanding to predict or create the appropriate local environments to favor the various phases of the healing process.

Finally, as we have seen and discussed, healing and repair can take place by either tissue regeneration or by connective tissue replacement. In an inflammatory injury, the ultimate outcome depends on a wide variety of factors, some host dependent and some agent dependent. In the case of a wound caused by an infectious agent or a wound contaminated by one, if the host destroys the invader and little tissue is lost, a return to normal is possible so long as the persistence of exudate (such as pus) does not promote scarring. If the invader is not promptly destroyed, the outcome depends most often on whether the tissue-supporting structures necessary to regeneration are intact or destroyed. Regeneration cannot occur satisfactorily in the absence of an intact connective tissue framework, and scarring is the usual result. Also recall that the nature of the host cells damaged is of importance, since permanent cells cannot regenerate well even if the connective tissue framework remains intact. The various options with respect to healing and repair are graphically summarized in Fig. 4-59. The unfortunate truth is that for most kinds of injury, some scarring almost inevitably results; even the most perfect surgical procedure leaves a scar, however small. The combination of ingredients and factors necessary for the restitution of complete tissue normalcy are much less likely to occur in a real-life setting than are the combination of ingredients and factors that lead to scarring. The result of tissue damage, therefore, usually includes some scarring rather than a complete restitution of normalcy. It may help to cushion our chagrin at the apparent

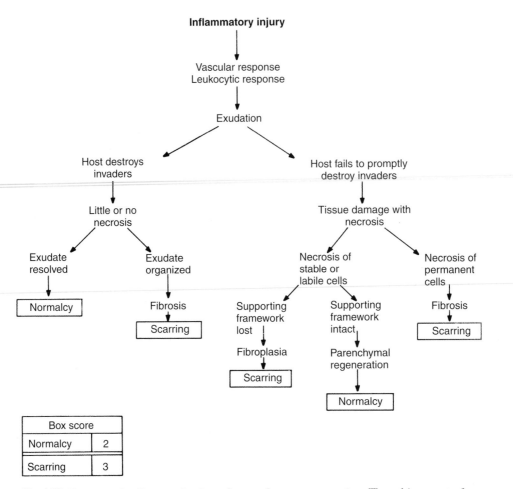

Fig. 4-59 Routes to healing: restitution of normalcy versus scarring. The achievement of normalcy at the end of a repair process depends on how well the host handles the invaders, how much necrosis occurs, how much exudate is present and how it is resolved, the nature of the injured tissue cells, and the condition of the supporting connective tissue framework. Scarring is more common than complete restitution of normalcy.

unfairness of this biological reality by reminding ourselves that the entire inflammation and repair process is survival oriented and that the other alternatives, dysfunction or death, are usually even less acceptable than scarring is.

RECOMMENDED READING

Abraham E: Corticosteroids and the neutrophil: cutting both ways, *Crit Care Med* 27:2583-2584, 1999.

Ahluwalia A, Perretti M: B$_1$ receptors as a new inflammatory target, *Trends Pharmacol Sci* 20:100-104, 1999 (kinins).

Alexander WS, Starr R, Metcalf D, Nicholson SE, Farley A, Elefanty AG, Brysha M, Kile B, Richardson R, Baca M, Zhang JG, Willson TA, Viney E, Sprigg NS, Rakar S, Corbin J, Mifsud S, DiRago L, Cary D, Nicola NA, Hilton DJ: Suppressors of cytokine signaling (SOCS): negative regulators of signal transduction, *J Leukoc Biol* 66:588-592, 1999.

Anderson JM: Multinucleated giant cells, *Curr Opin Hematol* 7:40-47, 2000.

Anstead GM: Steroids, retinoids, and wound healing, *Adv Wound Care* 11:277-285, 1998.

Bacher M, Meinhardt A, Lan HY, Mu W, Metz CN, Chesney JA, Calandra T, Gemsa D, Donnelly T, Atkins RC, Bucala R: Migration inhibitory factor expression in experimentally induced endotoxemia, *Am J Pathol* 150:235-246, 1997.

Baggiolini M: Proteinases and acid hydrolases of neutrophils and macrophages and the mechanisms of their release, *Adv Inflamm Res* 3:313-327, 1982.

Barrick B, Campbell EJ, Owen CA: Leukocyte proteinases in wound healing: roles in physiologic and pathologic processes, *Wound Repair Regen* 7:410-422, 1999.

Barton CH, Biggs TE, Baker ST, Bowen H, Atkinson PGP: *Nramp* 1: a link between intercellular iron transport and innate resistance to intracellular pathogens, *J Leukoc Biol* 66:757-762, 1999.

Bazzoni F, Beutler B: The tumor necrosis factor ligand and receptor families, *N Engl J Med* 334:1717-1725, 1996.

Belperio JA, Keane MP, Arenberg DA, Addison CL, Ehlert JE, Burdick MD, Strieter RM: CXC chemokines in angiogenesis, *J Leukoc Biol* 68:1-8, 2000.

Bertram TA: Neutrophilic leukocyte structure and function in domestic animals, *Adv Vet Sci Comp Med* 30:91-130, 1985.

Bhoola KD, Figueroa CD, Worthy K: Bioregulation of kinins: kallikreins, kininogens, and kininases, *Pharmacol Rev* 44:1-80, 1992.

Bistrian BR: Acute phase proteins and the systemic inflammatory response, *Crit Care Med* 27:452-453, 1999.

Böckman S, Paegelow I: Kinins and kinin receptors: importance for the activation of leukocytes, *J Leukoc Biol* 68:587-592, 2000.

Borregaard N: Development of neutrophil granule diversity, *Ann NY Acad Sci* 832:62-68, 1997.

Bowie A, O'Neill LA: The interleukin-1 receptor/toll-like receptor superfamily: signal generators for pro-inflammatory interleukins and microbial products, *J Leukoc Biol* 67:508-514, 2000.

Briskin M, Winsor-Hines D, Shyjan A, Cochran N, Bloom S, Wilson J, McEvoy LM, Butcher EC, Kassman N, Mackay CR, Newman W, Ringler DJ: Human mucosal addressin cell adhesion molecule-1 is preferentially expressed in intestinal tract and associated lymphoid tissue, *Am J Pathol* 151:97-110, 1997.

Broder CC, Collman RG: Chemokine receptors and HIV, *J Leukoc Biol* 62:20-29, 1997.

Brown E: Neutrophil adhesion and the therapy of inflammation, *Semin Hematol* 34:319-326, 1997.

Burns AR, Bowden RA, Abe Y, Walker DC, Simon SI, Entman ML, Smith CW: P-selectin mediates neutrophil adhesion to endothelial cell borders, *J Leukoc Biol* 65:299-306, 1999.

Butcher EC, Picker LJ: Lymphocyte homing and homeostasis, *Science* 272:60-66, 1996.

Calandra T, Bucala R: Macrophage migration inhibitory factor (MIF): a glucocorticoid counter-regulator within the immune system, *Crit Rev Immunol* 17:77-88, 1997.

Canonne-Hergaux F, Gruenheid S, Govoni G, Gros P: The Nramp1 protein and its role in resistance to infection and macrophage function, *Proc Assoc Am Physicians* 11:283-289, 1999.

Carmeliet P: Mechanisms of angiogenesis and arteriogenesis, *Nat Med* 6:389-395, 2000.

Clark RAF, Henson PM, editors: *The molecular and cellular biology of wound repair*, New York, 1992, Plenum Press.

Connor EM, Eppihimer MJ, Morise Z, Granger DN, Grisham MB: Expression of mucosal addressin cell adhesion molecule–1 (MAdCam-1) in acute and chronic inflammation, *J Leukoc Biol* 65:349-355, 1999.

Crockett-Torabi E: Selectins and mechanisms of signal transduction, *J Leukoc Biol* 63:1-14, 1998.

Czermak BJ, Friendl HP, Ward PA: Complement, cytokines, and adhesion molecule expression in inflammatory reactions, *Proc Assoc Am Physicians* 110:306-312, 1998.

Das AM, Flower RJ, Perretti M: Resident mast cells are important for eotaxin-induced eosinophil accumulation in vivo, *J Leukoc Biol* 64:156-162, 1998.

Davidson JM: Wound repair, *J Hand Ther* 11:80-94, 1998.

de Haas CJ, van der Zee R, Benaissa-Trouw B, van Kessel KP, Verhoef J, van Strijp JA: Lipopolysaccharide (LPS)-binding synthetic peptides derived from serum amyloid P component neutralize LPS, *Infect Immunol* 67:2790-2796, 1999.

de Haas CJ: New insights into the role of serum amyloid P component, a novel lipopolysaccharide-binding protein, *FEMS Immunol Med Microbiol* 26:197-202, 1999.

Dentener MA, Vreugdenhil AC, Hoet PH, Vernooy JH, Nieman FH, Heumann D, Janssen YM, Buurman WA, Wouters EF: Production of the acute-phase protein lipopolysaccharide-binding protein by respiratory type II epithelial cells: implications for local defense to bacterial endotoxins, *Am J Respir Cell Mol Biol* 23:146-153, 2000.

Deutschman CS: Acute-phase responses and SIRS/MODS: the good, the bad, and the nebulous, *Crit Care Med* 26:1630-1631, 1998.

Dickerson C, Undem B, Bullock B, Winchurch RA: Neuropeptide regulation of proinflammatory cytokine responses, *J Leukoc Biol* 63:602-605, 1998.

Dimmeler S, Zeiher AM: Endothelial cell apoptosis in angiogenesis and vessel regression, *Circ Res* 87:434-439, 2000.

Dvorak AM: New aspects of mast cell biology, *Int Arch Allergy Immunol* 114:1-9, 1997.

Dvorak HF, Brown LF, Detmar M, Dvorak AM: Vascular permeability factor/vascular endothelial growth factor, microvascular hyperpermeability, and angiogenesis, *Am J Pathol* 145:1029-1039, 1995.

Elangbam CS, Qualls CW Jr, Dahlgren RR: Cell adhesion molecules—update, *Vet Pathol* 34:61-73, 1997.

Elsbach P: The bactericidal/permeability-increasing protein (BPI) in antibacterial host defense, *J Leukoc Biol* 64:14-18, 1998.

Elsner J, Kapp A: Regulation and modulation of eosinophil effector functions, *Allergy* 54:15-26, 1999.

Etzioni A, Doerschuk CM, Harlan JM: Of man and mouse: leukocyte and endothelial adhesion molecule deficiencies, *Blood* 94:3281-3288, 1999.

Farsky SP, Sannomiya P, García-Leme J: Secreted glucocorticoids regulate leukocyte-endothelial interactions in inflammation: a direct vital microscopic study, *J Leukoc Biol* 57:379-386, 1995.

Fenton MJ, Golenbock DT: LPS-binding proteins and receptors, *J Leukoc Biol* 64:25-32, 1998.

Foletta VC, Segal DH, Cohen DR: Transcriptional regulation in the immune system: all roads lead to AP-1, *J Leukoc Biol* 63:139-152, 1998.

Gabay C, Kushner I: Acute-phase proteins and other systemic responses to inflammation, *N Engl J Med* 340:448-454, 1999.

Gabbiani G, Hirschel BJ, Ryan GB, Statkov PR, Majno G: Granulation tissue as a contractile organ: a study of structure and function, *J Exp Med* 35:719-734, 1972.

Galli SJ, Hammel I: Mast cell and basophil development, *Curr Opin Hematol* 1:33-39, 1994.

Gallin JI, Goldstein IM, Snyderman R: *Inflammation: basic principles and clinical correlates*, New York, 1988, Raven Press.

Giger U, Boxer LA, Simpson PJ, Lucchesi BR, Todd RF III: Deficiency of leukocyte surface glycoproteins Mo1, LFA-1, and Leu M5 in a dog with recurrent infections: an animal model, *Blood* 69:1622-1630, 1987.

Gilbert RO, Rebhun WC, Kim CA, Kehrli ME Jr, Shuster DE, Ackermann MR: Clinical manifestations of leukocyte adhesion deficiency in cattle: 14 cases (1977-1991), *J Am Vet Med Assoc* 202:445-449, 1993.

Goetzl EJ, An S, Smith WL: Specificity of expression and effects of eicosanoid mediators in normal physiology and human diseases, *FASEB J* 9:1051-1058, 1995.

Goppelt-Struebe M: Molecular mechanisms involved in the regulation of prostaglandin biosynthesis by glucocorticoids, *Biochem Pharmacol* 53:1389-1395, 1997.

Graham A: The use of growth factors in clinical practice, *J Wound Care* 7(9, part 1):464-466; 7(10, part 2):536-540, 1998.

Greenhalgh DG: The role of apoptosis in wound healing, *Int J Biochem Cell Biol* 30:1019-1030, 1998.

Grisham MB, Jourd'Heuil D, Wink DA: Nitric oxide. I. Physiological chemistry of nitric oxide and its metabolites: implications in inflammation, *Am J Physiol* 276:G315-G321, 1999.

Gudmundsson GH, Agerberth B: Neutrophil antibacterial peptides, multifunctional effector molecules in the mammalian immune system, *J Immunol Methods* 232:45-54, 1999.

Hallett MB: Controlling the molecular motor of neutrophil chemotaxis, *Bioessays* 19:615-621, 1997.

Hampton MB, Kettle AJ, Winterbourn CC: Inside the neutrophil phagosome: oxidants, myeloperoxidase, and bacterial killing, *Blood* 92:3007-3017, 1998.

Hayflick JS, Kilgannon P, Gallatin WM: The intercellular adhesion molecule (ICAM) family of proteins: new members and novel functions, *Immunol Res* 17:313-327, 1998.

Heidenreich S: Monocyte CD14: a multifunctional receptor engaged in apoptosis from both sides, *J Leukoc Biol* 65:737-743, 1999.

Hill PB, Martin RJ: A review of mast cell biology, *Vet Dermatol* 9:145-166, 1998.

Hobbs AJ, Higgs A, Moncada S: Inhibition of nitric oxide synthase as a potential therapeutic target, *Annu Rev Pharmacol Toxicol* 39:191-220, 1999.

Hochepied T, Van Molle W, Berger FG, Baumann H, Libert C: Involvement of the acute phase protein alpha 1-acid glycoprotein in nonspecific resistance to a lethal gram-negative infection, *J Biol Chem* 275:14903-14909, 2000.

Horadagoda NU, Knox KM, Gibbs HA, Reid SW, Horadagoda A, Edwards SE, Eckersall PD: Acute phase proteins in cattle: discrimination between acute and chronic inflammation, *Vet Rec* 144:437-441, 1999.

Horwitz MA: Phagocytosis of microorganisms, *Rev Infect Dis* 4:104-123, 1982.

Huang C, Sali A, Stevens RL: Regulation and function of mast cell proteases in inflammation, *J Clin Immunol* 18:169-183, 1998.

Hulten C, Tulamo RM, Suominen MM, Burvall K, Marhaug G, Forsberg M: A non-competitive chemiluminescence enzyme immunoassay for the equine acute phase protein serum amyloid A (SAA)—a clinically useful inflammatory marker in the horse, *Vet Immunol Immunopathol* 68:267-281, 1999.

Hulten C, Sandgren B, Skioldebrand E, Klingeborn B, Marhaug G, Forsberg M: The acute phase protein serum amyloid A (SAA) as an inflammatory marker in equine influenza virus infection, *Acta Vet Scand* 40:323-333, 1999.

Issekutz AC, Rowter D, Springer TA: Role of ICAM-1 and ICAM-2 and alternate CD11/CD18 ligands in neutrophil transendothelial migration, *J Leukoc Biol* 65:117-126, 1999.

Jaeschke H, Smith CW: Mechanisms of neutrophil-induced parenchymal cell injury, *J Leukoc Biol* 61:647-653, 1997.

Jones GE: Cellular signaling in macrophage migration and chemotaxis, *J Leukoc Biol* 68:593-602, 2000.

Jose PJ, Griffiths-Johnson DA, Collins PD, Walsh DT, Moqbel R, Totty NF, Truong O, Hsuan JJ, Williams TJ: Eotaxin: a potent eosinophil chemoattractant-cytokine detected in a guinea pig model of allergic airways inflammation, *J Exp Med* 179:881-887, 1994.

Karukonda SR, Flynn TC, Boh EE, McBurney EI, Russo GG, Millikan LE: The effects of drugs on wound healing: part 1, *Int J Dermatol* 39:250-257, 2000.

Kay AB, Barata L, Meng Q, Durham SR, Ying S: Eosinophils and eosinophil-associated cytokines in allergic inflammation, *Int Arch Allergy Immunol* 113:196-199, 1997.

Kehrli ME Jr, Schmalstieg FC, Anderson DC, Van Der Maten MJ, Hughes BJ, Ackermann MR, Wilhelmsen CL, Brown GB, Stevens MG, Whetstone CA: Molecular definition of the bovine granulocytopathy syndrome: identification of deficiency of the Mac-1 (CD11b/CD18) glycoprotein, *Am J Vet Res* 51:1826-1836, 1990.

Kim CH, Broxmeyer HE: Chemokines: signal lamps for trafficking of T and B cells for development and effector function, *J Leukoc Biol* 65:6-15, 1999.

Kinnula VL, Crapo JD, Raivio KO: Generation and disposal of reactive oxygen metabolites in the lung, *Lab Invest* 73:3-19, 1995.

Kjeldsen L, Calafat J, Borregaard N: Giant granules of neutrophils in Chediak-Higashi syndrome are derived from azurophil granules but not from specific and gelatinase granules, *J Leukoc Biol* 64:72-77, 1998.

Korade-Mirnics Z, Corey SJ: Src kinase–mediated signaling in leukocytes, *J Leukoc Biol* 68:603-613, 2000.

Kubes P: The role of shear forces in ischemia/reperfusion-induced neutrophil rolling and adhesion, *J Leukoc Biol* 62:458-464, 1997.

Kudravi SA, Reed MJ: Aging, cancer, and wound healing, *In Vivo* 14:83-92, 2000.

Kuijper PHM, Gallardo Torres HI, Houben LAMJ, Lammers J-W, Zwaginga JJ, Koenderman L: P-selectin and Mac-1 mediate monocyte rolling and adhesion to ECM-bound platelets under flow conditions, *J Leukoc Biol* 64:467-473, 1998.

Kunkel EJ, Ramos CL, Steeber DA, Müller W, Wagner N, Tedder TF, Ley K: The roles of L-selectin, β$_7$-integrins, and P-selectin in leukocyte rolling and adhesion in high endothelial venules of Peyer's patches, *J Immunol* 161:2449-2456, 1998.

Lacy P, Moqbel R: Eosinophil cytokines, *Chem Immunol* 76:134-155, 2000.

Lee B, Montaner LJ: Chemokine immunobiology in HIV-1 pathogenesis, *J Leukoc Biol* 65:552-565, 1999.

Leibovich SJ, Ross R: The role of the macrophage in wound repair: a study with hydrocortisone and anti-macrophage serum, *Am J Pathol* 78:71-100, 1975.

Leonard WJ, Lin JX: Cytokine receptor signaling pathways, *J Allergy Clin Immunol* 105:877-888, 2000.

Liaudet L, Soriano FG, Szabo C: Biology of ntiric oxide signaling, *Crit Care Med* 28(suppl):N37-N52, 2000.

Lien E, Means TK, Heine H, Yoshimura A, Kusumoto S, Fukase K, Fenton MJ, Oikawa M, Qureshi N, Monks B, Finberg RW, Ingalls RR, Golenbock DT: Toll-like receptor 4 imparts ligand-specific recognition of bacterial lipopolysaccharide, *J Clin Invest* 105:497-504, 2000.

Liles WC, Van Voorhis WC: Nomenclature and biologic significance of cytokines involved in inflammation and the host immune response, *J Infect Dis* 172:1573-1580, 1995.

Liu T, Stern A, Roberts LJ, Morrow JD: The isoprostanes: novel prostaglandin-like products of the free radical–catalyzed peroxidation of arachidonic acid, *J Biomed Sci* 6:226-235, 1999.

Luster AD: Chemokines: chemotactic cytokines that mediate inflammation, *N Engl J Med* 338:436-445, 1998.

Luster AD, Rothenberg ME: Role of the monocyte chemoattractant protein and exotoxin subfamily of chemokines in allergic inflammation, *J Leukoc Biol* 62:620-633, 1997.

MacMicking J, Xie QW, Nathan C: Nitric oxide and macrophage function, *Annu Rev Immunol* 15:323-350, 1997.

Majno G: Chronic inflammation: links with angiogenesis and wound healing, *Am J Pathol* 153:1035-1039, 1998.

Majno G: *The healing hand: man and wound in the ancient world,* Cambridge, Mass., 1975, Harvard University Press.

Martin LB, Kita H, Leiferman KM, Gleich GJ: Eosinophils in allergy: role in disease, degranulation, and cytokines, *Int Arch Allergy Immunol* 109:207-215, 1996.

Matzner Y: Neutrophil pathophysiology, *Semin Hematol* 34:265-266, 1997.

Meager A: Cytokine regulation of cellular adhesion molecule expression in inflammation, *Cytokine Growth Factor Rev* 10:27-39, 1999.

Medzhitov R, Janeway C Jr: Innate immunity, *N Engl J Med* 343(5):338-344, 2000.

Medzhitov R, Preston-Hurlburt P, Janeway CA Jr: The toll receptor family and microbial recognition, *Trends Microbiol* 8:452-456, 2000.

Medzhitov R, Preston-Hurlburt P, Janeway CA Jr: A human homologue of the *Drosophila* toll protein signals activation of adaptive immunity, *Nature* 388:394-397, 1997.

Metchnikoff E: *Lectures on the comparative pathology of inflammation,* 1893. Reprint by Dover Publications, New York, 1968.

Metz CN, Bucala R: Role of macrophage migration inhibitory factor in the regulation of the immune response, *Adv Immunol* 66:197-223, 1997.

Mollinedo F, Borregaard N, Boxer LA: Novel trends in neutrophil structure, function and development, *Immunol Today* 20:535-537, 1999.

Morrissette N, Gold E, Aderem A: The macrophage, a cell for all seasons, *Trends Cell Biol* 9:199-201, 1999.

Moshage H: Cytokines and the hepatic acute phase response, *J Pathol* 181:257-266, 1997.

Movat HZ: *The inflammatory reaction,* Amsterdam, 1985, Elsevier.

Muller WA, Randolph GJ: Migration of leukocytes across endothelium and beyond: molecules involved in the transmigration and fate of monocytes, *J Leukoc Biol* 66:698-704, 1999.

Nakagawa K, Chen YX, Ishibashi H, Yonemitsu Y, Murata T, Hata Y, Nakashima Y, Sueishi K: Angiogenesis and its regulation: roles of vascular endothelial cell growth factor, *Semin Thromb Hemost* 26:61-66, 2000.

Newton RA, Thiel M, Hogg N: Signaling mechanisms and the activation of leukocyte integrins, *J Leukoc Biol* 61:422-426, 1997.

Nicholson SE, Hilton DJ: The SOCS proteins: a new family of negative regulators of signal transduction, *J Leukoc Biol* 63:665-668, 1998.

O'Neill LAJ, Greene C: Signal transduction pathways activated by the IL-1 receptor family: ancient signaling machinery in mammals, insects, and plants, *J Leukoc Biol* 63:650-657, 1998.

Oberholzer A, Oberholzer C, Moldawer LL: Cytokine signaling: regulation of the immune response in normal and critically ill states, *Crit Care Med* 28(4 suppl):N3-N12, 2000.

Olchowy TWJ, Bochsler PN, Neilson NR, et al: Bovine leukocyte adhesion deficiency: in vitro assessment of neutrophil function and leukocyte integrin expression, *Can J Vet Res* 58:127-133, 1994.

Owen CA, Campbell EJ: The cell biology of leukocyte-mediated proteolysis, *J Leukoc Biol* 65:137-150, 1999.

Pawelec G, Solana R, Remarque E, Mariani E: Impact of aging on innate immunity, *J Leukoc Biol* 64:703-712, 1998.

Picker LJ: Control of lymphocyte homing, *Curr Opin Immunol* 6:394-406, 1994.

Pilcher BK, Wang M, Qin XJ, Parks WC, Senior RM, Welgus HG: Role of matrix metalloproteinases and their inhibition in cutaneous wound healing and allergic contact hypersensitivity, *Ann NY Acad Sci* 878:12-24, 1999.

Plager DA, Stuart S, Gleich GJ: Human eosinophil granule major basic protein and its novel homolog, *Allergy* 53(45 suppl):33-40, 1998.

Poltorak A, He X, Smirnova I, Liu MY, Huffel CV, Du X, Birdwell D, Alejos E, Silva M, Galanos C, Freudenberg M, Ricciardi-Castagnoli P, Layton B, Beutler B: Defective LPS signaling in C3H/HeJ and C57BL/10ScCr mice: mutations in Tlr4 gene, *Science* 282:2085-2088, 1998.

Premack BA, Schall TJ: Chemokine receptors: gateways to inflammation and infection, *Nat Med* 2:1174-1178, 1996.

Pretolani M: Interleukin-10: an anti-inflammatory cytokine with therapeutic potential, *Clin Exp Allergy* 29:1164-1171, 1999.

Ramadori G, Christ B: Cytokines and the hepatic acute-phase response, *Semin Liver Dis* 19:141-155, 1999.

Robinson DR: Regulation of prostaglandin synthesis by anti-inflammatory drugs, *J Rheumatol Suppl* 47:32-39, 1997.

Rothenberg ME: Eotaxin: an essential mediator of eosinophil trafficking into mucosal tissues, *Am J Respir Cell Mol Biol* 21:291-295, 1999.

Rotrosen D, Gallin JI: Disorders of phagocyte function, *Annu Rev Immunol* 5:127-150, 1987.

Rottman JB: Key role of chemokines and chemokine receptors in inflammation, immunity, neoplasia, and infectious disease, *Vet Pathol* 36:357-367, 1999.

Ryan GB, Cliff WJ, Gabbiani G, Irle C, Montandon D, Statkov PR, Majno G: Myofibroblasts in human granulation tissue, *Hum Pathol* 5:55-67, 1974.

Savill J: Apoptosis in resolution of inflammation, *J Leukoc Biol* 61:375-380, 1997.

Schuster JM, Nelson PS: Toll receptors: an expanding role in our understanding of human disease, *J Leukoc Biol* 67:767-773, 2000.

Scott KF, Bryant KJ, Bidgood MJ: Functional coupling and differential regulation of the phospholipase A_2–cyclooxygenase pathways in inflammation, *J Leukoc Biol* 66:535-541, 1999.

Selsted ME, Tang YQ, Morris WL, McGuire PA, Novotny MJ, Smith W, Henschen AH, Cullor JS: Purification, primary structures, and antibacterial activities of beta-defensins, a new family of antimicrobial peptides from bovine neutrophils, *J Biol Chem* 268:6641-6648, 1993.

Serhan CN, Haeggstrom JZ, Leslie CC: Lipid mediator networks in cell signaling: update and impact of cytokines, *FASEB J* 10:1147-1158, 1996.

Shapiro SD: Diverse roles of macrophage matrix metalloproteinases in tissue destruction and tumor growth, *Thromb Haemost* 82:846-849, 1999.

Shuster DE, Kehrli ME Jr, Ackermann MR, Gilbert RO: Identification and prevalence of genetic defect that causes leukocyte adhesion deficiency in Holstein cattle, *Proc Nat Acad Sci USA* 89:9225-9229, 1992.

Singer AJ, Clark RAF: Cutaneous wound healing, *N Engl J Med* 341:738-746, 1999.

Slocombe RF, Malark J, Derksen FJ, Robinson NE: Importance of neutrophils in the pathogenesis of acute pneumonic pasteurellosis in calves, *Am J Vet Res* 46:2253-2258, 1986.

Smith RE, Hogaboam CM, Strieter RM, Luckacs NW, Kunkel SL: Cell-to-cell and cell-to-matrix interactions mediate chemokine expression: an important component of the inflammatory lesion, *J Leukoc Biol* 62:612-619, 1997.

Smith RS, Smith TJ, Blieden T M, Phipps RP: Fibroblasts as sentinel cells: synthesis of chemokines and regulation of inflammation, *Am J Pathol* 151:317-322, 1997.

Smith SR, Manfra D, Davies L, Terminelli C, Denhardt G, Donkin J: Elevated levels of NO in both unchallenged and LPS-challenged C. *parvum*–primed mice are attributable to the activity of a cytokine-inducible isoform of iNOS, *J Leukoc Biol* 61:24-32, 1997.

Smith WL, Garavito RM, DeWitt DL: Prostaglandin endoperoxide H synthases (cyclooxygenases)-1 and -2, *J Biol Chem* 271:33157-33160, 1996.

Stadelmann WK, Digenis AG, Tobin GR: Impediments to wound healing, *Am J Surg* 176(2A suppl):39S-47S, 1998.

Standiford TJ: Anti-inflammatory cytokines and cytokine antagonists, *Curr Pharm Des* 6:633-649, 2000.

Steed DL: Modifying the wound healing response with exogenous growth factors, *Clin Plast Surg* 25:397-405, 1998.

Stickle JE: The neutrophil: function, disorders, and testing, *Vet Clin North Am Small Anim Pract* 26:1013-1021, 1996.

Styrt B: Species variation in neutrophil biochemistry and function, *J Leukoc Biol* 46:63-74, 1989.

Suffredini AF, Fantuzzi G, Badolato R, Oppenheim JJ, O'Grady NP: New insights into the biology of the acute phase response, *J Clin Immunol* 19:203-214, 1999.

Sutterwala FS, Mosser DM: The taming of IL-12: suppressing the production of proinflammatory cytokines, *J Leukoc Biol* 65:543-551, 1999.

Taichman NS, Young S, Cruchley AT, Taylor P, Paleolog E: Human neutrophils secrete vascular endothelial growth factor, *J Leukoc Biol* 62:397-400, 1997.

Tailor A, Flower RJ, Perretti M: Dexamethasone inhibits leukocyte emigration in rat mesenteric post-capillary venules: an intravital microscopy study, *J Leukoc Biol* 62:301-308, 1997.

Talbott GA, Sharar SR, Harlan JM, Winn RK: Leukocyte-endothelial interactions and organ injury: the role of adhesion molecules, *New Horizons* 2:545-554, 1994.

Tedder TF, Steeber DA, Chen A, Engel P: The selectins: vascular adhesion molecules, *FASEB J* 9:866-873, 1995.

Trowald-Wigh G, Hakansson L, Johannisson A, Norrgren L, Hard AF, Segerstad C: Leukocyte adhesion protein deficiency in Irish setter dogs, *Vet Immunol Immunopathol* 32:261-280, 1992.

Uhlar CM, Whitehead AS: Serum amyloid A, the major vertebrate acute-phase reactant, *Eur J Biochem* 265:501-523, 1999.

Ulevitch RJ, Tobias PS: Receptor-dependent mechanisms of cell stimulation by bacterial endotoxin, *Annu Rev Immunol* 13:437-457, 1995.

Urieli-Shoval S, Linke RP, Matzner Y: Expression and function of serum amyloid A, a major acute-phase protein, in normal and disease states, *Curr Opin Hematol* 7:65-69, 2000.

Vaday GG, Lider O: Extracellular matrix moieties, cytokines, and enzymes: dynamic effects on immune cell behavior and inflammation, *J Leukoc Biol* 67:149-159, 2000.

Venge P, Bystrom J: Eosinophil cationic protein (ECP), *Int J Biochem Cell Biol* 30:433-437, 1998.

Wagner JG, Roth RA: Neutrophil migration during endotoxemia, *J Leukoc Biol* 66:10-24, 1999.

Walker C: Cytokine inhibitor strategies, *Pulm Pharmacol Ther* 12:73-77, 1999.

Walton GS, Neal PA: Observations on wound healing in the horse: the role of wound contraction, *Equine Vet J* 4:1-5, 1971.

Watt SM, Gschmeissner SE, Bates PA: PECAM-1: its expression and function as a cell adhesion molecule on hemopoietic and endothelial cells, *Leuk Lymphoma* 17:229-244, 1995.

Weinberg JB: Nitric oxide production and nitric oxide synthase type 2 expression by human mononuclear phagocytes: a review, *Mol Med* 4:557-591, 1998.

Weiss SJ: Tissue destruction by neutrophils, *N Engl J Med* 320:365-376, 1999.

Weissmann G: *The Woods Hole cantata: essays on science and society*, New York, 1985, Raven Press.

Welle M: Development, significance, and heterogeneity of mast cells with particular regard to the mast cell–specific proteases chymase and tryptase, *J Leukoc Biol* 61:233-245, 1997.

Williams CS, DuBois RN: Prostaglandin endoperoxide synthase: Why two isoforms? *Am J Physiol* 270(3 pt 1):G393-G400, 1996.

Williams MA, Solomkin JS: Integrin-mediated signaling in human neutrophil functioning, *J Leukoc Biol* 65:725-736, 1999.

Winkler GC: Pulmonary intravascular macrophages in domestic animal species: review of structural and functional properties, *Am J Anat* 181:217-234, 1988.

Winn R, Vedder N, Ramamoorthy C, Sharar S, Harlan J: Endothelial and leukocyte adhesion molecules in inflammation and disease, *Blood Coagul Fibrinolysis* 9(suppl 2):S17-S23, 1998.

Wolfe MM, Lichtenstein DR, Singh G: Gastrointestinal toxicity of nonsteroidal antiinflammatory drugs, *N Engl J Med* 340:1888-1899, 1999.

Wu H, Zhang G, Ross CR, Blecha F: Cathelicidin gene expression in porcine tissues: roles in ontogeny and tissue specificity, *Infect Immun* 67:439-442, 2000.

Wynendaele W, van Oosterom AT, Pawinski A, de Bruijn EA, Maes RA: Angiogenesis: possibilities for therapeutic interventions, *Pharm World Sci* 20:225-235, 1998.

Yasukawa H, Sasaki A, Yoshimura A: Negative regulation of cytokine signaling pathways, *Annu Rev Immunol* 18:143-164, 2000.

Yong LC: The mast cell: origin, morphology, distribution, and function, *Exp Toxicol Pathol* 49:409-424, 1997.

Yount NY, Yuan J, Tarver A, Castro T, Diamond G, Tran PA, Levy JN, McCullough C, Cullor JS, Bevins CL, Selsted ME: Cloning and expression of bovine neutrophil beta-defensins: biosynthetic profile during neutrophilic maturation and localization of mature peptide to novel cytoplasmic dense granules, *J Biol Chem* 274:26249-26258, 1999.

Yu P-W, Schuler LA, Kehrli M, Mattocks L, Nonnecke BJ, Czuprynski CJ: Effects of dexamethasone treatment on IL-1 receptor mRNA levels in vivo, *J Leukoc Biol* 62:401-404, 1997.

Yuan C-J, Mandal AK, Zhang Z, Mukherjee AB: Transcriptional regulation of cyclooxygenase-2 gene expression: novel effects of nonsteroidal anti-inflammatory drugs, *Cancer Res* 60:1084-1091, 2000.

Zhang G, Wu H, Ross CR, Minton JE, Blecha F: Cloning of porcine NRAMP1 and its induction by lipopolysaccharide, tumor necrosis factor alpha, and interleukin-1 beta: role of CD14 and mitogen-activated protein kinases, *Infect Immun* 68:1086-1093, 2000.

Zhang G, Wu H, Shi J, Ganz T, Ross CR, Blecha F: Molecular cloning and tissue expression of porcine beta-defensin-1, *FEBS Lett* 424:37-40, 1998.

Zhang G, Ross CR, Blecha F: Porcine antimicrobial peptides: new prospects for ancient molecules of host defense, *Vet Res* 31:277-296, 2000.

Zwilling BS, Kuhn DE, Wikoff L, Brown D, Lafuse W: Role of iron in *Nramp1*-mediated inhibition of mycobacterial growth, *Infect Immun* 67:1386-1392, 1999.

CHAPTER 5

Immunopathology

Talmage T. Brown, Jr.
Maja M. Suter
David O. Slauson

The immune response is a critical host defense mechanism that serves to protect the body from exogenous threats. Normal immune responses are associated with the maintenance of good health, whereas immune responses that deviate from the normal may be the cause of a wide array of diseases. Generally these diseases are divided into three broad categories: (1) *hypersensitivity,* caused by an overreaction of the immune system to an antigenic stimulus, (2) *immunodeficiency,* caused by a congenital or acquired failure of some aspect of the immune system, and (3) *autoimmunity,* resulting from a breakdown in the ability of the immune system to distinguish self from nonself-antigens. *Immunopathology* encompasses the study of the disease mechanisms and lesions resulting from aberrant immune responses or a failure of the immune system.

Tissue injury associated with immunopathological reactions generally results from inflammation involving the same mediators and pathways associated with nonimmunological inflammatory reactions. The only difference is that the inflammatory process is stimulated by an immunological phenomenon such as allergy, autoimmunity, anaphylaxis, or immune complexes rather than by a microorganism or similar stimulus. Since the inflammatory processes evolving from immunopathological and nonimmunopathological reactions are similar, the focus of this chapter is on immunopathological mechanisms rather than on end points of immunopathological reactions.

Before the various mechanisms by which immune-mediated diseases develop are discussed, the immune cells and cytokines that are involved in immune-mediated diseases are briefly reviewed.

CELLULAR COMPONENTS OF THE IMMUNE RESPONSE

Pluripotential hematopoietic stem cells located in the bone marrow give rise to myeloid, lymphoid, and erythrocyte progenitor cells and megakaryocytes. Myeloid progenitor cells produce *monocytes* (destined to become tissue macrophages), *granulocytes,* and *mast cells,* and lymphoid progenitors give rise to *B and T lymphocytes.* Activated B cells differentiate into *plasma cells* that secrete antibodies, whereas T lymphocytes differentiate into *either cytotoxic T cells,* which kill virus-infected cells, or *helper T cells,* which activate B cells and macrophages.

Lymphocytes originate from the bone marrow. Differentiation and maturation occurs in either the bone marrow or thymus, which are referred to as the central lymphoid organs. Lymphocytes that remain in the bone marrow for development are called "B lymphocytes," or *B cells,* whereas those that leave to undergo development in the thymus are called "T lymphocytes," or *T cells.* After development in the bone marrow and thymus, B and T cells are nonactivated, or *naïve,* until they encounter specific antigen in one of the peripheral lymphoid organs, which includes lymph nodes, spleen, and mucosal lymphoid tissues. In lymph nodes, B cells localize in follicles, whereas T cells become more diffusely distributed in surrounding paracortical areas. Antigenic stimulation of B cells results in intense B-cell proliferation and the formation of large germinal centers within follicles. In the spleen, T cells localize around arterioles, forming periarteriolar lymphoid sheaths, and the B cells form primary follicles adjacent to the periarteriolar lymphoid sheaths. Other B and T cells locate in Peyer's patches of the small intestine, which are composed of large, central domes of B cells flanked by smaller zones of T cells. Similar mucosal lymphoid aggregates also may be found in other parts of the gastrointestinal tract and the upper and lower respiratory tracts.

B and T cells bear unique, highly diverse surface receptors necessary for antigen recognition. The receptors of individual lymphocytes are specific for only one antigen, but as a population, lymphocytes are capable of recognizing a wide array of antigens. The B-cell receptor is a membrane-bound immunoglobulin (Ig) molecule with the same antigenic specificity as the Ig or antibody molecule that will be secreted after B-cell activation. The T-cell receptor (TCR) is composed of two highly variable polypeptide chains that structurally resemble the Fab fragment of an antibody molecule.

T Lymphocytes

Antigen recognition by T lymphocytes occurs through a surface receptor that structurally resembles the Fab fragment of an antibody molecule. The T-cell receptor is formed by two highly variable polypeptide chains, designated α and β, that are bound together by a disulfide bond (Fig. 5-1). Each polypeptide chain contains a variable and a constant region, with the variable region of each chain forming the boundary of the antigen recognition site. The receptors of a small subpopulation of T cells are composed of γ and δ polypeptide chains rather and α- and β-chains. T cells bearing these receptors constitute only 1% to 5% of the total T-cell population and are most abundant in epithelial tissues. The function of γ:δ T cells remains obscure.

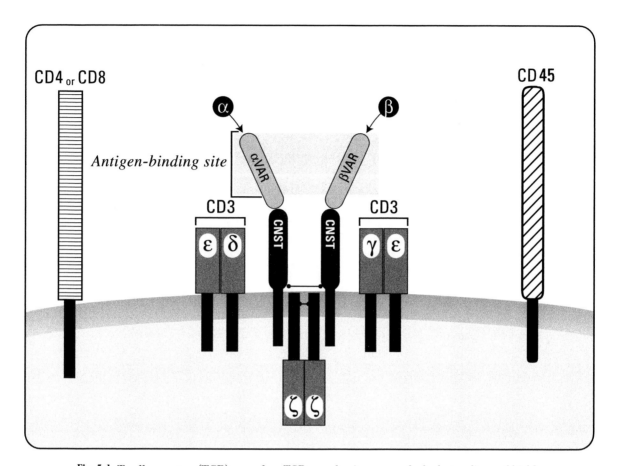

Fig. 5-1 T-cell receptor (TCR) complex. TCR complex is composed of a heterodimer of highly variable α and β polypeptide chains bound together by a disulfide bond, four nonvariable accessory polypeptide chains (CD3 complex), designated ε (two), δ, and γ, plus an intracytoplasmic nonvariable homodimer of two ζ (zeta) polypeptide chains. Variable region of α and β polypeptide chains forms the boundary of the antigen-binding site. For intracellular signaling to be stimulated after antigen recognition and binding, either the CD4 or the CD8 T cell coreceptor must bind to the TCR complex along with the tyrosine phosphatase, CD45. *(Adapted from Janeway CA et al, editors: Immunobiology: the immune system in health and disease, ed 4, New York, 1999, Current Biology Publications/Garland Publishing.)*

The T-cell α:β polypeptide chain complex, or heterodimer, can recognize and bind antigens presented by either MHC class I or II molecules. However, binding of antigen to the heterodimer is not a sufficient stimulus to activate intracellular signaling or cause the expression of additional α:β heterodimers on the cell surface. For this to occur, expression of 4 nonvariable, accessory polypeptide chains, termed the *CD3 complex,* and a nonvariable intracytoplasmic homodimer of ξ polypeptide chains are required. Association of these 6 polypeptide chains with the α:β heterodimer creates a complex of 8 polypeptide chains that form the complete T-cell receptor.

To facilitate signaling through the T-cell receptor complex, T cells express coreceptor surface proteins, *CD4* or *CD8*, which associate with components of the TCR complex during antigen recognition. T cells expressing the CD4 coreceptor bind antigens presented by MHC class II molecules on the surface of antigen-presenting cells, whereas T cells expressing CD8 coreceptors bind antigens presented by MHC class I molecules. Binding of either the CD4 or CD8 coreceptor to the TCR complex does not initiate intracellular signaling but requires the additional assistance of the transmembrane protein tyrosine phosphatase, *CD45 (leukocyte common antigen).* When CD45, either of the coreceptors, and the TCR complex bind, intracellular signaling is initiated.

To become activated, naïve T cells must encounter specific antigen expressed by either MHC class I or II molecules on the surface of antigen-presenting cells (APC). Although many cell types have the potential to present antigens, only a select group of cells can both present antigen and provide an activating secondary signal to naïve T cells. These cells are called *professional* (or functional) *APC* and include *dendritic cells, macrophages,* and *B cells.* Dendritic cells, whose only known function is the presentation of antigenic peptides through either MHC class I or MHC class II molecules, are found primarily in the T-cell zones of lymph nodes. Functionally diverse macrophages are scattered in all areas of the lymph node, whereas antigen-presenting B cells are concentrated in lymphoid follicles.

When the T-cell receptor and its CD4 or CD8 coreceptor bind an antigenic peptide:MHC complex on the surface of a professional (functional) APC, a signal is transmitted to the T cell that antigen has been recognized (Fig. 5-2). However, binding of the TCR and antigen:MHC complexes is not sufficient to activate the T cell. For this to occur, a second or costimulatory signal is required. This costimulatory signal is generated by the binding of *B7* molecules located on the surface of APC to *CD28* molecules on the surface of T cells. Binding of B7 and CD28 molecules triggers the secretion of interleukin (IL)-2, which stimulates the proliferation of activated T cells. Additionally, the IL-2 induces differentiation of the progeny T cells into fully functional effector T cells. The binding of B7 and CD28 molecules induces the expression of another receptor on T cells called *CTLA-4*, which binds B7 molecules with greater avidity than the CD28 receptor does. The binding of CTLA-4 and B7 generates inhibitory signals that suppress IL-2 production by activated T cells, thereby containing the clonal expansion of the activated T cells.

The importance of IL-2 production by activated T cells for the generation of a cellular immune response is dramatized by the immunosuppressive effect of two drugs, cyclosporin A and rapamycin. Cyclosporin A blocks production of IL-2, and rapamycin interferes with the response of activated T cells to IL-2. When given together, these drugs have a profound immunosuppressive effect caused by blocking clonal expansion of activated T cells.

Mature lymphocytes leaving the thymus are destined to become either CD4 or CD8 T cells. In the peripheral lymphoid tissues, naïve CD8 T cells become activated when they encounter specific antigenic peptide presented by MHC class I molecules expressed on the surface of a professional APC (Table 5-1). Antigenic peptides presented by MHC class I molecules are derived from pathogens, such as viruses and intracellular bacteria, that multiply and are degraded in the cytoplasm of the APC. Activated CD8 T cells, commonly called *cytotoxic T cells,* function by the release of cytotoxins and the secretion of cytokines (Fig. 5-3). Preformed cytotoxins, such as *perforin* or *granzymes,* are quickly released from cytotoxic T cells and are directly toxic to infected cells. At the same time that cytotoxins are being released, T cells begin synthesis of the cytokines, IFN-γ, TNF-α, and TNF-β, which are secreted a few hours later.

Naïve CD4 T cells arriving in peripheral lymphoid tissues have the potential to differentiate into one of two subclasses, either T_H1 or T_H2 cells. The type of differentiation stimulated by a specific antigen has significant immune functional ramifications because T_H1 cells promote cell-mediated immunity and T_H2 cells humoral immunity. Additionally, stimulation of

TABLE 5-1 Effector T-cell Role in Cell-mediated and Humoral Immune Responses to Different Pathogens

	CELL-MEDIATED IMMUNITY		HUMORAL IMMUNITY
Typical pathogens	Rabies virus	*Mycobacterium*	*Clostridium tetani*
	Influenza virus	*Pseudotuberculosis*	*Staphylococcus aureus*
	Listeria	*Corynebacterium*	*Streptococcus*
		Pseudotuberculosis	*Pneumocystis carinii*
		Leishmania	
		Pneumocystis carinii	
Pathogen location	Cytosol	Macrophage or other APC intracytoplasmic vesicles	Extracellular fluid
Effector T cell	Cytotoxic CD8 T cell	CD4 T_H1 cell	CD4 T_H1/T_H2 cell
Antigen recognition	Peptide:MHC class I on infected cell	Peptide:MHC class II on infected macrophage or other APC	Peptide:MHC class II on antigen-specific B cell
Effector action	Kill infected cells	Activation of infected macrophages	Activation of specific B cell to make antibody

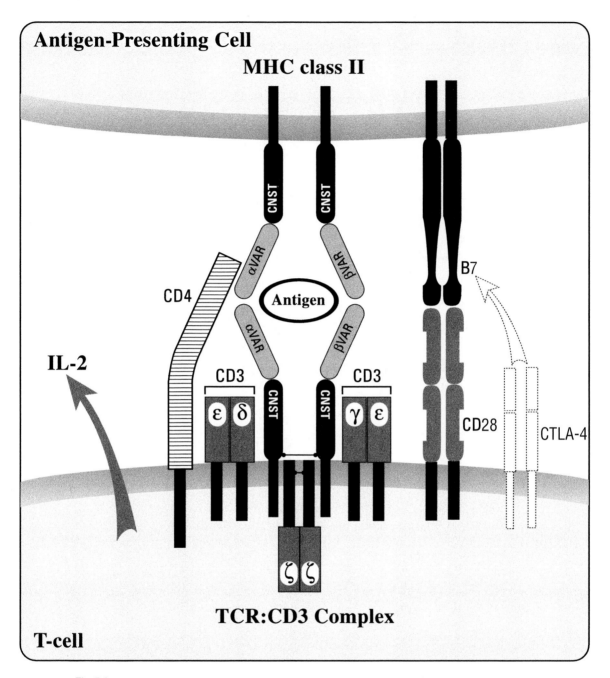

Fig. 5-2 Binding of CD4 T-cell receptor complex to antigen presented through an MHC class II molecule on the surface of an antigen-presenting cell. Antigen presented through a MHC class II molecule on the surface of an antigen-presenting cell is bound by the receptor complex of a T cell of the same antigenic specificity. For T-cell activation to occur, the CD4 coreceptor must bind the T-cell receptor complex, and the B7 molecule on the surface of the antigen-presenting cell must bind its CD28 receptor on the surface of the T cell. As a result, the T cell secretes IL-2, and there is expression of the CTLA-4 receptor that binds the B7 molecule with greater avidity than CD28 does. Binding of the CTLA-4 and B7 molecules generates an inhibitory signal, which suppresses further T-cell activation preventing an uncontrolled T-cell response to an antigen. *(Adapted from Janeway CA et al, editors: Immunobiology: the immune system in health and disease, ed 4, New York, 1999, Current Biology Publications/Garland Publishing.)*

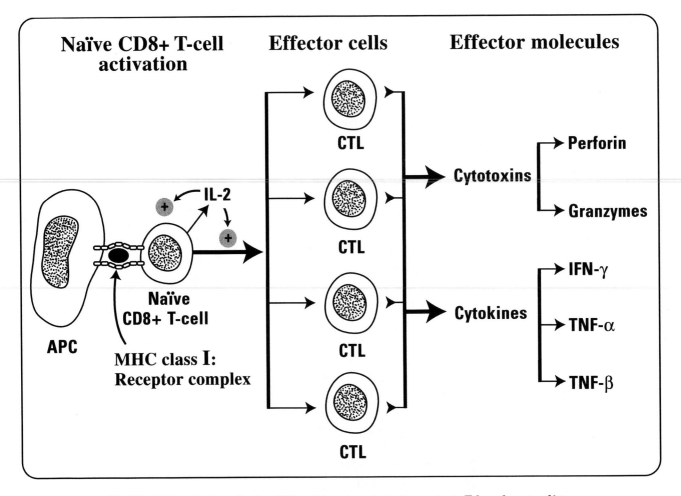

Fig. 5-3 Differentiation of naïve CD8+ T lymphocytes into cytotoxic T lymphocytes. Naïve CD8+ T lymphocytes receptors bind specific antigen complexed to MHC class I molecules on the surface of antigen-presenting cells. Receptor binding stimulates secretion of IL-2 by T lymphocytes, which acts in an autocrine and paracrine manner to stimulate proliferation and differentiation of CD8 T lymphocytes into effector cytotoxic T lymphocytes (CTL). Cytotoxic T lymphocyte effector functions are modulated by cytotoxins and cytokines.

naïve CD4 T cells to differentiate into one subclass tends to preclude differentiation of the other subclass because the cytokines produced by one subclass are inhibitory to the other subclass. The two factors that most influence the subclass differentiation of CD4 T cells are the *type of antigen* (see Table 5-1) encountered by the naïve CD4 T cells and the *cytokine environment* in which the stimulated CD4 T cells undergo differentiation. Pathogens such as *Mycobacterium* and *Leishmania* species are phagocytized by APC and localize in *intracellular vesicles,* where they grow and multiply. Antigenic peptides derived from these microorganisms are presented on the surface of APC complexed to MHC class II molecules. Naïve CD4 T cells recognizing these antigen:MHC complexes differentiate into T$_H$1 cells,

which promote cell-mediated immunity by stimulating activation of macrophages and the production of opsonizing IgG antibodies from B cells. Other pathogens, such as staphylococcal and streptococcal bacteria, which grow in the extracellular fluids, plus bacterial toxins, are taken into APC by endocytosis and localize in endocytotic vesicles, where they are degraded yielding antigenic peptides that bind to MHC class II molecules for presentation on the cell surface. Naïve CD4 T cells that recognize these antigen:MHC complexes differentiate into T$_H$2 cells, which promote activation of B cells and the production of neutralizing antibody and IgE, the initiator of immediate hypersensitivity. The other factor influencing the subclass differentiation pathway of naïve CD4 T cells is the cytokine environment in which

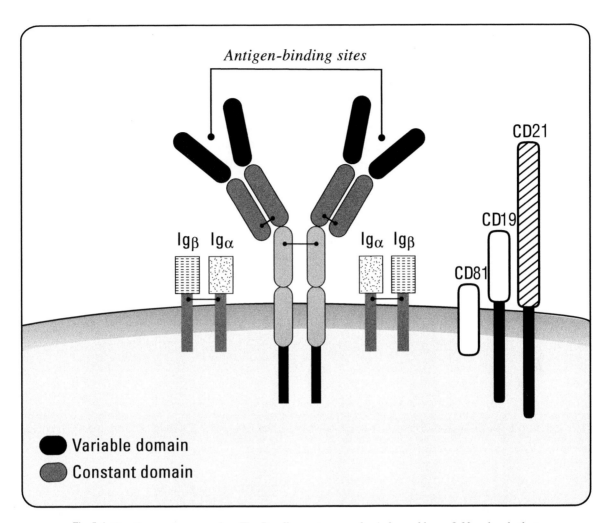

Fig. 5-4 B-cell receptor complex. The B-cell receptor complex is formed by an IgM molecule that binds antigen and two pairs of accessory proteins, Igα and Igβ, required for B-cell activation. A surface complex of 3 protein molecules, CD19, CD21 (complement receptor 2), and CD 81 (TAPA-1) colligates with the B-cell receptor complex to enhance the B-cell response to antigenic stimulation. *(Adapted from Janeway CA et al, editors: Immunobiology: the immune system in health and disease, ed 4, New York, 1999, Current Biology Publications/Garland Publishing.)*

differentiation occurs. During the early stages of viral or intracellular bacterial infections, dendritic cells, macrophages, and natural killer (NK) cells are stimulated to produce IL-12 and IFN-γ. IL-12 is a potent inducer of T_H1 cells, and IFN-γ, is an inhibitor of T_H2 cells. Thus the presence of both cytokines in the extracellular environment promotes T_H1 differentiation and inhibition of T_H2 differentiation. Additionally, newly formed T_H1 cells secrete IFN-γ, further promoting T_H1 subclass differentiation. By contrast, the activation of naïve CD4 T cells in the presence of IL-4 and IL-6 promotes T_H2 subclass differentiation and inhibition of T_H1 differentiation. Similar to T_H1 cells, newly formed T_H2 cells secrete a variety of cytokines including IL-4 and IL-

10, which promote additional T_H2 subclass differentiation and inhibition of T_H1 differentiation.

B Lymphocytes

B lymphocytes are the effector cells of the humoral immune response that terminally differentiate into antibody-producing plasma cells. B-cell development occurs primarily in the bone marrow where there is formed a receptor complex that includes IgM and two accessory proteins (Fig. 5-4). The antigen-binding part of the receptor complex is IgM, which provides the antigenic specificity of the receptor complex. Rearrangement of immunoglobulin heavy- and light-chain gene segments during B-cell development results in a genetically diverse population of B cells that have the potential to recognize 10^{11} or more different antigens. Antigen binding to surface IgM is not sufficient to activate B cells. Similar to the requirements for T-cell activation, activation of B cells requires the assistance of two accessory proteins, Igα and Igβ, which are associated in pairs with the heavy chains of the IgM molecule. These accessory proteins contribute to B-cell activation by stimulating surface expression of B-cell receptors and the initiation of intracellular signaling. The sensitivity of the B-cell response to antigenic stimulation is greatly enhanced by the presence of a B-cell surface complex of three protein molecules, CD19, CD21 (complement receptor 2), and CD81, that colligates with antigen and the B-cell receptor.

Naïve B cells leaving the bone marrow or just arriving in the peripheral lymphoid organs, express only IgM but are capable of binding antigens. However, antigen binding by these cells is a fatal mistake because many become inactivated and are lost whereas others become nonresponsive to additional antigenic stimulation or anergic. The positive aspect to the loss or paralysis of immature B cells is that many of the affected cells reacted to self-antigens. Depletion of immature B lymphocytes that react to self-antigens is an important part of an animal's development of tolerance to self. B cells further mature in peripheral lymphoid tissues, expressing IgD, in addition to IgM, on the cell surfaces.

The activation and differentiation of naïve B cells into antibody-producing cells usually requires the assistance of helper T cells but may occur by direct interaction with bacterial products, without the assistance of helper T cells. When the antigen activating naïve B cells is of protein origin, helper T-cell assistance is required. After receptor binding of a protein antigen, signaling within the B cell initiates receptor-mediated endocytosis of the antigen. The antigen is degraded intracellularly and antigenic peptides are presented on the B-cell surface by MHC class II molecules. Helper T cells with the same antigenic specificity as the B cells bind the antigen:MHC complex and are activated to express surface CD40 ligand molecules, which bind CD40 transmembrane proteins on B cells stimulating B-cell activation. In addition, the activated helper T cells secrete IL-4 locally in the region of contact with the B cell, further promoting B-cell activation. Initially, activated B cells proliferate and later differentiate into antibody-secreting cells or become memory cells. Antigens that require the assistance of helper T cells to activate naïve B cells are called *thymus dependent* because they do not stimulate antibody responses in animals unable to produce T cells because of the absence of the thymus.

Naïve B cells can be directly activated by some bacterial products, especially polysaccharide and lipopolysaccharide components of bacteria, without the assistance of helper T cells. Because T cells are not required for B-cell activation by these antigens and they may activate B cells in animals that do not have a thymus, these antigens are called *thymus-independent* antigens. The ability of selected B cells to respond to some bacterial pathogens, without the need for helper T-cell assistance, provides a rapid, specific defense mechanism against dangerous agents. However, the antibodies produced in response to direct activation by bacterial products are not so versatile as those produced by B cells activated with the assistance of helper T cells. In helper T cell–assisted activation of B cells, binding of the T-cell CD40 ligand to the B-cell CD 40 receptor promotes B cells switching from production of IgM to the production of IgA, IgG, or IgE antibodies *(isotype switching)* and the formation of antibodies with enhanced antigen affinity. In contrast, bacterial antigens that directly activate B cells stimulate limited isotype switching, cause diminished antibody-affinity maturation, and do not induce memory B cells.

Natural Killer Cells

Natural killer (NK) cells are large lymphoid cells with prominent intracytoplasmic granules providing the basis for these cells. Also being called *large granular lymphocytes*, NK cells are a key component of the innate or early nonspecific immune response to pathogens, being capable of reacting to an antigenic insult within hours in comparison to the specific immune response requiring days. NK cells destroy target cells by releasing the contents of their intracytoplasmic granules, which includes a membrane pore-forming molecule, *perforin*, and a group of serine proteases known as *granzymes*. NK cells are less numerous than T and B cells and are distinguished from other lymphoid cells by the presence of CD56 and CD16 (FcγRIII) surface molecules. They do not express antigen-specific T-cell receptor/CD3 complexes or immunoglobulin molecules on their surfaces but do express a variety of non–antigen specific activating and inhibitory receptors. The *activating receptors* that trigger killing by NK cells are poorly characterized but include C-type lectins, which recognize a wide variety of carbohydrate ligands found on many cells. NK cells also have *inhibitory receptors* that are biochemically different from T- and B-cell antigen-specific receptors but, like T- and B-cell receptors, bind MHC class I molecules present on all nucleated cells. Binding of these inhibitory receptors to MHC class I molecules prevents activation of NK cells and the destruction of normal self-cells, thereby protecting the healthy host from NK-cell attack. However, tumor or virus-infected cells are vulnerable to NK-cell attack because they do not express MHC class I molecules or express diminished numbers or structurally altered MHC class I molecules. As a result, these cells are unable to bind NK-cell inhibitory receptors and will be destroyed when bound by NK cell–activating receptors. A similar fate awaits any nucleated cell that fails to express MHC class I molecules. NK cells are also capable of killing antibody-coated cells. The CD16 surface molecule, or FcγRIII, which helps distinguish NK cells from other lymphoid cells, also is a receptor for IgG. Virus-infected cells and tumor cells express viral and tumor antigens on their surfaces that may bind IgG antibodies specific to these antigens. The FcγRIII receptor of NK cells recognizes and binds these antibody-coated cells, activating the NK cells to release their potent intracellular enzymes causing cell death. NK-cell destruction of such antibody-coated cells is called *antibody-dependent cell-mediated cytotoxicity* (ADCC).

NK cells secrete several cytokines including IFN-γ, TNF-α, and granulocyte/macrophage colony–stimulating factor. They are also sensitive to other cytokines that may be released at sites of tissue injury or infection. Included among these are IFN-α, IFN-β, and IL-12, which can increase NK-cell activity up to a hundredfold. In addition, IFN-α can synergize with IL-12 to stimulate the production of large amounts of IFN-γ from NK cells, which promotes macrophage activation and the preferential differentiation of T_H1 cells from naïve CD4 cells, thereby supporting both the innate and specific immune responses.

Macrophages

Macrophages are a phenotypically diverse population of cells that arise from myeloid progenitor cells in the bone marrow. Populations of macrophages constantly present in tissues as resident cells constitute the *mononuclear phagocytic system*. These include Kupffer cells, microglia, alveolar macrophages, Langerhans' cells, and osteoclasts, plus macrophages located in the red and white pulp and marginal zones of the spleen, the subcapsular and medullary sinuses of lymph nodes, and the lamina propria of Peyer's patches. In addition, inflammatory and immune stimuli may attract monocytes from the blood vascular system into tissues where they terminally differentiate into macrophages.

Macrophages are functionally multidimensional cells that express a variety of surface receptors and secrete a variety of cytokines and chemokines. They make important contributions to host defenses by participating in both the innate and adaptive immune responses and also may function as antigen-presenting cells. Macrophages provide a first line of defense against many invading microorganisms by nonspecially binding, phagocytizing, and destroying them. Participation in the nonspecific, innate response to infection is facilitated by nonopsonizing and opsonizing surface receptors present on macrophages. Nonopsonizing macrophage receptors, including complement receptor type 3 (CR3), lectins (mannose receptor), and class A scavenger receptor (SR-A), may bind one of the poorly defined ligands ubiquitous on the surface of many microorganisms. Microorganisms or other pathogens that become coated or opsonized by antibody or complement also may be bound by macrophage CR3 or Fc receptors. Many bacteria that are nonspecifically bound by macrophages are readily killed after being engulfed, thereby preventing disease and eliminating the need for an adaptive immune response. However, other ingested bacteria, including *Mycobacterium* and *Listeria* species, localize in intracellular lysosomes or endosomes of macrophages and persist, stimulating the macrophage to assume a new role as a professional (functional) antigen-presenting cell. As antigen-presenting cells, macrophages are able to present antigenic peptides on cell surfaces through either MHC class I or MHC class II molecules. The class of MHC molecule involved in antigen presentation is determined by the offending pathogen. Antigenic peptides released from bacteria that persist in intracytoplasmic vesicles of macrophages are bound and presented by MCH class II molecules, whereas antigenic peptides released from viruses and bacteria that localize in the cytosol of macrophages are bound and presented by MHC class I molecules.

In addition to functioning as APC, macrophages may function as effector cells in certain forms of cell-mediated and humoral immune responses. As has been previously discussed, naïve CD4 T cells that recognize antigens presented by MHC class II molecules on the surface of macrophages may differentiate into either T_H1 or T_H2 cells. T_H1 cells secrete chemokines and cytokines, which attract and activate macrophages. Macrophages attracted by T_H1-cell products function as effector cells by releasing inflammatory mediators that promote a delayed-type hypersensitivity response. Macrophages presenting antigens through MHC class I molecules stimulate the differentiation of naïve CD4 T cells into T_H2 cells, which promote activation of B cells and antibody production. Another effector function of macrophages in humoral immunity is the binding, phagocytosis, and killing of bacteria or other pathogens opsonized by antibody secreted from activated B cells.

Dendritic Cells

Antigen presentation through MHC class I or II molecules is essential for the development of humoral and cellular immune responses and one of the primary functions of macrophages, B lymphocytes, and *dendritic cells* (DCs). Macrophages and B cells have many other functions besides that of antigen presentation, whereas the only known function of DCs is the presentation of antigens to T cells. Similar to but independent of macrophages and lymphocytes, DCs originate from either myeloid or lymphoid progenitor cells in the bone marrow and migrate through the blood to peripheral, nonlymphoid tissues (Table 5-2). The primary function of immature DCs in tissues is antigen capture, which stimulates DC migration to T-cell areas of peripheral and mucosal lymphoid tissues. As DCs migrate to lymphoid tissues, they mature and gain the ability to present antigens through either MHC class I or MHC class II molecules. Additionally, they express high levels of B7 costimulatory molecules and become potent stimulators of naïve T cells. The dendritic cells abundantly present in the T-cell areas of lymphoid tissues are called *interdigitating dendritic cells*. Interdigitating DCs share many antigenic markers with other DCs and are believed to be composed of a subpopulation of DCs that have migrated from peripheral tissues to stimulate T-cell immunity and a resident subpopulation of DCs that are more involved in immune regulation and peripheral tolerance. Another population of DC is found in primary lymphoid follicles of lymph nodes and are called *follicular dendritic cells* (FDC). However, other than some morphological resemblance to interdigitating DCs, follicular DCs and interdigitating DCs have little in common. The exact origin and function of FDCs is unclear. Unlike bone marrow–derived DC, follicular DCs are believed to be of stromal origin, possibly of fibroblast lineage. Follicular DCs do not express MHC class II molecules but do express complement receptors and the Fc receptor for immunoglobulin. They provide signals essential for the survival and continued recirculation of naïve B cells and have a significant effect on the maturation of B-cell immunity by binding intact antigens on their surfaces for long periods of time.

Dendritic cells have two main functions that develop sequentially. First, immature DCs capture and process antigens in peripheral tissue sites, and this process stimulates DC maturation and migration to lymphoid tissues for antigen presentation and the expression of numerous membrane-bound glycoproteins that mediate T-cell binding and activation. Immature DCs that have captured and begun processing antigen lose their phagocytic capabilities and assume a new phenotype focused on T-cell activation. Immature DCs, such as *Langerhans' cells* of the skin and *interstitial DCs* of the heart and kid-

---

TABLE 5-2   **Dendritic System of Antigen-presenting Cells**

DENDRITIC CELLS (DC)	ORIGIN	DEVELOPMENT STAGE	TISSUE LOCATION OF DCs
Langerhans' cells	Bone marrow	Immature	Epidermis of skin and other stratified squamous epithelial tissues including vagina, cervix, anus, pharynx, and esophagus
Interstitial DC	Bone marrow	Immature	Heart, kidney, but not in brain
Veiled cells	Bone marrow	Immature	Afferent lymphatics; blood
Other DC	Bone marrow	Immature	Epithelial lining of respiratory tract, intestine, iris and ciliary body; subepithelial region of mucosal lymphoid tissues
Interdigitating DC	Bone marrow	Mature	T-cell areas of lymph nodes; thymic medulla
Follicular DC	Stroma (?Fibroblast)	Mature	B-cell areas of lymph node follicles

ney, are actively phagocytic by means of receptors such as DEC 205 and nonspecifically by macropinocytosis, a process of engulfment of large volumes of extracellular fluid. Processing of captured antigen for presentation complexed to either MHC class I or II molecules begins as the immature DCs begin migration to lymphoid tissues. Within the T-cell areas of lymphoid tissues, the now-mature DCs express high levels of antigen-complexed MHC class I and II molecules for prolonged periods. In addition, mature DCs express high levels of costimulatory B7 molecules and adhesion molecules ICAM-1, ICAM-2, LFA-1, and LFA-2 and secrete high levels of IL-12 and the chemokine T-cell chemotactic substance called "DC-CK."

Cytokines

When naïve T cells first encounter specific antigen bound to the surface of APC, they are stimulated to secrete a low-molecular-weight, soluble protein, interleukin (IL)-2, that promotes T-cell proliferation and differentiation into activated effector cells. IL-2 is a member of a large group of biologically active, small to medium-sized proteins and glycoproteins that are potent mediators of numerous physiological processes. These substances are called *cytokines* and include interleukins, interferons, monokines, chemokines, and certain growth factors (Table 5-3). Cytokines act on target cells that express surface receptors specific for one or more types of cytokines. Any given cytokine may be produced by more than one cell type and may be *pleiotropic,* having multiple effects on a variety of cell types. Cytokines generally function in a local microenvironment affecting the same cells secreting the cytokine (*autocrine* effect) or other cell types (*paracrine* effect). Some cytokines also behave in an *endocrine* manner affecting target cells in distant locations (for example, IL-1, IL-6, and TNF-α produced by macrophages stimulate the hypothalamus to elevate body temperature and liver cells to release acute-phase proteins as a part of the acute inflammatory response).

Naïve CD8 T cells stimulated by peptide:MHC class I complexes differentiate into cytotoxic T cells under the influence of IL-2. As previously described, cytotoxic T cells release cytotoxins and synthesize and secrete IFN-γ, TNF-α, and TNF-β. IFN-γ directly inhibits viral replication, activates macrophages, and stimulates the increased expression of MHC class I molecules. TNF-γ and TNF-β assist in macrophage activation by sensitizing macrophages to the activating stimulus of IFN-γ.

CD4 T-cell differentiation is more complex with the potential for naïve cells to evolve through intermediary immature T_H0 cells into either T_H1 cells, mediating cellular immune type 1 responses, or T_H2 cells, promoting type 2 humoral immune responses (Fig. 5-5). Type1 and type 2 responses are not mutually exclusive but usually occur simultaneously. Dominance of one type of response over the other is probably dependent, to a large extent, on the balance of cytokines in the microenvironment. Immune responses to facultative intracellular bacterial and protozoan infections are characterized by T_H1-cell differentiation. During early stages of infection with one of these infectious organisms, dendritic cells, macrophages, and NK cells secrete IFN-γ, IL-12, and IL-18, promoting T_H0-cell differentiation into T_H1 cells. Under the influence of IL-18, newly differentiated T_H1 cells produce high levels of IFN-γ, which further promotes differentiation of T_H0 cells into T_H1 cells while preventing the activation of T_H2 cells.

T_H2-cell differentiation is more characteristic of immune responses to extracellular bacteria, toxins, and other pathogens. During such infections, the local microenvironment is dominated by the secretion of IL-4, IL-6, and IL-10 from T_H2 cells or subsets of these cells. Both IL-4 and IL-6 promote T_H2 differentiation, whereas IL-4 and IL-10 inhibit T_H1-cell differentiation. The T_H1 inhibitory effect of IL-10 results from its negative effect on cytokine production by macrophages.

In type 1 responses, *effector T_H1 cells* promote the activation of macrophages and the recruitment of additional macrophages to tissue injury sites. The process of macrophage activation begins with the binding of CD40 ligand expressed on the surface of T_H1 cells to CD40 receptors on macrophages. This results in the sensitization of macrophages to activation by IFN-γ, which is secreted by effector T_H1 cells. In addition, effector T_H1 cells secrete the hematopoietic growth factors IL-3 and GM-CSF, which stimulate bone marrow production of additional macrophage precursor cells. T_H1 cells also secrete TNF-α and TNF-β, which increase the adhesiveness of endothelial cells for macrophages, thereby promoting additional macrophage accumulation in infected tissues. Once activated, macrophages may secrete a variety of cytokines including IL-1, IL-6, IL-8, IL-12, and TNF-α.

Activation and differentiation of B cells into antibody-producing cells is primarily a function of effector T_H2 cells, though a subset of T_H1 cells that may also assist in B-cell activation has been identified. Binding of effector T_H2 cells to peptide:MHC

TABLE 5-3 **Cytokines with Immunological Functions**—Selected cytokines and their immunologically related functions are included in the table. Many of these cytokines have other functions and there are many other cytokines not listed.

STRUCTURAL FAMILY	CYTOKINE	CELL SOURCES	ACTION
Hematopoietins	IL-2	T_H1 and T_H0 lymphocytes	T-cell proliferation, B-cell proliferation, NK-cell activation
	IL-3	T_H1, T_H2, and some cytotoxic lymphocytes	Stimulation of growth and differentiation of myelomonocytic progenitors
	IL-4	T_H2 lymphocytes, mast cells, eosinophils, basophils	B-cell proliferation and differentiation, B-cell isotype switching to IgG1 and IgE, promotion of T_H2-cell differentiation, inhibition of T_H1-cell differentiation, inhibition of macrophage activation
	IL-5	T_H2 lymphocytes, mast cells, eosinophils	B-cell differentiation, promotion of IgA secretion, eosinophil activation and growth, basophil activation
	IL-6	T_H2 lymphocytes, macrophages, fibroblasts, endothelial cells	T and B-cell growth and differentiation, stimulation of hematopoiesis, acute-phase protein production, fever
	GM-CSF	T cells, macrophages, fibroblasts, endothelium	Stimulates growth and differentiation of myelomonocytic progenitors
Interferons	IFN-γ	T_H1 and cytotoxic lymphocytes, NK cells	Macrophage activation and increased MHC expression, B-cell isotype switching to IgG2a and IgG3, inhibition of T_H2 lymphocytes, NK-cell activation
Tumor necrosis factors	TNF-α (cachectin)	Macrophages, NK cells, T lymphocytes	Tumor cytotoxicity; activities against viruses, bacteria, and parasites; acute-phase protein production; fever
	TNF-β (lymphotoxin)	T and B lymphocytes	Macrophage and neutrophil activation, B-cell inhibition, tumor and T-cell cytotoxicity
Unclassified	TGF-β	Most cells including T and B lymphocytes, macrophages, platelets, mesenchymal cells	B-cell isotype switching to IgG2 and IgA, immunosuppression, promotion of wound repair, inhibition of cell growth, tumor suppression, antiinflammatory
	IL-1	Monocytes and macrophages	Induction of cytokine production in many cell types, T-cell and macrophage activation, acute-phase protein production, fever
	IL-10	Activated T cells, B cells and macrophages	Potent inhibitor of proinflammatory cytokine secretion by macrophages, inhibition of MHC class II expression, inhibition of T_H1-cell differentiation
	IL-12	Monocytes, macrophages, and B lymphocytes	Activation of NK cells, promotion of development of T_H1 over T_H2 cells
	IL-18	Activated macrophages, epithelial cells	Stimulation of IFN-γ production by T cells and NK cells, promotion of T_H1 induction

GM-CSF, Granulocyte-macrophage colony-stimulating factor; *IL*, interleukin; *TGF*, transforming growth factor.

complexes located on the surface of B cells causes T_H2 cells to express CD40 ligand and secrete IL-4, which together induce B-cell proliferation. IL-5 and IL-6, also secreted by T_H2 cells, synergize with IL-4 to promote differentiation of proliferating B cells into antibody-producing cells or plasma cells. Initially, activated B cells produce IgM but are induced to switch production to different antibody isotypes under the influence of certain cytokines (Table 5-4). The cytokines promoting isotype switching inhibit

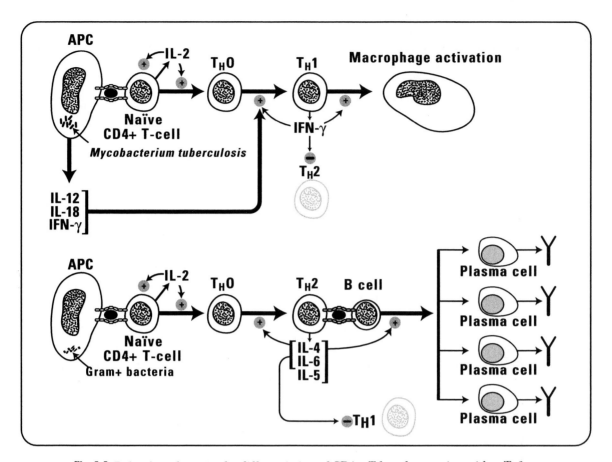

Fig. 5-5 Role of cytokines in the differentiation of CD4+ T lymphocytes into either T$_H$1 or T$_H$2 lymphocytes. Naïve CD4+ T lymphocyte receptors bind specific antigen complexed to MHC class II molecules on the surface of antigen-presenting cells. Receptor binding stimulates secretion of IL-2 from CD4+ T cells, which induces formation of T$_H$0 lymphocytes, which have the potential to differentiate into either T$_H$1 or T$_H$2 lymphocytes. The route of differentiation depends on cytokine stimulation. **T$_H$1 differentiation:** During mycobacterial infection, bacteria-stimulated macrophages secrete IL-12, IL-18, and IFN-γ, which promote differentiation of T$_H$0 lymphocytes to T$_H$1 lymphocytes. T$_H$1 lymphocytes secrete IFN-γ, which further promotes differentiation of T$_H$0 lymphocytes into T$_H$1 lymphocytes and inhibits the differentiation of T$_H$0 cells into T$_H$2 cells. The primary function of T$_H$1 cells is the activation of macrophages through the expression of the CD40 ligand and the secretion of IFN-γ. **T$_H$2 differentiation:** Toxins or gram-positive bacterial infections stimulate the preferential differentiation of T$_H$0 cells into T$_H$2 cells under the influence of IL-4. T$_H$2 cells produce IL-4, IL-5, and IL-6. The IL-4 and IL-6 further promote the differentiation of T$_H$0 cells into T$_H$2 cells. IL-4 also has an inhibitory effect on the differentiation of T$_H$0 cells into T$_H$1 cells. If T$_H$2 cells bind specific antigen complexed to MHC class II molecules on the surface of B cells, B cells are stimulated to become antibody-producing cells as a result of CD40 receptor ligation and the secretion of IL-4, IL-5, and IL-6 by T$_H$2 cells.

further production of IgM and inhibit production of other antibody isotypes.

Chemokines

Chemokines are a cytokine family of small, related proteins found in mammals, birds, and fish that are produced by leukocytes and a variety of other cell types (Table 5-5). All chemokines are secreted except for fractalkine, which is expressed in a membrane-bound form. Chemokines function primarily in inflammatory sites as chemoattractants for granulocytes, monocytes, immature dendritic cells, and activated T cells. The repertoire of cytokines released in an inflammatory site varies according to the causative agent and the type of tissue injured. As a result, the chemokines secreted are most likely to attract a subset of effector cells that will be most

TABLE 5-4 **Cytokine-induced Isotype Switching**—Cytokines produced by T_H2 and T_H1 cells inhibit further IgM production by B cells and promote switching to production of different antibody isotypes.

CYTOKINE	SOURCE	ISOTYPE SWITCHING
IL-4	T_H2 cells	IgM → IgG1 and IgE
TGF-β	T_H2 cells	IgM → IgG2 and IgA
IFN-γ	T_H1 cells	IgM → IgG2a and IgG3
IL-5	T_H2 cells	IgA secretion by IgA-producing cells

effective against a particular pathogen or type of tissue damaged. Chemokines, such as IL-8 and eotaxin, also activate neutrophils and eosinophils, respectively, to produce oxygen radicals and nitric oxide and to release enzymes from intracytoplasmic granules. Another important role for chemokines in immunoregulation has begun to emerge. Chemokines such as SLC (secondary lymphoid tissue chemokine), BLC (B-lymphocyte chemoattractant), MIP-3β, RANTES, IP-10, and TARC (thymus and activation-regulated cytokine) are constitutively expressed in primary and secondary lymphoid tissues. Evidence is accumulating to indicate that these chemokines form chemoattractant gradients required for the normal homeostatic trafficking of T and B cells in lymphoid tissues and in the trafficking of dendritic, T, and B cells that occurs in response to antigenic stimulation. Chemokines may also have a strong influence on tumor growth and metastasis through their angiogenic and angiostatic properties. Chemokines in the CXC subfamily in which the 3 amino acids preceding the first cysteine residue in the amino terminus are glucine, leucine, and arginine (Glu-Leu-Arg) (see Table 5-5) promote angiogenesis, whereas chemokines in the same subfamily that do not have the Glu-Leu-Arg arrangement of amino acids before the first cysteine promote angiostasis. Thus the balance of chemokines in a tumor that promote angiogenesis and angiostasis may be very important in determining the extent of tumor growth and its potential for metastasis. Similarly, angiogenic chemokines contribute to the healing process by promoting angiogenesis in granulation tissue.

Chemokines are subdivided into two major (CC, CXC) and two minor (C, CX3C) subfamilies according to the number and spacing of the two cysteine residues in the amino terminal region of the molecules (see Table 5-5). In the CC subfamily, the first two cysteine residues are adjacent to each other without an intervening amino acid. These cytokines promote migration of monocytes and other cell types and include *RANTES, MCP-1, MIP-1α,* and *eotaxin.* The CXC subfamily has an amino acid separating the first two cysteine residues and includes the prototype chemokine, *IL-8,* which is a potent attractant of neutrophils, plus *GRO-α, -β, -γ* and *NAP-2, ENA-78, IP-10,* and *SDF-1.* The two minor subfamilies include only one chemokine in each. The CXXXC (CX3C) subfamily is characterized by three amino acids intervening between the two N-terminal cysteine residues. *Fractalkine,* the only CX3C chemokine, is unique in that it is not secreted but rather is a large membrane-bound glycoprotein that mediates chemotaxis and firm adhesion of T cells, monocytes, and NK cells. The C subfamily of chemokines is missing the first N-terminal cysteine residue and is represented by *lymphotactin,* which is chemotactic for NK and T cells and possibly promotes epithelial integrity in mucosal immune responses.

Chemokines interact with target cells through one or more specific receptors expressed on target cell surfaces. Leukocytes are common targets for chemokines expressing one to numerous receptor types. Other cells also may express chemokine receptors, including epithelium, endothelium, neurons, astrocytes, and microglia. Chemokine receptors are a member of the seven–transmembrane domain G protein–coupled receptor family and consist of an extracellular N-terminus, three extracellular loops, three intracellular loops, and an intracellular C-terminus (Fig. 5-6). Similar to chemokines, the chemokine receptors are divided into four groups (CR, CCR, CXCR, CX3CR) based on the primary amino acid structure of the receptor (see Table 5-5).

Target cells may constitutively express functional receptors, or target cells may need activation before receptors become functional. For example, circulating or recently isolated neutrophils and eosinophils constitutively express functional chemokine receptors allowing them to vigorously respond immediately to chemokines without the need for additional stimulation. In contrast, nonactivated memory T cells express numerous receptor types, but these receptors do not become functional until the memory cells become activated as a result of interaction with specific antigen.

The N-terminus of chemokines binds to target cell receptors, whereas the carboxy (C)-terminus has a strong affinity for glycosaminoglycans and other negatively charged sugar moieties and, as a result, may bind endothelial cell surfaces and extracellular matrix glycoproteins found in connective tissues creating a fixed chemokine gradient. Thus, within an inflammatory site, the chemokine gradients that promote intravascular and extravascular

TABLE 5-5 Properties of Selected Chemokines

SUBFAMILY (N-TERMINUS)		CHEMOKINE	PRIMARY CHEMOKINE SOURCE	PRIMARY CHEMOKINE ACTION	CHEMOKINE RECEPTOR
CC (NH₂—CC—)		RANTES	T cells, endothelial cells, platelets	Attracts and activates T cells, NK cells, monocytes, eosinophils, and basophils	CCR1, 3, 4, 5, 9
		MCP-1	Monocytes and most other nonlymphocytes	Activates macrophages, promotes T_H2 immunity, basophil histamine release	CCR2
		MIP-1α	Monocytes, T cells, fibroblasts, mast cells	Antiviral host defense, promotes T_H1 immunity	CCR1, 3, 5
		Eotaxin	Endothelium, T cells monocytes, epithelium	Attracts eosinophils, monocytes, and T cells; involved in lung allergies	CCR3
CXC (NH₂—CXC—)	ELR⁺	IL-8	Monocytes, fibroblasts epithelial cells, endothelial cells	Attracts neutrophils and naïve T cells; neutrophil activation; angiogenesis	CXCR1, 2
		GRO-α, -β, -γ	Monocytes, fibroblasts, endothelial cells	Attract and activate neutrophils; fibroplasia; angiogenesis	CXCR2
		NAP-2	Platelets	Attracts and activates neutrophils; angiogenesis	CXCR2
		ENA-78	Epithelial cells, fibroblasts, endothelial cells	Attracts and activates neutrophils; angiogenesis	CXCR2
	ELR⁻	IP-10	Monocytes, T cells, keratinocytes	Attracts resting T cells, NK cells, and monocytes; immunostimulant; angiostasis	CXCR3
		SDF-1	Stromal cells	Attracts naïve T cells and B cells; stimulates B-cell development; angiostasis	CXCR4
C (NH₂—C—)		Lymphotactin	CD8 > CD4 T cells	Attracts thymocytes, dendritic cells, and NK cells; lymphocyte trafficking	CR1
CX3C (NH₂—CXXXC—)		Fractalkine	Monocytes, endothelium, microglia	Attracts and causes adhesion of T cells and monocytes to endothelium; brain inflammation	CX3CR1

ENA-78, Epithelial cell–derived neutrophil-activating factor; *IP-10*, interferon-inducible protein-10; *MCP-1*, monocyte chemoattractant protein-1; *MIP-1α*, macrophage inflammatory protein-1α; *NAP-2*, neutrophil-activating peptide-2; *RANTES*, regulated upon activation, normal T expressed and secreted; *SDF-1*, stromal cell–derived factor 1.
ELR⁺, 3 amino acids preceding first cysteine residue of CXC motif are Glu-Leu-Arg, and chemokines are chemotactic for neutrophils and promote angiogenesis.
ELR⁻, 3 amino acids preceding first cysteine residue of CXC motif are not Glu-Leu-Arg, and chemokines are chemotactic for lymphocytes and promote angiostasis.

directional movement of leukocytes are both soluble *(chemotactic)* and bound *(haptotactic)*.

The role of chemokines and receptors in infectious disease has received growing attention since the recognition that strains of human immunodeficiency virus (HIV) use many chemokine receptors as coreceptors to infect human CD4+ lymphocytes. Initially, CXCR4 was identified as a major coreceptor for T cell–tropic strains of HIV-1 and later CCR5 was identified as a major coreceptor for macrophage-tropic strains of HIV. The number of receptors with coreceptor activity for various

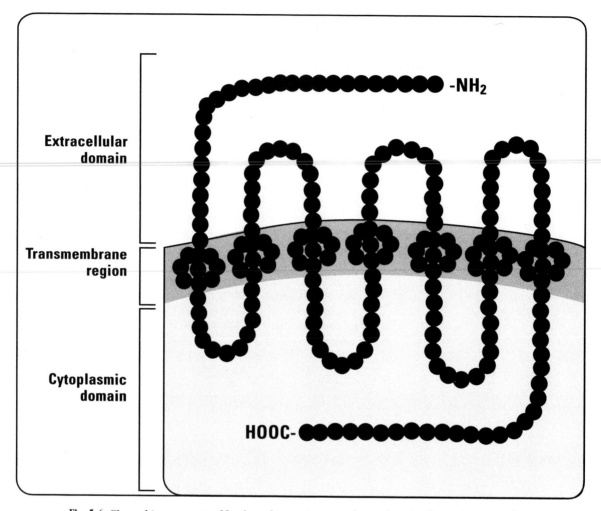

Fig. 5-6 Chemokine receptor. Member of seven-transmembrane domain G-protein—coupled receptor family. Receptor polypeptide composed of extracellular N-terminus, seven membrane hydrophobic domains, three extracellular loops, three intracellular loops, and an intracellular C-terminus. Receptor specificity determined by amino acid composition of receptor polypeptide chain.

strains of HIV-1 has grown to 11. Simian immunodeficiency virus uses several chemokine receptors as coreceptors, whereas feline immunodeficiency virus may use CXCR4 as a coreceptor. Other viruses produce their own chemokine receptors or secrete scavenger proteins capable of binding multiple CC and CXC chemokines.

IMMUNE-MEDIATED TISSUE INJURY

The immunological events that result in immune-mediated tissue injury are essentially the same as those that occur in protective immune responses. When the immune response has deleterious effects, it is termed a *hypersensitivity reaction*. As with all immune responses, hypersensitivity reactions are dependent on prior sensitization of the host with

specific antigen. Antigens that evoke hypersensitivity reactions in some individuals are harmless or cause only protective immune responses in many other individuals. The reasons for this dichotomy in responses to the same antigen by different individuals are still poorly understood but relate to the nature of the antigen, route of delivery, and host predisposition to hypersensitivity responses.

Hypersensitivity disorders are classified into *type I* to *type IV*, based on the classification scheme originally described by Coombs and Gell (Table 5-6). Types I to III are *antibody mediated* and develop rather quickly, whereas type IV is mediated by T cells and macrophages and is a *delayed reaction*. This classification scheme is based on the kinds of antibodies and cells involved. In most forms of naturally occurring immunological disease, however, multiple types of hypersensitivity responses may be

TABLE 5-6   Classification of Hypersensitivity Reactions

REACTION TYPE	IMMUNOLOGIC MEDIATOR	MECHANISM	DISEASE EXAMPLE
Type I	IgE	Mediator release	Anaphylaxis
Type II	IgG, IgM	Cytotoxic	Autoimmune hemolytic anemia
Type III	IgG, IgM	Immune complexes	Glomerulonephritis
Type IV	Sensitized T lymphocytes	Delayed-type hypersensitivity	Tuberculosis

occurring simultaneously in the pathogenesis of tissue injury.

Type I (Immediate) Hypersensitivity

Immediate hypersensitivity reactions occur within seconds to minutes after a previously sensitized individual is reexposed to an antigen. The absorbed antigen crosslinks antigen-specific IgE molecules bound to the surface of tissue mast cells or circulating basophils and eosinophils triggering the release of preformed mediators and stimulating the synthesis and secretion of other mediators. These released and synthesized mediators stimulate acute inflammatory reactions causing the signs and tissue damage associated with hypersensitivity reactions. The tissues most commonly involved in type I hypersensitivity reactions tend to reflect the tissue distribution of mast cells. Since the greatest concentrations of mast cells are in the skin and respiratory and gastrointestinal tracts, these are the most common sites for type I reactions. Examples of type I hypersensitivity include allergic rhinitis, hay fever, bronchial asthma, urticaria, atopy, and anaphylaxis. Of these, allergic rhinitis, caused by environmental antigens *(allergens),* such as ragweed, tree, and grass pollens, is the most common type of immediate hypersensitivity in humans, involving up to 50% of the population in North America and Europe. These are generally mild allergic disorders reasonably amenable to treatment. Less common but more severe type I reactions include bronchial asthma and urticaria, whereas even less common systemic hypersensitivity reactions result in circulatory collapse *(anaphylaxis)* and are life threatening.

Factors Contributing to Type I Hypersensitivity Responses

Like every immune response, type I reactions depend on initial contact of the host with an antigen that induces a primary immune response characterized by the production of IgE. The number of antigens that stimulate allergic responses is comparatively small, but they reproducibly elicit an IgE response in susceptible individuals. Type I reactions are most commonly elicited by delivery of an allergen to a mucosal or cutaneous surface. One of the most common human allergies, allergic rhinitis, is initiated by the deposition on respiratory mucosa of minute quantities of small, highly soluble proteins bound to desiccated particles, such as pollen grains or mite feces. On contact with the mucosa, the soluble allergens are eluted from the delivery particles and diffuse into the mucosa where mucosal DCs capture the allergens. Allergen capture by mucosal DC stimulates activation and migration of the DC to T-cell areas of regional lymph nodes, where they further differentiate and present allergenic peptides through MHC class I molecules. Because of the low dose of allergen delivered to mucosal surfaces, the density of allergenic peptides presented on the surface of dendritic cells complexed to MHC class I molecules is also low, favoring the stimulation of a T_H2 response by DC. One of the cytokines produced by activated T_H2 cells is IL-4, which further promotes T_H2-cell differentiation, B-cell proliferation and activation, and B-cell isotype switching to the production of IgE.

Another factor contributing to immediate hypersensitivity responses is the predisposition of certain individuals to respond to environmental antigens by the production of IgE. Among these individuals, some have exaggerated IgE responses to environmental allergens causing a condition called *atopy.* A genetic basis for atopy is well documented in humans and also believed to occur in animals. For example, atopic dermatitis commonly occurs in Cairn, Scottish, and West Highland white terriers, Dalmatians, and Irish setters. (For other examples of atopy, review Tizard 2000 concerning IgE.)

Role of IgE in Type I Hypersensitivity

IgE produced in response to initial allergen exposure is quickly bound by its Fc fragment to tissue mast cells and circulating basophils and eosinophils resulting in low serum levels of IgE. The circulating half-life of IgE is only about 2 days, whereas the half-life of IgE bound to mast cells, basophils, or eosinophils is 11 to 12 days, a period that helps explain prolonged sensitization, which may occur

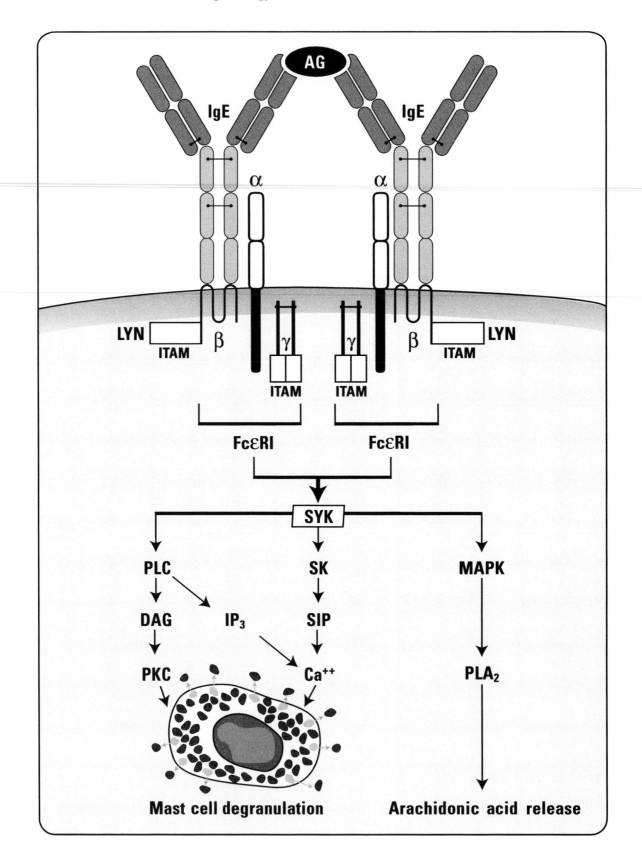

Fig. 5-7 Mast cell activation and degranulation. The FcεRI receptor is a tetrameric protein complex consisting of an IgE-binding α-chain, a single β-chain, and two disulfide-linked γ-chains. IgE molecules are bound to the high-affinity FcεRI receptors by two extracellular Ig-like domains of the α-chain. When two or more IgE molecules are cross-linked by antigen, *AG*, an SRC family kinase *(LYN)*, associated with the β-chain in the inactive receptor, becomes activated resulting in the phosphorylation of tyrosine residues located in immunoreceptor tyrosine-based activation motifs *(ITAM)* on the tails of the β- and γ-chains. Tyrosine phosphorylation promotes binding and activation of other kinases such as SYK. SYK activation stimulates activation of multiple pathways resulting in mast cell degranulation and the release of arachidonic acid. Phospholipase C *(PLC)* activation results in the generation of diacylglycerol *(DAG)* and inositol 1,4,5-triphosphate *(IP₃)*. DAG activates protein kinase C *(PKC)*, which in the presence of increased calcium causes mast cell degranulation. IP$_3$ may promote a transient release of calcium, but the principal pathway of calcium mobilization is through the activation of sphingosine kinase *(SK)*, resulting in the generation of the calcium second messenger, sphingosine-1-phosphate *(SIP)*. SYK also activates mitogen-activated protein kinase *(MAPK)*, which, in turn, activates phospholipase A$_2$ *(PLA₂)*, causing the release of arachidonic acid from cell membrane phospholipids. *(Adapted from Sánchez-Mejorada G, Rosales C: J Leukoc Biol 63:521-533, 1998.)*

after an initial exposure to an allergen. The Fc fragment of IgE preferentially binds high-affinity receptors (FcεRI) expressed on mast cells, basophils, and activated eosinophils without the need for accompanying bound antigen required by other antibodies for receptor binding. IgE may also bind low-affinity receptors (FcεRII or CD23) expressed on mast cells. The high-affinity FcεRI receptor is a member of the immunoglobulin superfamily, whereas unrelated CD23 is a selectin that is the only known antibody receptor not belonging to the immunoglobulin superfamily. Besides being expressed on mast cells, CD23 is also expressed on many other cell types, including B cells, activated T cells, monocytes, eosinophils, platelets, and follicular dendritic cells. The significance of IgE binding to CD23 in type I hypersensitivity is still not clear. The more important role of CD23 may be binding IgE- producing B cells to follicular dendritic cells, thereby preventing B-cell destruction by apoptosis and allowing their differentiation into IgE-secreting plasma cells.

Activation of Mast Cells and Mechanisms of Mediator Release

IgE binding to high-affinity FcεRI receptors occurs primarily on mast cells but also occurs to a lesser degree on circulating basophils and eosinophils that have been activated. Mast cells are derived from the bone marrow but originate from a different myeloid lineage than basophils and eosinophils do. They are widely distributed in tissues, with most being located near blood vessels and nerves in subepithelial sites where type I reactions are most likely to occur. Acti-

vation of mast cells in immediate-type hypersensitivity is initiated by the interaction of a multivalent antigen (allergen) with antigen-specific IgE bound to mast cell surfaces by means of high-affinity FcεRI receptors. Maximum histamine release occurs when 10% or more of the receptors are aggregated. The FcεRI receptor is a member of the immunoglobulin gene superfamily and is a tetrameric protein complex, consisting of the IgE-binding α-chain, a single β-chain, and two disulfide-linked γ-chains (Fig. 5-7). The α-chain has two extracellular Ig-like domains, and all chains have transmembrane domains plus cytoplasmic tails. Located in the cytoplasmic tail of both the β- and γ-chains is an immunoreceptor tyrosine-based activation motif (ITAM) that contains several tyrosine residues. Receptor aggregation causes activation of an Src family kinase (Lyn), which is associated with the β-chain in the inactive receptor, and phosphorylation of tyrosine residues located in β- and γ-chain ITAMs. The phosphorylated tyrosines serve as binding sites for other kinases, such as SYK. After SYK activation, multiple activation pathways contribute to mast cell degranulation and the generation of arachidonic acid. Phospholipase A2 activation and the release of arachidonic acid from cell membrane phospholipids are dependent on SYK-linked activation of mitogen-activated protein kinase (MAPK). SYK activation is also associated with activation of phospholipase C, which acts on the substrate phosphatidylinositol 4,5-biphosphate to form the second messengers inositol 1,4,5-triphosphate (IP$_3$) and diacylglycerol (DAG). IP$_3$ has long been believed to be the principal mediator of calcium mobilization after FcεRI aggregation. Although IP_3 may mediate a transient release of calcium after receptor aggregation, apparently the principal pathway of calcium mobilization is through SYK-induced activation of sphingosine kinase that results in the production of the calcium second messenger sphingosine-1-phosphate. DAG activates protein kinase C that in the presence of increased calcium promotes mast cell degranulation. Ultrastructurally, mast cell granules swell and fuse. The fused granules form tortuous cytoplasmic canalicular channels that fuse with the plasma membrane and open to the cell surface to permit the explosive release of mediators.

Mediators Released from Mast Cells

After activation of mast cells, there is a release of preformed mediators and the synthesis of additional mediators (Table 5-7) that are responsible for the inflammatory events characteristic of a type I hypersensitivity response. The immediate phase of type I hypersensitivity is characterized by dilatation and increased permeability of small blood vessels,

smooth muscle contraction, and increased secretion by nasal, bronchial, and gastric glands. These acute inflammatory events are primarily mediated by the biogenic amine *histamine,* which is present in high concentration in mast cells (see Chapter 4). Another amine that may contribute to the early inflammatory events of the type I response is *serotonin* (5-hydroxytryptamine), which is derived from the amino acid tryptophan and released from mast cell granules in rodents and cattle. Serotonin causes vasoconstriction and smooth muscle contraction in rodents but is a vasodilator in cattle. Among the other substances released from mast cell granules are two tetrapeptides that help mediate the accumulation of inflammatory cells characteristic of the late-phase reaction. *Eosinophilic chemotactic factor of anaphylaxis* promotes eosinophilia characteristic of type I reactions, whereas *neutrophil chemotactic factor* attracts neutrophils to reaction sites. Proportionally, mast cell granules contain abundant amounts of neutral proteases, represented primarily by the serine proteases *tryptase* and *chymase,* plus *carboxypeptidase.* The amounts and types of pro-

TABLE 5-7   **Preformed and Newly Synthesized Mediators Released from Mast Cells**

MEDIATOR	MEDIATOR CLASS	BIOLOGICAL ACTIVITY
PREFORMED		
Histamine	Biogenic amine	Vasodilatation and increased vascular permeability, smooth muscle contraction
Serotonin		Vasoconstriction and smooth muscle contraction
ECF-A	Chemotactic factor	Chemotaxis of eosinophils
NCF		Chemotaxis of neutrophils
Serine proteases (tryptase, chymase) and carboxypeptidase	Enzymes	Complement activation to form anaphylatoxins (C5a and C3a), degradation of extracellular matrix
Kallikreins		Kinin generation
Heparin, chondroitin sulfate	Proteoglycans	Protect mast cells by stabilizing mast cell proteases and altering biological activity of many enzymes; potent anticoagulant (heparin)
SYNTHESIZED AND RELEASED		
LTC_4, LTD_4, LTE_4	Lipids	Smooth muscle contraction, increased vascular permeability, mucus secretion
LTB_4		Neutrophil and eosinophil chemotaxis
PGD_2		Bronchospasm, vasodilatation, mucus secretion
PAF		Platelet aggregation and degranulation, neutrophil and eosinophil chemotaxis and activation; amplifies production of lipid mediators
IL-4, IL-13	Cytokines	Promote T_H2-cell responses
IL-3, IL-5, GM-CSF		Promote eosinophil production and activation
TNF-α		Promotes inflammation, stimulates cytokine secretion, promotes neutrophil adhesion to endothelial cells
MIP-1α	Chemokine	Attracts monocytes, lymphocytes, basophils, and eosinophils

ECF, Eosinophil chemotactic factor of anaphylaxis; *LT,* leukotriene; *MIP,* macrophage inflammatory protein; *NCF,* neutrophil chemotactic factor; *PAF,* platelet-activating factor; *PG,* prostaglandin.

teases vary from species to species and within populations of mast cells within a given species. Release of these proteases causes activation of components of complement resulting in the formation of C5a and C3a (anaphylatoxins), which stimulate smooth muscle contraction, increased vascular permeability, and the stimulation of additional mast cell degranulation. Additionally, these enzymes can trigger the generation of potent vasoactive kinins from serum kallikreins, and they may participate in extracellular matrix degradation. The proteoglycans *heparin* and *chondroitin sulfate* help prevent proteases contained in mast cell granules from being self-destructive by stabilizing and altering biological activity that might otherwise be harmful to the cells. Heparin also functions extracellularly as a potent anticoagulant.

As previously mentioned, one of the effects of mast cell degranulation after antigen binding of IgE is the rapid release of arachidonic acid from cell membrane phospholipids. Arachidonic acid metabolism by either the cyclooxygenase or the lipoxygenase pathways quickly results in the generation of prostaglandin and leukotriene metabolites respectively. *Leukotriene* (LT) C_4, LTD_4, and LTE_4 function similarly to histamine in stimulating dilatation and increased permeability of small blood vessels, smooth muscle contraction, and increased glandular secretions, but the LTs are up to 1000 times more potent in these functions than histamine is. Another product of the lipoxygenase pathway is LTB_4, which is a potent chemoattractant of neutrophils and eosinophils. The most abundant mediator derived from the cyclooxygenase pathway is PGD_2, which causes intense bronchospasm, vasodilatation, and the promotion of mucus secretion. Another lipid mediator triggered by the activation of phospholipase A2, but not a product of arachidonic acid metabolism, is *platelet-activating factor* (PAF). PAF causes platelet aggregation and degranulation and the release of histamine and has vasoactive properties similar to those of histamine. However, the more important function of PAF may be its contribution to the late phase of the hypersensitivity reaction through its attraction of neutrophils and eosinophils and, at higher concentration, the activation of these cells.

Mast cell activation also results in the synthesis of a variety of cytokines and some chemokines that tend to promote late-phase events. Among the cytokines secreted are *IL-4* and *IL-13*, which promote T_H2-cell differentiation, B-cell proliferation, and isotype switching to IgE production. In addition, *IL-3*, *IL-5*, and *GM-CSF* from activated mast cells stimulate growth and differentiation of eosinophil precursors in the bone marrow and activation of eosinophils, which accumulate in the inflammatory site. The proinflammatory cytokine *TNF-α* stimulates cytokine production by other cells and attracts eosinophils and neutrophils to the inflammatory site. In addition, TNF-α stimulates activation of vascular endothelial cells facilitating transmigration of leukocytes into the inflammatory site where they become activated by TNF-α. The chemokine, *MIP-1α* is also secreted by activated mast cells and contributes to the late-phase reaction by being an attractant for monocytes, lymphocytes, eosinophils, and basophils.

Treatment of type I hypersensitivity reactions is dictated by the severity of the response and the tissues involved. Systemic, life-threatening anaphylactic responses must be ablated quickly, most commonly by the systemic administration of epinephrine. The epinephrine promotes vasoconstriction in the skin and viscera and smooth muscle relaxation in shock organs. Antihistamines are the drugs of choice for treating less severe, immediate-phase type I reactions such as those occurring with pollen allergies. These reactions are mediated primarily by histamine, which has two general types of receptors, designated, H_1 and H_2, which can be competitively blocked by antihistamines. Most antihistamines are structured to bind H_1 receptors on target cells but have the objectionable side effect of causing sedation as a result of the antihistamine crossing the blood-brain barrier. More recently, antihistamines structured to bind the H_2 receptors have been developed and are less prone to cross the blood-brain barrier and therefore do not cause sedation. Late-phase type I reactions and chronic allergic diseases associated with antigen persistence are treated with topical or systemic corticosteroids, which are powerful antiinflammatory drugs.

Clinical Manifestations of Type I Hypersensitivity

Multiple factors determine the location and severity of the type I response. These include the number and location of mast cells stimulated, the amount of antigen-specific IgE antibody bound to mast cells, the dose of allergen initiating the response, and the route by which the allergen is delivered. The genetic composition of the host also influences the level of sensitivity of individuals to different allergens.

SYSTEMIC ANAPHYLAXIS

Systemic delivery of an allergen to tissues containing sensitized mast cells can result in life-threatening *anaphylactic shock*. The clinical manifestation of anaphylaxis varies from animal species to animal

TABLE 5-8 Anaphylactic Shock Organs

SPECIES	SHOCK ORGAN	PRIMARY CLINICAL SIGNS
Human	Respiratory tract	Urticaria, dyspnea (laryngeal edema)
Cattle and sheep	Lungs	Coughing, dyspnea (pulmonary edema)
Pigs	Lungs and intestines	Dyspnea, cyanosis
Horse	Lungs and intestines	Dyspnea, diarrhea
Dog	Liver (occlusion of hepatic veins)	Vomiting, diarrhea, collapse
Cat	Lungs and intestines	Dyspnea, vomiting, diarrhea

species related to which organs contain smooth muscle that is most highly sensitive to the mediators released from activated mast cells. The target organs for anaphylactic shock in different animals are listed in Table 5-8. Systemic anaphylaxis is typically mediated by histamine, though in cattle, serotonin, kinins, and leukotrienes are considered to be more important.

One of the most common causes of acute anaphylaxis in animals and humans is the systemic administration of a drug to which an individual has been previously sensitized. Penicillin and penicillin derivatives are most notorious for causing anaphylactic reactions, but many other drugs also have the potential to cause anaphylaxis. Another potential cause of systemic type I reactions are vaccines. Severe allergies have been associated with the administration of killed foot-and-mouth disease vaccines, rabies vaccines, and bovine pleuropneumonia vaccines. Anaphylactic reactions are also associated with the accidental or intentional rupture of subcutaneously encysted *Hypoderma bovis* (warble) larvae in cattle.

Milk Allergy

Milk allergy may be seen in high-producing Jersey cattle. The allergic reaction occurs to the milk protein α-casein, which is normally synthesized in the mammary gland and secreted in the milk. If milking is delayed, the increased intramammary pressure may force the α-casein into the bloodstream where it is recognized as a foreign antigen and stimulates an antibody response. If there is another incidence of delayed milking, α-casein may again be forced into the circulation and precipitate an immediate-type hypersensitivity reaction with signs ranging from localized urticarial skin lesions and multifocal cutaneous edema to acute systemic anaphylaxis and death.

Biphasic Type I Reactions

Restriction of allergen exposure to either the respiratory tract, intestinal tract, or the skin results in a more localized release of mediators from activated mast cells. The inflammation stimulated by these mediators is typically *biphasic* with an *immediate reaction* occurring within minutes after mast cell degranulation followed by a *late-phase reaction* that takes up to 8 to 12 hours to develop. The immediate reaction, characterized by a rapid increase in vascular permeability and the contraction of smooth muscle, is mediated primarily by histamine released from mast cell granules and PGD_2, LTB_4, LTC_4, and PAF, which are rapidly synthesized after mast cell activation. The late-phase reaction is less dramatic than the immediate reaction and is caused by mediators synthesized and released from activated mast cells including leukotrienes, cytokines, and chemokines. The late-phase reaction is characterized by sustained edema caused by increased vascular permeability, smooth muscle contraction, and the tissue accumulation of neutrophils, basophils, eosinophils, and T lymphocytes, which promote amplification and sustenance of the late-phase response, without the need for additional allergen exposure. Accumulation of eosinophils and T_H2 cells is especially important for the perpetuation of the late-phase inflammatory reaction because T_H2 cells promote synthesis of additional IgE and activated eosinophils synthesize LTC_4 and PAF. In addition, degranulation of eosinophils in the inflammatory site results in the release of *major basic protein* and *eosinophil cationic protein*, which further promote mast cell and basophil degranulation and are toxic to epithelial cells.

Canine Atopy

Atopy manifests as a triad of clinical conditions in humans including hay fever, asthma, and dermatitis but presents primarily as a *pruritic dermatitis* in dogs. Atopic dermatitis (AD) is one of the most common causes of chronic pruritus in dogs and may affect dogs of any breed including mongrels but occurs more commonly in certain breeds or families of dogs, an indication of a genetic predisposition. The number of breeds that have been incriminated as being genetically predisposed to atopy is substantial and varies according to geographic location. Those more commonly associated with atopy include Cairn terriers, West Highland white terriers, English and Irish setters, Dalmatians, boxers, and Labrador retrievers. The pathogenesis of canine atopy is complex and still poorly understood. Dogs with AD are frequently hypersensitive to more than one allergen. Some of the more common allergens include molds, tree, weed and grass pollens, and house dust mites. The route of allergen exposure is believed to be primarily epidermal resulting in a pattern of skin disease closely resembling that of allergic contact dermatitis. However, in some situations allergen exposure may be through the respiratory tract. Immunogenetic and breeding studies, though inconclusive, provide support for the genetic predisposition of AD. Tissue injury is considered to be a result of a type I reaction; however, the exact role of IgE in the disease process has not been clearly established. There is some evidence that other immunoglobulin isotypes, such as IgGd, also may be involved. Additional studies have suggested that the basis for the abnormal IgE response may actually lie in abnormalities of suppressor T-cell functions.

FELINE ATOPY

Feline atopy is less well characterized than atopy in dogs and may manifest as nonlesional or lesional pruritus. Lesions associated with feline atopy include miliary dermatitis, which may occur with lesions of the eosinophilic granuloma complex, plus otitis externa. Nonseasonal allergens are most commonly incriminated as the cause of feline atopy, and a genetic predisposition is suggested by a tendency for atopy to occur in some families of cats. Food allergens may be one of the more common causes of feline atopy. In one study, up to 70% of atopic cats improved when a change of diet was combined with hyposensitization.

Flea allergy is the most common cause of allergic skin disease in dogs and cats and may occur in both atopic and nonatopic individuals. Type I hypersensitivity is one of the pathogenic pathways involved in flea allergies, but type IV hypersensitivity and possibly other immune mechanisms are also involved.

RESPIRATORY HYPERSENSITIVITY

The best example of a type I respiratory allergic disorder in animals is *chronic obstructive pulmonary disease* (COPD), which affects horses housed in dusty conditions. COPD is characterized clinically by an insidious onset of exercise intolerance and dyspnea caused by mucinous or mucopurulent bronchiolitis. Allergens considered to be most important in the pathogenesis of COPD include the thermophilic molds *Micropolyspora faeni* and *Aspergillus fumigatus,* plus actinomycetes that grow in damp hay. Extracts of these allergens may cause positive skin reactions in horses suffering from COPD though a direct correlation between positive skin tests and clinical disease has not been established. Additionally, aerosol exposure of COPD horses to these allergens may precipitate an episode of respiratory distress. Type III hypersensitivity is also probably involved in the pathogenesis of COPD. *Feline asthma* is a clinical condition characterized by recurrent episodes of paroxysmal coughing, sneezing, and dyspnea that is believed to involve a type I reaction to inhaled allergens. A mucinous bronchiolitis, similar to that observed in the early stages of COPD in horses, is found in these cats, but a role for IgE in the pathogenesis of feline asthma has not been identified. An association between the chronic inhalation of mold and dust allergens has been suggested as the cause of chronic cough and allergic bronchiolitis in some dogs. Little is known regarding the pathogenesis of this clinical disorder in dogs, but the occasional finding of hyperplastic bronchiolitis, resembling that seen in horses and cats with allergic bronchiolitis, is suggestive that type I hypersensitivity may be involved.

Type II Hypersensitivity

Type II hypersensitivity reactions are classically referred to as cytotoxic in character because the result is lysis of target cells against which an antibody is directed. The reactions are mediated by antigen-specific antibodies (usually of the IgG or IgM isotypes), which react with antigens present on the surface of cells or other tissue elements. These antigens may be normal cell surface molecules that act like antigens *(self-antigens)* or exogenous antigens such as drug metabolites, viruses, or bacterial products that adhere to and alter cell surfaces or tissues. The two principle mechanisms involved in type II reactions are *complement-mediated cytotoxicity* and *antibody-mediated cellular cytotoxicity* (ADCC), which cause either cell death or other tissue changes, such as swelling or fragmentation of basement membranes (Fig. 5-8). Complement mediation of type II hypersensitivity may occur by two mechanisms: direct lysis and opsonization. Binding of antigen-specific IgM or IgG antibody to target-cell membrane antigenic determinants leaves the Fc portion of antibody molecules exposed. Complement binding of these exposed Fc components triggers complement activation and the assembly of the membrane attack complex that creates pores in cell

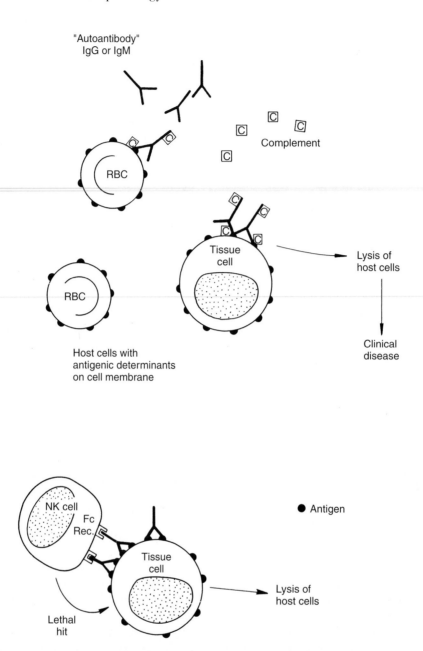

Fig. 5-8 Cytotoxic (type II) hypersensitivity. Antibody (IgG or IgM) directed at cell membrane components (often self-antigens) binds to the specific antigen on the cell surface. Two different mechanisms may be involved in the pathogenesis of cell injury: **A,** Complement-mediated cytotoxicity. Complement fixation and activation occurs after antibody binding, and cell lysis results. **B,** Antibody-mediated cellular cytotoxicity. NK cells bind the Fc fragment of antibodies (IgG) directed against cell surface antigens. After antibody binds to the cell, the "lethal hit" is executed by perforins and other cytotoxins. *C,* Complement; *RBC,* red blood cells.

membranes leading to cell death. The other mechanism involves adhesion of antibody or the C3b or C4b components of complement to target cell surfaces (opsonization) stimulating phagocytosis and destruction of target cells by macrophages, typically located in the spleen and liver. ADCC occurs when Fc receptors on cytotoxic cells bind to Fc components of IgG molecules that are adhered to the surface of target cells resulting in target cell lysis independent of phagocytosis. Cells with cytotoxic capabilities include monocytes, neutrophils, eosinophils, and NK cells. The ADCC form of type II hypersensitivity is believed to be involved in the destruction of certain kinds of targets that are

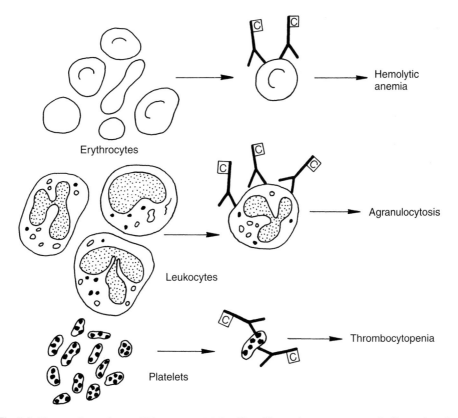

Fig. 5-9 Hematological type II hypersensitivity. Type II reactions are commonly directed against cellular elements in direct contact with plasma. *Hemolytic anemia* and *thrombocytopenia* are probably the most common and best documented naturally occurring examples. *C,* Complement.

too large to be phagocytosed, such as parasites and tumor cells, and also may be involved in graft rejection.

Cytotoxic reactions directed against self-antigens expressed on target cell membranes are referred to as *autoimmune,* and the antibody is thus termed an *autoantibody.* If an exogenous antigen or a hapten is adsorbed onto cell surfaces, a similar lytic reaction may ensue, also resulting in lysis. In this case, even though immune-mediated lysis of host cells occurs, the reaction is not autoimmune because the antigen is not native to the host. Such reactions occur in some of the drug-induced hemolytic anemias. Alternatively, destruction of host cells may occur if an exogenous antigen stimulates the production of antibodies that cross-react with self-antigens on the surface of the host cells *(molecular mimicry).* A typical example of such a reaction is the production of antibodies directed against β-hemolytic streptococci that cross-react with myocardial glycoproteins to cause human rheumatic heart disease.

Since the reactants (antibody, complement) for type II cytotoxic reactions are found primarily in the plasma, it is not surprising that many type II reactions occur against cells that are in the blood or exposed to blood (Fig. 5-9). Most of the hematological type II hypersensitivity diseases are caused by the production of antibodies against self-antigens and involve complement-mediated lysis. Examples of this form of hypersensitivity are reactions against red blood cells, white blood cells, platelets, and even endothelial cells.

One interesting variation of type II hypersensitivity is related to those diseases mediated purely by antibodies, without involvement of complement or cytotoxic cells. The involved antibodies are not necessarily cytotoxic, and the diseases involve other mechanisms leading to functional alterations. An important group of skin diseases, the bullous dermatoses, including the pemphigus complex and bullous pemphigoid, fits into this category. In these diseases, antibodies are formed that are directed against surface antigens of dermal and mucosal keratinocytes or the epidermal basement membrane. Complexing of antibodies with the keratinocytes leads to loss of cell-cell adhesion without actually causing keratinocyte death (pemphigus), whereas the anti–basement membrane antibodies cause a loss of cell–extracellular matrix adhesion (bullous pemphigoid). A second group of related diseases are the antireceptor antibody diseases such as myasthenia gravis and Graves' disease. In these diseases, antibodies are directed against specific receptors, and the binding of the antibody either increases or decreases receptor function. In myasthenia gravis, the antibody binds to the acetylcholine receptors in motor end plates of skeletal muscles impairing neuromuscular transmission and thereby causing muscle weakness. In Graves' disease, antibody binds to the TSH receptor on thyroid epithelial cells stimulating the secretion of excess thyroid hormone resulting in hyperthyroidism.

Immunohematological Diseases

By far the best studied and characterized clinical forms of type II hypersensitivity relate to the immunological destruction of cellular elements within the blood (Table 5-9). Clinical situations in which antibodies are directed against red blood cell antigens are probably the most common and are exemplified by transfusion reactions and by the various forms of acquired autoimmune hemolytic disease. Red blood cells, like nucleated cells, have surface molecules that can act like antigens. When red blood cells from a genetically dissimilar individual are transfused into an animal, one of two things may happen. If the recipient has "natural" antibodies against the red blood cells, a transfusion reaction may occur immediately resulting in agglutination or hemolysis or erythrophagocytosis, as a result of opsonization. Natural antibodies may be antibodies produced against antigenic determinants of unknown origin that are similar or identical to those on red blood cells, or they may be antibodies produced in response to exposure to infectious agents containing epitopes structurally similar to red blood cell antigens. If the recipient has not been previously exposed to transfused genetically dissimilar red blood cells and does not have natural antibodies, the transfused red blood cells will stimulate an immune response that will lead to their delayed destruction. Subsequent transfusion of the same red blood cells will elicit rapid destruction of the foreign cells with potentially serious pathological consequences. Transfusion reactions that result from circulating antibody causing destruction of erythrocytes from an incompatible donor are called *isoimmune*. These are not "autoimmune" diseases because the antigen is exogenous whereas the antibody is endogenous.

The antigens found on the surface of red blood cells are called "blood group antigens." The many and varied blood group antigens are used to classify blood group systems in humans and animals. In humans, ABO and Rh systems are the most important red blood cell antigenic determinants. The major blood groups of domestic animals are shown in Table 5-10.

TABLE 5-9   Immunohematologic Disorders

NAME	MECHANISM
Transfusion reaction	Blood group incompatibility
Erythroblastosis fetalis	Rh incompatibility
Neonatal isoerythrolysis	Blood group incompatibility
Autoimmune hemolytic anemia	Anti-RBC antibody
Neonatal leukopenia	Anti-WBC antibody
Acquired agranulocytosis	Anti-WBC antibody
Idiopathic thrombocytopenic purpura	Antiplatelet antibody
Hemolytic reactions to drugs	Drug acts as hapten

TABLE 5-10   Important Blood Groups of Domestic Animals

SPECIES	BLOOD GROUP SYSTEMS
Cattle	Eleven total; B and J most important; B group very complex and may be used to identify registered animals; J antigen is a serum lipid that passively adsorbs onto erythrocytes
Sheep	Seven total; B and R important; B group is complex and equivalent to bovine B group; R like bovine J group R antigen in serum, soluble and passively adsorbs onto erythrocytes
Pig	Fifteen total; A system most important and having two antigens, A and O
Horse	Seven total; antibodies against Aa, Qa, R, and S are most commonly involved in neonatal isoerythrolysis
Dog	Eight total; dog erythrocyte antigen (DEA)-1 through -8; DEA-1.1 and DEA-1.2 most antigenic and dogs expressing are group A positive; DEA-1.1 and -1.2 most commonly involved in transfusion reactions
Cat	Only one system: AB; A completely dominant over B; up to 95% cats are A positive

Hemolytic disease of the newborn or *neonatal isoerythrolysis* represents a special category of transfusion-like reaction in which transfer of antigens and antibodies between the fetus and the dam can lead to destruction of the red blood cells of the newborn. This situation occurs fairly commonly in horses and donkeys. Since the red blood cell antigenic makeup of the fetus is determined by genetic contributions from both the sire and the dam, the fetal red blood cells are antigenically distinct from those of the dam even though they have some common antigenic determinants. If, during fetal life, these red blood cells gain access to the circulation of the dam, they elicit an immune response in the dam in the same way that any incompatible blood transfusion would. That is, the dam makes antibodies against those fetal red blood cell antigens that are determined by the sire. Since the majority of maternal passive transfer of antibody in domestic animals takes place by the colostrum (in contrast to placental transfer), the antibodies reactive against the fetal red blood cells are not present in the fetal circulation until after birth, when they are transferred in the maternal colostral antibody supply. These antibodies then attack the antigenic determinants on the newborn's red blood cells derived from the sire's genetic material, and red blood cell destruction and hemolytic disease results.

In women, where transplacental transfer of antibody occurs, a similar situation results in the disease called *erythroblastosis fetalis*. Transplacental transfer of antierythrocyte antibody to the fetus results in infants being born with hemolytic anemia rather than developing it after birth. Neonatal isoerythrolysis is fairly common in newborn horses and mules but rarely occurs in dogs, cats, piglets, and calves. In piglets and calves it has occasionally been seen after vaccination of the dam with blood-containing vaccines (such as hog cholera, anaplasmosis, or babesiosis). Thrombocytopenia can develop by similar mechanisms when antibody against fetal platelets is transferred via the colostrum. Neonatal thrombocytopenia of this type has been described in puppies and piglets.

Autoimmune hemolytic anemia has been best characterized in dogs in which a fairly typical syndrome of anemia, spherocytosis, and a positive direct antiglobulin (Coombs') reaction develops. The Coombs test detects antibody coating the surface of the patient's red blood cells. The direct test is conducted by incubation of washed erythrocytes from the patient with antiimmunoglobulin antibody. The most puzzling aspect of the so-called autoimmune hemolytic diseases is that the factors responsible for initiating the production of antibody directed

against self-antigens are largely unknown. Animals that die of autoimmune hemolytic anemia have massive splenomegaly with pronounced hemosiderosis as a direct result of the splenic removal of large numbers of damaged red blood cells.

Autoimmune and immunologically mediated responses similar to those described for red blood cells have also been reported to occur against leukocytes. Although uncommon, immune-mediated responses against leukocytes are most likely to occur in association with the use of drugs, such as sulfonamides, phenylbutazone, phenothiazine, and chloramphenicol, which may bind to granulocytes and cause agranulocytosis mediated by a type II reaction.

Immune reactions against platelets can occur by means of mechanisms similar to those that occur against erythrocytes and leukocytes. The result is usually purpura or other manifestations of the coagulation defect produced by severe thrombocytopenia. Such immune reactions probably form the basis for much of what has been known as idiopathic thrombocytopenic purpura. Immune injury to platelets after antigen-antibody reactions on the platelet surface membrane can result in lysis or in accelerated removal of the injured platelets by the mononuclear phagocyte system of the liver and spleen. The pathogenesis of immune-mediated thrombocytopenia can include true autoimmune thrombocytopenia, with antibody directed against some structurally altered component of the platelet plasma membrane. Autoimmune thrombocytopenia is occasionally seen is association with autoimmune hemolytic anemia. The pathogenesis of other forms of immune-mediated thrombocytopenia have diverse mechanistic backgrounds. In addition to specific autoantibody directed against platelet membrane antigens, thrombocytopenia can result from the binding of antibodies to platelets bearing adsorbed viral, bacterial, rickettsial, or protozoal antigens. Similarly, the adsorption of drugs, such as sulfonamides, phenylbutazone, chloramphenicol, and quinine, to platelet surfaces may precipitate type II reactions resulting in platelet lysis and thrombocytopenia or the accelerated removal of the platelets from the circulation by means of the mononuclear phagocytic system.

Those diseases in which autoantibody is directed against receptors or other cell surface antigens are variations of type II hypersensitivity resulting from the interaction of autoantibodies with self-antigens. Examples include the bullous dermatoses and the antireceptor diseases such as myasthenia gravis. As such, they are truly autoimmune diseases, and we discuss them as examples of autoimmunity in the appropriate section of this chapter.

Type III Hypersensitivity (Immune-Complex Disease)

The type III hypersensitivity reaction is a complex process that includes a series of interdependent events involving antigen, antibody, complement, leukocytes and their products, platelets, and various other factors that contribute to a localized inflammatory reaction.

Immune complexes form by the binding of antigens and antibodies in the circulation or *in situ* as a result of circulating antibodies binding to tissue self-antigens or to exogenous antigens bound to tissues *(planted antigens)* (Fig. 5-10). Immune complexes formed within the circulation are generally removed by cells of the mononuclear phagocytic system and catabolized to harmless end products. However, a selected fraction of small to intermediate-sized immune complexes tend to evade phagocytosis. Sites of deposition of these complexes are governed by the anatomic and physiological character of the tissue rather than by an immunological relationship of the inducing antigen or antibody to the tissue. Immune complexes most commonly accumulate in locations that have a filtering function such as glomeruli, blood vessels, synovial membranes,

and the choroid plexus. Immune complex–related tissue injury does not result from the physical deposition of immune complexes but is caused by complement activation and the resulting inflammatory events triggered as a result of immune-complex deposition.

The pathogenicity of circulating immune complexes is determined primarily by the ratio of antigen to antibody and the isotype of antibody involved. Complexes formed in *antibody excess* tend to be large and insoluble and are rapidly removed from the circulation by cells of the mononuclear phagocyte system, thereby preventing their accumulation in sites where immune-complex injury characteristically occurs. Complexes formed in *extreme antigen excess* are usually too small to become trapped in physiological filters and do not contain an arrangement of immunoglobulin molecules capable of activating complement. Immune complexes formed in *slight antigen excess* are small to intermediate in size (about 19S) and are the most pathogenic because they are the right size for deposition in tissue. One of the differences between type I and type III hypersensitivity reactions is the amount of antigen required to stimulate each

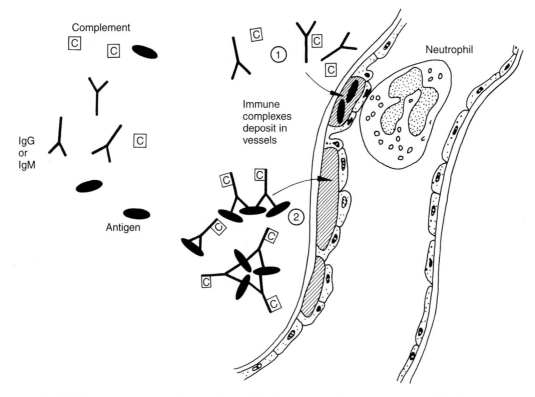

Fig. 5-10 Immune-complex disease (type III). *Immune complexes* may form *in situ (1)* or may form in the circulation and be deposited *(2)*. *Antigen* combines with *IgG* or *IgM* antibody and fixes *complement*, and the resulting activation generates the *C5a* for chemotactic attraction of *neutrophils*, which are responsible for much of the tissue damage.

of the reactions. Very small quantities of antigen (in microgram amounts) are required for type I reactions, whereas comparatively large quantities of antigen (in milligram amounts) are required for type III reactions. The pathogenicity of immune complexes is also influenced by the isotype of antibody involved, since some isotypes (IgM and IgG) are more capable of activating complement than other isotypes.

Pathogenesis of Lesions Resulting from Immune-Complex Deposition

Immune complex deposition in blood vessels and tissues must be preceded by a local *increase in vascular permeability* that is generally mediated by the vasoactive amines histamine and serotonin. Binding of the Fc fragments of immune-complex antibodies to cell membrane Fc receptors triggers release of va-

soactive amines from circulating basophils and platelets and tissue mast cells. In addition, the Fc fragments bind the C1 component of complement initiating the activation of the classical complement pathway leading to the generation of the anaphylatoxins C3a and C5a, which help perpetuate the type III reaction by directly activating basophils to release vasoactive amines and platelet-activating factor (PAF). The released PAF, in turn, is a potent platelet agonist that triggers the further release of vasoactive mediators. In addition to stimulating the release of vasoactive substances, anaphylatoxins also are capable of inducing smooth muscle contraction. The process by which the vasoactive amines increase vascular permeability and promote deposition of immune complexes in blood vessels and other tissues is termed the *"anaphylactic trigger"* (Fig. 5-11).

In addition to activating basophils, C5a as well as C5-7 are strong chemotactic agents for neutrophils,

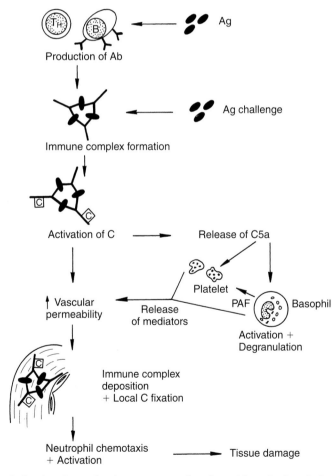

Fig. 5-11 Anaphylactic trigger for immune-complex deposition. Antigen induces synthesis of both IgG or IgM antibody, which leads to *immune-complex formation* within the circulation. The local *vascular permeability* increase necessary for their deposition is mediated by *C5a-basophil platelet activation and degranulation*, called the "anaphylactic trigger" mechanism. *Ab*, antibody; *Ag*, antigen; *PAF*, platelet-activating factor.

attracting large numbers of these cells to sites of immune-complex deposition. The membrane attack complex, C5-9, also formed as a result of complement activation, may cause cell membrane damage, contributing to tissue injury in sites of immune-complex deposition. Although C5a *attracts* neutrophils, tissue macrophages, activated by interacting with deposited immune complexes, *promote* accumulation of neutrophils at sites of immune-complex deposition by secreting TNF-α and IL-1, which upregulate the expression of the leukocyte adhesion molecules E-selectin and ICAM-1 on vessel endothelial surfaces.

The presence of neutrophils in sites of immune-complex deposition correlates directly with the occurrence of tissue injury. As neutrophils encounter and begin phagocytosis of immune complexes, they are stimulated to release and secrete large quantities of granule enzymes and *reactive oxygen species* (ROS). The destructive effects of these neutrophil products is intensified when neutrophil phagocyto-

sis is thwarted because immune complexes are attached to basement membranes, synovial membranes, or other tissue components resulting in *"frustrated phagocytosis."* The inability to phagocytize attached immune complexes results in the discharge of neutrophil enzymes and ROS into a confined space, concentrating their destructive effects in a small area

Included among the products released and secreted from neutrophils are myeloperoxidase, lysozyme, defensins, acid hydrolyases, and neutral proteases (elastase, cathepsin G, collagenase). Activated neutrophils also secrete a variety of ROS that contribute to tissue damage. These include superoxide anion (O_2^-), hydrogen peroxide (H_2O_2), hydroxyl radical (HO·), singlet oxygen ($^1O_2$), and hypochlorous acid (HOCl). These potent oxidants with strong microbicidal activity have been shown to be major participants in immune complex–induced tissue injury (Fig. 5-12). H_2O_2 can cause tissue damage by its reaction with myeloperoxidase

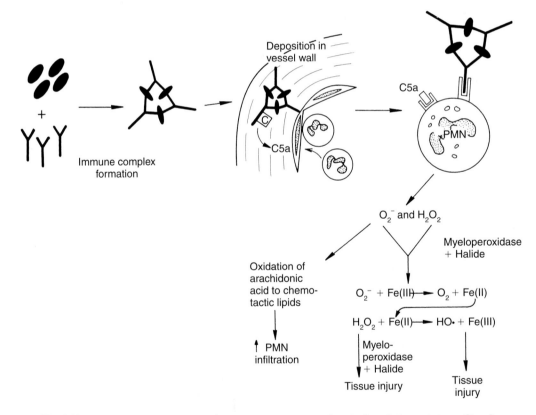

Fig. 5-12 Role of toxic oxygen products in immune complex–induced tissue injury. Circulating immune complexes are formed and deposited within the vascular wall. Activation of complement leads to formation of *C5a,* which is chemotactic for neutrophils, *PMN.* Release of toxic oxygen products by activated *PMN* causes direct tissue damage: hydroxyl radical *(HO·)* by direct oxidation of lipid membranes, hydrogen peroxidase *(H_2O_2)* by its interaction with myeloperoxidase and halides, and superoxide anion *(O_2^-)* by the production of chemotactic lipids, which further recruits neutrophils.

and halides, whereas HO· directly causes membrane damage. O_2^- may also enhance the inflammatory reaction by producing a chemotactic lipid from arachidonic acid. HOCl can inactivate antiproteases, which function to neutralize destructive enzymes released from neutrophils. In addition, nitric oxide released from activated tissue macrophages may interact with O_2^- to form peroxynitrite, thus also contributing to tissue damage.

Substantial neutrophil accumulation at immune-complex deposition sites requires 6 to 8 hours. The result of the effects of the enzymes and ROS secreted by neutrophils is tissue injury characterized by vascular necrosis, edema, hemorrhage, platelet aggregation, and thrombosis. If the type III reaction is extended, mononuclear cells appear in about 8 hours and may dominate the lesion by 24 hours.

Nature of Antigens Causing Type III Hypersensitivity

The antigen itself does not seem to be of great importance in immune-complex disease, and in many cases the exact antigen cannot be determined. However, a few types of antigens are known to be commonly involved in type III hypersensitivities and can be divided broadly into three groups: (1) repeatedly inhaled antigens, (2) self-antigens, and (3) antigens derived from persistent infectious agents.

Repeatedly inhaled allergens may encounter antibody at several levels of the respiratory tract and form immune complexes that are deposited in bronchiolar and alveolar walls resulting in hypersensitivity pneumonitis. A typical example is *extrinsic allergic alveolitis* of cattle. Inhalation of spores of the actinomycete *Micropolyspora faeni*, which grows in moldy hay, leads to induction of antibody production and, after repeated exposure, can cause an interstitial pneumonia. The histopathological lesion is lymphocytic interstitial pneumonia and bronchiolitis, a lesion that is suggestive that the pathogenesis of the disease probably involves both type III and type IV (delayed-type) hypersensitivities. A similar disease called *farmer's lung* occurs in farmers chronically exposed to dust from moldy hay containing the spores of *M. faeni*. The lung lesion of *chronic obstructive pulmonary disease* (COPD) of horses occurs initially as a result of a type I hypersensitivity reaction. With continual reexposure to barn dust containing *M. faeni* spores and a sustained antibody response, a type III response also contributes to the pathogenesis of the lung lesion.

The *self-antigens* most often implicated in immune-mediated tissue injury are those that are *persistently* available for interaction with circulating antibody. If appropriate levels of autoantibody are produced, immune-complex formation and deposition will occur. An example is *systemic lupus erythematosus* (SLE), a disease in which autoantibodies are produced against several self-antigens, including DNA. These diseases are, by definition, *autoimmune*.

A third group of antigens known to lead to immune-complex formation and deposition are derived from *persistent infectious agents*. Chronic staphylococcal dermatitis can lead to type III hypersensitivity with immune-complex deposition in vessel walls and dermal vasculitis. An occasional complication of infection or immunization of dogs with live adenovirus type I is an ophthalmic syndrome known as *blue eye*. A bluish corneal opacity in these dogs results from an anterior uveitis with corneal edema caused by inflammation induced by the deposition of virus-specific immune complexes in the eye. Again, we should point out that neither the antibody nor the antigen in this situation has any specificity for the eye. The eye is simply the site of immune-complex deposition. Other examples of persistent viral infections with immune-complex formation as an important part of the pathogenesis include feline infectious peritonitis, feline leukemia, Aleutian mink disease, equine infectious anemia, hog cholera, and African swine fever (Table 5-11). In each of these situations, the repetitive or persistent presence of moderate amounts of viral antigen accompanied by fairly low-level antibody production results in immune-complex formation, deposition, and subsequent tissue injury. Not all animals with these infections develop immune-complex disease. Very strong or very weak antibody producers may not develop suitable conditions for the formation of immune complexes of the proper size for deposition in tissue.

In Situ Immune-Complex Disease

The classical example of an *in situ* type III hypersensitivity reaction is the *Arthus reaction*. First demonstrated by Maurice Arthus in the early 1900s, the Arthus reaction is an immune-complex disease resulting from relatively large amounts of antigen and antibody precipitating in cutaneous vessel walls resulting in a localized, acute, necrotizing cutaneous vasculitis. In order for the reaction to occur locally, one of the reactants (antigen or antibody) must be circulating and the other injected locally. Usually, the Arthus reaction is studied by intracutaneous injection of antigen into animals having high circulating levels of precipitating antibody specific for the antigen. After injection, the antigen diffuses through the tissue and localizes in vessel walls where it forms immune complexes with

TABLE 5-11   Examples of Immune Complex Diseases of Domestic Animals

SPECIES	DISEASE	MAJOR LESIONS
Dog	Infectious canine hepatitis	Uveitis, corneal edema
	Pyometra	Glomerulonephritis
	Systemic lupus erythematosus	Glomerulonephritis, dermatitis, arthritis
	Lyme disease (*Borrelia burgdorferi*)	Glomerulonephritis
	Hereditary C3 deficiency	Glomerulonephritis
Cat	Feline infectious peritonitis	Phlebitis, uveitis, glomerulonephritis
	Feline leukemia virus infection	Glomerulonephritis
Pig	Hog cholera	Glomerulonephritis
	African swine fever	Glomerulonephritis
Horse	Equine infectious anemia	Glomerulonephritis
	Streptococcus equi	Purpura, glomerulonephritis
Sheep	Hereditary hypocomplementia in Finnish landrace lambs	Glomerulonephritis
Mink	Aleutian disease	Vasculitis, glomerulonephritis

circulating antigen-specific antibodies. The immune complexes bind and activate complement initiating the inflammatory events described previously. Immune complex–induced inflammation manifests as edema and erythema and eventually, if the reaction is severe enough, hemorrhage and necrosis of the skin at the site of antigen injection.

The type III Arthus reaction differs from a type I immediate hypersensitivity reaction in the type of cells that are involved and the time that it takes for the reaction to occur. In the type I reaction, mast cells and eosinophils are the major effector cells, and the reaction occurs almost immediately after re-exposure to an antigen against which the animal has previously been sensitized. In contrast, neutrophils are the primary effector cells in the Arthus reaction, and it takes 3 to 8 hours for the Arthus reaction to develop fully.

Systemic Immune-Complex Disease

Serum sickness is the prototype of a systemic immune-complex disease. Clinical serum sickness occurs less commonly today than when injections of large amounts of heterologous (usually equine) hyperimmune serum were the primarily treatment for individuals exposed to rabies virus or at risk for tetanus. Injection of the hyperimmune horse serum into these patients resulted in a humoral immune response and the production of antibodies against horse serum proteins. About 8 to 10 days after antiserum injection, some patients developed serious cardiovascular, joint, and renal disease, which occasionally was fatal. Subsequently, it was determined that these clinical disorders occurred as a result of tissue deposition of immune complexes.

Experimentally, serum sickness is induced by the intravenous infusion of a large dose of foreign serum or purified serum protein resulting in a series of fairly predictable events (Fig. 5-13). The antigen level in the serum declines in three distinct phases. The first decline results from equilibration of the injected protein between intravascular and extravascular protein pools. This is followed by slower loss caused by nonimmune catabolism of circulating free protein antigen at a rate characteristic for the particular protein injected and the recipient species. Last, a phase of rapid antigen loss from the circulation occurs as a result of specific antibody binding protein antigens to form immune complexes, plus antigen elimination by the host immune response. Initially there is extreme antigen excess with the formation of small soluble complexes that remain in the circulation. As the amount of specific antibody increases, a point is reached at which the antigen-antibody ratio is such that immune complexes are formed and deposited in tissues. This typically occurs about 7 to 10 days after antigen injection. Coincidental with the formation of antigen-antibody complexes in the circulation, there is a dramatic decrease in serum antigen, antibody, and complement levels that correlate with the appearance of acute inflammatory lesions in the kidneys, heart, arteries, and joints. In such lesions antigen, antibody, and host *complement components* can be detected immunohistochemically.

Experimentally, not all animals in a given study develop immune-complex disease. Animals that become sick are the ones that produce only moderate amounts of antibody resulting in the formation of large quantities of immune complexes of the appropriate size for tissue deposition. The strongest and

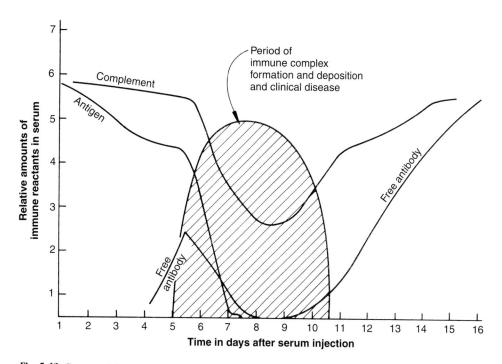

Fig. 5-13 Sequential events in acute serum sickness. After injection of antigen, it slowly decays from the circulation until specific antibody is formed, at which time rapid antigen elimination and complement consumption occur. After deposition, the lack of antigen allows free antibody to reappear and complement levels to return to normal. It is during the period of immune-complex formation and deposition that tissue injury occurs.

BOX 5-1 **Important Features of Diseases Caused by Circulating Immune Complexes**

- Immune reaction is not directed at target tissues; rather tissues are injured by virtue of being sites of immune-complex deposition.
- Occurrence of tissue injury is determined by amount of antibody produced by a given host for a given amount of antigen.
- The reaction is mediated largely by complement.
- Neutrophils are responsible for much of the tissue damage.
- The antigen may be totally innocuous of and by itself.

the weakest antibody producers do not become sick because they fail to produce sufficient *depositable* complexes of the right size. Thus it is apparent that the individuality of animals, not the scientists conducting the experiments, determines the outcome. *Animals determine their own fate by how much antibody they produce.* This is analogous to the clinical situation in which not all members of a given population will develop immune-complex disease

under like conditions of exposure. The central features of immune-complex disease caused by circulating immune complexes are shown in Box 5-1.

Immune-Complex Glomerulonephritis

Glomerular deposition of circulating, soluble immune complexes or the formation of immune complexes within the glomerulus are the principal causes of immune-complex glomerulonephritis. *In situ immune-complex glomerulonephritis* occurs when antibodies leave the circulation and complex with glomerular self-antigens or with endogenous or exogenous antigens that have become "planted" in some part of the glomerulus. An example of *in situ* immune-complex glomerulonephritis resulting from the complexing of antibody with a basement membrane antigen is *Goodpasture's syndrome.* This disorder occurs in humans when a virus infection or exposure to injurious agents, such as hydrocarbon solvents found in paints and dyes, causes a normally concealed glomerular basement membrane (GBM) antigen to be exposed. The basement membrane antigen exposed in Goodpasture's syndrome has recently been identified as *two discontinuous epitopes within the noncollagenous domain of the α3-chain of collagen type IV.* The pathogenesis of this type of immune-complex glomerulonephritis has been well characterized in a rat model of anti-GBM nephritis (Masugi, or nephrotoxic, nephritis). Rat anti-GBM antibodies produced in a rabbit are injected into rats. Circulating rat anti-GBM antibodies leave the bloodstream through glomerular capillaries and bind native (self) antigens located in the GBM to form immune complexes. Complement becomes activated by the immune complexes initiating a series of events resulting in inflammation and immune-complex glomerulonephritis. The anti-GBM antibodies also cross-react with basement membrane antigenic determinants in pulmonary alveoli resulting in immune complex–mediated lung lesions. The immune-complex glomerulonephritis and lung lesions closely resemble the lesions that occur in Goodpasture's syndrome in humans.

Another example of *in situ* immune-complex glomerulonephritis and a model of human membranous glomerulonephritis is *Heymann's nephritis*. Rats are inoculated with proximal tubular brush border preparations. The antibodies produced in response to the brush border antigen cross-react with an antigen complex located on the basal surface of glomerular visceral epithelial cells causing a membranous glomerulonephritis resembling the human lesion. The Heymann antigen within the proximal tubular brush border preparation has been identified as a 330 kD member of the low-density lipoprotein receptor superfamily called *megalin* that is located on both visceral epithelial cells and tubular brush borders. Antibody binding to the megalin antigen on visceral epithelial cells causes alternate-pathway activation of complement and subsequent shedding of the immune complexes from epithelial surfaces into the subepithelial spaces forming subepithelial deposits characteristic of human membranous glomerulonephritis.

In situ immune-complex glomerulonephritis also occurs when circulating antibodies bind endogenous or exogenous "planted" antigens that have become nonspecifically trapped or specifically bound to glomerular constituents. Factors affecting antigen trapping in the glomerulus include size, charge, molecular configuration, and carbohydrate content of the antigen. Examples of endogenous "planted" antigens include histone-DNA complexes, IgA and other Ig isotypes, whereas drugs and a variety of infectious agents are among the numerous exogenous antigens that may become planted in glomeruli.

Another cause of immune-complex glomerulonephritis is the *glomerular deposition of circulating immune complexes*. Potential sites of immune-complex deposition in the kidney are well characterized. These include sites between endothe-lial cells and the GBM (subendothelial), within the GBM (intramembranous), between epithelial cells and the GBM (subepithelial), and within the mesangium. Primary immune-complex deposition in one site is often accompanied by deposition of lesser amounts in other sites. Several factors influence the sites of immune-complex deposition in glomeruli. These are primarily the *molecular charge* of the soluble complexes and the strength of the bond between the antigen and antibody *(avidity)*. *Subendothelial* deposition of immune complexes is usually associated with highly anionic complexes that are excluded from the GBM and with highly avid antibodies that do not easily dissociate from bound antigen. In contrast, *subepithelial* deposition is more likely to occur with highly cationic complexes and antibodies of low avidity. Low-avidity antibodies may dissociate from immune complexes after initial subendothelial deposition and migrate independently of antigen through the basement membrane to reform immune complexes in a subepithelial location. *Intramembranous* deposition of immune complexes is less common and, in some cases, may represent a transitional stage of migration through the basement membrane. Immune complexes that tend to accumulate in the *mesangium* have a more neutral charge

Immune-complex glomerulonephritis is classified according to the site of immune-complex deposition within the glomerulus and the glomerular response to the immune complexes as either *membranous glomerulonephritis* (membranous nephropathy or glomerulopathy) or *membranoproliferative glomerulonephritis*. Membranous glomerulonephritis is the most common cause of the nephrotic syndrome in adult human patients. Histologically it is characterized by the presence of subepithelial deposits of electron-dense material along the GBM. As the lesions worsen, basement membrane material extends between and surrounds the deposits, eventually resulting in a considerably thickened capillary wall. Since cell proliferation and inflammatory cell infiltration is not a feature of membranous glomerulonephritis, the lesion is also referred to as either "membranous nephropathy" or "membranous glomerulopathy." Membranous glomerulonephritis may be idiopathic but most commonly occurs secondarily to other systemic diseases and a variety of etiological agents. As previously described, membranous glomerulonephritis may occur as a result of *in situ* immune-complex formation against self or "planted" antigens or as a result of the deposition of circulating immune complexes in subepithelial locations. In the latter incidence, immune complexes may also be deposited within the GBM and beneath endothelial cells.

Membranoproliferative glomerulonephritis (MPGN) is subdivided into two major types, I and II, with a third type, III, being relatively uncommon and controversial. Human type I MPGN is characterized by the presence of subendothelial glomerular deposits, an increased number of mesangial cells, expansion of the mesangial matrix, and diffuse enlargement of glomerular tufts. Glomerular capillary walls are thickened as a result of mesangial matrix becoming inserted between the GBM and the endothelium. The presence of immunoglobulins and components of complement in the capillary loops of some patients supports an immune-complex cause for some cases of type I MPGN. Examples of viral diseases of domestic animals that have immune-complex MPGN include feline infectious peritonitis, feline leukemia virus infection, equine infectious anemia, African swine fever, and Aleutian mink disease. Chronic bacterial infections and neoplasia may also be associated with type I MPGN.

In type II MPGN, electron-dense refractile deposits in the GBM create a ribbon-like thickening of the glomerular capillary wall. The composition of the dense deposits is not known but is probably *not* related to immune complexes because they do not contain immunoglobulins though they may contain C3.

Another type of immune-complex glomerulonephritis is *IgA nephropathy*. This is the most common form of human glomerulonephritis worldwide and a frequent cause of asymptomatic hematuria. It is characterized by mesangial deposition of IgA, proliferation of mesangial cells, and expansion of the mesangial matrix. Accordingly it is classified as a *mesangioproliferative glomerulonephritis*. Current evidence indicates that IgA nephropathy may result from an altered production or structure of IgA. Aberrant IgA production may be triggered by mucosal exposure to foreign antigens during respiratory or gastrointestinal infections because patients with these illnesses often are hematuric. Circulating IgA immune complexes are present at levels that correlate with disease severity. The IgA within glomerular mesangial deposits is primarily an aberrantly glycosylated IgA1. Therefore, circulating IgA1 immune complexes may escape asialoglycoprotein receptor–mediated phagocytosis by fixed macrophages of the mononuclear phagocytic system promoting their mesangial deposition in glomeruli. The presence of C3 and the terminal components of complement but not C1 and C4 in mesangial deposits is suggestive that IgA-mediated activation of the alternative complement pathway is important in the pathogenesis of this form of mesangioproliferative glomerulonephritis. Diagno-

sis of IgA nephropathy is based on demonstrating mesangial IgA deposits by immunofluorescence microscopy. IgA nephropathy is not recognized as a clinically important disease of domestic animals. Some dogs suffering from enteritis or liver disease have glomerular IgA deposits, and a high percentage of IgA positive glomerulonephritides have been found in mink with Aleutian mink disease.

These various models and examples of glomerulonephritis focus attention on the importance of the process by which immune complexes are deposited in tissue, since it is abundantly clear that if immune complexes *are not* deposited, tissue injury does not occur.

Immune complex glomerulonephritis occurs in a variety of domestic animals (see Table 5-11). Recognition and diagnosis of immune-complex disease is often based on the history, clinical observations, and light and electron microscopic findings. A history of increased water consumption and increased frequency of urination (polydipsia and polyuria) should immediately alert one to possible renal glomerular disease. Hematuria might be the earliest sign of glomerular disease. Later, more profound proteinuria would be more suggestive of a protein-losing renal disease. Proteinuria in combination with an elevated blood urea nitrogen, hypoalbuminemia, and hypercholesterolemia would indicate that the nephrotic syndrome may be caused by either glomerulonephritis or amyloidosis. Light microscopically, diffuse capillary basement membrane thickening with or without increased cellularity in the glomerular tufts would be suggestive of immune-complex glomerulonephritis (Fig. 5-14). The diagnosis of immune-complex glomerulonephritis is confirmed by demonstration of immunoglobulins and complement components, usually C3, in the glomerular lesions (Fig. 5-15). Ultrastructurally, immune-complex deposits should be seen as electron-dense deposits in the glomerular basement membranes or other locations in the glomerulus (Fig. 5-16). Even though a morphological diagnosis of immune-complex glomerulonephritis is made, identification of the causative antigen may be more elusive and often is never made.

Type IV Hypersensitivity (Delayed-Type Hypersensitivity)

Type IV delayed-type hypersensitivity (DTH) reactions differ in many respects from the other forms of hypersensitivity, the major difference being the *lack of dependence on antibody*. DTH cannot be transferred with serum but can be adoptively transferred by T lymphocytes. These are cellular

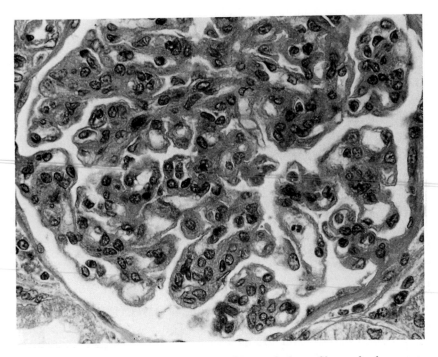

Fig. 5-14 Immune-complex glomerulonephritis: histopathology. Glomerular basement membranes are thickened, and there are adhesions to Bowman's capsule

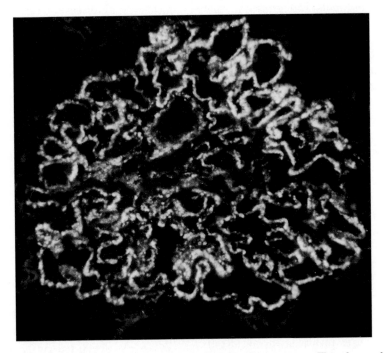

Fig. 5-15 Immune-complex glomerulonephritis: immunofluorescence. This glomerulus shows irregular, lumpy deposits of host IgG. Similar results could be obtained by staining for C3. The immunofluorescence results indicate glomerular deposition of immune complexes. *(Courtesy Dr. R.M. Lewis, Ithaca, N.Y.)*

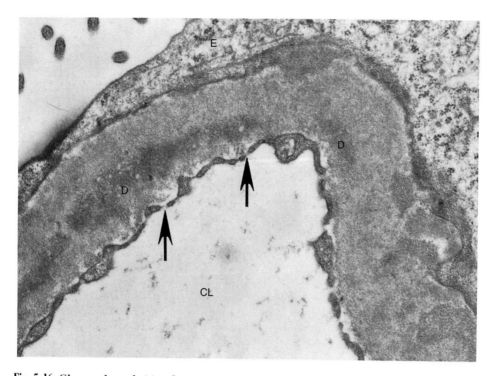

Fig. 5-16 Glomerulonephritis: electron microscopic findings. In this micrograph, there are irregular dense deposits, *D*, within the glomerular basement membrane. These correspond to the irregular pattern seen by immunofluorescence. The epithelial foot processes, *E*, are fused over the basement membrane, a common change in proteinuria. Typical fenestrated glomerular endothelium, *arrows*, lines the capillary lumen, *CL*.

hypersensitivity reactions, with immunological specificity lying in the *sensitized T lymphocyte* rather than in the antibody. The cells and factors central to this type of hypersensitivity are those of a normal immune response and inflammation; as such, many of the mechanisms involved are already familiar. It is not always easy to visualize a clear distinction between delayed-type hypersensitivity (DTH) as an immunopathological process and cell-mediated immunity (CMI) as an expression of host defense. The mechanisms involved are almost identical. It is important to reemphasize that if a reaction proves deleterious to the host it is referred to as a "hypersensitivity reaction" but if the outcome is beneficial it is called an "immune reaction."

The classical example of a DTH response is the tuberculin reaction, which was first demonstrated by Robert Koch in the late 1800s. In trying to develop a vaccine for tuberculosis Koch discovered that a killed tuberculin preparation was not effective in preventing tuberculosis in previously unexposed individuals but could be used in a diagnostic test. Individuals injected intradermally with the tuberculin preparation developed a delayed inflammatory reaction at the injection site if they had been previously exposed to *Mycobacterium tuberculosis*

whether or not they were symptomatic. Since that time, the tuberculin reaction has been extensively studied as a prototypic type IV reaction, and it provides a basis for understanding the molecular and cellular events constituting DTH. Of more clinical importance, however, are the type IV hypersensitivity reactions that lead to chronic granulomatous inflammation, such as infections with mycobacteria, fungi, and protozoa. Allergic contact dermatitis and graft-versus-host disease are other type IV hypersensitivities of clinical importance. The complexity of these immune-mediated mechanisms makes it increasingly difficult to provide a cohesive and workable definition of DTH, but three features are worthy of attention: (1) DTH reactions are antigen-specific immune reactions characterized by tissue infiltration of blood-derived mononuclear cells (lymphocytes, monocytes); (2) DTH reactivity can be transferred between animals or individuals with viable lymphoid cells but not with immune serum; (3) DTH reactions are dependent on T lymphocytes. As the name indicates, DTH reactions usually exhibit a maximum intensity at a delayed time (24 to 72 hours or even more), rather than within a few minutes (type I reactions) or a few hours (type III reactions).

Initiation and Causes of Type IV Hypersensitivity

Initiation of a type IV reaction is dependent on an individual first being sensitized to the offending antigen. The type of antigen and the molecular mechanism of antigen processing within the APC determines whether the antigenic peptides will be presented by MHC class I or class II molecules, which in turn will determine whether the type IV reaction will be mediated primarily by CD4 T cells or CD8 T cells. After initial exposure to an antigen, sensitized T cells remain in a pool of memory cells for months or even years. After reexposure to the antigen, APC cells interact with memory T cells initiating a type IV hypersensitivity reaction resulting in a characteristic inflammatory response.

Antigens that stimulate DTH reactions are often infectious agents that escape killing by the immune system, survive, and multiply in macrophages. Of these, *Mycobacterium tuberculosis* and other *Mycobacterial* spp. are the best recognized. Many other bacteria, nonbacterial infectious agents, and noninfectious agents also may cause type IV hypersensitivity reactions (Table 5-12).

Cells Involved in Type IV Hypersensitivity

CD4 T cells have long been recognized as the primary mediator of type IV reactions, but in recent years it has become clear that CD8 T cells are also important participants. Both CD4 and CD8 T cells have similar capabilities in DTH responses, with both subsets having the potential to be cytotoxic and also capable of secreting cytokine patterns characteristic of CD4 T_H1 and T_H2 cells. The major difference between CD4 and CD8 T cells in DTH responses is that CD4 T cells recognize antigens presented through MHC class II molecules, whereas CD8 T cells recognize antigens presented through MHC class I molecules. Additionally, CD4 T cells tend to secrete higher levels of certain cytokines, especially those that promote antibody production by B cells (IL-4 and IL-5).

The specific type of T cell that is the primary mediator of a DTH reaction is determined by which class of MHC molecules present the offending antigen on the surface of APCs. As previously described, the mode of antigen presentation on the surface of APC is determined by the mechanism of

TABLE 5-12 Antigens and Cellular Mediators of Type IV Hypersensitivity

ANTIGEN	MEDIATOR CELL
Bacteria	
Mycobacterium spp.	**CD4*** and CD8 T cells
Brucella spp.	**CD4** and CD8 T cells
Listeria monocytogenes	**CD4** and CD8 T cells
Fungi	
Blastomyces dermatitidis	CD4 T cells
Cryptococcus neoformans	CD4 T cells
Histoplasma capsulatum	CD4 T cells
Protozoa	
Toxoplasma gondii	CD4 T cells
Leishmania spp.	**CD4** and CD8 T cells
Bacterial toxins	CD4 T cells
Viruses	
Lymphocytic choriomeningitis virus	CD8 T cells
Allergens	
Pollen	CD4 T cells
House dust mites	CD4 T cells
Contact allergens	
Poison ivy (urushiol)	**CD8** and CD4 T cells
Haptens of drugs and industrial and household chemicals	**CD8** and CD4 T cells
Transplantation antigens	**CD8** and CD4 T cells
Tumor-associated antigens	CD8 T cells

*Bold indicates primary T cell involved.

intracellular antigen processing. *Antigens that will be presented through MHC class II molecules* are taken into APC by pinocytosis or phagocytosis and become localized in *intracellular vesicles* that fuse with lysosomes. Included in this group of antigens are extracellular and facultative intracellular bacteria, bacterial toxins, fungi, protozoa, and some allergens. Microorganisms and other antigenic proteins trapped in these intracellular vesicles are degraded by endosomal and lysosomal proteases releasing antigenic peptides that bind to MHC class II molecules for transportation to the cell surface for presentation and recognition by CD4 T cells. *Antigens that will be presented through MHC class I molecules* enter APC and locate in the *cytosol*, where they are degraded by the proteosome complex into antigenic peptides suitable in size for binding to MHC class I molecules. Viruses, some bacteria, transplantation antigens, and tumor-associated antigens are processed in this manner. The antigenic peptides generated by action of the cytosolic proteosome complex are translocated into the lumen of the endoplasmic reticulum where they bind MHC class I molecules and are transported to the cell surface for presentation and recognition by CD8 T cells.

After sensitization of either CD4 or CD8 T cells, reexposure to the sensitizing antigen results in stimulation of memory T cells and the initiation of an inflammatory response characteristic of DTH. The cellular events that characterize a DTH response are best exemplified in the *tuberculin reaction.* By 2 hours after tuberculin injection of a previously sensitized animal, neutrophils begin accumulating around postcapillary venules located in the injection site. Neutrophil accumulations subside by 12 hours and are replaced by perivenular accumulations of a mixture of CD4 and CD8 T cells, blood monocytes, and basophils. Endothelial cells lining the venules swell and become leaky allowing exudation of plasma macromolecules including fibrinogen, which is converted to fibrin. Tissue swelling and induration at the injection site result from edema, fibrin deposition, and infiltrating cells and reach a maximum in 24 to 72 hours. Many of the cells infiltrating DTH lesions are macrophages derived from blood monocytes that are attracted to the site and activated by cytokines. In areas of a chronic DTH response, macrophages become the dominant cell type present with lesser numbers of lymphocytes, most of which are nonspecific but with a few being antigen-specific CD4 or CD8 T cells. The morphological appearance of macrophages in these areas may change as their primary

function changes from phagocytosis to secretion. Secreting macrophages become elongated with eccentric nuclei and more abundant eosinophilic cytoplasm causing them to resemble epithelial cells. These cells are called *epithelioid cells,* but it is important to remember that they are really modified macrophages. Other macrophages may fuse to form multinucleated giant cells. A DTH lesion resulting from the focal accumulation of epithelioid cells, giant cells, macrophages, and lymphocytes is called a *granuloma* (Fig. 5-17).

Allergic contact dermatitis (ACD) is a typical example of a cutaneous type IV hypersensitivity that has been recognized in dogs, horses, and rarely cats. The initiating substances are haptens, which by themselves are not immunogenic but may bind to cell-associated or extracellular proteins in the epidermis to initiate an allergic reaction. Poison ivy is a well-recognized cause of ACD in humans, whereas relatively simple chemicals such as formaldehyde, aniline dyes, organophosphate insecticides, topical medications such as neomycin, and chemicals, such as the salts of nickel and cobalt, may cause ACD in humans and animals. The understanding of the pathogenesis of allergic contact dermatitis has shifted in recent years, with more and more evidence being presented indicating that CD8 T cells, rather than CD4 T cells, are the primary cellular mediators. Langerhans' cells are generally considered to be the primary APC in the epidermis and typically present antigens through MHC class II molecules. However, in ACD reactions, hapten-modified self-proteins are presented in the context of MHC class I molecules resulting in the activation of CD8 T cells. It is not clear which APC is responsible for ACD antigen presentation through MHC class I molecules. Langerhans' cells may present antigens through both MHC class I and II molecules, or alternatively an epidermal cell functions as an APC. The *keratinocyte* is the candidate epidermal APC because it is capable of presenting antigens through both MHC class I and II molecules.

The involvement of CD8 T cells in ACD is best exemplified in the human T-cell response to urushiol, the immunogen of poison ivy. Oxidation of urushiol results in formation of intermediates that bind to extracellular or intracellular proteins making them antigenic and promoting their processing for presentation through MHC class I and II molecules. The urushiol hapten is small and lipid soluble allowing it to cross the cell membrane for cytosol processing and presentation by MHC class I molecules. This ability of urushiol to cross cell membranes and enter the cytosol of epidermal cells for

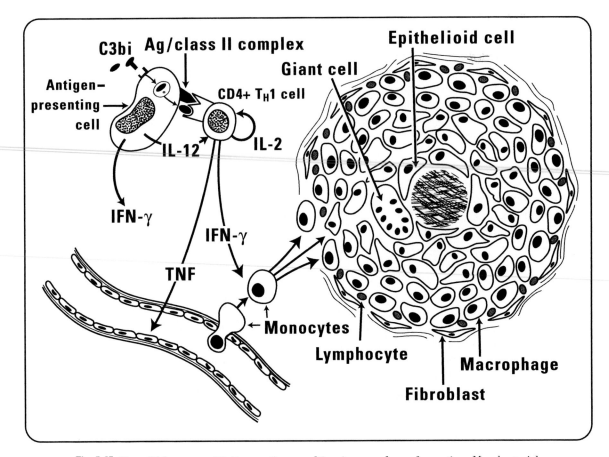

Fig. 5-17 Type IV hypersensitivity reaction resulting in granuloma formation. Mycobacterial or similar bacterial antigen is presented through MHC class II molecules to sensitized CD4 T_H1 cells. Antigen-presenting cells secrete IL-12 and IFN-γ. IL-12 promotes T_H1 differentiation, and IFN-γ inhibits T_H2 differentiation. CD4 T_H1 cells secrete self-promoting IL-2 and IFN-γ. In addition, CD4 T_H1 cells secrete TNF-α and -β, which act in concert with IFN-γ to promote vasodilatation, increased vascular permeability, and leukocyte recruitment. Recruited monocytes differentiate into macrophages, which may further differentiate into epithelioid cells or fuse to form multinucleated giant cells. The focal collection of macrophages, epithelioid cells, and giant cells with accompanying lymphocytes is called a "granuloma." *(Adapted from Cotran RS et al, editors: Robbins pathologic basis of disease, ed 6, Philadelphia, 1999, Saunders.)*

processing and presentation in a MHC class I context is the most likely explanation for IFN-γ secreting CD8 T cells, rather than CD4 T cells being the primary mediators of poison ivy dermatitis. In somewhat of a role reversal, CD4 T cells apparently function more as inhibitory than stimulatory cells in the poison ivy reaction, secreting a T_H2 cytokine profile than tends to dampen the ACD reaction. Besides secreting T_H2 cytokines in the ACD reaction, CD4 T cells may also function as cytotoxic cells potentially destroying any cell expressing MHC class I molecules.

Graft rejection is another disease in which DTH contributes significantly to the disease process and is most typically encountered after allogeneic (genetically dissimilar individuals of same species) tissue grafts. The primary histocompatibility antigens stimulating the rejection reaction are MHC class I and II molecules and the major blood group glycoproteins. The microscopic appearance of a rejected allograft often is similar to that of a tuberculin reaction. Graft rejections may be mediated by CD8 T cells, CD4 T_H1 cells, or both cell types. If the graft recipient has been previously exposed to donor antigens (such as regraft of tissue from the same donor), antibodies can also contribute to the rejection reaction.

Presentation of transplant alloantigens to the recipient's T lymphocytes is believed to occur in two ways. First, donor APC expressing alloantigens migrate from the graft to the recipient's regional lymph nodes, where they interact with host T cells expressing alloreactive receptors. Recipient T cells activated by the alloantigens migrate back to the graft directly attacking the graft tissue. Secondly, recipient APC take up and process alloantigens from the graft and present these antigens through self MHC class I and II molecules. Recipient T cells expressing alloreactive receptors interact with the alloantigens presented by APCs and become activated. These activated T cells migrate to the graft to participate in graft rejection. The immune response in most instances will be directed against MHC class I alloantigens resulting in CD8 T cells being the primary mediator of most rejection reactions.

Mediators of Type IV Hypersensitivity

When a sensitized animal is reexposed to an antigen, dendritic cells in the area of exposure will capture and process antigen for presentation through either MHC class I or II molecules. Antigen capture and processing stimulates DCs to migrate to T-cell areas of mucosal and peripheral lymphoid tissues. Within the lymphoid tissues, the dendritic cells interact with antigen-sensitized memory CD8 or CD4 T cells. When a bacterial or similar antigen is presented through MHC class II molecules, the DCs secrete IL-12 and IFN-γ just as macrophages and NK cells do in the area. IL-12 is a potent inducer of T_H1 cells, whereas IFN-γ inhibits T_H2-cell differentiation. Additionally, newly formed activated T_H1 cells secrete IL-2 and IFN-γ, further promoting T_H1 differentiation (see Fig. 5-17). If a viral antigen initiates the DTH response, presentation of antigen to CD8 T cells occurs through MHC class I molecules on the surface of APC. Similar to CD4 T_H1 cells, the naïve CD8 T cells, under the influence of IL-12 and IFN-γ, differentiate into a CD8 T-cell subset that secretes a cytokine profile similar to that produced by CD4 T_H1 cells. Further, if naïve CD8 T cells are exposed to IL-4, IL-6, and IL-10, they will differentiate into a subset of CD8 T cells that secrete a cytokine profile similar to that of CD4 T_H2 cells. In summary, the type of T cell that mediates a hypersensitivity reaction is determined for the most part by the type of antigen causing the reaction and the profile of cytokines released during the T- cell differentiation stage. Antigens normally presented through MHC class I molecules sometimes also can be presented through MHC class II molecules and vice versa. Therefore, in some type IV reactions both CD4 T cells and CD8 T cells can participate in the reaction with one or the other cell type dominating. In some cases, this results from antigen processing through both intracytoplasmic vesicles and the cytosol, and in other situations the reason is unknown. Regardless, such redundancy is typical of the immune system.

Although activated T cells and DCs secrete a variety of cytokines that can attract neutrophils and monocytes to the inflammatory sites, it is more likely that *endothelial cell activation* and secretion is responsible for the early inflammatory events of a DTH response. T-cell secretion of TNF-α and TNF-β stimulates endothelial cells in postcapillary venules to produce prostacyclin, which in turn causes vasodilatation and increased blood flow promoting delivery of immune cells to the DTH site. TNF-α and IFN-γ acting in concert stimulate remodeling of endothelial cell basement membranes allowing extravasation of plasma proteins, especially fibrinogen. As a result of fluid and protein loss plus vasodilatation, blood flow slows allowing leukocytes in the bloodstream greater opportunity to interact with endothelial cell surfaces. There is an upregulation of the adhesion molecules E-selectin, VCAM-1, and ICAM-1 on endothelial cells, promoting adhesion of neutrophils, lymphocytes, and macrophages. In addition, the activated endothelial cells secrete IL-8 and MCP-1, which attract neutrophils and macrophages to the inflammatory site. Once cells have been recruited to a DTH site, the cause-and-effect relationships are less clear. Numerous cytokines and inflammatory mediators may participate in DTH reactions. Included are IL-1 to -6, IL-8, IL-10, IL-12, GM-CSF, PGE₂, TNF-α, TGF-β, and IFN-α, -β, -γ. Of these, IFN-γ and TNF-α are the most important.

DISEASES OF THE IMMUNE SYSTEM

Not all diseases associated with the immune system result from immune-mediated tissue injury. Equally important are diseases that result from the immune system failing to provide normal protective functions. These diseases may be inherited or acquired or result from the immune system inappropriately reacting against self-antigens. The inability to mount an appropriate immune response after antigenic stimulation can result from defects of any part of the delicately balanced immune system. Defects in antigen presentation may occur if mononuclear phagocyte function is altered; disturbances of antigen recognition and stimulation of B cells or cytotoxic cells can result from defective T cells; and insufficient or inappropriate antibody production may ensue if B-cell function is modified. Immunodeficiency diseases are subdivided into primary disorders that are *inherited*, or have a genetic predisposition, and secondary disorders that are *acquired* as a result of infections or exposure to certain environmental toxins and drugs. When the normally functioning immune system is tricked into reacting against autoantigens (self-antigens), an *autoimmune disease* ensues.

Primary Immunodeficiency Diseases

The *Chédiak-Higashi syndrome* (CHS) is a potentially fatal autosomal recessive genetic disorder that is associated with severe immunological deficiency, partial albinism, ocular abnormalities, and a mild bleeding tendency. Giant intracellular granules, which are abnormal lysosomes or secretory granules, are present in neutrophils and other granulocytes, monocytes, and lymphocytes. In addition, melanocytes contain giant, abnormal melanosomes. CHS affects humans, cattle (Hereford, Japanese black, Brangus), Persian cats, Aleutian mink, beige mice, rats, foxes, white tigers, and killer whales. Immunological deficits in animals with CHS are multiple. The neutrophils and monocytes of affected animals have decreased migration and chemotactic responses. Phagocytosis by leukocytes is normal, but the intracellular killing of microorganisms is delayed. NK-cell function is also impaired as a result of defective cytotoxic activity. There is a loss of CD8 T-cell cytotoxicity, but B-cell functions remain normal. As a result of these defects, there is a heightened susceptibility to microbial infections and an increased incidence of lymphoproliferative disorders. The biological defect responsible for CHS is not known, but the tendency for the abnormal lysosomes and melanosomes to be located in the perinuclear region of cells rather than being more widely distributed in the cytoplasm indicates that there may be a defect in the maturation of these organelles. The molecular basis for CHS has been shown to be one or more mutational defects in the CHS1 gene in humans, beige mice, and Japanese black cattle. CHS1 gene products are believed to be required, in some common way, for the genesis, structure, and function of a variety of intracellular organelles including lysosomes, intracellular secretory granules, and melanosomes. Presumably, CHS1 gene defects are also responsible for CHS in other animals.

Leukocyte adhesion deficiency (LAD) is an autosomal recessive disorder that occurs in Irish setters, Holstein cattle, and humans. The clinical syndrome in dogs and cattle is characterized by persistent neutrophilia, recurrent infections associated with poor growth performance, poor wound healing, and a deficiency or absence of pus in inflammatory sites despite a striking blood neutrophilia. Affected calves

usually die before 1 year of age. The biochemical basis of LAD is an inherited deficiency of the cell-surface adhesion molecule belonging to the *integrin* family. Each integrin consists of a noncovalently linked, heterodimeric α- and β-chain. The genetic defect responsible for LAD occurs in the β_2-integrin subfamily. There are three heterodimeric glycoproteins within this subfamily that share a common β subunit designated β_2 (CD18). The α subunits of each of the heterodimers are lymphocyte function–associated antigen-1 (LFA-1), macrophage antigen-1 (Mac-1), and p150,95, designated CD11a, CD11b, and CD11c respectively. LAD results from point mutations in the gene coding CD18 resulting in diminished or failed expression of CD18 and therefore failure of formation of the CD18/CD11a-c heterodimers. Of these, the lack of CD18/CD11a and CD18/CD11b are most important for normal leukocyte responses to infectious diseases. In cattle, the point mutation in CD18 results in an absence of CD18/CD11b. As a result, the neutrophilic response to infection is impaired because circulating neutrophils cannot bind to the intercellular adhesion molecules expressed on the surface of endothelial cells and therefore are unable to leave the bloodstream. Additionally, since CD11b (Mac-1) is a receptor for C3bi, opsonized particles cannot be properly phagocytized.

Severe combined immunodeficiency (SCID) is a disorder of humans, Arabian foals, dogs, and mice caused by a complete failure of antigen-specific immune responses. The most thoroughly documented example of SCID in domestic animals is an autosomal recessive disorder that occurs in both male and female Arabian foals. Affected foals are clinically normal at birth and remain so until 1 to 3 months of age when they lose protection provided by colostral maternal immunoglobulins. The loss of passive immunity combined with the inability to immunologically respond to antigens makes foals highly vulnerable to infectious agents that primarily target the respiratory system or the gastrointestinal tract. Equine adenovirus is the most significant pathogen of SCID foals, with *Cryptosporidium parvum*, *Pneumocystis carinii*, and *Rhodococcus equi* also being commonly involved. Foals infected with one of these agents usually die by 5 months of age. The immunologically deficient foals have severe lymphopenia (<1000 lymphocytes/μl blood), and IgM cannot be detected in the serum after 26 days of age. The molecular basis of SCID in Arabian foals recently was determined to be related to defective receptor gene rearrangements in B and T cells. During maturation of B and T cells, a programmed series of receptor gene rearrangements is required for the development of mature B and T cells, which have functional antigen-specific receptors. One of the enzymes that is required for receptor gene rearrangement is DNA-dependent protein kinase (DNA-PK). This enzyme is composed of three subunit proteins, one of which is the DNA-PK catalytic subunit (DNA-PK$_{cs}$). A mutation in the gene encoding DNA-PK$_{cs}$ results in a five-base-pair deletion causing a frame shift and premature formation of a stop codon. Without functional DNA-PK$_{cs}$, there is a lack of DNA-PK activity preventing receptor gene rearrangement in precursor B and T cells resulting in the absence of mature, functional T and B cells.

X-linked SCID has been described in Bassett hounds and a Cardigan Welsh corgi. The disease is characterized by a failure to grow normally, hypogammaglobulinemia, thymic dysplasia, T cells that do not respond to mitogenic stimuli, and increased susceptibility to infection. The X-chromosome inherited defect results from a mutation in the gene encoding the γ-chain of the IL-2 receptor (IL-2Rγ). The same γ-chain is also a component of the IL-4, IL-7, IL-9, and IL-15 receptors. T-cell numbers may be nearly normal in affected dogs, and their ability to produce IL-2 is not impaired. However, the genetically induced receptor defect renders T cells unable to bind and respond to IL-2. The genetic defect causing X-linked SCID in Bassett hounds and Welsh corgis involves the same gene, but the site of mutation in the γ-chain gene is different in each breed.

Agammaglobulinemia has been described in male horses (Thoroughbred, Quarter Horse, and Standardbred) that lack mature B cells and plasma cells and do not produce antibodies after antigenic stimulation. A defect in the differentiation of B cells has been suggested to be the cause of this disorder. Affected foals have recurrent bacterial infections but survive up to 19 months of age with passive antibody and antibiotic therapy because T cells functions are intact.

Selective immunoglobulin deficiencies also have been observed in several animal species. Included is a selective IgG2 deficiency in red Danish cattle, a selective IgA deficiency in dogs (German shepherd, beagle, shar pei), and a selective IgM deficiency in foals.

Thymic hypoplasia and *altered lymphocyte functions* have been described in black pied Danish cattle of Frisian descent with autosomal recessive zinc deficiency *(lethal strain A 46)*. Affected calves are normal at birth but develop diarrhea and later severe parakeratotic skin lesions as plasma zinc levels diminish below 0.5 ppm at 2 to 6 weeks of age.

Lymphocyte numbers and function in these calves are normal at birth and remain so until plasma zinc levels decrease below normal. Zinc supplementation can prevent or partially restore the lymphocyte disorders in affected calves. Zinc deficiency is caused by the inability to absorb zinc from the gastrointestinal tract possibly as a result of a mutation in a gene that encodes a cysteine-rich intestinal protein that is involved in zinc absorption from the intestinal tract. Thymic hypoplasia and altered lymphocyte functions are believed to evolve from a zinc deficiency manifest as an induced deficiency of a zinc-containing DNA polymerase that is found primarily in the thymus and thymocytes and required for their normal development and function.

Acquired Immunodeficiency Diseases

Intense interest in acquired immunodeficiency diseases of animals has evolved from the worldwide attention focused for the past 20 years on the devastating effects of acquired immunodeficiency syndrome (AIDS) in humans. AIDS occurs as a consequence of infection with the *human immunodeficiency virus* (HIV), a lentivirus in the Retroviridae family that specifically infects cells expressing CD4 cell-surface molecules. These include T cells, the monocyte/macrophage lineage of cells, and dendritic cells. HIV infection of these cells begins with the binding of HIV envelope glycoprotein 120 (gp120) to CD4 molecules on the surface of susceptible cells. However, this initial interaction of HIV gp120 with CD4 molecules does not result in fusion of the viral and cellular membranes. For this to occur, a second molecule or *coreceptor* on the surface of cells being infected must interact with gp120 as it binds CD4 molecules. Recently, two chemokine receptors have been identified as the primary coreceptors for gp120 on CD4+ cells. The chemokine receptor CXCR4 is the coreceptor for gp120 on T cells, and the chemokine receptor CCR5 serves a similar coreceptor function on monocytes/macrophages. These two chemokine receptor molecules are not only critical for HIV infection of cells but also define the tropism of different strains of HIV for specific cell types. Some strains of HIV-1 selectively bind CXCR4 receptors specifically expressed on T cells (T-tropic), whereas other strains bind CCR5 receptors expressed on monocytes/macrophages (M-tropic). Some M-tropic strains of HIV can also infect T cells. Although CXCR4 and CCR5 are the primary coreceptors for HIV, the list of other chemokine receptors that have coreceptor functions grows. The importance of the coreceptor function of chemokine molecules in facilitating HIV infection of susceptible cells is emphasized by the finding that individuals who carry a mutation in the gene encoding CCR5 have a defective receptor protein and are resistant to HIV infection.

HIV may adversely affect lymphocytes in a variety of ways. HIV may directly kill CD4+ T cells, progenitor CD4+/CD8+ cells and immature CD8+ thymocytes. Infected CD4+ T cells may be trapped in lymphoid tissues or killed by CD8+ HIV–specific T cells. Uninfected T cells may be killed as a result of fusing with infected cells resulting in the formation of short-lived multinucleated syncytial giant cells. In addition, HIV infection may cause downregulation of CD4 expression on infected T cells.

Clinical expression of AIDS may not occur for years after HIV infection. In the first few days after infection, large quantities of HIV are produced in activated lymphocytes in lymph nodes possibly causing lymphadenopathy in addition to "flulike" symptoms. An asymptomatic phase of infection ensues for variable time periods. Some individuals will show signs of disease progression and develop AIDS in the first 2 to 3 years after HIV infection. Those who survive longer usually develop AIDS by 10 years after infection, with a few surviving even longer. The onset of fatal illnesses is associated with an increased virus burden and a decline in CD4+ T-cell numbers to below 200 cells/μl of blood. Opportunistic infections and neoplasms emerge and are usually the cause of death. Some of the infections more commonly encountered in AIDS patients include *Pneumocystis carinii*, *Toxoplasma gondii*, adenovirus, cytomegalovirus, *Cryptosporidium* spp., *Candida*, *Cryptococcus neoformans*, *Histoplasma*, *Bartonella*, and *Legionella*. An increased incidence of Kaposi's sarcoma, B-cell lymphomas, cervical carcinomas, and other forms of malignancy is also observed

The identification of HIV as the cause of a devastating immunodeficiency syndrome in humans has stimulated considerable interest in research on animal retroviral diseases that can produce immunodeficiency and potentially serve as models for the human disease (Table 5-13). Some of the best-characterized acquired immunodeficiencies in domestic animals occur in cats infected with either the feline leukemia virus (FeLV), the feline immunodeficiency virus (FIV), or both viruses. Dual infections are common in cats and cause more severe and rapid disease than caused by infection with either virus alone. *Feline leukemia virus* is a mammalian type C retrovirus responsible for the development of several different diseases in cats including immunodeficiency, aplastic anemia, and neoplasia. Lymphoma, myeloproliferative diseases, and fibrosarcoma are the most common neoplastic disorders encountered in FeLV-infected cats, whereas the more common immune dysfunctions include lymphopenia, neutropenia, and impaired T- and B-lymphocyte functions. FeLV is grouped into three related, genetically nonidentical interference subgroups (FeLV-A, -B, and -C). There have recently been identified T cell–tropic cytopathic variants of FeLV (FeLV-T) that induce immunological deficiencies and possibly belong to a fourth subgroup. An inorganic phosphate transporter protein (PiT-1) functions as a viral receptor for FeLV-B and -T. In addition, a coreceptor, which may be fixed or soluble, has been identified for FeLV-T and named FeLIX (FeLV infectivity X-essory [accessory] protein).

TABLE 5-13 Animal Models of Acquired Immune Deficiency Syndrome

VIRUS	RECEPTOR	CORECEPTOR	HOST INFECTED	PRIMARY CELL TYPE INFECTED	CLINICAL DISORDER
Feline immuno-deficiency virus	CXCR4		Cat	T lymphocytes	Immune deficiency Encephalopathy
Feline leukemia virus			Cat	T lymphocytes	Immune deficiency Anemia
FeLV-B	PiT-1				Neoplasia
FeLV-T	PiT-1	FeLIX			
Murine leukemia virus			Mouse	T and B lymphocytes	Immune deficiency Hypergamma-globulinemia
Ecotropic	mCAT-1				Lymphadenopathy
Simian immuno-deficiency virus	CD4	CCR5	Primate	T lymphocytes	Immune deficiency Encephalopathy

Adapted from Levy JA: *HIV and the pathogenesis of AIDS*, ed 2, Washington, DC, 1998, ASM Press.
FeLIX, FeLV infectivity X-essory [accessory] protein; *mCAT-1*, mouse cationic amino acid transporter; *PiT-1*, nonorganic phosphate transporter.

Feline immunodeficiency virus is a lentivirus that preferentially infects CD4+ T cells during primary infection. In later stages of infection, FIV targets B cells and can also infect CD8+ T cells and macrophages. Unlike HIV, the feline immunodeficiency virus does not apparently use the CD4 molecule as a receptor for infecting cells because FIV readily infects non-CD4+ immune cells as well as CD4+ cells. Recent findings indicate that the CXCR4 chemokine receptor is the primary cellular receptor for FIV. Signs of primary FIV infection are more commonly seen in young cats and include lymphadenopathy, fever, and neutropenia associated with high levels of viral RNA in the plasma and diminished CD4+ T-cell numbers. Cats surviving primary infection enter a stage of chronic, asymptomatic infection that may last for several years. The onset of terminal stages of FIV infection are associated with a decline in CD4+ cell numbers, a decrease in the CD4:CD8 T-cell ratio, and functional abnormalities of T and B cells. Signs of chronic disease resulting from FIV infection include appetite and weight loss, recurrent fever, increased incidence of opportunistic infections, bone marrow disorders, neurological disorders, and an increased incidence of neoplasia, especially of B-cell lymphomas and myeloproliferative diseases.

Other Acquired Immunodeficiencies

In addition to the retroviral diseases, which cause AIDS-like immunodeficiency syndromes, many other infectious agents have been shown to be immunosuppressive. Organisms that belong to this group are canine distemper virus (in dogs), infectious bursal disease virus and Newcastle disease virus in chickens, feline parvovirus, bovine viral diarrhea virus (in cattle), African swine fever virus (in pigs), equine herpesvirus 1, and the ectoparasite *Demodex*. Certain environmental toxins may also have a suppressive effect on the immune system. These include polychlorinated biphenyls, polybrominated biphenyls, dieldrin, iodine, lead, cadmium, methylmercury, and DDT. Additionally, the T2 toxin from the fungus *Fusarium* that grows in moldy hay depresses the immune system. Many drugs including corticosteroids, cyclosporin A, and cyclophosphamide have been used to induce immunosuppression as part of the therapy for certain diseases.

AUTOIMMUNE DISEASES

Autoimmunity is defined as an antigen-specific immune response *against self-tissue antigens (autoantigens),* which can lead to an *autoimmune disease* characterized by chronic inflammation and severe tissue injury. Autoimmune diseases are severe, often crippling, or even fatal diseases that occur in many different species. The number of self-antigens involved in the pathogenesis of autoimmune diseases is small but consistent from disease to disease. Much has been learned about disease pathogenesis, but in most circumstances a specific cause of an autoimmune disease cannot be identified.

Immune responses to foreign antigens usually result in the elimination of antigen. However, when immune responses are directed against self-antigens, it is almost impossible to completely eliminate these autoantigens, resulting in sustained responses that manifest as chronic inflammatory disease. Like most diseases, the mechanisms of tissue injury in autoimmune diseases are not unique but involve cellular functions and biochemical pathways that are involved in normal immune responses and hypersensitivity diseases.

The immune system of healthy individuals is considered to be *self-tolerant* because it can distinguish between self- and nonself-antigens and does not mount an immune response against self-antigens. When this normal state is somehow perturbed, humoral or cell-mediated immune responses can develop against self-antigens. However, autoimmune disease does not always occur as a result of immune responses to self-antigens. Of all the proteins that may serve as self-antigens, few do so because most are not produced in sufficient quantities to stimulate effector lymphocyte responses. As a result, many clinically normal animals may have autoantibodies present in their serum or experience transient autoimmune responses unassociated with disease expression.

When sufficient quantities of self-antigens are produced, self-reactive lymphocytes that might participate in autoimmune responses against them are either eliminated during development in the central lymphoid organs or rendered nonfunctional, or *anergic,* in the peripheral lymphoid tissues. Most self-reactive lymphocytes are eliminated in the thymus or bone marrow by clonal depletion. Clonal depletion occurs when the receptors of developing self-reactive lymphocytes bind self-antigens presented through self-MHC molecules on the surface of APCs. In the thymus, developing T cells bind self-antigens expressed on bone marrow–derived dendritic cells and macrophages and less frequently, thymic epithelial cells. Receptor binding of these self-peptides triggers the onset of apoptosis leading to thymic lymphocyte death. Similarly, binding of self-peptides to newly expressed IgM on developing B lymphocytes in the bone marrow causes these cells to either die immediately as a result of apoptosis or become nonfunctional.

Not all self-reactive T and B cells are eliminated during development in the thymus and bone marrow. Most of those that escape the central lymphoid organs are rendered anergic when they encounter self-proteins in peripheral tissues. Outside of the central lymphoid organs, self-peptides are presented through MHC class I molecules on the surface of the tissue cells in which they are made. Since these antigen-presenting tissue cells are unable to provide the costimulatory signals needed to activate naïve cells, the self-reactive T cells are not stimulated to produce IL-2 and as a result do not proliferate and differentiate into effector cells. These anergic T cells remain nonfunctional even when they subsequently encounter antigen presented by professional APC with costimulatory capabilities.

Self-reactive naïve B cells that arrive in the peripheral lymphoid tissues can be eliminated or inactivated by several mechanisms. B cells that recognize self-antigens without the assistance of activated helper CD4 T cells become unable to migrate out of the T-cell zone in peripheral lymphoid tissues and eventually die as a result of apoptosis. Other self-reactive B cells may complex with activated T cells having specificity for the same self-peptide facilitating the binding of Fas ligand on T cells with Fas on B cells triggering apoptosis of the B cells. Additionally, self-reactive B cells that bind soluble circulating self-proteins may be rendered nonfunctional as a result of the downregulation of surface IgM expression and the blockage of B cell–signaling pathways.

Mechanisms of Injury Associated with Autoimmunity

As previously mentioned, the presence of autoantibodies does not always correlate with the occurrence of autoimmune disease. A variety of disease processes may result in the formation of autoantibodies, and the clinician and pathologist often struggle to determine if the autoantibodies are part of an autoimmune disease response or are clinically insignificant. For example, in any disease with tissue damage there may be secondary development of autoantibodies. Post–myocardial infarction patients often develop antimyocardial autoantibodies, but a "heart attack" is not considered to be an autoimmune disease. Similarly, patients with severe burns may develop antibodies directed against previously hidden keratinocyte epitopes in the skin. Another example of this type of "autoimmunity" occurs in vasectomized males who develop antisperm antibodies after surgery. These examples emphasize that autoantibodies produced in association with a disease process are not always a cause of the disease

but can be an effect of the disease. In a true autoimmune disease, autoantibodies bind self-antigens precipitating disease mechanisms that result in lesions characteristic of the disease; that is, a cause-and-effect relationship can be demonstrated. Despite the difficulties associated with establishing such a cause-and-effect relationship, the demonstration of circulating or *in vivo* bound autoantibodies by immunohistochemical or immunofluorescence techniques remains an important diagnostic tool for autoimmune diseases, especially when used in combination with appropriate clinical signs and histopathological lesions (Figs. 5-18 to 5-20).

Mechanisms of Autoimmune Diseases

The clonal depletion of T and B cells in the central lymphoid organs and the inactivation or elimination of self-reactive lymphocytes in peripheral lymphoid tissues are very efficient processes. Autoimmune diseases do not result from a failure of these protective processes but rather involve other complex processes for which several induction mechanisms have been proposed (Table 5-14). The situation *in vivo* may be even further complicated by the fact that the tissue injury in any given autoimmune disease may actually result from multiple mechanisms and multiple pathogenetic schemes.

One induction mechanism for which there is substantial evidence involves the *exposure of anatomically or molecularly sequestered antigens*, that is, antigens that do not normally encounter circulating lymphocytes and therefore are not recognized as self-antigens. Tissue damage caused by inflammation or trauma may disrupt cell or tissue barriers exposing antigens previously *anatomically* hidden from the immune system. Such an example is post-traumatic uveitis that can result from rupture of the lens capsule releasing previously sequestered lenticular proteins. Another example is the formation of antisperm antibodies in vasectomized men, even though they do not necessarily cause autoimmune disease. Milk allergy that has been described in Jersey cattle and the demyelination in human multiple sclerosis may be caused, at least in part, by exposure of previously sequestered antigens.

Even more commonly, inflammatory or traumatic tissue damage causes exposure of self-antigens *molecularly sequestered* in proteins. The tertiary structure of self-proteins allows exposure of only a few epitopes that participate in the clonal deletion or inactivation of self-reactive lymphocytes. Configurational alteration of such proteins as a result of tissue damage or other unknown factors may result in the *exposure of molecularly hidden epitopes*. These

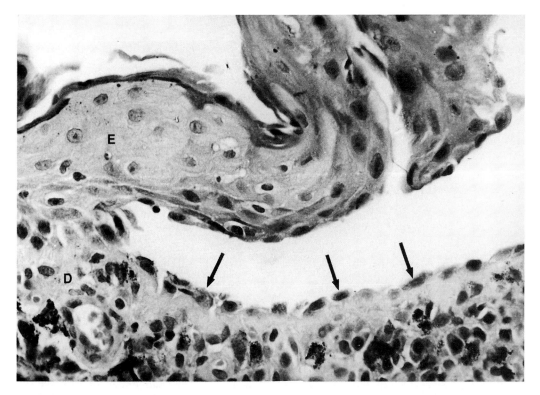

Fig. 5-18 Pemphigus vulgaris. Seven-year-old male poodle with a 4-month history of crusting, ulcerative lesions at mucocutaneous junctions and in the oral cavity. Histological section of skin with cleft formation above the basal cell layer. Basal cells on the basement membrane, *arrows*, are intact, whereas suprabasilar epithelial cells have lifted off forming a suprabasilar vesicle. *D*, Dermis; *E*, epidermis.

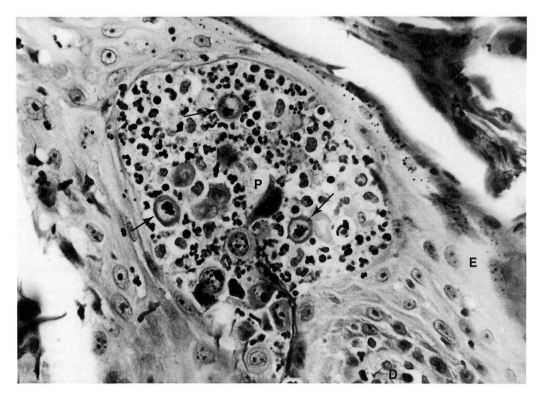

Fig. 5-19 Pemphigus vulgaris. Same dog as Fig. 5-18. Histological section of an intraepidermal pustule, *P*, containing many acantholytic cells (detached, rounded epidermal cells), *arrows*, and abundant neutrophils. *D*, Dermis; *E*, epidermis.

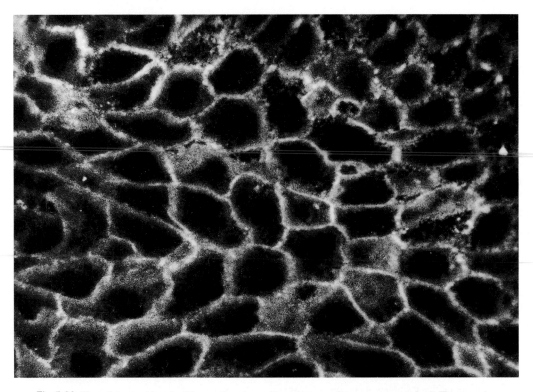

Fig. 5-20 Pemphigus vulgaris. Diagnosis using a direct immunofluorescence method. Fluorescein-labeled rabbit anticanine IgG reveals autoantibody bound to desmosomal desmoglein-3 of keratinocytes creating a distinct pattern of immunofluorescence staining in the perilesional epidermis.

TABLE 5-14 Proposed Induction Mechanisms for Autoimmunity

MECHANISM	MEDIATORS
Exposure of anatomically sequestered antigens	Brain, spermatozoa, and lenticular antigens Milk α-casein
Exposure of molecularly sequestered antigens	IgG molecule in rheumatoid arthritis, immunoconglutinins, erythrocyte band 3 protein
Molecular mimicry	*Streptococcal* antibodies against kidney, joint, heart antigens *Mycoplasma hyopneumoniae* antibodies against normal pig lung *Mycoplasma mycoides* antibodies against normal bovine lung T cells against self-peptides
Induced expression of costimulatory activity by antigen-presenting cells	Various infectious agents
Polyclonal activation of T cells	Bacterial, viral, and mycoplasma-induced superantigens
Loss of suppressor T cells	Unknown

newly exposed epitopes may incite novel autoimmune reactions or perpetuate ongoing autoimmune responses. Molecular exposure of previously sequestered epitopes is one of the mechanisms proposed for the continual formation of antibodies to IgG in human rheumatoid arthritis.

Another mechanism for inducing autoimmune diseases is *molecular mimicry* in which antibodies and T cells generated in response to viral, bacterial, or mycoplasmal infections cross-react with peptides of self-proteins. A well-known example of molecular mimicry occurs in humans when antibodies produced in response to infection with some streptococcal species cross-react with kidney, joint, and heart antigens to produce rheumatic fever. In enzootic pneumonia of swine, antibodies to *Mycoplasma hyopneumoniae* have been shown to cross-react with porcine lung tissue. Similar cross-reactivity has also been demonstrated in contagious bovine pleuropneumonia between *Mycoplasma mycoides* antibodies and normal bovine lung tissue. In these latter examples, it is not clear, however, if these antibodies are involved in the development of lesions. More recently, an increasing body of evidence has been presented to indicate that some natural infections may stimulate the generation of destructive T cells that cross-react with self-peptides to cause tissue injury.

Another possible mechanism for breaking tolerance is *the induction of costimulatory activity* by tissue antigen-presenting cells that do not normally provide this function. Induced expression of costimulatory activity may occur as a result of inflammation and tissue damage caused by infectious agents or by other unknown mechanisms. *Polyclonal activation of T cells by superantigens* may be another mechanism that triggers autoimmune disease. Superantigens are molecules produced by a variety of pathogens including bacteria, mycoplasmas, and viruses that are capable of nonspecifically binding MHC class II molecules on antigen-presenting cells to antigen receptors on selected populations of T cells. Superantigen binding activates these T cells to produce large quantities of cytokines. If anergic, self-reactive T cells are among the population of T cells stimulated by a given superantigen, it is possible that an autoimmune reaction might ensue. Such a pathogenesis is proposed for some cases of type I diabetes in humans. The *loss of suppressor T cells* that can limit the activity of self-reactive T and B cells is another proposed mechanism for autoimmune diseases. However, definitive proof that such a mechanism contributes to autoimmune diseases is still lacking.

Clearly, multiple complicated pathways can lead to autoimmune reactions, but the factors truly important in initiating these aberrant responses remain largely unknown. Viruses and other infectious agents may trigger autoimmune diseases, but it is still not clear why and under what circumstances they may cause autoimmune disease in one individual but not in another individual of the same species. One of the factors influencing the occurrence of autoimmune diseases is *genetics*. In both humans and domestic animals, there is a tendency for familial clustering of selected autoimmune diseases indicating a genetic component in their pathogenesis. The most important genes that regulate the development of autoimmunity are located within the major histocompatibility complex. Of these, the ones that encode the MHC class II molecules are the most important in determining the genetic predisposition of an individual to autoimmune diseases. The occurrence of autoimmune diseases is linked to the expression of certain alleles on the MHC class II locus or to combinations of alleles in different regions of the same locus or different loci. However, gene expression is only one factor contributing to the occurrence of autoimmune diseases because many individuals expressing a susceptibility-related gene never develop disease, whereas other individuals that do not express susceptibility-related genes develop autoimmune diseases. Systemic lupus erythematosus (SLE), autoimmune hemolytic anemia, autoimmune thyroiditis, rheumatoid arthritis, myasthenia gravis, and pemphigus are linked to certain genes or combinations of genes in humans, whereas diabetes mellitus, SLE, and autoimmune polyarthritis are associated with certain genes in dogs.

Classification of Autoimmune Diseases

Autoimmune diseases can be classified in several ways. One approach is to subdivide them into two distinct groups according to the distribution of self-antigens involved in the diseases. One group includes organ-specific autoimmune diseases in which the self-antigens and lesions are essentially localized to a given organ or cell type. Examples include autoimmune thyroiditis, pemphigus, myasthenia gravis, and autoimmune hemolytic anemia. In the other group, self-antigens are widespread throughout the body and may actually circulate in the bloodstream. As a result, there is systemic deposition of immune complexes resulting in type III hypersensitivity reactions that involve characteristic target tissues such as the kidneys, joints, and skin. The prototypes of systemic autoimmune diseases are *systemic lupus erythematosus* and *rheumatoid arthritis*. In SLE, antibodies against a variety of nuclear and cytoplasmic self-antigens are produced including antibodies against DNA, histone, and other nuclear antigens, plus antierythrocyte, antilymphocyte, and antiplatelet antibodies.

Another approach is to classify autoimmune diseases according to the structure of self-antigens. These include (1) *cell membrane receptors* such as the TSH receptor in Graves' disease, the insulin receptor in some diseases in man, and the acetylcholine receptor of the motor end plate in myasthenia gravis; (2) *cell surface proteins* such as the

TABLE 5-15 Types of Hypersensitivity and Antigens involved in Autoimmune Disease

HYPERSENSITIVITY	DISEASE	ANTIGEN
Type II (antibody to cell surface or matrix proteins)	Autoimmune hemolytic anemia	Erythrocyte cell membrane
	Autoimmune thrombocytopenia	Platelet cell membrane
	Acute rheumatic fever	Streptococcal cell wall (antibodies cross-react with kidney, joint, and heart antigens)
	Pemphigus vulgaris	Desmoglein-3 (desmosomes)
	Pemphigus folliaceus	Desmoglein-1 (desmosomes)
	Bullous pemphigoid	Desmoplakins (hemidesmosomes)
	Myasthenia gravis	Acetylcholine receptor
	Graves' disease	Thyroid-stimulating hormone receptor
	Autoimmune thyroiditis	Thyroid peroxidase, thyroglobulin
	Autoimmune diabetes mellitus	Glutamic acid decarboxylase and other intracellular islet cell antigens
Type III (immune-complex disease)	Systemic lupus erythematosus	DNA, histones, nonhistone proteins bound to RNA, nucleolar antigens; erythrocyte, lymphocyte, and platelet cell membrane antigens
	Rheumatoid arthritis	IgG (rheumatoid factor)
Type IV (T cell–mediated disease)	Insulin-dependent diabetes mellitus	Pancreatic β-cell peptide
	Goodpasture's syndrome	Noncollagenous domain of α3-chain of collagen type IV
	Rheumatoid arthritis	Unknown synovial membrane antigen
	Multiple sclerosis	Myelin basic protein

pemphigus antigen on keratinocytes and certain red blood cell antigens in autoimmune hemolytic anemia; (3) *nuclear components* like DNA, histones, nonhistone proteins bound to RNA, and nucleolar antigens in SLE; and (4) *immunoglobulins* like IgG in rheumatoid arthritis.

As has been emphasized before, the mechanisms of tissue damage in autoimmune diseases are essentially the same as those occurring in protective immune responses and hypersensitivity diseases. Therefore, another approach to classifying autoimmune diseases is according to the type of hypersensitivity triggered by the autoimmune reaction (Table 5-15).

RECOMMENDED READING

Anderson MM, Lauring AS, Burns CC, Overbaugh J: Identification of a cellular cofactor required for infection by feline leukemia virus, *Science* 287:1828-1830, 2000.

Banchereau J, Steinman RM: Dendritic cells and the control of immunity, *Nature* 392:245-252, 1998.

Benacerraf B: Antigen processing and presentation: the biologic role of MHC molecules in determinant selection, *J Immunol* 141:817-820, 1988.

Black CA: Delayed type hypersensitivity: current theories with an historic perspective, *Dermatol Online J* 5:1-7, 1999.

Brown TT, Shin K: Effect of bovine herpesvirus-1 or parainfluenza-3 virus on immune receptor mediated functions of bovine alveolar macrophages in the presence of absence of virus-specific serum or pulmonary lavage fluids collected after virus infection, *Am J Vet Res* 51:1616-1622, 1990.

Cibrik DM, Sedor JR: Immunopathogenesis of renal disease. In Greenberg A, Cheung AK, Falk RJ, Coffman TM, Jennette JC, editors: *Primer on kidney diseases,* ed 2, San Diego, 1998, Academic Press.

Cohen IR: The self, the world and autoimmunity, *Sci Am* 258:52-60, 1988.

Cotran RS, Kumar V, Collins T, editors: Diseases of immunity and the kidney. In *Robbins pathologic basis of disease,* ed 6, Philadelphia, 1999, Saunders, pp 188-259, 930-996.

Cox E, Mast J, MacHugh N, Schwenger B, Goddeeris BM: Expression of β2 integrins on blood leukocytes of cows with or without bovine leukocyte adhesion deficiency, *Vet Immunol Immunopathol* 58:249-263, 1997.

Cyster JG: Chemokines and cell migration in secondary lymphoid organs, *Science* 286:2098-2102, 1999.

Flint SJ, Enquist LW, Krug RM, Racaniello VR, Skalka AM: *Principles of virology,* Washington, D.C., 2000, ASM Press, pp 101-142, 632-650.

Gallo RC, Montagnier L: AIDS in 1988, *Sci Am* 259:41-48, 1988.

Gerardi AS: Bovine leukocyte adhesion deficiency: a review of a modern disease and its implications, *Res Vet Sci* 61:183-186, 1996.

Gershwin LJ, Krakowka S, Olsen RG: *Immunology and immunopathology of domestic animals,* ed 2, St. Louis, 1995, Mosby.

Gordon S: Macrophages and the immune response. In Paul WE, editor: *Fundamental immunology,* ed 4, Philadelphia, 1999, Lippincott-Raven.

Gordon S, Keshav S, Chung LP: Mononuclear phagocytes: tissue distribution and functional heterogeneity, *Curr Opin Immunol* 1:26-35, 1988.

Ho DD, Pomeran RJ, Kaplan JC: Pathogenesis of infection with human immunodeficiency virus, *N Engl J Med* 317:278-286, 1987.

Hoover EA, Mullins JI, Quackenbush SL, Gasper PW: Experimental transmission and pathogenesis of immunodeficiency syndrome in cats, *Blood* 70:1880-1892, 1987.

Hricik DE, Chung-Park M, Sedor JR: Glomerulonephritis, *N Engl J Med* 339:888-899, 1998.

Janeway CA, Travers P, Walport M, Capra JD: *Immunobiology: the immune system in health and disease,* ed 4, New York, 1999, Current Biology/Garland Publishing.

Jennette JC, Falk RJ: Glomerular clinicopathologic syndromes. In Greenberg A, Cheung AK, Falk RJ, Coffman TM, Jennette JC, editors: *Primer on kidney diseases,* ed 2, San Diego, 1998, Academic Press.

Kalish RS, Askenase PW: Molecular mechanisms of CD8+ T cell–mediated delayed hypersensitivity: implications for allergies, asthma, and autoimmunity, *J Allergy Clin Immunol* 103:192-199, 1999.

Kovacs EM, Baxter GD, Robinson WF: Feline peripheral blood mononuclear cells express message for both CXC and CC type chemokine receptors, *Arch Virol* 144:273-285, 1999.

Krakauer T, Vilcek J, Oppenheim JJ: Proinflammatory cytokines: TNF and IL-1 families, chemokines, TGF-β, and others. In Paul WE, editor: *Fundamental immunology,* ed 4, Philadelphia, 1999, Lippincott-Raven.

Leonard WJ: Type I Cytokines and interferons and their receptors. In Paul WE, editor: *Fundamental immunology,* ed 4, Philadelphia, 1999, Lippincott-Raven.

Leung DYM: Molecular basis of allergic diseases, *Mol Genet Metab* 63:157-167, 1998.

Levy JA: *HIV and the pathogenesis of AIDS,* ed 2, Washington, D.C., 1998, ASM Press.

Machen M, Montgomery T, Holland R, Braselton E, Dunstan R, Brewer G, Yuzbasiyan-Gurkan V: Bovine hereditary zinc deficiency: lethal trait A 46, *J Vet Diagn Invest* 8:219-227, 1996.

Metcalf DD, Baram D, Mekori YA: Mast cells, *Physiol Rev* 77:1033-1067, 1997.

Mire-Sluis AR, Thorpe R, editors: *Cytokines,* San Diego, 1998, Academic Press.

Mosier DE: Animal models for retrovirus-induced immunodeficiency disease, *Immunol Invest* 15:233-261, 1986.

Mosmann TR, Li L, Hengartner H, Kagi D, Fu W, Sad S: Differentiation and functions of T cell subsets, *Ciba Found Symp* 204:148-158, 1997

Murphy PM: Chemokine receptors: structure, function, and role in microbial pathogenesis, *Cytokine Growth Factor Rev* 7:47-64, 1996.

Murray JS: How the MHC selects Th1/Th2 immunity, *Immunol Today* 19:157-163, 1998.

Pedersen NC, Ho EW, Brown ML, Yamamoto JK: Isolation of a T-lymphotropic virus from domestic cats with an immunodeficiency-like syndrome, *Science* 235:790-793, 1987.

Perryman LE: Primary immunodeficiencies of horses, *Vet Clin North Am Equine Pract* 16:105-116, 2000.

Puck JM: X-Linked severe combined immunodeficiency. In Ochs HD, Smith CIE, Puck JM, editors: *Primary immunodeficiency diseases: a molecular and genetic approach,* New York, 1999, Oxford University Press.

Roitt IM: The production of effectors. In *Roitt's essential immunology,* ed 9, London, 1997, Blackwell Science.

Rottman JB: Key role of chemokines and chemokine receptors in inflammation, immunity, neoplasia, and infectious disease, *Vet Pathol* 36:357-367, 1999.

Sanchea-Mejorada G, Rosales C: Signal transduction by immunological Fc receptors, *J Leukoc Biol* 63:521-533, 1998.

Schwartz K, Notarangelo LD, Spanopoulou E, Vezzoni P, Villa A: Recombination defects. In Ochs HD, Smith CIE, Puck JM, editors: *Primary immunodeficiency diseases: a molecular and genetic approach,* New York, 1999, Oxford University Press.

Scott DW, Miller WH, Griffin CE: Immunological skin diseases. In *Miller and Kirk's small animal dermatology,* ed 5, Philadelphia, 1995, Saunders.

Slauson DO, Lewis RM: Comparative pathology of glomerulonephritis in animals, *Vet Pathol* 16:135-164, 1979.

Somberg RL, Robinson JP, Felsburg PJ: T lymphocyte development and function in dogs with X-linked severe combined immunodeficiency, *J Immunol* 153:4006-4015, 1994.

Somberg RL, Tipold A, Hartnett BJ, Moore PF, Henthorn PS, Felsburg PJ: Postnatal development of T cells in dogs with X-linked severe combined immunodeficiency, *J Immunol* 156:1431-1435, 1996.

Steinman RM: Dentritic cells. In Paul WE, editor: *Fundamental immunology,* ed 4, Philadelphia, 1999, Lippincott-Raven.

Suter MM, Wilkinson JE, Dougherty EP, Lewis RM: Ultrastructural localization of pemphigus antigen on canine keratinocytes in vivo and in vitro, *Am J Vet Res* 51:507-511, 1990.

Tizard IR: *Veterinary immunology: an introduction,* ed 6, Philadelphia, 2000, Saunders.

Wells TNC, Powe CA, Proudfoot AE: Definition, function, and pathophysiological significance of chemokine receptors, *Trends Pharmacol Sci* 19:376-380, 1998.

Willett BJ, Hosie MJ: The role of the chemokine receptor CXCR4 in infection with feline immunodeficiency disease, *Mol Membr Biol* 16:67-72, 1999.

Williams TJ, Hellewell PG, Jose PJ: Inflammatory mechanisms in the Arthus reaction, *Agents Actions* 19:66-72, 1986.

Yamamoto JK, Sparger E, Ho EW, Andersen PR, O'Connor TP, Mandell CP, Lowenstine L, Munn R, Pedersen NC: Pathogenesis of experimentally induced feline immunodeficiency virus infection in cats, *Am J Vet Res* 49:1246-1258, 1988.

CHAPTER 6

Disorders of Cell Growth and Cancer Biology

Gary L. Cockerell
Barry J. Cooper

Many diseases involve abnormalities of tissue growth, including both nonneoplastic and neoplastic disorders. Interestingly the study of these diseases has led not only to an increased understanding of the mechanisms of these diseases themselves but also to elucidation of a wide variety of other processes in cell biology. The study of disorders of cell growth has produced numerous convergent observations in areas such as control of the cell cycle, angiogenesis, the origin and function of genes that regulate cell proliferation, tissue growth factors, and immunological recognition of altered cells. In this chapter we consider these diseases and how recent advances in cell biology have derived from and contributed to an increased understanding of their pathogenesis.

NONNEOPLASTIC DISORDERS OF GROWTH

Throughout the embryonic and postnatal development of an individual, tissues grow as a result of a coordinated combination of cellular proliferation and differentiation. We must admit that tissue mass also can be increased by an increase in cell size, but, as a component of growth, this mechanism is relatively unimportant. Many tissues retain the capacity for cellular proliferation throughout the life of the individual, and in some there is continual mitotic division to replace cells that are lost. In the skin, for example, there is continual loss of keratinized epithelial cells requiring replacement by proliferation of basal cells. Similarly, in the bone marrow there is continual cell proliferation to replace cells of the peripheral blood whose lifetime is limited. Other cells, such as those of the renal tubular epithelium or of the liver, do not continually proliferate but retain the capacity for mitotic division as a mechanism for repair.

Most of the daughter cells that result from cell proliferation undergo differentiation, adopting the structural and functional characteristics of the tissue they are destined to become. Although somatic cells are believed to retain all the individual's genetic information, at some point differentiation involves the regulated expression of particular genes, providing the commitment to a particular course of development and specialization. Thus cells committed to be epidermal cells reproduce only epidermal cells, liver cells produce liver cells, and so on. In most cases fully differentiated cells lose the capacity to divide, and so loss of this capacity may be regarded as one feature of the process of differentiation. Although differentiation apparently involves alteration, or restriction, of genetic expres-

sion, the exact mechanisms by which it is accomplished are poorly understood. The most important point to be made here is that these modifications of cell behavior apparently are accomplished by regulation of the expression of the genetic information in each cell and not by any process analogous to mutation.

The final adult tissue therefore can be regarded as containing a mixture of cells, some continually dividing, some that are not dividing but fully differentiated to postmitotic cells. It is useful to think of nonneoplastic disorders of growth as representing deficiencies, excesses, or abnormal patterns of cellular proliferation and differentiation. For convenience, these are often divided into developmental (congenital) and acquired (postnatal) disorders.

Developmental (Congenital) Defects

These defects of growth and development of a tissue or organ are present at birth as congenital lesions. Although the cause is often unknown and may be attributable to genetic defects, such abnormalities also may be caused by toxins (including drugs used for therapeutic purposes), infections, and other factors. Therefore, isolated cases of developmental anomalies cannot be assumed to be inherited. These defects usually result in decreased function or functional reserve and, depending on the organ involved, may be subclinical or a cause of fetal or neonatal morbidity or mortality. In most cases, they result in an irreversible change in tissue structure.

APLASIA

Aplasia indicates a failure to grow but is usually accompanied by the presence of a rudimentary organ (the term *agenesis* indicates a complete failure of that tissue to develop). The term "aplasia" also is used to refer to the failure of a tissue to renew itself, with one example being aplastic anemia in which there is failure of renewal of hematopoietic cells in the bone marrow.

HYPOPLASIA

Hypoplasia refers to the failure of an organ to reach normal size. It is therefore a developmental defect occupying the spectrum between aplasia and normal development. Examples that are seen regularly are renal hypoplasia (Fig. 6-1) and testicular hypoplasia. A prominent histological feature of this lesion is the presence of immature or "embryonal" tissue as a result of interruption in differentiation to normal mature cell types.

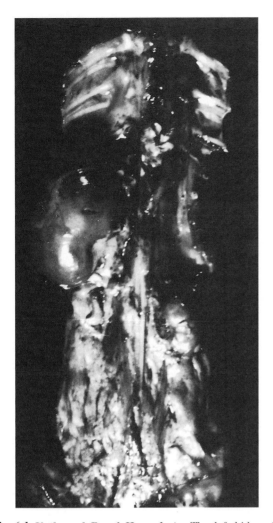

Fig. 6-1 Unilateral Renal Hypoplasia. The left kidney in this 2-week-old goat was approximately one-third normal size (compare to normal-sized right kidney). This was a congenital but not necessarily heritable lesion. Because the right kidney was normal, no signs of renal failure were present in the animal.

MISCELLANEOUS DEVELOPMENTAL ANOMALIES

Many tissue or organ malformations may occur during growth and development and are detected as congenital lesions. The types of defects include failure to close or fuse (such as palatoschisis, interventricular cardiac septal defects), failure to canalize or separate (such as atresia ani, horseshoe kidney), vestigial remnants (such as cystic Rathke's pouch), accessory or supernumerary tissues (such as polydactyly), and ectopic location of tissues (such as ectopic thyroid or ectopic pancreas).

Also included in this category are the relatively rare *hamartomas* (abnormal overgrowth of tissue normal to the location in which they are found)

and *choristomas* (normal tissue in an abnormal location).

Acquired Defects

Acquired lesions are often a compensatory or protective change in response to demands for increased or decreased function. As compared to developmental defects, these changes are usually reversible if the causative agent or process is eliminated.

ATROPHY AND HYPERTROPHY

Atrophy, defined as decreased size of an organ or tissue after it has achieved normal size caused by loss of cells or decreased cell size, and hypertrophy, defined as increased size of an organ or tissue caused by increased cell size, are discussed in Chapter 2. Although not truly disorders of growth, these disorders are mentioned again here as a reminder that they are processes that can result in alterations in tissue mass or organ size.

HYPERPLASIA

Hyperplasia is defined as an increase in organ size or tissue mass caused by an increase in the number of constituent cells. Hyperplasia therefore occurs only in cells capable of mitotic division. It may occur concurrently with hypertrophy, but under similar demands for increased function, postmitotic cells undergo hypertrophy but not hyperplasia. Some cell types, such as bone marrow and intestinal epithelium, remain mitotically active throughout life and are therefore capable of undergoing hyperplasia in response to the demand for increased function. Other cell types, such as neurons and muscle, lose their mitotic potential before or soon after birth and can respond to similar demands only by undergoing hypertrophy.

Organs or tissue undergo hyperplasia in response to an increased level of a normal stimulus, such as a hormone or as a regenerative or compensatory response. For example, the mammary gland undergoes hyperplasia in response to increased hormonal stimulation during pregnancy and lactation, and the adrenal cortex undergoes hyperplasia in response to increased ACTH levels. In response to the loss of one kidney, the contralateral kidney undergoes enlargement caused by hyperplasia (as well as cellular hypertrophy) as a compensatory response. The liver or bone marrow, in which there has been loss of functional reserves of hepatocellular or hematopoietic tissue, undergoes regenerative hyperplasia. Extreme examples of hyperplasia frequently occur as a

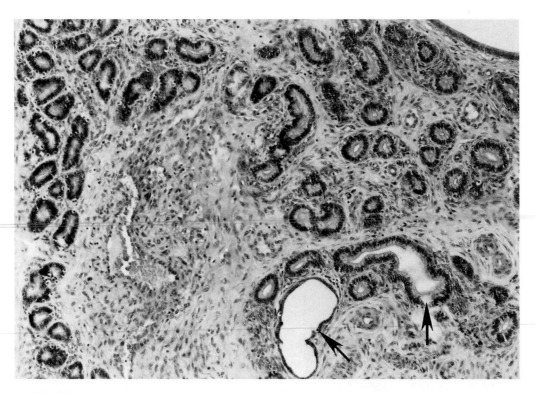

Fig. 6-2 Endometrial Hyperplasia. In the dog, hyperplasia of the endometrium occurs during the estrus cycle in response to stimulation by progesterone. Continued stimulation may lead to cystic dilatation of the endometrial glands, *arrows*, and eventually to infection and inflammation of the uterus.

result of excessive stimulation or chronic irritation. For example, prolonged progesterone secretion results in endometrial hyperplasia (Fig. 6-2), and prolonged stimulation of the thyroid gland in iodine deficiency results in hyperplastic goiter. Examples of hyperplasia caused by irritation are usually associated with inflammation such as chronic otitis externa, in which there is hyperplasia of the ceruminous glands, or chronic bronchitis, in which the bronchial epithelium becomes hyperplastic (Fig. 6-3, *A*). Infection (and presumably chronic irritation) of biliary epithelium by *Eimeria stiedai* in rabbits causes profound epithelial hyperplasia (Fig. 6-3, *B*).

In general, hyperplasia is a relatively orderly process, but under some conditions it can become difficult to distinguish from benign neoplasia. For example, *nodular hyperplasia* occurs commonly in the liver and pancreas of dogs and consists of variably sized nodules of well-differentiated parenchymal cells within the tissue, similar to hepatomas or pancreatic exocrine adenomas. This raises a critical point in the definition of hyperplasia and its differentiation from neoplasia. Hyperplasia, by definition, remains responsive to control and, in the absence of the causative stimulus, will not progress and in fact may regress. Unfortunately the stimuli

for hyperplastic lesions, in particular nodular hyperplasia, are not always known, making it sometimes impossible to definitively distinguish between benign neoplastic nodules and hyperplastic nodules.

METAPLASIA

Metaplasia is an adaptive response in which one type of mature differentiated cell is replaced by a different type that is not normal to that tissue or organ. It may be thought of as a redirection of differentiation. In natural disease settings, it occurs within and is limited to a given tissue type; that is, one type of epithelial tissue is replaced by another type of epithelial tissue and similarly for mesenchymal tissue. Metaplasia does not occur as the result of alterations in existing mature cells, but rather it depends on proliferation of germinal, or stem, cells whose progeny undergo modified differentiation.

Metaplasia, especially within epithelia, is usually a response to chronic irritation, including inflammation. Under these conditions, a highly specialized epithelial tissue is commonly replaced by less specialized but more resistant epithelium. For example, the respiratory epithelium lining the trachea, bronchi, and bronchioles may be replaced by strati-

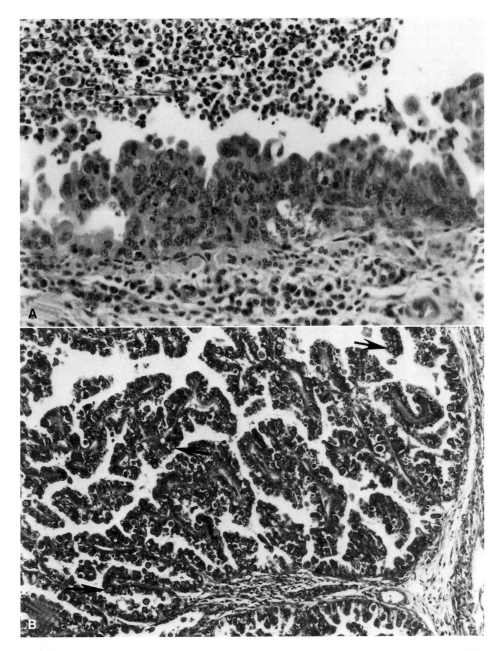

Fig. 6-3 A, Hyperplasia of the bronchiolar epithelium associated with bronchiolitis caused by parainfluenza-3 virus infection in a cow. Instead of normal columnar epithelial cells, the bronchiole is lined by multiple layers of immature epithelial cells that lack specialized structures such as cilia. This lesion would be expected to result in abnormal clearance of material from the airways. Inflammatory cells are present in the lumen of the bronchiole, *top.* **B,** Hyperplasia of the biliary epithelium in hepatic coccidiosis in a rabbit. Severe proliferation of biliary epithelium has resulted in folded, papillary epithelial ingrowths into the lumen of the bile duct. The causative organism *Eimeria stiedai* is visible, *arrows,* as small spherules in many of the cells.

fied squamous epithelium (Fig. 6-4). Although this change is an adaptive host response to cover and protect damaged mucosal surfaces, it has the undesirable consequences of decreased mucus secretion, loss of cilia, and consequently loss of clearance mechanisms from the airways. In metaplasia of mesenchymal tissue, fibrous tissue may be replaced by bone or cartilage (Fig. 6-5). This change is less easily regarded as an adaptive response, and the cause is usually unknown.

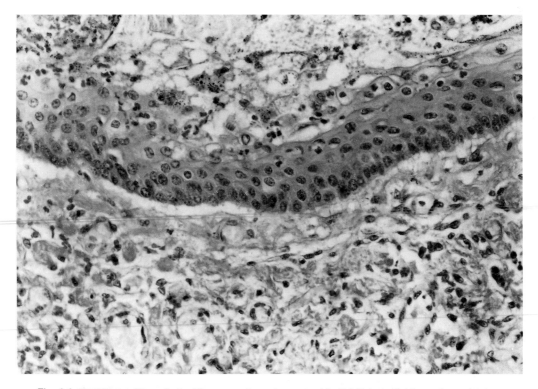

Fig. 6-4 Squamous Metaplasia. The normal respiratory epithelial lining of this trachea of a cow has been replaced by stratified squamous epithelium that lacks specialized ciliated and goblet cells. As a result, clearance of material from the trachea is impaired. Inflammatory cells and debris resulting from chronic tracheitis are present in the lumen, *top*.

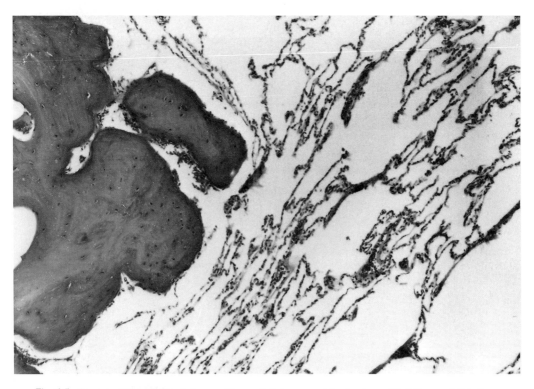

Fig. 6-5 Osseous Metaplasia. A focus of bone, *left*, is present in the interstitial tissue of this lung from a dog. This is a common lesion in dogs and is usually of no functional consequence. Its cause is unknown.

Stable metaplastic conversion of epithelia, such as that from pancreatic exocrine cells to hepatocytes, has been reported after treatment with low doses of carcinogens. However, in most naturally occurring disease settings epithelial metaplasia is reversible, with the normal tissue being restored if the stimulus is removed.

DYSPLASIA

Dysplasia is a somewhat generic term (sometimes used interchangeably but imprecisely with the term "dystrophy"), which literally means 'abnormal growth' and sometimes is used in that sense in terms such as "chondrodysplasia" or "hip dysplasia." Commonly, however, it is used in a more restricted sense to describe a proliferative response accompanied by loss of regular differentiation and orderliness and by cellular atypia—it may be thought of as disorderly or atypical hyperplasia. Cellular atypia is characterized by *pleomorphism* (variation in size and shape) and *hyperchromicity* (increased staining). There is a loss of the normal regular progression from germinal to fully differentiated cells, and mitoses are found in abnormal positions (Fig. 6-6).

By definition, dysplasia is a nonneoplastic lesion and therefore is reversible if the cause is removed. Morphologically, however, it is difficult to distinguish a severely dysplastic lesion from a neoplastic one. Studies of large numbers of cases do, however, support the conclusion that many such lesions are, in fact, incipient carcinomas. They are therefore often regarded as "preneoplastic." When the features of disorderliness and cellular atypia become evident enough to conclude that the lesion is in fact neoplastic but there is no invasion of the adjacent tissue and the changes are confined to the epithelial layer, the term *"carcinoma in situ"* often is applied. These lesions are most frequently observed in epithelia in association with chronic irritation or inflammation. For example, dysplastic lesions occur commonly in the prepuce of horses, presumably caused by constant local irritation by smegma, and squamous cell carcinomas frequently occur at this site. The term, of course, implies neoplasia and malignancy, but it should be emphasized again that there is no way to be certain that such a lesion is neoplastic. To the clinician then, the importance of dysplastic lesions is the increased risk of an invasive carcinoma developing at the site if the lesion or its cause is not removed.

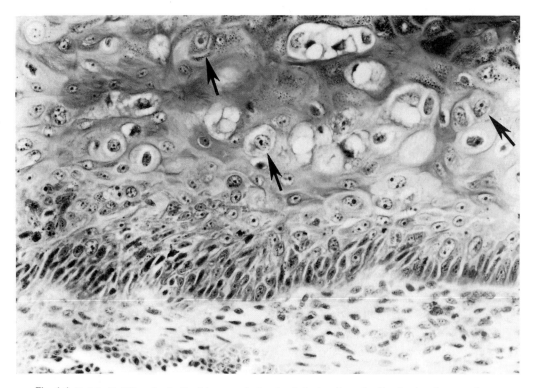

Fig. 6-6 Epithelial Dysplasia. In this severely dysplastic lesion from the lip of a dog there are large poorly differentiated cells in the spiny layer of the mucosa, *arrows.*

NEOPLASTIC DISORDERS OF GROWTH

Neoplasia literally means 'new growth', but this is as insufficient as defining "pathology" as the 'study of disease'. Many definitions have been applied, and these continue to change as we learn more about the disorder, but the definition given by Willis a half century ago provides several important criteria: "A neoplasm is an abnormal mass of tissue, the growth of which exceeds and is uncoordinated with that of normal tissues and persists in the same excessive manner after cessation of the stimulus which evoked the change." Included in this definition are three key features of neoplasia that distinguish it from other forms of disorders of growth:

1. Excessive tissue growth
2. Lack of responsiveness to control mechanisms
3. Lack of dependence on the continued presence of the stimulus

In this section we examine these and other salient features of neoplastic disorders of growth.

Epidemiological Considerations

Neoplasia is a disease that affects ~~most if not~~ all vertebrate species. With some exceptions, it tends to be a disease associated with aging. It is presumably partly for this reason that neoplasia is seen more frequently in dogs and cats than in other domestic animals because dogs and cats are allowed to live out their natural life span, that is, to age. It is generally considered that aging *per se* is not a direct factor in the induction of tumors but presumably allows increased opportunity to develop neoplasia, including cumulative exposure to environmental carcinogens. Furthermore, the development of neoplastic disease is a very prolonged process, often requiring half the normal lifetime of the animal. This alone would bias the occurrence of neoplasia to older animals.

Neoplastic disease is a major cause of morbidity and mortality in domestic animals as well as in humans. Although comparable data are not readily available for animals, cancer ranks second only to cardiovascular disease as a cause of death in humans. The most common sites for tumor development in humans are the breast, prostate, lung, and colon. In domestic animals, the most frequently occurring types of tumors varies considerably between species. For example, tumors of the eye are the most common type of tumor in cattle, and most of these are malignant (squamous cell carcinoma). Dogs and horses most commonly develop tumors of the skin, and the majority of these are benign; a large percentage of skin tumors in horses represent "sar-

coids," a unique locally aggressive tumor of dermal fibroblasts. Malignant tumors of the hemolymphatic system, leukemias and lymphomas, are the most common type of tumors in cats, most of which are attributable to infection with feline leukemia virus. Some naturally occurring tumors of domestic animals serve as excellent models of their human counterparts, such as osteosarcomas in dogs, but no single species mirrors the array and frequency of tumors that occur in humans.

Nomenclature and Classification

There are several commonly used synonyms for neoplasia. By strict definition, the term *tumor* means a tissue swelling or mass but by common usage has come to mean a *neoplasm*. The term *cancer* should be reserved for reference to a malignant neoplasm.

Neoplasms are named according to a binomial system denoting their *histogenetic origin* and *biological behavior*. Histogenetic origin refers to the tissue or cell type from which the tumor arose and can generally be divided into *epithelial* and *mesenchymal* types. Biological behavior includes the degree of tumor cell differentiation and pattern of growth and is divided into *benign* and *malignant*. As shown in Table 6-1, benign tumors originating from either epithelial or mesenchymal cells are denoted with the suffix "-oma." In contrast, malignant tumors arising from epithelium end with the suffix "[adeno]carcinoma," whereas those originating from mesenchymal tissue end with "-sarcoma." The tissue of origin is indicated by the addition of an appropriate prefix or simply the name of the tissue. Table 6-2 lists commonly encountered neoplasms, their tissue of origin, and the names of their benign and malignant counterparts. Notice that, in

TABLE 6-1 Binomial Classification of Tumors		
BIOLOGICAL BEHAVIOR	**HISTOGENETIC ORIGIN***	
	EPITHELIAL	**MESENCHYMAL**
Benign	"-oma" suffix (*e.g.*, papilloma)	"-oma" suffix (*e.g.*, osteoma)
Malignant	"-carcinoma" suffix† (*e.g.*, squamous cell carcinoma)	"-sarcoma" suffix (*e.g.*, osteosarcoma)

*"Mixed" tumors originate from more than one germ layer.
†"Adeno-" may be added to the start of these to denote a benign ("adenoma") or malignant ("adenocarcinoma") tumor that forms glands, ducts, or acini.

some cases, such as tumors of hematopoietic tissue, benign tumors are not recognized.

This system of nomenclature and classification are important because they form the basis of the language by which pathologists and clinicians communicate the nature and significance of the lesion to one another. Because many forms of treatment are specific to a particular type or even subtype of neoplasm, it is imperative that the pathologist be able to convey to the clinician the nature of the neoplastic lesion involved. This classification system continues to serve us well, but as more and more tools become available to help in classifying neoplasms, it becomes apparent that there are difficulties with it. The major problem is that oncogenesis does not always mimic embryogenesis, and neoplastic cells may not closely resemble their parentage either morphologically or functionally. Classifications of tumors continue to change as new information and technology becomes available, but from the clinical point of view, the most important thing is that classification be based on consistent criteria and, whenever possible, correlated with clinical behavior. Further, despite these rules and regulations for classifying and naming neoplasms, inconsistencies persist. For example, melanoma is used to describe tumors arising from melanocytes but does not indicate the malignancy of these neoplasms. Pathologists often use the term "malignant melanoma" to overcome this problem. Some tumors are referred to by the name of the investigator principally responsible for their study (such as Burkitt's lymphoma, Wilms' tumor, Rous sarcoma, Marek's disease), which unfortunately does not indicate the histogenetic origin or biological behavior of the tumor.

HISTOGENETIC ORIGIN: EPITHELIAL VERSUS MESENCHYMAL

Classification of tumors as "epithelial" or "mesenchymal" relates to their origin from cells from one of the three primary germ layers, ectoderm,

TABLE 6-2   **Classification of Some Common Neoplasms**

TISSUE OF ORIGIN	BENIGN	MALIGNANT
MESENCHYMAL		
Fibrous tissue	Fibroma	Fibrosarcoma
Bone	Osteoma	Osteosarcoma
Cartilage	Chondroma	Chondrosarcoma
Adipose tissue	Lipoma	Liposarcoma
Endothelium of blood vessels	Hemangioma	Hemangiosarcoma
Endothelium of lymphatics	Lymphangioma	Lymphangiosarcoma
Skeletal muscle	Rhabdomyoma	Rhadomyosarcoma
Smooth muscle	Leiomyoma	Leiomyosarcoma
Mast cells	Mastocytoma	Malignant mast cell tumor
Synovium	Synovioma	Synovial cell sarcoma
Meninges	Meningioma	Malignant meningioma
Mesothelium	Mesothelioma	Malignant mesothelioma
Lymphocytes		Malignant lymphoma
Plasma cells		Myeloma
Monocytes		Monocytic leukemia
Granulocytes		Granulocytic leukemia
Erythrocytes		Erythroleukemia
EPITHELIAL		
Squamous epithelium	Papilloma	Squamous cell carcinoma
Bronchial epithelium	Bronchogenic adenoma	Bronchogenic carcinoma
Basal cells	Basal cell tumor	Basal cell carcinoma
Liver	Hepatoma	Hepatocellular carcinoma
Biliary epithelium	Biliary adenoma	Biliary adenocarcinoma
Transitional epithelium	Transitional cell papilloma	Transitional cell carcinoma
Spermatogenic epithelium	Seminoma	Malignant seminoma
Sertoli cell	Sertoli cell tumor	Malignant Sertoli cell tumor
Adrenal cortex	Adrenocortical adenoma	Adrenocortical carcinoma
Adrenal medulla	Pheochromocytoma	Malignant pheochromocytoma
Pancreatic islets	Islet cell adenoma	Islet cell carcinoma

[Handwritten annotation spanning Lymphocytes, Plasma cells, Monocytes, Granulocytes, Erythrocytes: "Normally circulate in blood so if neoplastic = automatically metastic ∴ only malignant"]

mesoderm, and endoderm. Whereas epithelial cells derive from all three germ layers, mesenchymal cells are predominately derived from the mesoderm, including the primitive filling tissue known as "mesenchyme." Derivatives of mesenchyme include connective tissue, cartilage, bone, blood, smooth muscle, and endothelium, all being the cell types from which the majority of mesenchymal tumors arise. This histogenetic origin is reflected in the histological patterns of epithelial versus mesenchymal tumors (see below) and is therefore generally useful; however, it is not entirely precise and does not follow strict embryological definitions. Particularly problematic are tumors derived from the neural crest (neuroectoderm). For example, it remains unclear whether tumors of melanin-producing cells (melanocytes) should be classified as epithelial or mesenchymal. Pathologists frequently encounter this dilemma when confronted with melanomas that have histological characteristics of both epithelial and mesenchymal cells. Further, tumors may occasionally derive from more than one embryonic germ layer; these are called *mixed neoplasms*. The most common example of this is mixed mammary tumors of dogs, in which proliferating epithelial tissue occurs intermixed with mesenchymal components such as myoepithelium, bone, and cartilage. Another example is teratomas, which occur most commonly in the testes or ovaries and contain any number of tissues of any type including bone, skin, nervous tissue, intestinal epithelium, muscle, and hair.

BIOLOGICAL BEHAVIOR: BENIGN VERSUS MALIGNANT

Several criteria are used to judge the biological behavior of tumors to classify them as benign or malignant. Many of these criteria are based on histological characteristics (Table 6-3). Generally the pathologist

and the clinician are attempting to predict the behavior of a particular neoplasm, and the classification as either benign or malignant is one way to express this. It must be realized, however, that neoplasms do not always fall neatly into one or the other category but that a range from completely benign to highly malignant exists and errors are bound to occur in trying to predict the future behavior of a neoplasm. In addition, the features on which we judge malignancy, which are discussed below, do not always hold true. Some neoplasms, though having histological features suggestive of malignancy, characteristically behave in a benign fashion. It is therefore very important for the pathologist and the clinician to be aware not only of the usual clinical and histological features of neoplasms, which indicate their likely behavior, but also of the characteristic behavior of particular types of neoplasms in each species. As an example, basal cell tumors of the skin in dogs may show histological features, such as a high mitotic index, that usually are suggestive of malignancy. Despite this, these neoplasms are almost invariably benign. Species differences can be illustrated when mammary neoplasms in dogs and cats are contrasted. In dogs, mammary tumors vary greatly in behavior, and although malignant tumors certainly occur, most are relatively benign, whereas in cats most mammary tumors are carcinomas and metastasize very readily.

Benign tumors usually grow slowly, whereas malignant tumors grow rapidly. Both types of tumors grow by expansion, frequently compressing adjacent normal tissue; however, benign tumors remain more clearly delineated from normal tissue and may be encapsulated (Fig. 6-7, *A* and *C*). In contrast, malignant tumors are poorly delineated from surrounding nonneoplastic tissue and often infiltrate it. This makes it difficult for the surgeon to visualize the junction of malignant neoplasm with normal tissue and to achieve total surgical excision.

TABLE 6-3 Biological Behavior of Benign and Malignant Tumors

CRITERIA	BENIGN	MALIGNANT
Rate of growth	Slow	Rapid
Mode of growth	Expansive, encapsulated, circumscribed	Expansive, infiltrative, poorly delineated
Cellular differentiation	Uniform, well differentiated	Pleomorphic, poorly differentiated (anaplastic)
Mitotic figures	Rare	Common
Recurrence after treatment	Rare	Frequent
Invasion of vessels	Uncommon	Frequent
Metastasis	Absent	Frequent

Benign tumors usually are well differentiated and resemble the tissue from which they arose both cytologically and architecturally. Nuclear and cytoplasmic morphology is similar to that in the precursor tissue (Fig. 6-7, *B* and *D*). Malignant tumors, on the other hand, vary greatly in the degree to which they differentiate, but generally they exhibit some degree of *anaplasia* (Fig. 6-8, *A* and *C*). Anaplasia means 'failure to differentiate' or 'loss of differentiation' and is one of the most important morphological features of malignancy. Anaplasia should not be thought of as dedifferentiation, which would imply that cells already differentiated revert to a more primitive form—it is generally accepted that this does not

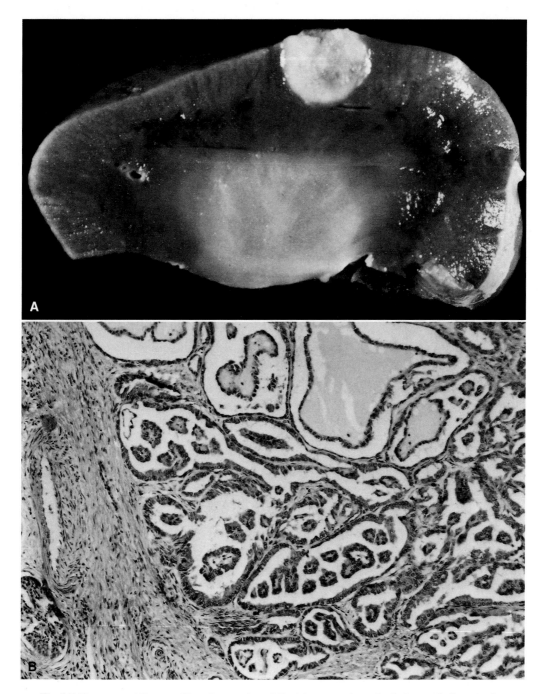

Fig. 6-7 Features of Benign Neoplasms. A and **B,** Adenoma of renal tubular epithelium in the kidney of a horse. The neoplasm is discrete and has sharply delineated borders, **A.** Histologically the neoplasm is made up of uniform, well-differentiated cells arranged in a papillary pattern, **B.**

continued

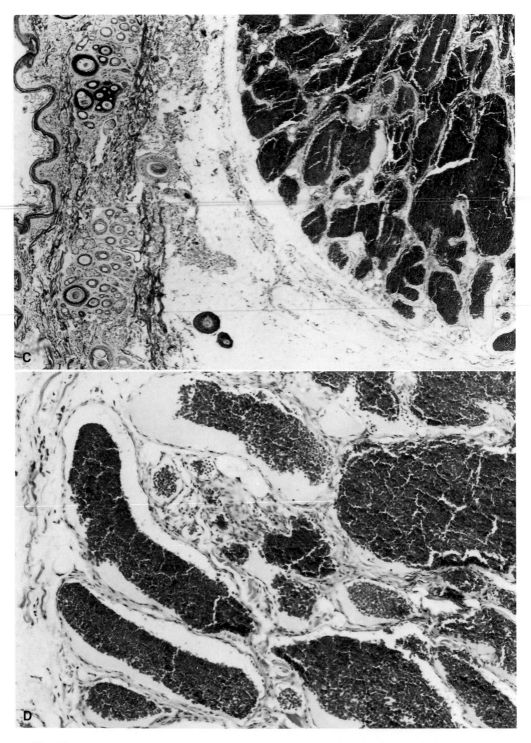

Fig. 6-7, cont'd. C and **D,** Hemangioma in the skin of a dog. The neoplasm is discrete and has sharply demarcated borders. It forms large blood-filled spaces lined by neoplastic endothelium, **C.** The neoplastic cells are well differentiated and closely resemble normal endothelial cells. They are supported on a fibrous stroma, **D.**

occur. Anaplastic cells usually exhibit *pleomorphism,* meaning 'variable morphology'. The nuclei of such neoplasms are often large, hyperchromatic or vesicular, have an abnormal shape, and may contain one or more prominent nucleoli (Fig. 6-8, *B* and *D*).

Well-differentiated neoplasms may retain the functional characteristics of the parent tissue. Logically enough, functional capacity is retained best in highly differentiated, benign neoplasms. Thus, glandular adenomas may secrete mucus, and endocrine

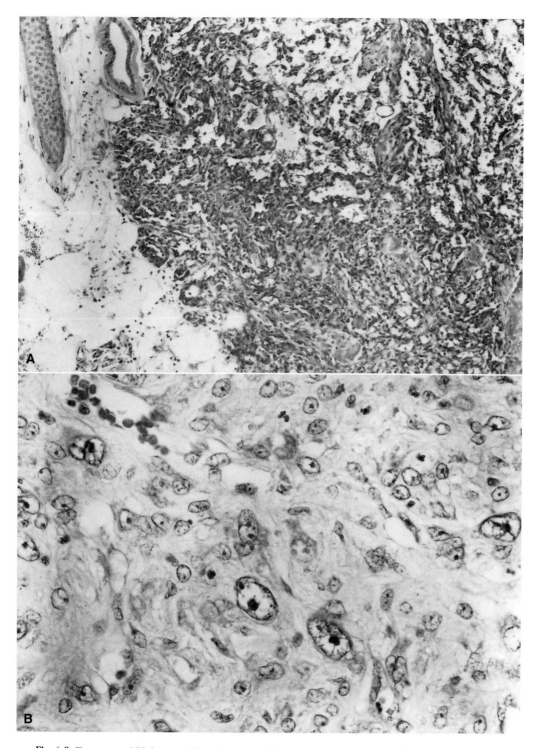

Fig. 6-8 Features of Malignant Neoplasms. A, Hemangiosarcoma in the skin of a dog. The neoplasm is relatively poorly differentiated, but in some areas it forms recognizable blood-filled spaces. In other areas it forms solid cellular masses. It is poorly demarcated from the surrounding normal tissue. **B,** Anaplastic sarcoma. This neoplasm is very poorly differentiated, and its tissue of origin is not recognizable. There is severe nuclear pleomorphism, and many of the nuclei are vesicular and contain prominent nucleoli.

continued

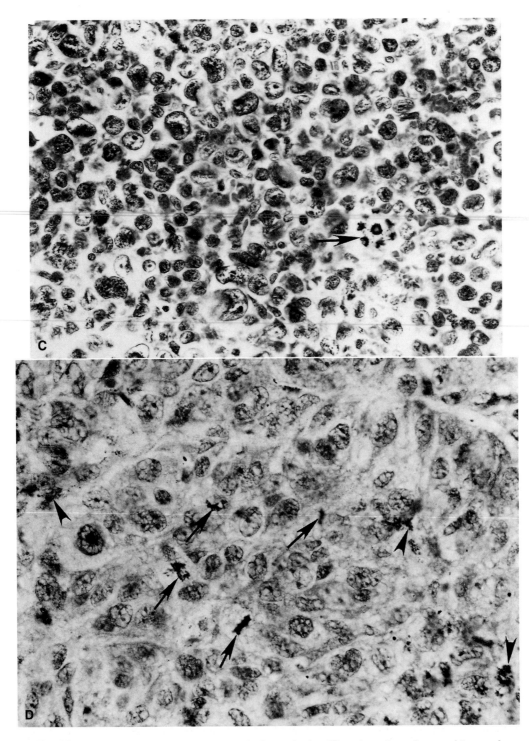

Fig. 6-8 cont'd. C, Anaplastic neoplasm in the lung of a dog. There is nuclear pleomorphism, and the neoplastic cells are anaplastic. A bizarre, abnormal mitotic figure is present, *arrow.* **D,** Malignant melanoma from the skin of a horse. There are many mitotic figures, *arrows.* Although this neoplasm is poorly differentiated, many cells contain melanin granules, *arrowheads,* allowing it to be classified as a melanoma.

adenomas may secrete hormones. Malignant neoplasms may retain some functional capacity, and in some cases these functions may be very deleterious to the host, as discussed later. Functional activity is in fact the basis on which the origin of many neoplasms may be recognized. For example, melanomas produce melanin, osteosarcomas produce osteoid, and adenocarcinomas of the thyroid gland produce colloid. Some neoplasms, of course, fail to mimic their tissue of origin sufficiently for it to be recognized. In such a case, the neoplasm is said to be a *poorly differentiated* sarcoma or carcinoma, as the case may be. Also, malignant neoplasms may be highly cellular. This is an important feature in classifying mesenchymal neoplasms in which the high cellular density may partly reflect the failure of the neoplastic cells to differentiate and produce extracellular matrix.

Failure to differentiate may make it difficult to classify a malignant neoplasm, but often a careful search will reveal the evidence of an attempt to mimic the tissue from which the neoplasm is derived, thus allowing a definitive diagnosis (Fig. 6-8, *D*). Sometimes it is necessary to resort to special techniques to demonstrate the differentiation that allows classification of a neoplasm, with light microscopy being only one tool by which the nature of neoplastic cells can be identified. More and more sophisticated techniques such as electron microscopy, immunohistochemistry, biochemical analysis, and identification of specific receptors are being used to detect evidence of specific features of differentiation not discernible by light microscopy. Immunohistochemical techniques are now widely used in the study and diagnosis of neoplasms. A particular example is the use of antibodies against different types of intermediate filaments to identify poorly differentiated neoplasms. Carcinomas are expected to express cytokeratins, most sarcomas express vimentin, and tumors of smooth or skeletal muscle origin express desmin. In the central nervous system, the expression of glial fibrillary acidic protein can be used to differentiate neoplastic astrocytes from other cell types.

Mitotic figures, including abnormal forms, are more commonly observed in malignant than in benign tumors (Fig. 6-8, *B* and *D*). The number of mitotic figures per microscopic field (mitotic index) is a frequently used criterion to assess tumor cell proliferation and therefore the degree of malignancy. However, as discussed later under the subject of the cell cycle, caution should be used in interpreting the mitotic index, since this method measures the shortest period of the proliferating tumor cell population and lacks reproducibility.

From a clinical standpoint, the most important differences between benign and malignant tumors are their frequency of recurrence after surgical resection, invasion of vessels, and spread to distant sites, or metastasis. As mentioned above, because of their infiltrative mode of growth, it is difficult to identify the junction between a malignant tumor and normal adjacent tissue at surgery. As a result, the tumor recurs at the surgical site because of incomplete excision. Of even greater effect is the tendency for malignant tumors to invade lymphatic or blood vessels leading to systemic distribution and development of

the same tumor type at distant sites. Whether attributable to local invasion or systemic spread, the development of metastatic disease is the ultimate criterion of malignancy. Because metastasis is such a major clinical feature of malignant tumors, this subject is discussed in greater detail later in this chapter.

The following case illustrates many of these features of the biological behavior of tumors and the problems associated with diagnosing particularly undifferentiated malignant neoplasms.

CASE 6-1: HISTOGENETIC ORIGIN AND BIOLOGICAL BEHAVIOR

Mickey, a 10-year-old male mixed-breed dog, was presented because of a steadily enlarging mass on the third digit of the right front foot. The lesion had first been noticed by the owners about 1 month previously, but, because it was not unduly troubling the dog, no immediate attention had been sought. On clinical examination the dog was normal in all respects except for the mass, which was about 1.5 cm in diameter, covered with ulcerated haired skin, and firm to palpation. No discomfort was apparently associated with its presence. The clinician advised the owners to have the mass removed and submitted for histological examination.

The mass was submitted in neutral buffered formalin. Its cut surface was firm and white, but no clear demarcation between the mass and surrounding normal tissue could be seen. Histologically (Fig. 6-9) the cells making up the mass were very pleomorphic. They had large, vesicular nuclei that varied from round to elongate in shape and contained very prominent nucleoli. There was a high mitotic index, with one to six mitoses visible in each high-power field. The cytoplasm was faintly basophilic and moderate in amount. The cells were arranged in cords and clusters separated by strands of fibrous tissue. In some areas elongate cells were arranged in parallel arrays. Similar cells were present in the basal layer of the epidermis and extended deep into the dermis.

No definitive evidence of differentiation was found, and, based on the arrangement of the cells, a diagnosis of *anaplastic carcinoma* was made. In an attempt to obtain a definitive diagnosis small pieces of tissue were processed for electron microscopy.

Ultrastructurally (Fig. 6-10) the neoplastic cells were tightly packed with closely apposed plasma membranes that sometimes displayed specialized intercellular junctions. The nuclei contained abundant euchromatin, less heterochromatin, and prominent nucleoli. The cytoplasm contained mitochondria, a moderate amount of rough endoplasmic reticulum (RER), and abundant free polysomes. In addition, there were relatively rare electron-dense organelles that, at high magnification, had an appearance consistent with that of melanosomes. Based on this evidence the diagnosis was amended to malignant melanoma.

Comments on Case 6-1

In this particular case, at the light microscopic level, the neoplasm exhibited many features indicative of malignancy. The cells were anaplastic and pleomorphic, had

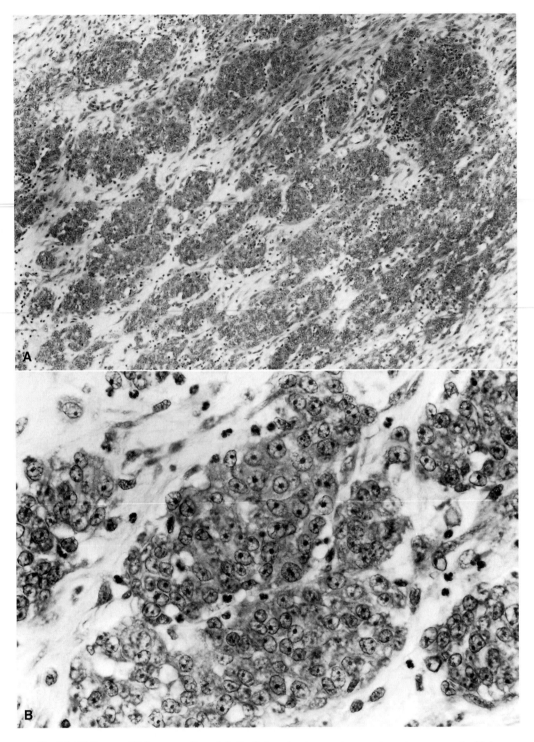

Fig. 6-9 Malignant Melanoma, Case 6-1. By light microscopy, the neoplasm is composed of lobules and clumps of closely apposed tumor cells separated by a cellular fibrous stroma, **A.** At higher magnification, **B,** the cells have large vesicular nuclei and usually one prominent nucleolus. Occasional neutrophils are present in the stroma.

vesicular nuclei with prominent nucleoli, and produced a high mitotic index. In addition, there was evidence of tissue invasion. Two types of neoplasm would be likely to occur in this area. One is squamous cell carcinoma, and the other is melanoma. Together these tumors make up

most of the malignant tumors occurring on the toe of the dog. In this case it was considered to be important to determine which tumor, if either, this represented because the prognosis would differ in each case. Squamous cell carcinomas in this site are very locally invasive but metas-

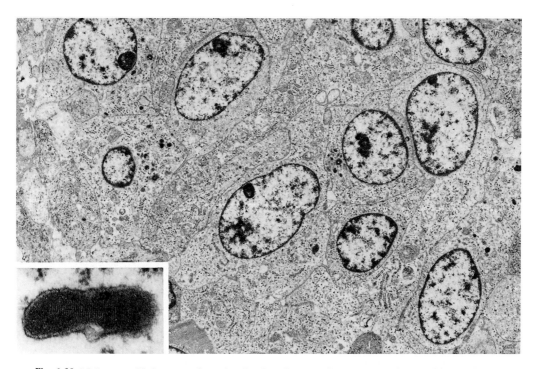

Fig. 6-10 Malignant Melanoma, Case 6-1. In this electron photomicrograph, neoplastic cells are closely apposed and form interwoven cytoplasmic processes. The cytoplasm contains a variety of organelles, including electron-dense structures that, at higher magnification, *inset,* can be seen to have features consistent with premelanosomes. *(Micrograph courtesy R.M. Minor and L. Barr, Ithaca, N.Y.)*

tasize less rapidly than malignant melanomas. Melanomas in dogs vary in malignancy, depending, for one thing, on their site of occurrence. When on the toe, they are often extremely malignant and metastasize widely and rapidly. After the diagnosis of malignant melanoma therefore, a very poor prognosis was offered. Two months later the dog was subjected to euthanasia because of general malaise believed to be related to the neoplasm. At postmortem examination multiple metastases were found in the local lymph nodes and in the lung.

This case demonstrates several principles. The neoplasm had histological features on which a diagnosis of malignancy could be based. Although no evidence of differentiation was present at the light microscopic level, the application of a special technique was able to show definitive features of differentiation characteristic of melanocytes. In addition, the case illustrates that a knowledge of the usual behavior of specific neoplasms in particular species is valuable in formulating a prognosis over and above that suggested by the histological features and observed clinical behavior.

Morphological Characteristics

Gross Pathology

Grossly, neoplasms manifest as abnormal masses of tissue. Depending on the degree of malignancy there is associated replacement of normal tissue architecture (sometimes referred to as "effacement"). A variety of adjectives is used to describe the gross appearance of neoplasms, including papillary, sessile, pedunculated, ulcerative, circumscribed, fungating, multicentric, and annular. Some tumors have a characteristic gross appearance that permits a specific diagnosis to be made. Examples include pigmented melanomas in the perineal region of gray horses and mast cell tumors in the skin of dogs producing a "pin-feather" appearance because of the aggregates of hair follicles separated by dermal infiltrates of neoplastic mast cells. These are the exception, however, rather than the rule, and most tumors cannot be definitively diagnosed grossly.

Microscopic Pathology

The basic distinguishing feature of neoplasms at the light microscopic level is the monotony of the cell populations, with all cells resembling one another to some degree. Of course, the more malignant the tumor is, the more pleomorphic the cells may be, but close inspection reveals an underlying resemblance between cells.

Importantly, all tumors are accompanied by varying amounts of nonneoplastic supportive fibrovascular stromal tissue that provides the vascular supply necessary for the tumor to survive. Malignant

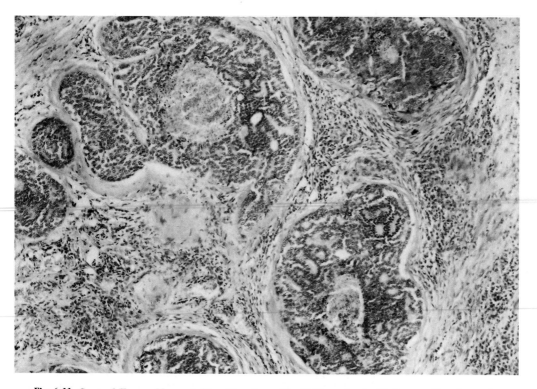

Fig. 6-11 Central Tumor Necrosis Resulting from Rapid Growth of a Malignant Neoplasm. In this carcinoma from the mammary gland of a dog, central areas of necrosis are present in the larger lobules of neoplastic tissue.

not so ↗

tumors frequently contain central areas of necrosis. This is at least partially attributable to the rapid growth rate of the tumor that exceeds that of the vascular supply to central portions of the tumor, resulting in ischemia (Fig. 6-11). Some carcinomas have a propensity to induce extraordinary proliferation of the stroma in excess of that associated with a supportive function. Such neoplasms are referred to as *scirrhous carcinomas*. The excessive fibroblastic response makes these neoplasms characteristically firm to palpation. This stromal induction appears to be a property of the neoplastic cells and is characteristic of certain neoplasms, such as carcinomas of the stomach or intestine.

As a result of their resemblance to the tissue from which they arose, epithelial and mesenchymal neoplasms have characteristically different microscopic features. Epithelial tumors generally grow as nests or cords of cells, reflective of intercellular junctions or orientations along basement membranes, characteristic of many epithelial cells. In contrast, mesenchymal cells appear as sheets of cells in tissue sections without organization into subanatomical structures, characteristic of epithelial neoplasms.

The microscopic features of epithelial versus mesenchymal neoplasms and benign versus malignant neoplasms are reflected not only in tissue sections

but also as cytological characteristics in touch preparations from tumor masses or in smears of effusions or aspirates from neoplasms (Fig. 6-12). This technique sometimes can provide a rapid diagnosis and assure prompt treatment. Cytological criteria that are particularly useful to establish a diagnosis of malignancy include anaplasia and pleomorphism, irregular or angulated cells, changes in nuclear to cytoplasmic (N:C) ratio, variable thickness of the nuclear membrane, multiple nuclei with multiple and angular nucleoli, and abnormal figures.

Grading and Staging

The criteria for malignancy discussed above are of obvious prognostic significance, and attempts have been made to quantitate them to more precisely define the prognosis. *Grading* of neoplasms represents an attempt to *quantitate* characteristics, such as anaplasia and mitotic activity, that form the basis of our subjective evaluation of malignancy. *Staging* of neoplasms represents an attempt to classify them according to their progression, with the size of the primary lesion, the presence of lymph node involvement, and the presence of metastasis being taken into account. Unfortunately these systems are not

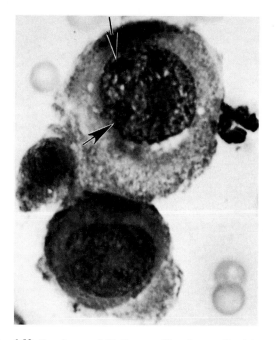

Fig. 6-12 Cytology of Malignant Neoplasms. In this imprint from a malignant squamous cell carcinoma from the skin of a dog, there are nests of large, cohesive, hyperchromatic cells with nuclei that contain prominent nucleoli, *arrows.*

so well developed for domestic animals as they are for humans, largely as a result of the difficulty of obtaining good follow-up information on animal patients. Such systems are useful only if their ability to correlate morphological characteristics with clinical behavior is established for each type of neoplasm in each animal species. For example, useful grading and staging systems have been developed for canine mast cell tumors and lymphomas. Clear differences in survival have been shown between low-grade and high-grade canine mast cell tumors, and responses to different chemotherapeutic regimens have been shown to depend on the stage of disease in dogs with lymphoma. Clinicians and pathologists should strive to develop additional systems for other tumor types.

Pathogenesis

The pathogenesis of neoplasia is sometimes referred to as *oncogenesis* or *carcinogenesis*. It is common to refer to a neoplastic cell as a *transformed* cell and the associated event as *transformation*. In this section, current knowledge of the mechanisms that underlie the development and subsequent behavior of neoplastic cells are discussed. It should be stated from the outset that there is no generally accepted, unified concept of the biological mechanisms that underlie the development of neoplastic disease. The student will probably feel some frustration in reading this material because of a certain lack of dogma. That lack simply reflects the changing nature of our understanding of pathogenetic mechanisms in neoplasia. In view of this, it would be unrealistic to attempt to synthesize a single viewpoint that could, in only too few years, be proved to be wrong. Therefore we will continue to outline the major theories that presently form the basis of our understanding of the biology of neoplasia.

MATURATIONAL ARREST VERSUS DEDIFFERENTIATION

Because of the relative lack of differentiation of neoplastic cells as compared to their normal counterparts, there is a tendency to assume that neoplastic cells arise by dedifferentiation from a more mature cell type. It has now been shown that this is not the case and rather that tumors arise as a result of a partial or complete arrest in differentiation. Further, the point of maturation arrest of target cell and the degree of subsequent inhibition of differentiation determine the degree of malignancy (Fig. 6-13). Immature, undifferentiated cells that undergo neoplastic transformation result in malignant tumors, whereas mature, differentiated (albeit mitotically active) target cells result in benign tumors. Since the degree of inhibition of differentiation of the transformed cell is not necessarily complete, some neoplastic cells are capable of differentiating into mature, postmitotic cells. Nonetheless, a tumor results because of the preponderance of undifferentiated transformed target cell population. Neoplasia therefore represents a pathology of cells involved in tissue renewal. Tumors are composed of neoplastic stem cells and their well-differentiated progeny, which form a "caricature" of their tissue of origin.

During carcinogenesis, this block in the maturation process allows neoplastic cells to accumulate. The microscopic appearance of the tumor reflects the stage of maturation at which the majority of the tumor cells are blocked. For example, squamous cell carcinomas consist of a predominance of undifferentiated basilar epithelial stem cells (the target cell that has undergone neoplastic transformation) admixed with cells in various stages of squamous differentiation, with some proceeding to fully differentiated keratinocytes that form keratin pearls (Fig. 6-14). It is the presence of this differentiated end product that permits a definitive diagnosis of squamous cell carcinoma to be made. Studies have shown that these differentiated, postmitotic, end-stage cells no longer behave as neoplastic cells upon transplantation,

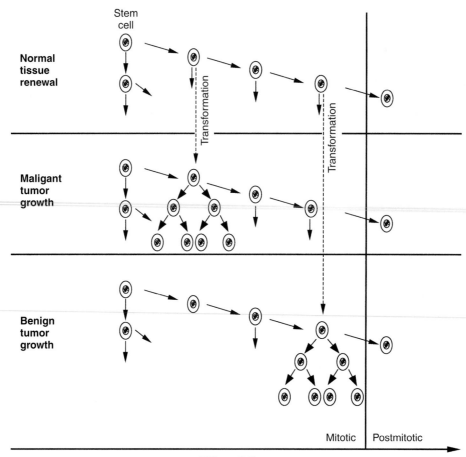

Fig. 6-13 Tumors Arise Because of a Partial or Complete Arrest in Differentiation. During normal tissue renewal, *top panel*, normal stem cells undergo division and differentiation to produce a mature tissue type. During neoplastic growth, *lower two panels*, a maturation arrest leads to an accumulation of the tumor cells at the stage of differentiation of the transformed target tumor cell, *vertical arrows*. The stage of differentiation of the target cell and the subsequent maturation arrest determine the biological behavior (benign or malignant) of the tumor. Some portion of tumor cells escape the arrest and go on to differentiate and become mature, postmitotic cells. Thus, tumors are composed of neoplastic stem cells and their well differentiated progeny, which form a caricature of their tissue of origin.

whereas their less well-differentiated precursors retain the capacity to reform tumors. Thus, once a tumor, not always a tumor. This property is exploited in cancer therapy with the use of growth factors to induce neoplastic cells in the undifferentiated, transformed population to undergo differentiation to more mature, postmitotic, nonneoplastic end-stage cells.

CLONALITY

The question here is whether a given abnormal mass of tissue is the result of proliferation of a single target cell, in which case the growth would be *monoclonal*, or multiple cells in the same area each gave rise to

their own subpopulation, in which case the growth would be *polyclonal*. The answer to this question may reveal important clues about the underlying pathological process. For example, from the foregoing discussion, one might assume that a hyperplastic response associated with chronic inflammation would result in the proliferation of numerous cells in the field and thus a polyclonal growth. Alternatively, as we shall see later, if tumors result from rare somatic mutations and if multiple "hits" are necessary, only rarely should an initially normal target cell acquire the changes that result in a neoplasm. To answer the question, it is necessary to identify and examine certain cell markers that are capable of differentiating between these two alternatives.

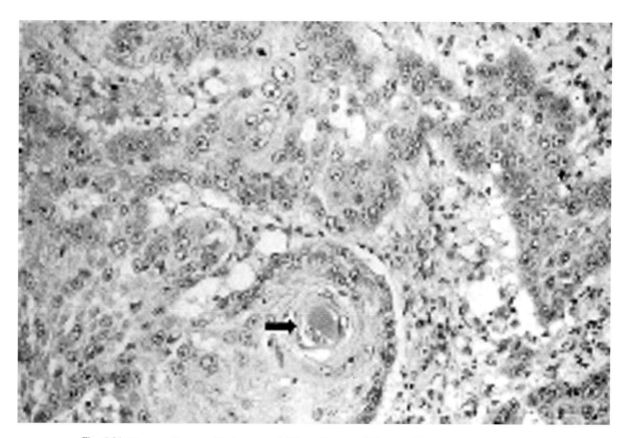

Fig. 6-14 Tumors Form a Caricature of Their Tissue of Origin. Photomicrograph of a squamous cell carcinoma from the ear of a cat. Tumor cells form interconnecting islands composed of a preponderance of poorly differentiated precursor basal cells that have accumulated as a result of a maturational block. Some of the tumor cells have escaped this block and have gone on to form mature, keratinized squamous epithelial cells that form keratin pearls, *arrow.*

Because B and T lymphocytes have unique markers, neoplasms of these cells provide excellent models for such investigations. For example, multiple myelomas, neoplasms of B lymphocytes that have differentiated to plasma cells, secrete a single class of immunoglobulin, resulting in a typical spike in the gammaglobulin region of the serum electrophoretogram, the so-called monoclonal gammopathy. This would not be expected to be so if the tumors were derived from multiple plasma cells. Similar results have been obtained at the molecular level by analysis of immunoglobulin gene rearrangements in neoplastic B cells or analysis of T-cell receptors in neoplastic T cells.

Another marker system that has been used results from the process of *X-inactivation mosaicism.* In each somatic cell, during the early growth of the female embryo, one X chromosome of each pair is randomly inactivated. Some enzymes that occur in two forms (that is, isoenzymes) are encoded by genes carried on the X chromosome. If an individual is heterozygous for such an enzyme, the form carried by any particular cell will be either one or the other, depending on which X chromosome is inactivated, but not both. In humans, one such enzyme is glucose-6-phosphate dehydrogenase (G6PD). The two forms may be designated G6PD^a and G6PD^b. In any given cell, if the X chromosome carrying the gene for G6PD^a is inactivated, the cell will contain G6PD^b, and *vice versa.* Because X-chromosome inactivation is random and tissues are made up of many cells, all tissues of females contain both enzyme forms, though each cell contains only one or the other. If a neoplasm arises in a heterozygous individual from a single altered cell, the neoplastic tissue should contain only one isoenzyme (Fig. 6-15). With this system being used in humans, many types of tumors have been examined, and, in almost all cases, tumors have proved to be monoclonal. In the case of multiple tumors, such as multiple leiomyomas of the uterus, any one tumor has a single enzyme type, though different tumors in the same organ may have different isoenzymes. Similar studies, using chimeric animals produced in the laboratory, have yielded similar

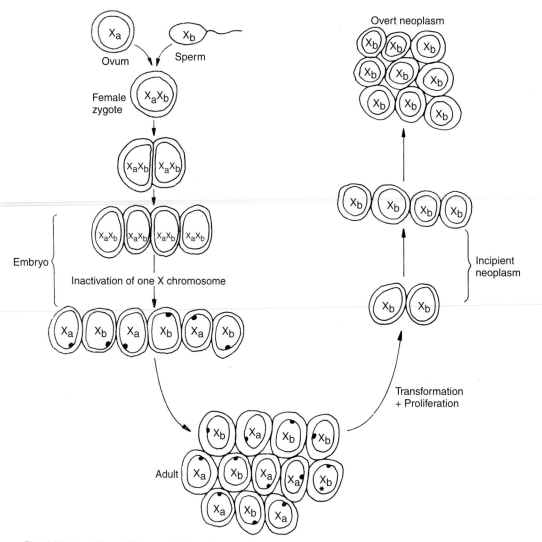

Fig. 6-15 The Clonal Nature of Neoplasms. The phenomenon on X-inactivation mosaicism can be used to test the hypothesis that neoplasms are clonal, or derived from a single transformed cell. During development of the female embryo, one X chromosome is randomly inactivated in all somatic cells. If the individual is heterozygous for an isoenzyme (indicated here as X_a and X_b) coded for by genes on the X chromosome, each cell in the adult will contain one or the other isoenzyme form. If only one cell, indicated by an *asterisk* (*), undergoes neoplastic transformation, all of the cells in the resultant tumor will bear the same isoenzyme. Results of studies such as this have shown that most tumors are monoclonal in origin.

findings. These results imply that most tumors are derived from a single altered cell and are thus monoclonal. This is compatible with the "multiple-hit" model of carcinogenesis. It also argues against the idea, suggested in the past, that normal cells may be recruited into neoplasms. The possibility that tumors arise as polyclonal populations with subsequent elimination of all but the "fittest" clone must be considered; however, there is little or no evidence for this.

Occasional neoplasms that contain cells of both G6PD isoenzymes are found in humans. In particular, hereditary neurofibromas and trichoepithe-

liomas are usually of mixed-enzyme pattern. This indicates that, in these cases, tumors may be derived from many altered cells. One could explain this finding by arguing that the genetic defect carried by all the patient's cells would make it more likely that several cells in a given area could undergo additional events leading to polyclonal neoplasms. Similarly, it has been shown in mice, using the marker enzyme phosphoglycerate kinase, that tumors induced by the carcinogen 3-methylcholanthrene are polyclonal. This effect is dose related, with very low doses of carcinogen tending to produce monoclonal tumors. Therefore it seems likely that the production of polyclonal tumors by high doses of chemical carcinogen are attributable to the initiation of many cells, making progression to multiple neoplasms relatively likely.

Analysis of retrovirus-induced tumors for sites of viral integration into tumor cells provides evidence for both monoclonal and polyclonal derived tumors. Some acute transforming oncogenic viruses, such as feline sarcoma virus, may produce polyclonal tumors as the result of infection of multiple cells at different sites and independent transformation of individual infected cells. However, analysis of tumors resulting from the more common chronic transforming viruses, such as bovine leukemia virus, indicate integration of one or several copies of the provirus in the same site in all tumors from the same animal. This finding is suggestive of monoclonal transformation of a single cell to produce the primary tumor and spread of those cells to establish metastatic foci of the same monoclonal population of tumor cells.

MULTISTEP PROCESS OF ONCOGENESIS

Whatever the fundamental cellular changes underlying carcinogenesis are, certain observations can be made about the process. It is, at least in the case of chemical carcinogenesis, a dose-dependent and cumulative process. Therefore the quantity of chemical that will cause neoplasia may be administered singly or as multiple sequential doses. This implies that progressive changes occur in the target cells during exposure to the substance. Whatever these changes are, they are retained in affected cells after cessation of treatment and may be expressed many cell generations later as neoplasia. It has been shown in several experimental systems that the changes brought about in cells exposed to a dose of a chemical carcinogen that is insufficient to produce tumors are retained. Therefore the exposed individuals retain a higher-than-normal risk of developing neoplasia if again exposed to the same substance. This is of obvious importance to individuals who have been exposed to a carcinogen.

Cellular proliferation enhances the process of carcinogenesis and probably is necessary for carcinogenesis. This may well reflect a necessity for changes to progress or become fixed in the altered cells. It is known that cells that are transformed either *in vivo* or *in vitro* must evolve in some way before they can express themselves as neoplasms. For example, if cells are transformed *in vitro* and immediately implanted into an experimental animal, they usually are not tumorigenic. However, if they are transformed and allowed to proliferate *in vitro* be-

fore implantation, they do produce tumors. There is also evidence that some carcinogens interact preferentially with DNA in proliferating cells and at certain stages of the cell cycle.

Carcinogenesis is a chronic process, requiring long periods of time, sometimes amounting to more than half the life span of the animal. It is now generally believed that in most cases carcinogenesis involves changes in a small number of cells occurring in many steps. The process is progressive, with each step increasing the probability of the emergence of a malignant neoplasm. The appearance of recognizable neoplastic cells therefore occurs as a late event. Much of the evidence for this concept has come from the detailed study of chemical carcinogenesis in the skin, the liver, and other tissues. In these models it has been possible to dissect some of the steps involved.

Some of the first evidence that more than one process, or step, is involved in carcinogenesis was provided by experiments carried out years ago that led to the concept of two-stage induction of neoplasia. More recently this concept has been extended to include progressive changes that occur in transformed foci and in established neoplasms. In the original experiments it was found that a single dose of a carcinogen, such as benzo[a]pyrene, could sensitize skin to which it was applied without actually producing tumors. When a second agent, such as croton oil, was applied repeatedly to the same area, tumors appeared. These processes were called *initiation* and *promotion* respectively, with the first agent being the *initiator* and the second being the *promoter*. Initiation and promotion have been shown to occur in many organs *in vivo*, notably in the skin, liver, colon, and urinary bladder, as well as *in vitro*. These processes are summarized in Fig. 6-16.

Initiation

Initiation involves a change in a target tissue caused by a carcinogen such that the altered cells can be induced (by a promoter) to develop focal proliferations, which in turn can act as sites for the further development of malignancy. Initiation is a rapidly occurring, heritable, essentially irreversible change that produces no permanent morphological changes or autonomous growth in the tissue. It is induced by a single exposure to the initiator. Although it is generally regarded as irreversible, there is some evidence that tumor yield may decrease after long periods, with such a decrease indicating slow reversibility. Initiation therefore resembles direct carcinogenesis in that it apparently induces a change in the treated cells that is passed on from one generation of cells to

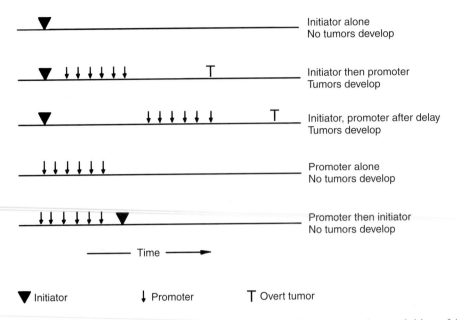

Fig. 6-16 Actions of Initiators and Promoters. Production of tumors requires an initiator followed by a promoter. Initiator alone, promoter alone, or initiator preceded by promoter fail to produce tumors. Tumors may develop even when there is considerable delay between the initiator and the promoter.

the next. Initiation, itself, is believed to involve at least two steps. The first is the induction of a molecular lesion (or lesions) in a rare target cell. The second is the fixation of such lesions by a round of cell proliferation. In models of carcinogenesis in the liver, for example, it is possible to show that the molecular lesion relevant to initiation has a relatively short duration, unless cell proliferation occurs. Thus, to induce initiation in the liver, the administration of the initiator must be accompanied or shortly followed by something that causes cell proliferation.

The nature of the molecular lesion responsible for initiation is unknown. Most initiators, like carcinogens in general, bind to DNA, RNA, and proteins, and it is generally held that DNA is a major molecular target in initiation. The stable nature of initiation, together with the requirement for a round of cell proliferation to "fix" the change, indicates that permanent genetic alterations in DNA are important. On the other hand, there are many known carcinogens that do not seem to interact chemically with DNA. Whether these compounds can induce more subtle genetic changes is yet to be established. The general question of the genetic basis of neoplasia is discussed later in this chapter.

Promotion

Promotion is the process by which an initiated tissue is induced to develop focal proliferative lesions, some of which may later be the site of further changes leading to the development of full-fledged malignant neoplasms. After initiation, no proliferative lesions are present. Under the influence of the promoter, such lesions appear. These lesions result from the expansion by growth of cells phenotypically altered by initiation, and their constituent cells can be shown to have increased mitotic activity. At least in the liver these proliferative lesions have been shown to be clonal in origin; that is, each nodule is derived from a single initiated cell. Promoters may therefore be regarded as providing a selection pressure allowing the emergence of clones of initiated cells.

Again, the molecular basis of promotion is uncertain, but several observed effects of promoters may be important. Promoters exhibit a wide variety of effects on normal tissues. They can cause inflammation, induce hyperplasia, alter patterns of differentiation, or induce a variety of biochemical changes. Unlike initiation, promotion appears to be a prolonged process that requires continual or repeated applications of the promoter over a certain period of time to produce tumors in the initiated tissues. After their application there is a minimal latent period before tumors appear that is independent of the dose of promoter used. Because interruption of treatment with a promoter can result in the failure of development of tumors, promotion is reversible. Although this is true, it is also apparent that at some point the process of promotion is complete and the development of tumors, after the latent period, is irrevocable. Different promoters, with comparable effects in terms of inflammatory or hyperplastic responses, can produce different tumor yields. Promotion is therefore a complex phenomenon, and its mechanisms may vary with different promoters. As compared to initiation, which usually involves a permanent genetic alteration, promotion can be viewed as an epigenetic change involving altered gene expression without a change in the DNA sequence. Promotion should be distinguished from *cocarcinogenicity*, that is, a simple additive effect with the initiator. Some substances that do act as cocarcinogens are not promoters, and some weak promoters are in fact anticarcinogenic when applied together with the initiator.

Progression

From this discussion of initiation and promotion it is evident that several sequential events are necessary for the development of preneoplastic proliferative lesions. Furthermore, these clones, though homogeneous at first, generally become progressively more heterogeneous with respect to a variety of phenotypic features, including proliferative capacity. As already discussed, these lesions eventually develop into malignant neoplasms. This evolution, which has been termed *tumor progression*, can be considered a third stage after initiation and promotion.

At first glance, the evolution of malignant tumors from benign tumors would seem to be incompatible with the stem cell theory of tumorigenesis. However, neoplastic cells have greater genetic instability than normal cells have and continually change by evolution of clonal variants throughout their natural history. In other words, progression arises from a series of discrete changes in a population of cells, with initiation being the earliest. Subsequent changes take place in the population of cells altered during the early events of tumor initiation. Evidence for this concept comes from changes in the nature of some neoplasms observed with time. Relatively benign tumors may gradually show more and more anaplasia and become more malignant in behavior. Other features change progressively as well. For example, the karyotype of neoplastic cells may become increasingly abnormal with time. It is still debated whether all malignant neoplasms evolve through a transient benign focal proliferative lesion, as described in these experimental systems, or some malignant neoplasms arise without such an intervening benign phase. Certainly some malignant neoplasms seem to arise from dysplastic lesions. In other cases without

apparent preneoplastic changes, it is difficult to rule out unobserved changes.

Included within the concept of tumor progression is *tumor cell latency*. Latent tumor cells are those that have undergone some inherent change that makes them neoplastic but that, at least for a while, fail to express this potential for one reason or another. Initiated cells, for example, can be regarded as latent tumor cells that, under appropriate circumstances (in the initiation-promotion model, brought about by the promoter), progress to form overt neoplasms. Latency also has been documented in other experimental tumor systems, in particular the murine mammary tumor model. In this system, carcinogens such as oncogenic viruses, chemical carcinogens, or hormonal influences initially induce multiple hyperplastic nodules that fail to grow beyond a few millimeters in diameter. It has been shown that this failure to grow is attributable to control exerted by normal epithelial cells in nearby mammary ducts. The hyperplastic nodules are capable of more extensive growth when removed from this influence and therefore represent latent tumors. Autonomously growing neoplasms apparently arise as a result of subsequent changes, or progression, which occur in some of these cells. In the murine mammary tumor system, these occur as multiple, morphologically distinct variants. The fact that such distinct lesions develop implies that a variety of changes may occur in numerous cells, with each one different from the next. However, only those with changes enabling the cell to escape from growth controls are able to proliferate. Each of these then gives rise to a clone of heritably stable subtypes. Most such changes appear to be random and independent of selection pressures. There is some evidence, however, that, at least in some cases, heritable changes in the neoplastic cell population can be induced by changes in the local environment.

The basis of progression, like that of carcinogenesis itself and initiation and promotion, is at present unknown. Arguments can be advanced to support multiple mutations (multiple "hits") or epigenetic phenomena (that is, abnormalities of regulation and differentiation) as the explanation for these changes.

Latent, or *dormant*, tumor cells are well known in clinical medicine. It sometimes happens, years after the surgical excision of a primary neoplasm, that tumors recur at the original site or that metastases appear, presumably derived from cells "left behind" at the time of surgery. The emergence of these tumors usually is explained as being attributable to some poorly defined local environmental changes that allows them to grow. An equally viable explanation is that random changes equivalent to tumor progression have occurred in the dormant cells allowing them to escape the constraints to which they had been subjected for all those years.

It also is possible that changes can occur that result in reduced tumorigenicity in initiated cell populations. It is been mentioned that hyperplastic nodules induced in the liver by carcinogens can regress by differentiating to morphologically normal cells. Similarly, dysplastic lesions induced in tracheal mucosa by carcinogens also can regress to a morphologically normal state. What is not known at present is whether these regressed lesions retain an increased susceptibility to neoplasia. Certainly in the tracheal mucosa system regression of the dysplastic lesions is not accompanied by a reduced risk of neoplasia, but it is not clear whether this retained susceptibility resides in the cells derived from the original dysplastic lesions or in other altered cells.

TUMOR CELL GROWTH AND THE CELL CYCLE

Most tissues can be regarded as containing a mixture of cells, some continually dividing, some that are not dividing but are capable of returning to the mitotic pool, and some that are terminally differentiated and no longer able to undergo mitosis. The sequence of events composing mitosis is called the *cell cycle*. Since neoplastic disease represents uncoordinated cell growth, one might expect that derangements in the cell cycle are involved. Recent studies have greatly increased our understanding of the cell cycle and abnormalities in this process that lead to tumors (Fig. 6-17).

The cell cycle is divided into four distinct phases: the *S phase*, when DNA is synthesized; the *M phase*, when mitosis or actual cell division occurs; and two gap phases, G_1 and G_2, preceding the S and M phases respectively. The time required to complete this cycle varies widely between cell types; however, a typical cycle of cultured cells lasts about 24 hours, including about 12, 6, 6, and 0.5 hours for G_1, S, G_2, and M respectively. After mitosis, cells may leave the cycle to differentiate and become "postmitotic." In addition, some types of cells, such as lymphocytes, may enter a resting G_0 pool, where they remain until there is a stimulus for cell proliferation, at which time they may reenter the G_1 phase of the cycle.

The orderly progression of cells through this cycle is controlled by protein complexes composed of *cy-*

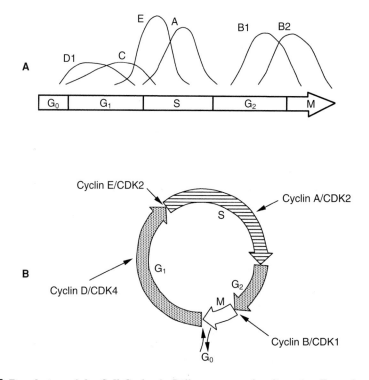

Fig. 6-17 **Regulation of the Cell Cycle. A,** Different types of cyclins, *A* to *E*, reach maximum expression during different phases of the cell cycle (G_0, resting; G_1, gap 1; S, DNA synthesis; G_2, gap 2; *M*, mitosis). **B,** As cyclins reach maximum expression during specific phases of the cycle, they form complexes with more stably expressed cyclin-dependent kinases (CDKs), which then regulate transition of cells from one phase to the next by phosphorylating different protein targets. *(Modified from Cordon-Cardo C: Am J Pathol 147:545-560, 1995.)*

clins and *cyclin-dependent kinases (CDK)*. Different cyclins are synthesized at specific phases of the cell cycle, at which time they complex with and activate more stably expressed CDKs. Activated cyclin–CDK complexes then phosphorylate critical proteins involved in transition from one phase of the cell cycle to another. Five major classes of cyclins (referred to as *A* to *E*) have been described in mammalian cells. Cyclins C, D, and E are maximally expressed from G_1 to S. This is a critical transition in the cycle; once cells pass a *"restriction point"* in late G_1 they become refractory to extracellular signals and are committed to divide. By comparison, cyclins A and B are maximally expressed during S and G_2 respectively and regulate the transition to mitosis. Different types of CDKs have also been identified, and each appears to complex with a specific cyclin to fulfill its specific function in the cycle. For example, cyclin D/CDK4 regulates progression through G_1, cyclin E/CDK2 controls entry into S phase, cyclin A/CDK2 regulates progression through S phase, and cyclin B/CDK1 controls entry into mitosis. More recently, a family of negative regulators of the cycle that further control the cell cycle have been identified. These *CDK-inhibitory (CDKI) proteins* appear to act by binding to and inactivating specific cyclin/CDK complexes. The first and best characterized CDKI protein is p21, which inactivates cyclin E/CDK2, cyclin A/CDK2, and cyclin D/CDK4 complexes.

Abnormalities in any one of these components, that is, cyclins, CDKs, cyclin/CDK substrates, or CDKIs, would thus be expected to disrupt the cycle and lead to uncontrolled cell proliferation and neoplastic disease. For example, studies in humans have shown that cyclin D or its catalytic partner CDK4 are commonly overexpressed in a variety of tumor types. However, the cell cycle regulatory pathways that have received the most attention and are most frequently disrupted in cancer cells involve two genes, *Rb* and *p53*. The role of Rb and p53 as so-called tumor-suppressor genes is discussed later in this chapter, but it is important to discuss them here because of their role in regulating the cell cycle.

The Rb protein is a critical substrate for cyclin/CDK complexes. The level of the Rb protein does not change during different phases of the cell cycle; however, its degree of phosphorylation does and is an important determinant for the G_1-S transition. During G_0 to middle G_1, Rb protein is hypophosphorylated and exists in a complex with DNA-binding transcriptional activation factors, the best studied of which is the E2F family. After phosphorylation of Rb by cyclin D/CDK4, E2F is released and activates the transcription of several genes implicated in the induction of the S phase, such as dihydrofolate reductase and c-*myc*. Thus, in the absence or mutation of Rb or with overexpression of cyclin D/CDK4, the activity of E2F is unrestrained and the G_1-S transition becomes nonrestricted.

The p53 protein is another prototypical cell cycle checkpoint regulator. One of its roles is to arrest the cell cycle in G_1 after genotoxic damage—the so-called p53-dependent G_1 checkpoint. This characteristic has led to p53 being dubbed "guardian of the genome." Depending on subsequent signals, cells either then undergo apoptosis or are allowed time to repair their DNA damage before proceeding through the cycle. p53 protein is a transcription factor, and its DNA binding activity is critical for its ability to mediate the expression of a wide variety of important cellular genes. The ability of p53 to mediate G_1 arrest is at least partially attributable to its activation of the p21 CDKI protein, which inhibits the formation of complexes between cyclins A, E, and D and CDK2, 4, and 6. Thus mutations in p53 destroy its ability to transcriptionally activate p21, relieving a negative regulatory constraint on the G_1 checkpoint.

Interestingly and further demonstrating the importance of Rb and p53 in regulating the cell cycle, the oncogenic properties of several viruses appear to be mediated by effects of viral oncogenes (discussed later in this chapter) on these molecules. Additional studies have shown that the activities of Rb and p53 genes are closely interconnected such that loss of activity of one tumor-suppressor gene is compensated by the other. Oncogenic viruses with especially potent cellular transformation activity have been shown to inactivate both Rb and p53.

Tumor Growth as a Balance of Cell Proliferation and Cell Loss

In general, benign tumors grow slowly, and malignant tumors grow rapidly. At first glance it would seem logical that the growth rate of neoplasms is exponential and a function of the length of the mitotic cycle; however, this is not generally true. The actual growth rate of a neoplasm, like that of a normal tissue, is determined not only by the length of the mitotic cycle but also by the growth fraction (or proportion of cells in mitosis) and the rate of cell loss.

It is now known that the length of the mitotic cycle for neoplastic cells is in fact frequently longer than that of the normal germinal cells from which they are derived. Human bone marrow precursor cells, for example, have a cell cycle time of about 18 hours, whereas the neoplastic cells of acute myeloblastic leukemia have a cell cycle time of about 80 hours. In the case of chronic myelogenous leukemia, the cell cycle time has been measured at about 120 hours. The length of the mitotic cycle, then, is relatively unimportant in determining the rate of growth of neoplasms. Of more importance is the growth fraction, which can vary widely. The factors determining the proportion of cells in mitosis are not well defined, but the most important may be the degree of differentiation of the neoplasm. In many cells, full differentiation precludes further mitotic division. Therefore, well-differentiated neoplasms contain a high proportion of cells unable to divide and so grow slowly. On the other hand, poorly differentiated neoplasms often contain a high proportion of cells in the growth fraction and usually grow rapidly. The immune response, which is discussed in more detail later in this chapter, apparently also can influence the number of cells in the growth fraction. At least, in some experimental systems, interference with the immune response allows an increased number of undifferentiated neoplastic cells to become mitotically active. Even the growth fraction, however, is not the only important factor in determining the rate of growth of neoplasms. The *mitotic index,* or proportion of cells in mitosis at any one time, is also an undependable measure of growth rate. Mitoses may take two or three times as long in some neoplasms as in normal tissues, producing a high mitotic index without a commensurate increase in cell growth rate.

The extent to which cells are lost from neoplasms, by death or exfoliation, is the most important factor determining their overall rate of growth. In neoplasms the rate of cell death may be very high, approaching 100% of those produced in some cases. Although this may seem unlikely at first glance, it can be put into perspective by comparison with tissues that are normally continually replaced, where the rate of cell loss *is* 100% of those produced. Any rate of loss below 100% therefore represents actual growth. Tumor cells may die because of differentiation and cell aging, chromosomal and biochemical abnormalities, ischemia, inadequate nutrition, or immunological attack. Ischemia is one of the most important causes of tumor cell death. Cells further than about 100 to 150 μm from a small blood vessel will die. In addition, although the cell cycle length is not influenced by relative ischemia, the proportion of cells in the growth fraction is. Neoplastic tissue near a zone of ischemia therefore will have fewer cells in mitosis than that in a well-oxygenated area.

Apoptosis and Tumor Growth

In addition to the well-recognized loss of tumor cells as a result of necrosis, several examples of which have already been described, it is apparent that many tumor cells may also be lost as a result of programmed cell death, or apoptosis. This normal physiological process is discussed in greater detail in Chapter 2; however, it is important to mention here because recent studies indicate that apoptosis may be dysregulated in neoplastic cells and may play a role in the overall rate of growth of tumors.

Apoptotic cells can be detected either simply by their characteristic morphological appearance in routinely stained tissue sections or by the use of more-specialized techniques to detect apoptosis-specific biochemical changes or expression of apoptosis-associated proteins in tissue sections. When this is done, an *apoptotic index,* defined as the percentage of apoptotic cells per all tumor cells, can be calculated and applied, similar to the more commonly used mitotic index as a measure of tumor growth and prognosis. Studies in humans have shown that, although there is a wide variation in the apoptotic index between and within different tumor types, apoptosis is generally increased in cancer. This seems counterintuitive because it might be reasoned that increased accumulation of cells and increased tumor growth would be associated with decreased rather than increased apoptosis. The explanation probably is attributable, at least in part, to the activation of oncogenes that influence cell death pathways. Further, there seems to be a consistent positive correlation between apoptosis and proliferation, implying that these processes are mechanistically linked. This is supported by the fact that many proteins that influence the cell cycle (discussed above) are also involved in the regulation of apoptosis (discussed in Chapter 2), prime examples of which are p53 and Rb. It must also be remembered that increased apoptosis in cancer has desirable features. For example, it is well established that most chemotherapeutic agents eliminate tumors by apoptosis, leading to the suggestion that resistance to chemotherapy is attributable to the inactivation of apoptotic machinery in tumor cells.

Telomeres and Cell Division

Recent studies of *telomeres* have provided important new information on cellular longevity and the number of times a cell can traverse the cell cycle before undergoing senescence. Human telomeres are specialized DNA hexameric repeat sequences that are believed to stabilize the ends of chromosomes. However, because conventional DNA polymerases cannot fully replicate the ends of linear DNA, telomeres become progressively shortened with successive cell divisions. In the absence of a mechanism to maintain telomere length, progressive shortening occurs with each cell division, eventually leading to cessation of cell proliferation and the onset of cellular senescence. To compensate for this loss, a ribonucleoprotein with reverse transcriptase activity, *telomerase*, stabilizes telomere length by adding hexameric DNA repeats to the telomeric ends of chromosomes. In agreement with expected cell-replicative capacities, telomerase is expressed in embryonic and adult male germline cells but not in adult somatic cells, except those that retain replicative capacity throughout life, such as hematopoietic stem cells, basal epidermal cells, and intestinal crypt cells. In other words, in the absence of telomerase, progressive shortening of telomeres may serve as the "molecular clock" that determines cellular proliferative potential. In support of this concept, it has recently been demonstrated that the life span of normal human cells can be extended and telomere length can be maintained by transfecting the cells with vectors encoding the human telomerase catalytic subunit.

Since cancer involves aberrations in cell cycle control and excessive cell proliferation, it is of obvious interest to study telomeres in tumor cells. It has now been shown that, in contrast to normal cells, tumor cells do not show a loss of telomere length with cell division, and this correlates with the expression of telomerase in 85% to 95% of the most common types of human cancers, including prostate, breast, colon, lung, and liver. It is unlikely, however, that maintenance of telomerase in tumor cells is causally linked to tumorigenesis. Not all cancers express telomerase, and, in contrast, telomerase activity is maintained in normal renewal tissue and has been detected in some cases of hyperplasia. Nonetheless, these findings have important implications in cancer and make telomerase an attractive target for anticancer therapy.

VASCULARIZATION OF NEOPLASMS

Neoplastic cells, like all other cells, need a supply of nutrients and oxygen and a way to rid themselves of waste products to survive. Diffusion of oxygen and other substances can occur over a range of only about 150 μm, and so cells need to be within this distance of capillary vessels. Tumors therefore need to become vascularized to grow to a significant size. It has been known for many years that proliferation of blood vessels occurs in tissues adjacent to tumors and that capillaries from those tissues penetrate and vascularize the neoplasm. Only more recently, however, has this process, known as *tumor angiogenesis*, been recognized to be a specific biological phenomenon.

Several lines of evidence support the contention that the degree of vascularization determines the rate of growth and biological behavior of neoplasms. For example, when fragments of tumors are transplanted to avascular sites such as the anterior chamber of the eye, they do not grow beyond about 2 mm in diameter. At this stage, cells near the surface still proliferate, but the mass does not enlarge because of loss of cells that die in the center of the mass. Moreover, if neoplastic tissue is transplanted to the cornea, it grows as a thin plate between the layers of corneal stroma until it nears the vascular bed at the limbus. At that stage, when neoplastic cells are within about 2 mm of the vascular supply, small vessels begin to grow into the cornea toward the mass, which they eventually reach and penetrate. After vascularization, the rate of growth of the mass increases dramatically. Endothelial cells within tumors divide at an accelerated rate and express greatly elevated levels of cell adhesion proteins such as α_v-integrins, which are involved in angiogenesis, as compared to normal endothelial cells. Increased intratumor microvessel density is associated with increased tumor aggressiveness and a poorer prognosis. This correlates with the fact that shedding of tumor cells into the circulation begins only after the tumor has become vascularized, and the number of cells entering the circulation is related to the degree of tumor vascularization. In addition, as compared to normal capillaries, tumor microvessels are leaky and contain fragmented basement membranes, which increases the likelihood of tumor embolization and metastasis.

Several steps are involved in the vascularization of tissue *in vivo*. New capillaries are formed by sprouting, mainly from venules. The basement membrane of the venule is locally degraded, probably because of secretion of collagenase and plasminogen activator by endothelial cells. Endothelial cells migrate toward the angiogenic stimulus, in this case a developing tumor, align to form sprouts, and then develop lumens. Continued growth of the budding capillaries is accompanied by mitosis of cells near the leading edge of the sprout. The formation of anastomotic capillary loops is followed by the establishment of blood flow. The discovery of this orderly sequence of events was followed by a search for signals that might initiate this process in both physiological and pathological situations, including neoplasia.

Based on these concepts, tumors can be considered to grow in two phases (Fig. 6-18). Avascular growth precedes tumor vascularization, and during this phase a tumor can reach only 1 to 2 mm in diameter before it becomes dormant in terms of total tumor growth. This might provide one explanation for the clinical observation of dormancy in which metastatic lesions develop many years after the removal of the primary mass. Carcinoma *in situ* also might be regarded as an example of growth in the avascular phase. It has been suggested that such

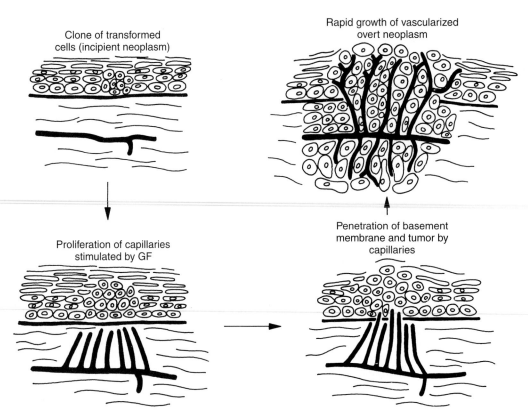

Fig. 6-18 Effect of Angiogenesis on Tumor Growth. Before vascularization, the incipient tumor is limited in its ability to grow. Neoplastic cells produce endothelial growth factors, *GF*, which stimulate the growth of blood vessels toward the tumor. Once the tumor is vascularized the neoplastic cells are able to proliferate to produce an overt tumor.

lesions are limited in size until the basement membrane is breached and the neoplasm becomes vascularized. Whether the basement membrane is breached by tumor cells or by proliferating vessels is not yet established. Preneoplastic lesions have also been shown to have increased angiogenic capabilities. The vascular phase of growth results from an "angiogenic switch" and is signalled initially by the exponential growth of tumor cells. The growth of large tumors is, however, limited by necrosis, as we have already discussed. It is often said that rapidly growing malignant neoplasms "outgrow their blood supply," but more plausible explanations are provided by the observations that the surface area of the vascular network relative to tumor mass decreases as the tumor grows, and that tumors develop high interstitial fluid pressure, which compresses capillaries within the mass. Necrosis then is probably largely attributable to ischemia resulting from these phenomena.

The process of tumor vascularization shares many of the features of vascularization associated with normal wound healing. The difference is that in neoplasia, angiogenesis is persistent and excessive, re-sulting in continued growth of the tumor. It is now known that tumor angiogenesis is stimulated by diffusible substances secreted by neoplastic cells or other cells associated with the neoplasm, in particular macrophages. Many such substances have been demonstrated in tumor extracts. An initial angiogenic substance extracted from tumors was called *tumor angiogenesis factor* (TAF), but it is now recognized that a variety of endothelial growth factors, which may be produced by neoplastic or normal cells, is involved in angiogenesis (Table 6-4). Many of these growth factors are potent mitogens for endothelial cells and are angiogenic *in vivo*, whereas others may act through an intermediate mechanism, perhaps by causing release of other angiogenic factors from tissue cells such as macrophages.

The discovery of the importance of tumor angiogenesis in converting latent tumors to overt tumors has led to a search for antiangiogenic factors. The significance of possibly being able to inhibit vascularization of tumors is obvious. Without vascularization, the growth of neoplasms, in particular metastases, would be limited, and much of their clinical significance might possibly be avoided. Sim-

TABLE 6-4 **Naturally Occurring Regulators of Angiogenesis**

ANGIOGENESIS-STIMULATING FACTORS

Acidic and basic fibroblast growth factor (aFGF, bFGF)
Angiogenin
Granulocyte colony-stimulating factor (G-CSF)
Heparinase
Hepatocyte growth factor
Insulin-like growth factor-1 (IGF-1)
Interleukin-8 (IL-8)
Placenta growth factor
Platelet-derived growth factor (PDGF)
Pleotropin
Prostaglandins E_1, E_2
Transforming growth factors α and β (TGF-α, TGF-β)
Tumor necrosis factor α (TNF$-\alpha$)
Vascular endothelial growth factor (VEGF)

ANGIOGENESIS-INHIBITING FACTORS

Angiostatin
Cartilage-derived inhibitor
Endostatin
Heparinase
Interferon-α, -β, and -γ (IFN-α, IFN-β, IFN-γ)
Interleukin-1 and -12 (IL-1, IL-12)
Platelet factor 4 (PF4)
Prolactin fragment
Protamine
Thrombospondin-1 (TSP-1)
Tissue inhibitor of metalloproteinase (TIMP)

ilar to efforts to identify factors that stimulate angiogenesis, numerous naturally occurring factors that inhibit angiogenesis have now been identified (see Table 6-4). Early experiments concentrated on cartilage as a source of such factors for several reasons. Normal hyaline cartilage is of course devoid of blood supply in the adult animal. Furthermore, cartilage is known to resist invasion by neoplasms. For example, osteosarcomas rarely invade across joint spaces (Fig. 6-19), apparently as a result of resistance to invasion by the articular cartilage. Experimentally it has been shown that fragments of viable cartilage can inhibit the vascularization of transplanted tumors, as in the cornea. If the cartilage is first boiled, this inhibitory effect is lost, and such a loss indicates that viable cartilage may secrete an inhibitory substance or substances. A 27 kD peptide that inhibits mammalian collagenase has been purified from cartilage. The antiangiogenic activity of this molecule is likely related to its ability to prevent degradation of basement membranes,

which are one of the important barriers to tumor cell invasion.

Another rewarding line of tumor antiangiogenesis investigation was stimulated by the interesting clinical observation that some cancer patients suddenly experience rapid and widespread growth of distant tumors after removal of the primary mass. These patients do not have clinical evidence of metastatic disease before surgery, indicating that removal of the primary tumor may remove a constraint on preexisting but clinically silent metastatic tumors. Two factors, *angiostatin* and *thrombospondin-1*, which inhibit angiogenesis *in vitro* and *in vivo* have now been characterized. Angiostatin is a 38 kDa protein that is 98% homologous to an internal fragment of plasminogen. The *in vivo* source of angiostatin remains unclear. There is evidence that proteases from macrophages and tumor cells cleave plasminogen to yield angiostatin. As another example of converging lines of investigation in tumor biology, it has been shown that the tumor-suppressor gene p53 (see later) controls the expression of thrombospondin-1. Loss of p53 function associated with neoplasia results in decreased expression of thrombospondin-1 and thus loss of the constraint on tumor vascularization.

In summary, it appears that primary tumors produce factors that both promote angiogenesis (as angiogenin does) and inhibit it (as angiostatin does). The balance of production and release of these opposing sets of factors determines the extent of angiogenesis of the primary tumor and its ability to invade and metastasize. In some cases, removal of the primary tumor, the largest source of angiogenesis-inhibitory factors, removes the constraint on vascularization and thus the growth of preexisting micrometastases. Inhibition of angiogenesis provides a novel target for tumor cytostatic therapy aimed at constraining tumor growth, invasion, and metastasis.

CHANGES IN TUMOR CELL SURFACES

Neoplastic cells, particularly those of malignant neoplasms, differ in many ways from normal cells. Some of these differences can be appreciated by clinical presentations of tumor-bearing patients, whereas other differences can be demonstrated by analysis of the tumor cells themselves. When normal cells are grown *in vitro*, they spread out to form a single sheet, or monolayer, of cells. Growth ceases when the cells reach a certain density, and the cells remain quiescent but healthy. This process is known as *cell density–dependent inhibition*, or *contact inhibition* of growth. In contrast, malignant cells

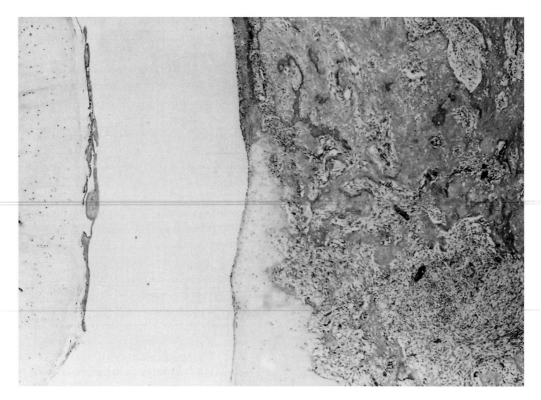

Fig. 6-19 Resistance of Articular Cartilage to Neoplastic Invasion. The osteosarcoma at the right of the micrograph has compressed but not invaded the articular cartilage, leaving the joint space in this cat free of tumor. This is the usual finding in osteosarcomas and presumably reflects the general resistance of cartilage to neoplastic invasion.

grow in a haphazard way, pile up into multiple layers, and are much less responsive to cell density–dependent mechanisms of growth control. Biochemical changes, such as the absence of normal enzymes or the presence of abnormal ones, can occur in neoplastic cells. Very anaplastic cells tend to revert to glycolytic energy metabolism even in the presence of oxygen. Many of these changes probably represent epiphenomena, or "noise," resulting from the fundamental changes underlying neoplastic transformation but not causing it. This problem has made the analysis of the molecular basis of transformation extremely difficult.

Changes in the cell membrane in transformed cells have been studied extensively in an attempt to discover the basic defect in cellular control that underlies neoplasia. Numerous biochemical changes in the surface of transformed cells have been described. Among the most prominent is the consistent loss of a protein once referred to as LETS (large external transformation–sensitive) protein, now called *fibronectin*, from transformed cells. In addition, other proteins and polypeptides may be lost from or reduced on the cell surface. The mechanism of loss of these molecules is unknown but probably includes failure of synthesis and shedding from the cell sur-

face. Other proteins, especially glycoproteins, may be increased in amount or appear *de novo* in transformed cells. This is important because some of these presumably include new antigens that appear on the surface of some transformed cells. Variable changes in sialic acid content, glycosylation of surface glycoproteins and length of glycosyl chains on cell membrane gangliosides also may occur. Changes in the cell surface may result in increased *agglutinability* of transformed cells by plant agglutinins. This apparently is attributable to the synthesis or unmasking of receptors for these substances. Many of these changes also occur in normal cells during mitosis. However, in transformed cells at rest there is no switch to the normal pattern. Therefore, there appears to be a loss of ability to carry out cell density–dependent modulation of the cell membrane in transformed cells.

Cell surface enzyme activities also may be altered in transformed cells. In particular there is usually an increase in activity of proteases and glycosidases. These may be of some pathogenetic importance because treatment of normal cells with proteases induces in them many of the characteristics of transformed cells. Also, some of the altered growth properties of transformed cells *in vitro* and some of their altered surface characteristics can be modified by protease inhibitors.

Thus a variety of cell membrane changes that appear related to mechanisms of control of growth occurs in neoplastic and transformed cells. The various surface changes described in transformed cells may lead to failure to establish functional contact between cells that, through transmembrane cytoskeletal linkages, normally results in modulation of DNA synthesis and cell movement. The exact mechanism or mechanisms involved, however, remain to be fully elucidated.

Genetic Aspects of Oncogenesis

Genetic versus Epigenetic Changes

In the recent past there has been considerable controversy concerning the genetic basis of carcinogenesis and neoplastic transformation. For a single abnormal cell to give rise to a monoclonal tumor, it must be *heritable* in the sense that it must pass its abnormality on to its daughter cells. The controversy is whether the heritable abnormality is *genetic,* that is, the result of somatic mutation in the DNA sequence, or *epigenetic,* that is, the result of an alteration in gene expression without a change in the DNA sequence. Further, mutational and epigenetic factors are not mutually exclusive, and both types of change can contribute to the development of a neoplasm. For example, both mechanisms are involved in the two-stage initiation-promotion model of carcinogenesis discussed previously. Initiators usually induce a genetic alteration resulting in a permanent somatic mutation, whereas promoters produce an epigenetic alteration in the pattern of gene expression.

Although it seems quite logical that genetic changes are heritable (passed from cell to cell through mitosis), it is not so intuitively obvious that epigenetic changes may also be heritable and responsible themselves for the neoplastic transformation. However, it may be argued that characteristics reflecting "cell memory" such that, for example, liver cells produce liver cells, represent heritable epigenetic changes. The argument may be extended to implicate epigenetic change in oncogenesis when one notices the similarities between the behavior of some normal tissue cells and those of neoplastic cells. For example, trophoblastic cells are invasive and endometrial cells may implant in abnormal sites. Furthermore, there is evidence that the loss of control of growth and differentiation that is characteristic of neoplasia may, in some circumstances, be reversible. There are documented cases of neoplasms undergoing terminal differentiation with the loss of a further capacity to grow. The most striking evidence of this type comes from studies that have been carried out using teratocarcinomas of mice. These malignant neoplasms are believed to arise from primitive stem cells and show multiple pathways of differentiation. If teratocarcinoma cells are implanted into developing blastulas from normal mice, the baby mice that result are mosaics composed of cells from the blastula and cells from the implanted neoplastic cells. These mice do not develop teratocarcinomas; thus it appears that the neoplastic cells can be induced to undergo normal differentiation if subjected to the appropriate environment. In this particular case epigenetic control mechanisms apparently underlie neoplastic transformation.

Hormonal control of tumor growth is another example an epigenetic change. Hormones are known to be involved in the cause of many tumors in domestic animals, rodents, and humans. In many cases these arise in the target tissue of the hormone as a consequence of continual hormonal stimulation. For example, if ovarian tissue is implanted into the spleen of ovariectomized animals, the implanted ovary will eventually become neoplastic. In this experimental situation, continued stimulation of the ovary occurs because of the hepatic destruction of the estrogens secreted by the implanted tissue and consequent loss of feedback on the pituitary gland. Another example is the occurrence of mammary tumors in dogs receiving long-term administration of progesterone. Other neoplasms in the dog also are known to be hormone dependent, and knowledge of this fact may be important to the clinician. For example, multiple adenomas of the circumanal glands occur frequently in old, male dogs. These are influenced by testosterone, and castration of the affected animal will greatly reduce the incidence of recurrence of neoplasms in the animal.

Overall, however, there is compelling evidence that most forms of neoplasia are attributable to genetic alterations in the host DNA sequence. There is now a large body of evidence supporting somatic mutation as the cause of neoplastic transformation, and there is no doubt that damage to the host genome and mutations in certain genes result in tumor formation.

Most chemical carcinogens or their metabolites react with DNA in various ways and can, in suitable test systems, be shown to be mutagenic. Because of the potential hazards of any new chemical, including drugs and many other compounds used in modern society, methods are required to test for carcinogenicity. Some of the testing is done in animals, but this is obviously time consuming and expensive and raises important concerns related to the humane use of animals. The idea that most carcinogens are also mutagens has led to alternative methods of testing *in vitro* such as the *Ames test*. This test uses specific mutant strains of *Salmonella typhimurium* bacteria that are incubated with the test chemical. Liver microsomes are included to provide for metabolic activation of the test chemical, and mutagenicity is measured by detection of the number of bacterial revertants, or reverse mutations. The validity of this test depends on the assumption that a chemical, if proved mutagenic in a bacterial system, will be carcinogenic in animals. Compilation of data collected over many years has shown that the majority of chemicals that are carcinogenic in rodents are mutagenic in the Ames test and conversely that the majority of mutagens are carcinogens. On this basis the Ames test has assumed a dominant role in short-term genotoxicity testing of chemicals. Tests similar to the Ames test but using animal cells instead of bacteria also have been utilized to detect mutagenicity. However, there are exceptions to the axiom that all carcinogens are mutagens, as discussed below.

Radiation also is known to be mutagenic. UV irradiation, for example, is known to cause DNA damage, including the formation of pyrimidine dimers. Normally cells try to repair damage to DNA (see Chapter 7), but some of the mechanisms are error prone, and altered sequences may become incorporated permanently. There is evidence, in mammalian cells, that such errors may be significant in carcinogenesis. For example, if these error-prone mechanisms of repair are inhibited, the toxicity of mutagens is increased. However, the carcinogenicity of skin irradiation is *reduced* by the same treatment. In this situation, it seems that no repair is better than incorrect repair.

Individuals with mutations resulting in defective repair of DNA are prone to neoplastic disease. The most instructive of these diseases is *xeroderma pigmentosum* of humans. This syndrome is known to be attributable to a specific defect in the ability of patients to repair damage to DNA induced by UV irradiation. Affected individuals can repair other types of damage to DNA, such as that caused by x irradiation, indicating an exquisite level of specificity in these repair mechanisms. Patients with xeroderma pigmentosum have a very high incidence of skin neoplasms associated with exposure to sunlight. These tumors occur at an early age, and the relative frequency of the various types of neoplasms parallels that of normal people with excessive exposure to sun. The absolute frequency is, however, about 10,000 times that of normal individuals. This strongly indicates that faulty repair of DNA can result in neoplasia. Additional evidence for the mutational basis of neoplasia is provided by the high frequency of cancer in humans with other hereditary chromosomal fragility syndromes. Some of these are associated with DNA repair deficiencies. Furthermore, there is now overwhelming evidence that chromosomal abnormalities are consistently found in neoplastic cells. The evidence that these are involved in the development of neoplasia are discussed below.

In addition to the syndromes referred to above, there are several well-known instances of hereditary neoplasia, or hereditary predisposition to neoplasia. These include retinoblastoma, Wilms' tumor, and others in man and a hereditary form of renal carcinoma in rats. In the case of hereditary *retinoblastoma* it has been shown quite clearly that individuals at risk are heterozygous (that is, are carriers) for deletions or some other defect in a particular segment of chromosome 13. All cells of their body therefore carry one defective chromosome. It has also been shown that tumors in most of these individuals are homozygous or hemizygous for the defective chromosome, with the normal one having been lost or replaced by duplication of the defective one. Thus it seems that some gene and its product have been lost from these cells. The role that such a gene might play in the development of neoplasia is discussed further below. This disease not only contributes to the evidence for a mutational basis of neoplasia but also provides a compelling example of the "multiple-hit" phenomenon, whereby more than one genetic event is required to induce a neoplasm. Here, the first event is a germline mutation, and the second event is a somatic mutation, often brought about by chromosomal rearrangement.

Another excellent example of genetic alterations and the multiple-hits phenomena of neoplasia is provided by colorectal cancer in humans. Colon cancer, a portion of which are familial in origin, now represents the second leading cause of cancer deaths in the United States. It has been studied in depth at the molecular level, in part because, as compared with most malignancies, stages that represent the progression from normal mucosa, to hyperplasia, to adenoma, to carcinoma *in situ*, through to carcinoma and metastasis are readily identifiable. These stages parallel the sequential and progressive accumulation of alterations in different genes. One of the first to be involved is the *adenomatosis polyposis coli* (APC) gene. Germline mutations in the APC gene on chromosome 5 are responsible for an inherited form of human colon cancer known as *familial adenomatosis coli* (FAP). APC gene defects are also common in nonfamilial sporadic cases of colon cancer in humans. FAP patients develop hundreds to thousands of polyps in the large intestine at a young age, a portion of which will progress to colonic carcinomas if not removed. Progression to malignancy is associated with 7 to 10 subsequent additional alterations in more than a half dozen other genes. The function of each of these genes is not completely known. Some act as *oncogenes*, whereas others, such as the APC gene, clearly act as *anti-oncogenes* or *tumor suppressors*. These two important categories of genes are discussed more fully below.

In summary, there are compelling arguments for the role of somatic mutation and genetic abnormalities in the cause of neoplasia. The fact that most neoplasms are clonal in origin (see above) also is consistent with a mutational basis for neoplasia. One could ask why more varied manifestations of somatic mutation do not become apparent. For the results of a mutation to be evident, however, a clone of recognizable size must develop, and only those events that confer a proliferative advantage, that is, cause a tumor, would become manifest. The most impressive arguments against mutation depend on the fact that the neoplastic phenotype can sometimes be reversed. However, it is now apparent that the normal control of cellular growth and differentiation is extremely complex, involving many interactive processes, some of which counter others. There is accumulating evidence that the products of different genes can augment or counteract those of others, such that the final phenotype depends on the relative contributions of each.

CHROMOSOMAL ABNORMALITIES AND NEOPLASIA

The fact that cancer cells have karyotypic abnormalities, involving alterations in chromosome number or morphology, has been known for many years. However, it was generally believed that many of these changes represented secondary events occurring during the progression of the neoplasm. The advent of high-resolution cytogenetic banding techniques changed our view of the significance of chromosomal abnormalities in neoplasia. It is now recognized that nonrandom chromosomal abnormalities are a consistent feature of many neoplasms. Over 90% of human malignancies have clonal cytogenetic alterations. In many cases the abnormalities are specific and characteristic for a particular type of neoplasm. Several chromosomal abnormalities, in particular human lymphomas and leukemias, have been especially instructive in understanding the genetic events that may underlie the development of neoplasia.

An example is the so-called *Philadelphia chromosome* (Ph[1]), a cytogenetic marker for chronic myelogenous leukemia in humans. This marker chromosome, resulting from a translocation between chromosomes 9 and 22, provided an early exception to the belief that karyotypic abnormalities in cancer were secondary events. Ph[1] is present in most patients with the disease and has been observed in normal individuals who later developed the disease. It was therefore believed to play some causative role in this neoplasm. This was subsequently shown to be the case when it was found that the Ph[1] chromosome represents a transposition of a specific oncogene (see below), c-*abl*, from chromosome 9 to chromosome 22, near a particular locus called *bcr*. The juxtaposition of *abl* and *bcr* results in the transcription of a hybrid mRNA that in turn encodes a fusion protein containing parts of each parent protein. This protein has a high level of protein kinase activity.

Another instructive example is Burkitt's lymphoma, an aggressive B-cell neoplasm usually affecting children. It is endemic in Africa, where it is associated with infection with Epstein-Barr virus (EBV), and occurs sporadically in other parts of the world unassociated with the virus. All cases of Burkitt's lymphoma have translocations between chromosome 8 and either chromosome 14, 22, or 2. Each of the latter three chromosomes carries a locus for parts of the immunoglobulin molecule. The breakpoint on chromosome 8 is close to the cellular oncogene c-*myc*, and the result is that c-*myc* becomes juxtaposed to one of the immunoglobulin loci, and the oncogene comes under the influence of tissue-specific genetic enhancers at these sites. The net result of these translocations is believed to be that the transcription of the c-*myc* oncogene is deregulated, contributing to the neoplastic phenotype. The *myc* oncogene is discussed more fully later in this chapter. Further weight is added to the significance of these findings by the fact that analogous translocations, involving immunoglobulin loci and *myc*, are associated with plasmacytomas in the mouse and the rat and that translocations the breakpoints of which interrupt the T-cell receptor are involved in T-cell neoplasms in humans. Molecular analysis of chromosomal breakpoints in other lymphoid neoplasms has now been used to identify and clone putative new oncogenes.

Chromosomal abnormalities tend to become progressively more extensive as tumors progress, contributing additional changes in the genetic makeup of the neoplastic cell population—part of the multiple-hit hypothesis, as already mentioned. The changes may include addition or loss of chromosomes. The former may cause increased expression of important genes, whereas the latter could lead to the loss of important genes, similar to that occurring in retinoblastoma. Particularly as tumors progress, particular parts of the genome may become amplified and are seen as abnormal banding regions, so-called double minutes, or homogeneous staining regions revealed during cytogenetic examination. In some cases, these amplified regions have been shown to involve oncogenes leading to increased gene expression. This is believed to contribute to progressive increase in malignancy.

Unfortunately, specific chromosomal defects have not been studied in detail in most naturally occurring neoplasms of animals. In dogs, consistent chromosomal abnormalities occur in the transmissible venereal tumor (TVT), where tumor cells have an abnormal number of chromosomes, usually 59, rather than the normal 78. Interestingly, this particular karyotypic abnormality is associated with another unusual feature of this neoplasm: transplantability between dogs. Despite numerous abnormalities in tumor cells, including chromosomal defects, most tumors cannot be transplanted between different outbred hosts because the tumor cells retain major histocompatibility antigens on their surface, which stimulate immune rejection by a heterologous host. For reasons that are not fully understood, TVT cells escape this immune rejection when they are transferred to a new canine host.

The well-understood examples from human neoplasms that we have discussed above document the significance of chromosomal abnormalities in the pathogenesis of neoplasia and provide compelling evidence for the role of specific "cancer genes," the oncogenes.

ONCOGENES

The explosion in understanding of the genetic basis of neoplasia is attributable to dramatic advances in the identification and characterization of specific genes believed to be important in control of growth and differentiation and in the generation of the neoplastic phenotype. These genes are the *oncogenes*. The first indications of the existence of such genes came from the study of oncogenic retroviruses, which are discussed in more detail elsewhere in this chapter. Typical retroviruses contain three genes, *gag*, encoding capsid proteins; *pol*, encoding reverse transcriptase; and *env*, encoding envelope proteins. Viruses containing these genes are replication competent and include some slowly transforming retroviruses, such as murine leukemia virus (MuLV), avian leukosis virus, and feline leukemia virus (FeLV). These are infectious viruses capable of producing lymphomas or leukemias in their host. Characteristically they require a long incubation period

to produce neoplastic disease. In contrast, the acutely transforming retroviruses are capable of inducing tumors very rapidly. They do not occur widely as infectious viruses but are typically isolated from tumors. The archetype of this group is Rous sarcoma virus, originally isolated from a sarcoma in a chicken. In addition to the three genes already described, this virus was found to contain an additional gene, dubbed *src*. Since this gene was shown to be necessary and sufficient for cellular transformation, it was referred to as a *viral oncogene* (v-*onc*). It is one of about 20 v-*onc*s known to be associated with acutely transforming retroviruses. These viruses are replication defective, in that parts of the usual genome are deleted and replaced by the v-*onc*. They are therefore able to replicate only if cells are coinfected with a competent "helper" virus that supplies the missing functions.

Knowledge of the viral oncogenes led to the discovery that tissue cells of normal animals contain homologous genomic sequences known as *proto-oncogenes*, to connote their potential transforming capability. These are highly conserved, ubiquitous genes found in organisms widely separated on the evolutionary scale. It is now known that oncogenes originally described in acutely transforming retroviruses are actually proto-oncogenes captured ("transduced") by the virus and converted into v-*onc*s. In addition, the structure or function of proto-oncogenes may be altered while they remain within the host genome, as by the action of chemical carcinogens, such that they acquire transforming capability. Such altered proto-oncogenes are referred to as *cellular oncogenes* (c-*onc*s). More than 100 proto-oncogenes have now been characterized. Not all of these are associated with viral homologs. Alternative approaches, such as cloning chromosomal breakpoints and DNA transfection assays, have identified these additional oncogenes.

What then, is the normal function of these genes, and how are they involved in the development of neoplasia? The term "oncogene" is really, in the light of current understanding, a misnomer. Obviously these genes are not present to cause cancer. Rather, it is generally believed that proto-oncogenes encode proteins that play important roles in normal cellular functions, including regulation of growth and differentiation. Normal growth mediated by proto-oncogenes versus cellular transformation mediated by viral or cellular oncogenes is attributable to qualitative or quantitative differences in the expression of the encoded protein products. Table 6-5 summarizes some of the better-characterized oncogenes and groups them according to their subcellular location and function. As can be seen from the

Cell Division only

TABLE 6-5   Some Oncogenes, Their Gene Product, and Subcellular Location

FUNCTIONAL GROUP	ONCOGENE	ASSOCIATED RETROVIRUS	ASSOCIATED TUMOR	GENE PRODUCT*	SUBCELLULAR LOCATION
PROTEIN KINASES					
	src	Rous sarcoma	Fibrosarcoma	TK	Plasma membrane
	yes	Avian sarcoma	Sarcoma	TK	Plasma membrane
	ros	Avian sarcoma	Sarcoma	TK; related to GF receptor	Plasma membrane
	abl	Abelson murine leukemia	Leukemia	TK	Plasma membrane
	fes	Feline sarcoma	Fibrosarcoma	TK	Plasma membrane
	kit	Feline sarcoma	Fibrosarcoma	TK	Plasma membrane
	fms	Feline sarcoma	Fibrosarcoma	TK; CSF-1 receptor	Plasma membrane
	erb-B	Avian erythro-blastosis	Erythroleukemia	TK; EGF receptor	Plasma membrane
	neu (erb-B2)	None	Breast carcinoma (humans)	TK; related to EGF receptor	Plasma membrane
	mos	Moloney murine sarcoma	Sarcoma	S/TK	Cytoplasm
GTP-BINDING PROTEINS					
	H-ras	Harvey murine sarcoma	Many types (humans)	GTP-binding protein	Plasma membrane
	K-ras	Kirsten murine sarcoma	Many types (humans)	GTP-binding protein	Plasma membrane
	N-ras	None	Many types (humans)	GTP-binding protein	Plasma membrane
GROWTH FACTORS					
	sis	Simian sarcoma	Sarcoma	PDGF	Secreted
NUCLEAR PROTEINS					
	c-myc	Avian myelocy-tomatosis	Murine myeloma; Burkitt's lympho-ma (humans)	DNA-binding transcription factor	Nucleus
	L-myc	None	Small cell lung carinoma (humans)	DNA-binding transcription factor	Nucleus
	N-myc	None	Neuroblastoma (humans)	DNA-binding transcription factor	Nucleus
	myb	Avian myelo-blastosis	Leukemia	DNA-binding transcription factor	Nucleus
APOPTOSIS REGULATORS					
	bcl-2	None	Follicular lympho-mas (humans)	Antiapoptosis regulator	Mitochondrial membrane
	bax	None	Follicular lympho-mas (humans)	?	Mitochondrial membrane

*CSF-1, Colony-stimulating factor-1; EGF, epidermal growth factor; GF, growth factor; GTP, guanine triphosphate; PDGF, platelet-derived growth factor; S/TK, serine/threonine-specific protein kinase; TK, tyrosine-specific protein kinase.

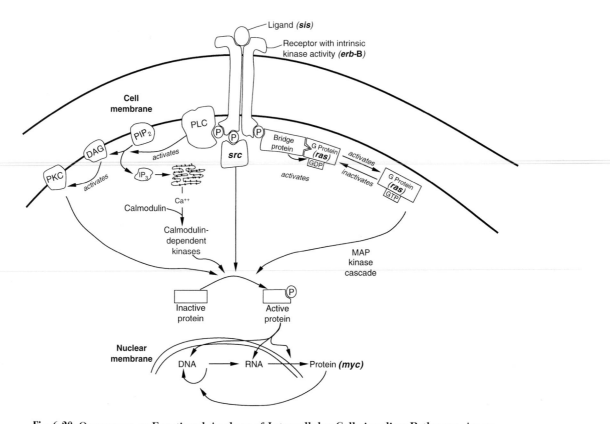

Fig. 6-20 Oncogenes as Functional Analogs of Intracellular Cell-signaling Pathways. An example of normal signaling through a tyrosine kinase receptor and how oncogene products serve as analogs in signal-transduction pathways. After binding with its ligand, the cell surface receptor becomes autophosphorylated and develops tyrosine (or less commonly serine/threonine) kinase activity. The autophosphorylated cytoplasmic extension of the receptor binds a series of cytoplasmic proteins, which in turn activate distinct signaling systems. Examples of binding to three different types of proteins are shown. (1) The receptor can bind directly to a member of the SRC family of tryosine kinases, *center.* (2) Bridge proteins couple the receptor to guanine-binding proteins *(G proteins), right.* Activated G proteins exchange guanosine diphosphate *(GDP)* for guanosine triphosphate *(GTP),* which then become activated and signal through the so-called mitogen-activated protein *(MAP)* kinase cascade. (3) The receptor can activate phospholipase C *(PLC), left.* PLC cleaves phosphatidylinositol 4,5-biphosphate *(PIP₂)* to inositol 1,4,5-triphosphate (IP_3) and 1,2-diacylglycerol *(DAG).* IP_3 causes release of calcium ions from the endoplasmic reticulum, whereas DAG activates protein kinase C *(PKC).* Notice that in each case the final effect is mediated by protein kinases that phosphorylate critical cytoplasmic proteins. Oncogene protein analogs depicted in this example *(shown in bold-faced type)* include **sis,** acting as a ligand (homologous to platelete-derived growth factor); **erb-B,** as a growth factor receptor with kinase activity (related to epidermal growth factor receptor); **src,** as a cytoplasmic protein kinase; **ras,** as a guanine-binding protein; and **myc,** as a DNA-binding transcription factor.

table, the product of many onocogenes are functional analogs of proteins involved in normal cell signaling pathways beginning with receptor-ligand binding at the cell membrane and culminating in cell proliferation and other cell functions (Fig. 6-20).

Oncogenes with protein products that are located in the nucleus are involved in regulation of transcription and gene expression. These include the *myc* family (c-*myc,* N-*myc,* and L-*myc*), c-*myb,* c-*fos,* which bind to DNA and regulate the transcrip-

tion of many genes. It is interesting to note that *myc* and *myb* share sequence homology with the E1a transforming gene of adenovirus, which also acts as a DNA-binding transcription-regulating factor. The products of *myc* and *fos* are also associated with small nuclear ribonucleoproteins in the nucleus that are involved in posttranscriptional splicing of RNA. These genes may therefore also play a role in regulating these events. Both *myc* and *fos* are expressed during the transition of cells from the G_0 to the G_1

phase of the cell cycle. Although the exact mechanisms are still not clear, all this evidence indicates that these genes are involved in the regulation of expression of other genes important in mitotically active cells.

The picture is a little clearer concerning the probable functions of oncogenes forming protein products that are expressed in the cytoplasm or at the cell membrane. Most of these code for proteins with protein kinase activity, phosphorylating their targets on either tyrosine or threonine-serine residues. As discussed in Chapter 4, such protein phosphorylation is known to be an important mechanism of regulation of a wide variety of cellular functions. This group of oncogenes can be grouped in the *src* gene family, all showing some homology with the tyrosine kinase domain of *src*. Some of these oncogenes code for receptors for growth factors. For example, *erb*-B encodes the epidermal growth factor receptor, and *fms* encodes the CSF-1 receptor. The sequence of others, such as *kit, neu,* and *ros* indicates that they may also encode similar membrane-spanning receptors. Each of these also demonstrates protein kinase activity in its cytoplasmic domain. The normal gene product of the *sis* oncogene is platelet-derived growth factor that is secreted into serum and is a potent mitogen for fibroblasts and endothelial and other cells.

The *ras* family of oncogenes also forms a special group. It includes three genes, H-*ras* (related to the Harvey murine sarcoma virus), K-*ras* (related to the Kirsten murine sarcoma virus) and N-*ras* (a cellular oncogene discovered in neuroblastoma cells). These genes are very closely related and, again, are highly conserved, being found in yeast, for example. The proteins encoded by the *ras* genes are closely related to the G proteins. These are GTP-binding proteins located on the cytoplasmic side of the plasma membrane that have intrinsic GTPase activity and are important in the transduction of signals from certain receptors to cytoplasmic second messengers.

The *bcl*-2 family of oncogenes is one of the more recently discovered groups and has been localized in the mitochondrial membrane. The protein products encoded by these genes regulate the rate of apoptosis, or programmed cell death. Through interaction with the products of other oncogenes such as *bax*, *bcl*-2 protein products determine whether cells undergo apoptosis or survive and contribute to tissue growth.

Thus an intriguing thread begins to emerge with respect to the oncogenes that have been implicated in the pathogenesis of neoplastic transformation. Various oncogenes encode growth factors, known or putative receptors for growth factors, G proteins involved in transduction of surface signals to the interior of the cell, nuclear factors involved in regulation of gene expression, and regulators of apoptotic cell death. They form an interactive network of regulatory mechanisms involved in controlling many aspects of cellular function, only part of which is control of growth and differentiation. If these genes or their products function abnormally in neoplastic cells, it is not surprising that the latter show a bewildering variety of phenotypic changes, even without the alterations of other genes that also presumably contribute. What then is the evidence that these genes contribute to the development of neoplastic disease?

There is a massive literature pertaining to the role of oncogenes in the causation of cancer. Discussion of a few well-studied oncogenes will serve to illustrate that there is strong reason to believe that they can indeed act as cancer-causing genes. A primary piece of evidence, of course, comes from the fact that acutely transforming viruses, such as Rous sarcoma virus, are capable of transforming cells *in vitro* and of causing tumors *in vivo*. Fibroblasts transformed by RSV, for example, are tumorigenic when inoculated into chickens. The specific role of the v-*src* gene in this case has been documented by the fact that mutations, such as deletions, within the gene result in loss of transforming capability. Furthermore, cloned v-*src* DNA has been shown to be capable of transforming cells into which it is introduced by transfection. The very rapid development of tumors that characterizes the acutely transforming viruses, however, is in strong contrast to the slow and progressive development of most naturally occurring neoplasms. Despite this, there are several lines of evidence that oncogenes play a role in natural tumorigenesis.

Transfection assays, in which DNA from tumor cell lines, or tumor tissue, is introduced into rodent cells have shown that about 15% to 20% of human tumors contain "activated" oncogenes, capable of transforming the recipient cells. Most of these have turned out to be members of the *ras* family.

In many cases it has been shown that oncogenes such as *myc* are expressed as high levels in certain neoplasms. We have already discussed the example of Burkitt's lymphoma where translocation of the *myc* gene to immunoglobulin loci is associated with the development of lymphoid neoplasms. Two points related to this phenomenon argue for a causative role of the oncogene in the development of the neoplasm: (1) consistency between the deregulation of *myc* transcription and juxtaposition to the immunoglobulin enhancers and (2) the development of neoplasms in the particular types of cells in which the immunoglobulin enhancers would be expected to be active. The *myc* gene is expressed in high levels in several other kinds of tumor, such as small cell lung carcinoma in humans. It is interesting that this amplification of expression, which may be 20 to 80 times normal, is usually associated with the more highly malignant forms of the tumor. It is also importnat to note that amplification is often a late event in the progression of the tumor, an indication that other factors must be involved in its development.

In many other cases, mutations in the oncogene seem to be important in endowing transforming capacity. One of the best examples is provided by the *ras* oncogene family. The *ras* genes most commonly acquire their transforming capabilities by point mutations involving particular amino acids. As already mentioned, the *ras* protein product shares sequence homology with G proteins and shares their ability to bind and hydrolyze GTP. Normal G proteins are activated by binding of GTP and inactivated by its hydrolysis to GDP. The mutations that activate *ras* oncogenes block or greatly reduce the ability to hydrolyze GTP. In this way the transducing functions of the *ras* G protein are continually active, leading to activation of cellular functions that apparently affect the growth and differentiation of the cell. Further support for the role of activated *ras* genes in tumor development comes from studies of carcinogen-induced neoplasms in animals. In a high percentage of these, including mammary tumors, skin carcinomas, thymomas, and kidney tumors, one of the *ras* family of genes has been found to be activated. Furthermore, specific mutations in the gene have been found. Activated *ras* genes have also been found in early papillomas resulting from typical initiation-promotion protocols. This indicates that activation of *ras* may contribute to the initiation of the tumor.

Other examples of activation of an oncogene by structural abnormalities is provided by the *abl* and the viral *erb*-B genes. As explained previously, the transposition between chromosomes 9 and 22, which is common in chronic myelogenous leukemia in humans, results in a hybrid gene that produces a fusion protein. The v-*abl* gene product is a tyrosine kinase, whose activity is greatly enhanced in the fusion protein. Again, a structural abnormality in the gene product drives an important cell-regulatory mechanism at abnormally high levels. The v-*erb*-B gene encodes a truncated form of the receptor for epidermal growth factor lacking its extracellular domain. In this case, it is believed that the tyrosine kinase activity of the cytoplasmic domain is constitutively activated.

It is generally accepted that, except for the acutely transforming retroviral oncogenes, activation of a single oncogene is insufficient for complete tumorigenesis. Several pieces of evidence support this view. For example, mutated *ras* oncogenes transform rodent fibroblastic cell lines but not primary rat embryonic fibroblasts. To explain this it is argued that the cell lines have already undergone some genetic changes accounting for their immortality. Activation of the *ras* gene is apparently sufficient for initiation of tumor development but not for complete carcinogenesis. Similarly, activation of the *myc* gene alone does not seem to be sufficient for tumorigenesis. For example, in transgenic mice carrying an activated *myc* gene driven by an immunoglobulin enhancer, the gene is expressed constitutively in the target lymphoid tissue. However, the neoplasms that develop are clonal, indicating that additional events may be required for complete transformation. Similar results have been obtained with *myc* genes constitutively expressed in mammary tissue. It has been proposed that cooperation between nuclear and cytoplasmic oncogenes is particularly important, the former contributing immortalization of the cells, the latter contributing changes in growth control, reflected *in vitro* by properties such as anchorage-independent growth. In agreement with this concept, transformation of primary rat fibroblasts can be achieved by cotransfection with *ras* and a nuclear oncogene such as one of the *myc* genes. As well, several human tumors have been found to contain two activated oncogenes, one from each of these groups.

Elegant experiments in a reconstituted organ system have further elucidated the cooperative role of *ras* and *myc* in tumorigenesis. When progenitor cells were infected with a retrovirus containing only the *ras* oncogene, the resultant tissue was either normal or, if sufficient numbers of cells were infected, showed dysplastic changes. On the other hand, infection with a virus carrying only *myc* produced hyperplastic changes. Neither oncogene alone produced any tumors. In contrast, infection with a virus carrying both *ras* and *myc* resulted in the development of malignant tumors. Most of the tumors were clonal, indicating that even in this situation further genetic changes had contributed to development of malignancy. Nevertheless, these studies confirm the potential for oncogenes, particularly multiple oncogenes acting in concert, to induce neoplastic disease.

ANTI-ONCOGENES: THE TUMOR SUPPRESSOR GENES

The oncogenes that we have just discussed are often referred to as "dominant genes," or "dominantly acting genes," because they encode a protein that, *when present,* has a positive action in the induction of cancer. In other words, their gene products promote abnormal cell proliferation or differentiation. Since the original description of these dominant oncogenes, evidence has now accumulated for the another set of genes the gene product of which, *when absent,* contributes to the development of neoplasia. These genes have therefore come to be known as *anti-oncogenes,* or *tumor-suppressor genes.*

Although both oncogenes and anti-oncogenes undergo mutations in cancer, there are fundamental differences in the properties of the mutant genes and the resultant development of tumors (Table 6-6). A single mutational event in an oncogene produces a critical change that contributes to the neoplastic phenotype. The reason is that the mutant allele expresses a dominant-acting *gain of function.* These mutations are not heritable because the dominant-acting gain of function is lethal in the developing fetus. Mutant oncogenes are thus not involved in inherited predispositions to cancer but rather develop as a result of somatic mutations in otherwise normal proto-oncogenes. Although specific mutations in specific proto-oncogenes are associated with several tissue-specific types of tumors (see above discussion of chromosomal abnormalities in cancer), in most cases, many proto-oncogenes are activated in tumors arising from a wide variety of tissues.

In comparison, two independent mutations in anti-oncogenes are required before the mutant allele can contribute to tumorigenesis. The reason is that the mutant allele incurs a *loss of function* that acts in a recessive manner to the wild type of allele. Since mutant alleles act in a recessive manner, they do not harm the fetus, are heritable through the germline, and are a major cause of inherited predisposition to cancer. Similar to oncogenes, anti-oncogenes are subject to somatic mutations. Somatic mutations of the wild type of allele are responsible for the characteristic *loss of heterozygosity* of anti-oncogenes in tumor cells. Finally, in heritable forms of cancer the type of somatic mutation in specific anti-oncogenes

is usually associated with tumors in specific types of tissue.

Early evidence for the existence of tumor-suppressor genes came from work in which transformed, tumorigenic cells were fused with normal cells. When this is done, the hybrid cells that result often lose their tumorigenicity. Furthermore, some of these, if maintained in culture, can regain tumorigenicity, and it has been found that this phenomenon is associated with the loss of particular chromosomes derived from the normal parent cell, implying that suppression is the property of particular genes. Subsequent to these seminal observations, modern concepts of cancer-suppressor genes have been based on the study of inherited cancers associated with chromosomal deletions, the best example of which is hereditary retinoblastoma.

Hereditary retinoblastoma is a rare tumor affecting infants and children less than 6 years of age. The age distribution of this tumor is explained by the fact that once retinoblasts differentiate to specialized retinal cells and become postmitotic in early childhood, they can no longer serve as a target for neoplastic transformation. Thus the tumor is not seen in older children or adults. Newborns at risk for retinoblastoma are heterozygous for a defect in a particular locus on chromosome 13. In some cases this is attributable to a deletion. Such individuals therefore carry the defect in all of their somatic (and germ) cells. In contrast, analysis of the karyotype of the tumor cells has shown homozygosity for the defect on chromosome 13. This results from either recombinational events leading to loss of the normal chromosome 13 or replacement of the normal chromosome by duplication of the defective one. This is consistent with a model for inherited cancer predisposition where the first "hit" is an inherited mutation and the second inactivates the remaining normal allele. In these patients therefore, the first genetic event is the inheritance of a mutation in a particular locus (termed the *Rb* locus) through the germ cells. The second is a loss of the normal chromosome in

TABLE 6-6   **Comparison of Mutant Alleles in Oncogenes and Anti-oncogenes**

PROPERTY OF MUTANT ALLELE	ONCOGENE	ANTI-ONCOGENE
Number of mutant alleles required for tumorigenesis	One	Two
Function of mutant allele	Dominant; gain of function	Recessive; loss of function
Heritability through germ line	Not reported	Frequent
Somatic mutation contributes to tumorigenesis	Yes	Yes
Tissue specificity of resultant tumors	Minimal; tumors in wide variety of tissues	Pronounced (heritable forms)

one cell or a few cells such that the latter become homozygous for the defective gene. This phenomenon is strongly suggestive that the product of the Rb gene is somehow important in suppressing neoplastic development, but again, the Rb gene presumably is not present just to prevent cancer. As discussed previously, it is now known that the Rb protein is an important regulator of the cell cycle, and aberrations in the expression of this protein lead to unregulated cell proliferation characteristic of cancer. Since the Rb gene is widely expressed in all tissue cells, carriers of retinoblastoma are also at high risk for the development of other types of tumors, such as osteosarcoma. In this case too, the tumors are homozygous for the *Rb* locus.

Observations similar to those for retinoblastoma have been made in certain other tumors in humans, suggesting the existence of a diverse group of genes that act to suppress tumor development. However, as compared to the more than 100 known oncogenes, only a dozen or so putative anti-oncogenes have been identified to date in humans. Table 6-7 lists some of the better characterized candidates. Amongst these, Rb and p53 are the best known. As compared to Rb, which has already been discussed, p53 is the most frequently mutated gene in human tumors. More than 50% of human cancers, including more than 50 different cell and tissue types, contain mutations in p53. As previously discussed, the p53 protein is a DNA-binding transcription factor that enhances the transcription of a half dozen or more genes that subsequently carry out, at least in part, the function of p53 in the cell. p53 mutations in human cancers result in p53 proteins that fail to bind to DNA and thus fail to enhance transcription. Several characteristics of p53 differentiate it from other tumor-suppressor genes. For example, many mutant p53 alleles act in a dominant fashion. That is, mutant p53 alleles can induce neoplastic transformation in cells carrying a wild-type p53 allele. This is apparently attributable to the unusual biochemistry of its encoded protein, which again unlike other suppressor proteins, assembles into multimeric structures. Under such conditions, mutant p53 molecules complex with wild-type molecules and disrupt the function of the complex as a whole.

Finally, recent findings have provided important new insights on the mechanism of action of the adenomatosis polyposis coli (APC) tumor-suppressor gene. As previously mentioned, defects in the APC gene are associated with familial as well as some cases of nonfamilial colon cancer in humans. It has been known for sometime that the APC protein, together with serine-threonine glycogen synthase kinase, binds β-catenin, a multifunctional protein involved in cell-cell adhesions and developmental pathways. In mutant *APC*-containing colon tumor cells, free β-catenin levels are dramatically increased. β-Catenin was thus believed to be involved in the pathogenesis of colorectal cancer, but the underlying mechanism was unknown. It has now been shown that β-catenin also binds a family of transcription factors known as T-cell factor–lymphoid enhancer factor (Tcf-Lef). In colon tumor cells containing mutant APC protein, β-catenin is free to bind Tcf-Lef, which then binds to DNA and enhances the expression of genes that cause cell proliferation. Other studies have shown that mutations in β-catenin rather than the APC protein also lead to increased cell proliferation, implying that β-catenin is itself an oncogene.

To recapitulate, there is now overwhelming evidence that genetic mechanisms, including somatic mutation and chromosomal rearrangements, play an important basic role in the genesis of neoplastic disease. In many cases, these mechanisms involve the activation or mutation of oncogenes, which promote the development of neoplasia. However, another group of genes having products that suppress

---

TABLE 6-7   **Examples of Putative Tumor-Suppressor Genes in Humans**

GENE*	ASSOCIATED TUMOR	GENE FUNCTION
Rb	Retinoblastoma, osteosarcoma	Binds E2F family of transcription factors
p53	Wide variety	Transcription factor
p16	Wide variety	Cyclin-dependent kinase inhibitor
WT-1	Wilms' tumor (nephroblastoma)	Transcription factor
NF-1	Neurofibromatosis	GTPase activating protein
APC	Colorectal tumors	Binds β-catenin
DCC	Colorectal tumor	Cell adhesion molecule
BRCA-1	Breast cancer	?

*APC, Adenomatosis polyposis coli; *BRCA*, breast cancer; *DCC*, deleted in colon cancer; *NF*, neurofibromatosis; *Rb*, retinoblastoma; *WT*, Wilms' tumor.

the development of cancer are also important. Since only about 20% of human tumors have been shown to contain activated oncogenes, it is likely that these so-called tumor-suppressor genes play a role at least equal in importance to that of oncogenes.

Mechanisms of Metastasis

The spread of neoplastic cells by metastasis is the ultimate criterion of malignancy and the most serious and life-threatening characteristic of malignant cells. More cancer-treatment failures and deaths result from the consequences of metastatic disease than from the primary tumor. This is partly attributable to the high probability of metastasis, especially via lymphatic or blood vessels, of the primary tumor before such spread can be detected clinically. For example, it has been estimated that surgical resection of the primary neoplasm fails to be curative in nearly 50% of patients because metastases, many of which are microscopic, have occurred by that time. It is important therefore to understand the mechanisms by which cancer cells are able to metastasize. Metastasis is a complex biological process and has formed the basis of intensive research.

Metastasis is defined as the transfer of *disease* from one organ to another; however, the term is usually reserved clinically to refer to the transfer of *tumor* cells. The initial tumor is referred to as the *primary* tumor and site, whereas metastatic tumors are referred to as *secondary* tumors and sites.

Routes of Metastasis

Malignant tumors may metastasize by three different routes; direct *invasion* of the surrounding tissue, *implantation,* or through *lymphatic* and *blood vessels.*

Direct Invasion

As previously discussed, a general feature of malignant neoplasms is their ability to invade and infiltrate local tissue. In the process, infiltrating portions of the tumor may remain contiguous with the primary tumor or become free from this connection and appear as closely located secondary sites. Considerable destruction of surrounding tissue may occur during the process of local invasion (Fig. 6-21). Some types of neoplasms are known to be characteristically locally invasive yet do not usually spread far from their original site. Examples are neurofibromas and hemangiopericytomas of the skin of the dog and sarcoid of the skin of horses. Clinical knowledge of this property prompts the surgeon to attempt wide excision to avoid leaving foci of neoplastic cells in the tissue. However, such tumors are difficult to completely remove and tend to recur locally, thus necessitating a cautious prognosis.

Intraorgan spread represents a unique form of metastasis by infiltration and invasion. It is typical of certain primary tumors of certain organs, such as biliary carcinomas of the liver and bronchogenic carcinomas of the lung. In these cases, secondary tumors develop as a result of cells from the primary tumor gaining access to subanatomical structures within the organ by which they then spread throughout the organ. As a result, in the examples cited, biliary carcinomas spread via bile ductules and bronchogenic carcinomas spread via bronchioles, frequently present as multifocal masses in the primary organ.

Implantation

Neoplasms also may metastasize by exfoliation and implantation. This occurs when neoplastic cells, usually from a carcinoma, penetrate a serosal surface and desquamate. These cells may spread throughout the body cavity, implant, and proliferate. This process is commonly encountered in cases of gastric or intestinal carcinoma (Fig. 6-22) and in canine ovarian adenocarcinomas, where it may be referred to as *carcinomatosis.* Direct transplantation of neoplastic cells by means of surgical instruments, gloved hands, or hypodermic needles may lead to the establishment of metastasis. For example, the use of a scalpel to first excise a tumor and then to perform a biopsy of a lymph node could lead to the growth of neoplastic tissue in the second surgical site. Surgeons also take this into consideration by shielding normal tissue with sterile drapes to prevent contact with neoplastic tissue being resected at surgery.

Vascular Spread

Metastasis by invasion of lymphatic or blood vessels is the most unequivocal characteristic and dangerous property of malignant neoplasms. When metastatic transport occurs via *lymphatics,* secondary sites are influenced by the lymphatic drainage of the primary lesion and the site of the primary tumor (Figs. 6-23 and 6-24, *A*). For example, adenocarcinomas of the mammary gland tend to spread to superficial inguinal and mammary lymph nodes, whereas malignant neoplasms of the mouth tend to spread to the submandibular and cervical lymph nodes. Further dissemination can occur along the secondary pathways of lymphatic drainage. Metastasis via *blood vessels* is equally important and perhaps even more serious because the draining lymph node that might at least provide some barrier

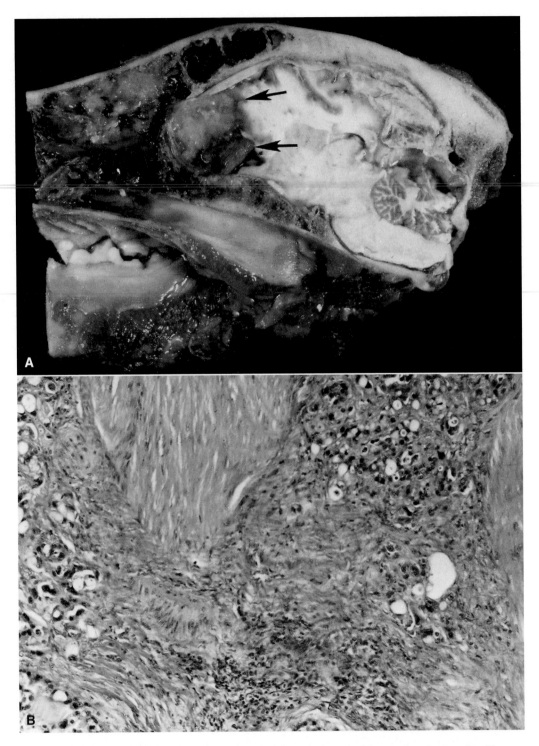

Fig. 6-21 Invasion of Malignant Neoplasms. A, Adenocarcinoma of the nasal cavity in a dog. Notice that the neoplasm has invaded through the cribriform plate into the parenchyma of the brain, *arrows.* **B,** Transitional cell carcinoma of the urinary bladder in a dog. Groups of neoplastic cells have invaded the muscular wall of the bladder. *At left,* The primary mass.

to widespread dissemination is not available. Invasion of blood vessels, a prelude to hematogenous spread, occurs most commonly via veins, venules, and capillaries because the thick walls of arteries are more resistant to penetration (Fig. 6-24, *B*). The pattern of spread again reflects, at least to some extent, the distribution of the affected vessels. Thus, intestinal tumors may gain access to the portal circulation and spread to the liver. Many blood-borne tumor emboli metastasize to the lung because it is the first

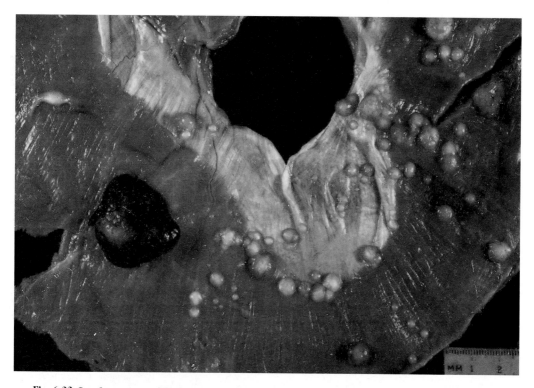

Fig. 6-22 Implantation of Malignant Neoplasms. Neoplastic cells from a gastric carcinoma in a dog have implanted and are growing on the abdominal surface of the diaphragm. One mass is dark as a result of intratumoral hemorrhage.

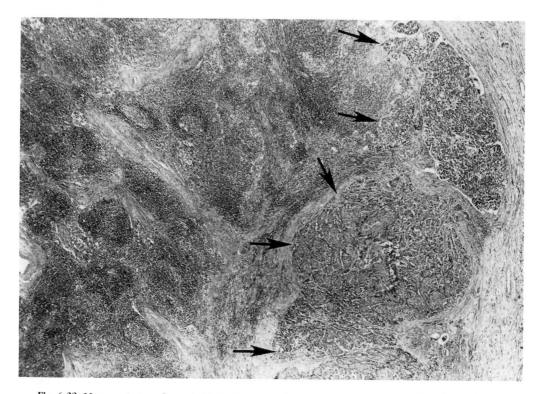

Fig. 6-23 Metastasis to a Lymph Node. A metastatic carcinoma is present in the subcapsular sinus and adjacent cortical tissue of the lymph node, *arrows*. The primary neoplasm was a carcinoma of the mammary gland.

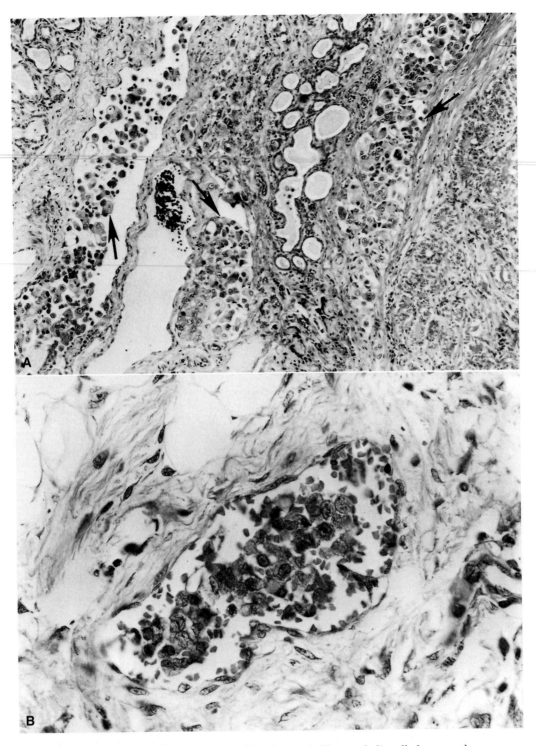

Fig. 6-24 Vascular Invasion by Malignant Neoplasms. A, Many embolic cells from an adenocarcinoma of the mammary gland are present in lymphatic vessels, *arrows.* Part of the primary neoplasm is visible on the *right.* **B,** Embolic cells from a carcinoma of the esophagus are present in a venule. Erythrocytes are also present in the lumen of the vessel.

major capillary bed encountered (Fig. 6-25). For this reason, radiographic examination of the lung often is carried out when metastasis is suspected, as it might be, for example, in the case of an osteosarcoma of the long bones. The histopathological detection of vascular invasion (shown in Fig. 6-24) is therefore of great prognostic significance. Vascular invasion is definitive evidence of malignancy; however, although it indicates a strong potential for metastasis, it does not confirm that metastasis has occurred or even that it will occur. For example, in some neoplasms such as canine seminoma, vascular tumor emboli often can be detected if a careful histopathological search is made, but these neoplasms rarely metastasize. Experimental studies in which embolization of tumor cells can be measured indicate that many tumors continuously release neoplastic cells into the circulation, but <0.01% of these cells actually result in metastatic disease.

TUMOR CELL INVASION

Tissue invasion is important as a mechanism of local spread of neoplastic tissue and as a mechanism of local tissue destruction. It is also a prerequisite for development of systemic metastases, being necessary for neoplastic cells to gain access to and to leave the vasculature. In general, poorly differentiated neoplasms demonstrate more aggressive invasiveness than those that are well differentiated. Three basic mechanisms, *mechanical pressure, tumor cell motility,* and *enzymatic destruction of local tissue barriers,* have been proposed to account for the ability of malignant cells to invade normal tissues. It is likely that all three contribute.

Mechanical Pressure

Rapid tumor growth results in neoplastic cells being forced into the surrounding tissues by mechanical pressure. This is certainly an oversimplification because some neoplasms that grow rapidly are noninvasive, and, oppositely, some of which are highly invasive grow slowly. It is possible also to inhibit tumor cell proliferation without preventing invasion. Furthermore, such a mechanism does not account for the fact that individual or small groups of neoplastic cells are commonly observed in the stroma removed from the main mass.

Tumor Cell Motility

In studying malignant neoplasms histologically, one often observes cords of neoplastic cells insinuating themselves between surrounding tissue elements, or individual tumor cells in the surrounding tissue completely detached from the main mass. Such appearances indicate that the neoplastic cells can actively migrate through the tissue. In fact, tumor cells have been directly observed, under experimental conditions, to migrate through tissues. This includes vessel walls, either between endothelial cells or through gaps created by endothelial cell necrosis. Ultrastructurally, invading neoplastic cells are seen to possess long, thin processes squeezing between tissue structures. Thus it seems reasonable to assume that active migration by tumor cells is an important part of invasion. Unfortunately, there is conflicting evidence regarding the role of active cell motility in neoplastic invasion. Detailed studies of particular neoplastic cell lines show poor correlation between invasiveness and motility *in vitro,* and treatment with inhibitors of cell motility, such as cytochalasin B, apparently does not reduce tissue invasion or the rate of metastasis. We will proceed on the assumption, however, that neoplastic cells are able to be translocated from the primary mass into the surrounding tissue. Part of this process seems to involve detachment of tumor cells from the main mass, a phenomenon consistently observed in malignant neoplasms. The mechanisms of cell detachment have not been well characterized, but the process seems to occur most readily in poorly differentiated tumor cells. It may involve changes in intercellular junctions, such as desmosomes, or in *cell adhesion molecules* (CAMs) expressed on the cell surface. CAMs are exemplified by neural cell adhesion molecule (N-CAM) and liver cell adhesion molecule (L-CAM), the latter of which is found on a variety of epithelial cells. CAMs are now recognized to play an important role in intercellular recognition, inductive events during development, and maintenance of adult tissues. They are tempting targets therefore for speculation concerning some of the altered behavior of neoplastic cells. Little information is available on changes in CAMs on transformed cells. However, in certain cells transformed by the Rous sarcoma virus there is a dramatic reduction in the expression of N-CAM with a concomitant reduction in cellular adhesiveness. These cells also display increased motility, but whether the two events are related is unclear. This seems not to be a generalized phenomenon either, because a different, chemically transformed cell line does not show any reduction in the expression of N-CAM.

Enzymatic Destruction of Local Barriers

There are considerably more data to support the role of various enzymes in the localized destruction of

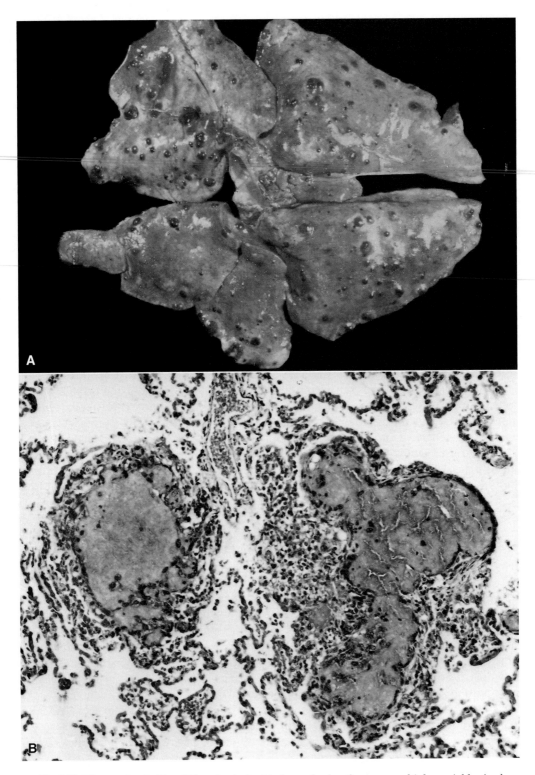

Fig. 6-25 Metastasis via Blood Vessels. A, In this lung of a dog there are multiple, variably sized nodules of metastatic neoplastic tissue that, when fresh, were bright red. **B,** Histologically the neoplastic tissue formed spaces filled with blood, thus indicating a diagnosis of hemangiosarcoma.

tissue surrounding a neoplasm. The main barriers that invading tumor cells need to overcome are basement membranes, cell-cell junctions, and the *extracellular matrix* (ECM). The composition of these barriers varies depending on location but includes different forms of collagen, glycoproteins, proteoglycans, and glycosaminoglycans. A common mechanism by which tumors breach each of these barriers during invasion is the elaboration of proteolytic enzymes by either tumor cells themselves, host stromal cells, or both. The most important family of such enzymes are the *matrix metalloproteinases* (MMPs), a family of zinc endopeptidases responsible for degradation of the ECM as well as nonmatrix proteins during normal embryo development, morphogenesis, and tissue remodeling. Further, the proteolytic activity of the MMPs is carefully regulated by naturally occurring *tissue inhibitors of metalloproteinases* (TIMPs). Disruption of the balance of activity between MMPs and TIMPs enhances not only cancer invasion, angiogenesis, and metastasis, but also the development of diseases characterized by excessive or deficient degradation of the ECM, such as arthritis and atherosclerosis.

MMPs are secreted as proenzymes that require extracellular activation involving interruption of an interaction between cysteine and zinc, characteristic of the inactive molecule. A total of 17 MMPs have been sequenced up to now in humans and can be divided into three general classes: interstitial collagenases, stromelysins, and gelatinases. Interstitial collagenases degrade triple helical regions of fibrillar collagens types I, II, III, VII, VIII, and X. The stromelysins cleave fibronectin, proteoglycans, and nonhelical regions of type IV collagen. The gelatinases (type IV collagenases) cleave degraded collagen (gelatin) and native collagen types IV, V, VII, IX, and X as well as fibronectin and elastin.

All three classes of MMPs are regulated by the action of TIMPs. Three TIMPs have been identified and found to bind to and inhibit either the proenzyme or the activated form of the MMP in humans. TIMP-1 specifically binds and inhibits activated interstitial collagenase, stromelysin-1, and both the activated and latent forms of gelatinase B. TIMP-2 binds to either the latent or the activated form of gelatinase A. TIMP-3, unlike TIMP-1 and -2, which are soluble proteins, is associated with the ECM and inhibits both gelatinase A and B.

Overexpression of each class of MMPs is associated with malignant transformation both *in vitro* and *in vivo*. Importantly, *in situ* hybridization studies have shown that expression of MMP is not limited to tumor cells but is frequently associated with stromal cells in proximity to tumor cells. Stromal cells such as activated fibroblasts, macrophages, neutrophils, and endothelial cells have been shown to express a variety of MMPs in a wide variety of human tumors, especially carcinomas. This likely explains the frequent expression of MMPs in normal tissue adjacent to a tumor. It has been suggested that the release of MMPs from stromal cells may be induced either as a result of direct contact with tumor cells or by tumor cell–derived soluble factors.

The mechanism by which MMPs enhance tumor invasion and metastasis is probably a direct effect of degradation of basement membranes and components of the ECM. However, there is also evidence that once tumors cells have gained access to the stroma as a result of this process, the MMPs subsequently promote their growth. It has been suggested that this is an indirect effect of latent growth factors, such as basic fibroblast growth factor (bFGF) and vascular endothelial growth factor (VEGF), released from dissolved basement membranes. On the opposing side, it has been demonstrated that TIMPs have antiangiogenic properties and can thus inhibit tumor growth. This may be the result of TIMPs either blocking the effect of angiogenic factors such as bFGF or inhibiting endothelial cell invasion by regulating the proangiogenic proteolytic activity of MMPs.

The recent increased understanding of the critical role of MMPs and TIMPs in cancer progression has made them attractive targets for cancer therapy. Traditional cytotoxic chemotherapeutic drug regimens are intended to cause a reduction in tumor mass. In contrast, drugs targeting the MMPs and TIMPs would be expected to behave as *cytostatic* agents by inhibiting or halting tumor growth, vascularization, invasion, and metastasis without absolute reduction in tumor burden. Three approaches are available: inhibit the conversion of inactive pro-MMP to the active MMP, directly inhibit the activity of MMP, or enhance the activity of TIMP. There is experimental evidence to support each of these approaches, and several low-molecular-weight MMP inhibitors have been tested in clinical trials.

Another enzyme system worthy of specific mention is *plasminogen activator* (PA). There is evidence that urokinase-PA (uPA) is involved in matrix degradation in the tumor invasion zone. uPA converts plasminogen to plasmin, an enzyme with broad proteolytic activity and capable of activating latent collagenase. In at least one experimental system it has been shown that inhibition of uPA by specific antibodies reduced metastasis, presumably by interfering with invasion by neoplastic cells.

Interaction of certain tissues with the tumor is also important in limiting invasive behavior. This is particularly apparent in the case of hyaline cartilage and may be attributable to mechanical barriers provided by the tissue or to specific mechanisms such as inhibition of angiogenesis, as previously discussed. Inflammation in tumors may either increase or reduce their ability to invade, depending on the balance between destruction of surrounding tissue and destruction of tumor cells.

STEPS IN THE METASTATIC PROCESS

It should now be evident that metastasis is an extremely complex but inefficient process. This is especially true in the case of the most clinically important form of metastasis, that occurring by vascular dissemination. Even in a tumor capable of metastasis, only a fraction of a percentage of neoplastic cells released into the circulation survive to form new growths. However, tumors are capable of shedding literally millions of neoplastic cells into the circulation each day, and so if even a tiny fraction survive, many metastases can be formed. To produce metastases, tumor cells must successfully accomplish several steps. They must detach from the primary mass, invade local tissue, penetrate blood vessels or lymphatics, and release emboli. The embolic tumor cells must survive in the circulation, be arrested in small vascular channels in distant sites, again penetrate the vessel wall and invade locally, proliferate, and become vascularized (Fig. 6-26). Metastasis is therefore a stepwise process. Because only those cells able to accomplish *all* these criteria can produce metastasis, it is generally referred to as being selective.

Vascular Invasion

We have already discussed in some detail the mechanisms that are believed to be involved in invasion of local tissue. Here we will simply reinforce some concepts that are particularly related to ways in which tumor cells penetrate vessels to gain entrance to the circulation.

A distinction is often made between the lymphatic and the hematogenous routes of metastatic dissemination. This concept is convenient for the purposes of discussion, but the final consequences are similar. Although tumor cells initially may enter either lymphatics or blood vessels, they readily exchange between the two systems. Lymph, of course, eventually drains into the vena cava, and venolymphatic anastomoses have been demonstrated in other tissues. Cells have been shown to pass from lymphatics to blood vessels and the reverse course, sometimes migrating through tissue spaces to do so.

Despite these strictures, the early pattern of metastasis can be influenced by the route of dissemination. Neoplastic cells entering the lymphatic system tend to be carried to the regional lymph node. It is a common belief that, once there, tumor emboli will be filtered out. Although this can occur, the lymph node can be bypassed, either by cells moving through the lymph node to the efferent lymphatics or by passing through anastomosing vessels in the perinodal tissue. When embolic neoplastic cells do reach the draining lymph node, they enter the subcapsular sinus where they may be arrested and grow (Fig. 6-27). As the metastatic lesion develops, cells grow into the cortical sinuses and medullary sinuses and eventually destroy and replace (efface) the normal nodal tissue. Well before the latter occurs, however, neoplastic cells are present in the efferent lymphatics, and these may establish metastatic lesions in more distant lymph nodes or in other organs.

The importance of the regional lymph node as a barrier to the dissemination of neoplastic cells is of more than academic interest because of clinical disagreement as to whether apparently normal lymph nodes should be removed during surgical treatment of neoplasms. Proponents argue that they should be removed and examined for the presence of micrometastases. Antagonists argue that they should be left to act as a filter. Current evidence indicates that the role of the lymph node as a filter in neoplasia is variable and, at best, may serve only to delay dissemination of the neoplasm.

The lymph node draining a neoplasm may undergo hyperplasia of both T-lymphocytic and B-lymphocytic components, suggestive of a possible immune response to the neoplasm. Experimental studies, however, fail to demonstrate a specific role for the regional lymph node compared to other lymphoid tissues. For example, in dogs with naturally occurring tumors, no difference in cytotoxicity to tumor cells could be demonstrated between lymphocytes from the regional lymph node, distant lymph nodes, and circulating lymphocytes. In addition, removal of the regional lymph nodes has not affected the rate of metastasis of neoplasms in other experimental studies. The subject of tumor immunology, including the role of immunological events in limiting metastasis, is discussed later in this chapter.

Metastasis by the hematogenous route occurs when competent neoplastic cells invade blood vessels or gain access to the bloodstream via the lymph. Direct penetration of blood vessels usually involves the capillaries and venules (as well as lymphatics, of course). Invasion of arterial vessels to gain access to the circulation is quite rare. However

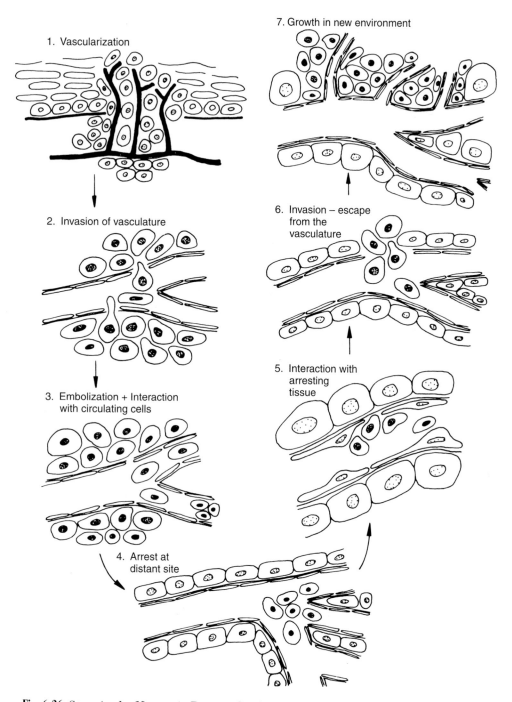

Fig. 6-26 Steps in the Metastatic Process. Graphic summarization of the several processes that neoplastic cells must accomplish to undergo metastasis through the vascular system.

tumor cells gain access, when dissemination occurs by the hematogenous route, metastatic lesions can occur in a variety of organs. Factors affecting patterns of metastatic spread are discussed below.

One of the first steps in the metastatic process, then, is the release of cells from the primary mass to form emboli (Fig. 6-28). Many of the same mechanisms that apply to tumor cell invasion of local tissue

(discussed above) are involved in tumor cells gaining access to the vasculature. In addition, vascularization of the tumor is clearly a prerequisite for tumor cell embolism. In experimental studies, tumor emboli are never detected in the effluent blood before proliferating vessels penetrate the mass. Furthermore, lesions diagnosed as carcinoma *in situ* very rarely if ever metastasize before vascularization

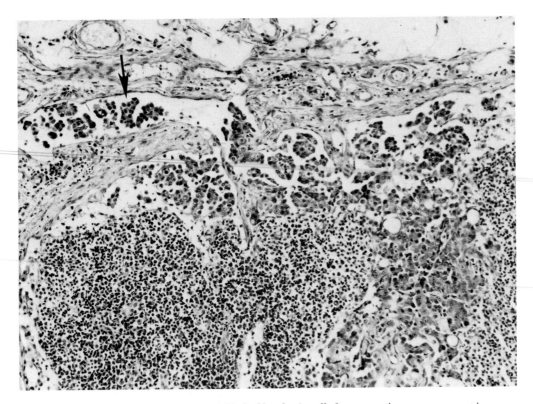

Fig. 6-27 Early Metastasis to a Lymph Node. Neoplastic cells from a carcinoma are present in an afferent lymphatic duct, *arrow*, and in the subcapsular sinus. Proliferating cells have invaded the cortical tissue.

occurs. The penetration of vessels by neoplastic cells is probably influenced by factors similar to those involved in local invasion. The basement membrane of endothelial cells presents a particular barrier to the entry of neoplastic cells to the vasculature. As has been discussed, some tumor cells produce specific collagenases capable of attacking type IV collagen. It is worthy of note that several neoplastic cell lines show a positive correlation between this ability and the capacity to metastasize. Blood turbulence and manipulation of the tumor mass also are known to increase the number of cells released into the circulation. This observation has obvious potential clinical significance; however, it should be noted that such manipulation has never been proved to result in increased numbers of metastases.

Dissemination of Embolic Tumor Cells

Embolism of tumor cells, when it occurs, is probably a continuous process, and large tumors can release enormous numbers of neoplastic cells into the circulation. Quite obviously, not all of these cells result in metastatic neoplasms, and other factors must affect the success of the metastatic process. Most cells released from the primary tumor die, many of them in the circulation. Factors involved in killing embolic tumor cells include mechanical shear forces, oxygen toxicity (mediated by reactive oxygen species), attack by host immune cells, and unfavorable nutritional environment, including lack of growth factors, which might be present in the environment of the primary tumor but not in the bloodstream. From this and discussions below, it is quite clear that the presence of tumor emboli in the circulation does not necessarily mean that metastatic lesions will develop. In fact, in humans, careful comparisons of patients with otherwise comparable tumors show no difference in prognosis between those observed to have vascular invasion and those who do not. The presence of emboli is, however, definitive evidence of malignancy and hence affects the prognosis adversely.

Arrest of Embolic Tumor Cells

Most of the tumor cells that do survive the journey through the vasculature are arrested in the first capillary bed they encounter. Commonly this is in the lungs, but for intestinal neoplasms, for example, the primary site of arrest is the liver. The arrest of tumor emboli is partly dependent on their size, and

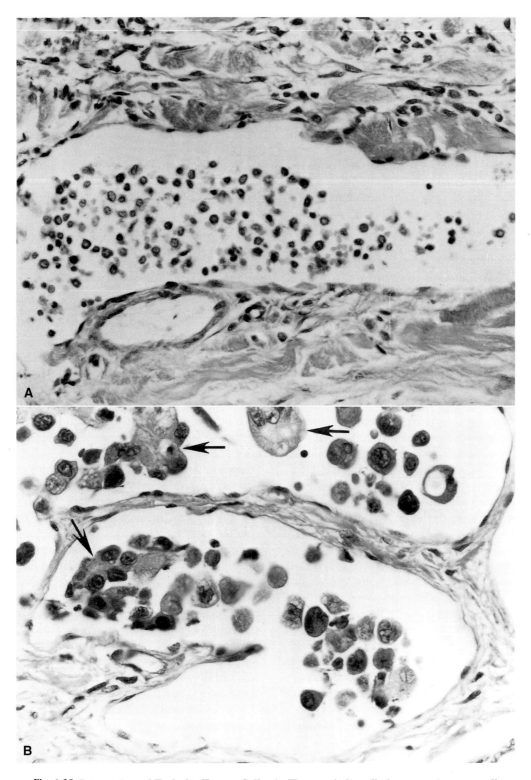

Fig. 6-28 Interaction of Embolic Tumor Cells. A, These embolic cells from a canine mast cell tumor are individualized and therefore less likely to become arrested within the vasculature. **B,** Some of these embolic cells from a canine mammary carcinoma are present as single cells, but many have formed multicellular clumps, *arrows*. The clumped cells are more likely to be arrested in a distant capillary bed.

aggregates of cells (such as those shown in Fig. 6-28, *B*) survive longer at the site of arrest and are more likely to result in metastases than single cells. Neoplastic cells can be released in groups, or single cells may form aggregates in the circulation as the result of adhesive interactions among themselves or by interaction with platelets, lymphocytes, monocytes, or fibrin. Despite these interactions, experimental studies have demonstrated that most metastases are clonal in origin; that is, they originate from single arrested embolic cells.

Endothelial damage may favor metastasis by providing a site at which platelets, fibrin, and tumor cells can interact. Experimental studies have shown that depletion of platelets can reduce the incidence of metastasis, and inhibition of fibrin formation or stimulation of fibrinolysis has had similar effects. Platelet aggregation by tumor cells may also result in secretion of important mediators. These include potential adhesion factors, such as fibronectin, vasoactive substances that may enhance entrapment of embolic cells, and growth factors, in particular PDGF.

The fate of circulating cells has been studied by injection of labeled tumor cells into experimental animals, usually by the intravenous route. As observed in clinical cases, most of these cells are arrested in the first capillary bed they encounter, typically the lung. Depending on the nature of the cells, including their deformability, some of them fail to be arrested and continue to circulate. The majority of the cells that are arrested quickly die. There also is evidence that some of the arrested cells later are released and recirculate. Pulmonary metastases develop from the relatively few cells that become arrested and *remain* in the lung. Of those that escape arrest and those that recirculate, some may be arrested in other tissues, a proportion of which may develop into metastases at those sites. Some of the arrested cells apparently also can remain dormant, though still viable. The main evidence for this is that patients may develop metastatic disease years after the removal of a primary tumor, but the phenomenon has been reproduced experimentally, albeit on a shorter time scale. Dormancy can result from failure of arrested cells to become vascularized, lack of appropriate growth factors, or immunological restraint. We have already discussed the possible role of tumor progression in altering the constituent cells such that these constraints would be overcome, releasing them from dormancy.

Growth at the Secondary Site

Once the neoplastic cells have arrested in the vasculature at a distant site, they must then reverse the process and escape from the vasculature and grow in the new environment. Many of the same considerations that apply for primary tumors to become established and gain entrance to the vasculature also apply for exit of metastatic tumor cells from the vasculature and growth at secondary sites. This includes tumor invasion and establishment of an adequate vascular supply. There is abundant evidence that the arrest and retention of embolic neoplastic cells in distant capillary vessels and subsequent escape from the vasculature and successful growth at a metastatic site are not chance events. Rather, this frequently involves specific interactions between the surface of the tumor cell and endothelial cells, the underlying basement membrane, and the new environment. Because these interactions can influence the site of arrest and metastatic growth, they are discussed separately below.

ORGAN PREFERENCE OF METASTASIS

It is obvious from the study of clinical material that certain types of neoplasms show a characteristic distribution of metastatic lesions. In other words, they show organ preference for development of metastases. Recognition of this type of behavior is of obvious importance in evaluation of a patient with neoplastic disease. For example, osteosarcomas in the dog metastasize frequently and, when they do, most commonly to the lung. Therefore, follow-up evaluation of a canine patient with an osteosarcoma always should include assessment of the possible existence of pulmonary metastases. Similarly, some lymphomas in cats preferentially involve the thymus, some the intestine, and some the cortex of the kidney. In the cow, lymphoma commonly involves the wall of the abomasum, the uterus, or the right atrium of the heart. In humans, the high proportion of bone metastases in breast, prostate, and lung cancer are examples of selective homing of tumor cells to a specific organ.

It has been estimated that 60% of cases of human metastatic disease patterns can be explained by *hemodynamic* and *anatomic factors*. This mechanism indicates that embolic tumor cells are distributed according to patterns of lymphatic or venous drainage. It is consistent with the fact that the lung or regional lymph nodes, the first organs encountered by most circulating neoplastic cells, are often the first sites of metastatic involvement. However, this mechanism does not explain organ-specific metastases. In these cases, the so-called *seed-and-soil theory*, proposed by Paget in 1889, has been invoked. This century-old theory states that peculiar properties of the embolic neoplastic cells (the "seed") and their preferred tissue (the "soil") may determine preferred patterns of metastasis. Direct evidence in support of Paget's view is provided by experimental studies of metastasis to ectopic tissue. For example, if neoplastic cells with a known propensity for pulmonary metastasis are injected into an animal bearing lung tissue implanted subcutaneously, the cells will colonize the ectopic lung as well as the normal lung but not similarly implanted kidney tissue used as a control. In the following discussion we address several specific types of interactions between neoplastic cells and normal tissue components that support the seed-and-soil theory as an explanation for organ preference of metastasis.

Cellular adhesion events are now recognized as being of importance in the pathogenesis of metastasis. In the current context, interactions between circulating neoplastic cells and endothelial cells, basement membrane, and parenchymal cells in the arresting tissue are of interest. There is clear experimental evidence correlating adhesion between tumor cells and endothelial cells with capacity and site preference of metastasis. Highly metastatic cell lines have been shown to adhere avidly to microvascular endothelium, whereas low metastatic lines do not. Furthermore, B16 melanoma cells selected for high lung-colonizing capability (see below) adhere preferentially to lung microvascular endothelium, whereas brain-colonizing variants prefer brain microvascular endothelium. Similar results have been obtained with several other tumor cell systems.

The cell surface components responsible for these interactions have been studied extensively in recent years. Four major families of cell surface adhesion receptors have been identified: the *integrins*, the *immunoglobulin superfamily*, the *cadherins*, and the *selectins*. Integrins frequently bind to extracellular matrix proteins such as fibronectin, whereas others mediate cell-cell attachments through heterophilic interaction with members of the immunoglobulin family. Members of the latter are also involved in cell-cell adhesion by homophilic interaction. Cadherins typically mediate homophilic interaction between cells and are linked to the cytoskeleton through catenin molecules. Selectins are involved in interactions between endothelial cells, leukocytes, and platelets. As compared to other adhesion molecules, selectins are unique in that they bind to carbohydrates rather than other proteins. Specific interactions between these surface receptors on tumor cells and their ligands on endothelial cells and the extracellular matrix are likely major determinants for adhesion as well as organ-specific patterns of metastasis. This involves a complex series of interactions and varies depending on the stage of tumor cell growth. For example, experimental studies have shown that, when tumor cells are injected intravenously, increased tumor cell adhesiveness corre-

lates with increased metastatic behavior. Alternatively, when tumors are implanted experimentally and allowed to invade naturally, there is an inverse relationship between cohesiveness and metastatic behavior.

Neoplastic cells have also been shown to be able to bind to the basement membrane underlying endothelial cells. Such interaction can occur when endothelial cells are injured or when they retract after interaction with tumor cells. Several components of the basement membrane, including fibronectin, laminin, proteoglycans, and type IV collagen may be involved. Antibodies to laminin binding cell surface moieties or peptide fragments of laminin, for example, interfere with binding of certain neoplastic cells to basement membrane and can reduce metastatic capability. We should stress, also, that laminin is certainly not the only important recognition molecule in the basement membrane.

There is also evidence that components of the extracellular matrix can modulate interactions between tumor cells and endothelial cells. When endothelial cells from bovine aorta are grown on extracellular matrix from particular organs, they adopt characteristics that allow them to selectively interact with metastasizing tumor cell lines specific for the organ from which the extracellular matrix was derived. For example, tumor cells that metastasize to the lung adhere preferentially to aortic endothelial cells grown on lung matrix. Similarly, tumor cells preferring the liver adhere to endothelium grown on liver matrix. Nonmetastasizing tumor cells show no such preference. These findings indicate that the expression of components on the surface of endothelial cells that are recognized by metastatic neoplastic cells is modulated by the extracellular matrix. Finally, interactions between neoplastic cells and parenchymal cells are also probably important in determining metastatic preference, but less firm data are available.

TUMOR CELL HETEROGENEITY

A series of benchmark experiments conducted more than two decades ago provided important new information on the effect of phenotypic heterogeneity on the metastatic capabilities of neoplastic cells. These experiments are still worth considering today because they have contributed significantly to our understanding of the properties that influence the behavior of malignant cells.

The hypothesis upon which these experiments were based was that primary tumors were a heterogeneous population of cells, differing in a number of characteristics, including their metastatic capability. If this is the case, it should be possible to select a line of cells that is more highly metastatic than those of the primary tumor. To do this, the B16 melanoma, which arose in a syngeneic strain of mice, was used. When unselected tumor cells were injected into mice, some of the cells produced metastatic lesions in the lung. Cells were harvested from pulmonary lesions, passaged *in vitro*, and then again injected into mice. In this way cells that metastasized to the lung were repeatedly selected (Fig. 6-29). The cells resulting from ten such passages (B16 F10) were then compared with B16 F1 cells. The results indicated that B16 F10 cells had a much greater capacity to metastasize than B16 F1 cells. Furthermore, the B16 F10 cell line metastasized exclusively to the lung, in contrast to B16 F1 cells, which formed metastases in multiple organs. Following similar procedures, another B16 melanoma line that metastasized preferentially to the rhinal fissure of the brain was developed. These experiments supported the hypothesis that the primary tumor contained cells with an enhanced ability to metastasize and that the *in vivo* passage procedure had merely allowed for their selective enrichment.

Other interpretations are possible, however. In particular it could be argued that the cells that come to rest in the lung or brain might adapt to growth in those tissues, thus producing a population better able to survive at those sites. This possibility was ruled out by serial transplanting of cells directly to the brain. When cells were directly passaged in this way, rather than passaging metastases, no selection occurred. That cells with special capabilities for metastasis preexist in the primary tumor was confirmed by the production of clones from single, unselected cells. When cloned-cell suspensions were injected into recipient mice, a wide variation in the number of metastases resulted, with some lungs having only a few and some having hundreds (Fig. 6-30). In contrast, cells from the original tumor not subjected to cloning produced a relatively constant intermediate number of pulmonary metastases.

These experiments, which have now been repeated with other tumor cells, provide strong evidence that the component cells within a primary neoplasm differ in their capacity to metastasize and to colonize particular tissues. The question then can be asked: what are the differences between neoplastic cells that determine their ability to do this? Many factors probably contribute. Highly metastatic selected cell lines have been shown to be more invasive in the subcutaneous tissue, to form clumps more readily, and to be more easily entrapped in the lung. They also are better able to adhere to cell culture monolayers, whether of the same or of different cell type. More importantly B16 F10 cells, which metastasize preferentially to the lung, adhere

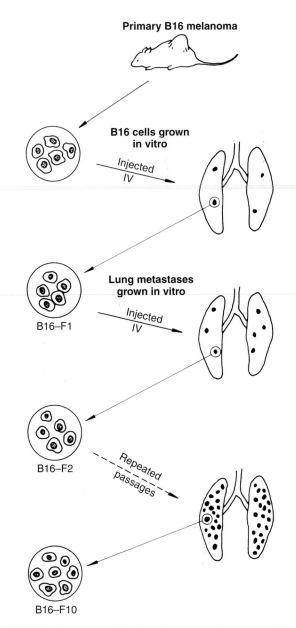

Fig. 6-29 Selection of Highly Metastatic Neoplastic Cells. Cells from a primary tumor, in this case a B16 melanoma, are grown *in vitro* and then injected intravenously. Cells harvested from pulmonary metastases are again cultured to produce a B16 F1 population. After the 10th passage, the B16 F10 cells metastasize much more readily and preferentially to the lungs, as compared to the unselected B16 F1 cells. *(Modified from Nicholson GL: Sci Am 240:66-76, 1979.)*

rapidly and strongly to lung cells but less readily to cells of other tissues. In contrast, B16 F1 cells are less adherent and nonselective. In addition, highly metastatic cell lines of several types, when compared to the corresponding low metastatic lines, adhere more avidly to pulmonary endothelial basement membrane. As already discussed, they also adhere to the appropriate microvascular endothelial cells. Highly metastatic B16 cell lines also produce

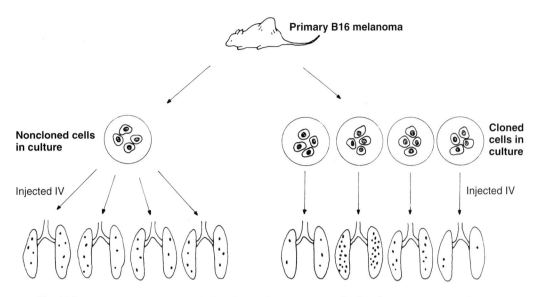

Fig. 6-30 Cloning of Neoplastic Cells. If cells from a primary B16 melanoma are injected intravenously, they produce a relatively uniform number of pulmonary metastases in different mice. If clones are produced from single neoplastic cells, they will produce widely divergent numbers of pulmonary metastases. This is evidence that, within the original tumor cell population, there are cells that have a variable ability to metastasize. *(Modified from Nicholson GL: Sci Am 240:66-76, 1979.)*

relatively high levels of type IV collagenase, indicating an enhanced ability to lyse subendothelial basement membranes.

There is also evidence that these properties are associated with differences in the surfaces of the neoplastic cells. When maintained in tissue culture, highly metastatic B16 F10 cells shed vesicles that can be fused with the plasma membranes of low metastatic B16 F10 cells. When this is done, an enhanced capacity to metastasize to the lung is conferred on the B16 F10 cells. Other properties of the F10 cells, such as resistance to cytotoxic lymphocytes, also can be conferred on the F1 cells. Because the transferred vesicles persist in the recipient cells for only 18 to 24 hours, it appears that the properties transferred from the donor cells are important early in the metastatic process, probably in the process of arrest or early invasion. Presumably then, some of the surface components discussed earlier in this chapter are important in determining their ability to metastasize. Despite all these advances, no general property has been found that explains the metastatic ability of all malignant cells. In fact, given the wide variation in metastatic ability and the complexity of interactions between the host and the neoplastic cells, it is unlikely that any single property will explain the ability of some cells or oppositely the inability of others to metastasize. Undoubtedly, however, our increasing knowledge of the biology of malignant cells eventually will lead to more effective control of the disease.

It should now be obvious that not all the cells making up a neoplasm are identical, but rather there

is considerable cellular heterogeneity within a given tumor. In retrospect, as empirical as it may seem, such variability is clearly evident from histopathological examination of tumors; recall that cellular pleomorphism is one of the standard criteria for malignancy. In addition, from the foregoing discussions it is also evident that tumor cells vary considerably in a wide variety of characteristics, including biochemical properties, cell surface antigens and receptors, growth rate, susceptibility to therapeutic interventions and susceptibility of immune attack.

It may be confusing to try to reconcile the fact that the majority of tumors arise from single altered cells with the fact that all tumors contain a heterogeneous cell population. Perhaps the best way to rationalize this is to consider that the whole organism arises from a single cell and is a clone yet is made up of cells with considerably different characteristics. This analogy can be taken further because the properties that characterize tumor cell heterogeneity are heritable in the sense that they are passed on as cells divide. Differences between tumor cells in a single neoplasm therefore arise during the evolution of the tumor, that is, during tumor progression.

As we have already discussed, tumor progression is generally considered to be the result of accruement of genetic alterations, and neoplastic cell populations are regarded as being genetically unstable. However, variants can arise very rapidly in tumors, and epigenetic mechanisms, rather than true mutations, are likely to play an important role. Particular attention has been drawn to methylation of DNA, a mechanism of inactivation of gene expression that is heritable from cell to cell. Conversely, demethylation can reactivate genes. It has been proposed that progressive hypomethylation of DNA in tumors results in altered gene expression. This is not to exclude mutation as a means of generating tumor heterogeneity. Since neoplastic cell populations are generally recognized as having high mutation rates and many genes can contribute to the characteristics that we are discussing, accumulated mutations in many genes could occur quite quickly.

A fascinating aspect of tumor heterogeneity concerns the interaction of subclonal cell populations within a neoplasm to stabilize the population as a whole. When clones have been isolated from heterogeneous tumor cell populations, they have been found to be highly unstable. Passage either *in vivo* or *in vitro* generates variant cell populations much more quickly than such variants emerge in polyclonal, or heterogeneous, populations. When several clones are cultured together, however, the phenotype of the constituent cells is stabilized. This indicates that interactions between the tumor cells in polyclonal tumors is important in establishing an equilibrium in which the generation of new variants is limited. The mechanisms underlying these interactions are unknown, but they have some important implications. As mentioned previously, individual metastases are believed to arise from single cells that become established at a distant site; that is, they are clones. Although these clones are initially homogeneous, cellular heterogeneity quickly arises. It appears that the same phenomena occur *in vivo*, driving the emergence of new variants. Another implication is that the reduction of tumor cell burden by therapeutic means presumably reduces tumor cell heterogeneity, again driving the generation of new variants. Some of these may acquire increased resistance to the treatment, a possibility that forms part of the rationalization for the use of multiple drugs in the treatment of cancer.

Effects of Tumors on the Host

INTERFERENCE WITH VITAL FUNCTION

Tumors interfere with vital organ function to produce a variety of detrimental effects on the host. Obviously malignant neoplasms, because of their invasive nature and ability to metastasize, will cause more harm to the host than benign tumors will. Even benign tumors, however, can have devastating effects. Any *space-occupying* lesion can lead to dysfunction of an organ. For example, a mass compressing the common bile duct can cause obstruc-

tion to bile flow, icterus, and eventually extensive liver damage. Tumors in the brain, even when histologically benign, cause local destruction of the parenchyma and can produce severe clinical illness and eventually death. Another example occurs in horses in which benign, pedunculated lipomas become twisted around a segment of intestine producing intestinal obstruction or infarction and death. Malignant neoplasms can cause similar problems. For example, adenocarcinomas of the intestine, especially scirrhous adenocarcinomas associated with abundant sclerosis, often cause obstruction. Malignant neoplasms also have the ability to *invade* and *destroy* adjacent tissue, which is obviously detrimental to the host (see Fig. 6-21).

PARANEOPLASTIC SYNDROMES

Apart from their ability to injure host tissues directly, as just described, many neoplasms can cause illness by indirect mechanisms. An example of this are tumors that produce *biological substances* resulting in so-called *paraneoplastic syndromes*. In some of these (examples of which are included in Table 6-8) the underlying mechanisms are well understood. In others they are unknown. Benign tumors, being well differentiated, retain functions characteristic of normal cells, and excessive secretion of these products can cause clinical disease. This occurs most commonly in animals with tumors of endocrine origin. A well-known example is provided by tumors of the beta cells of the pancreatic islets, which occur relatively commonly in dogs. These tumors, when functional, secrete insulin and cause severe hypoglycemia, which results in syncope and seizure-like activity. Other neoplasms of endocrine origin also can secrete hormones. For example, functional tumors of the adrenal cortex or of the adenohypophysis can cause hyperadrenocorticism, and tumors of the alpha cells in the pancreatic islets can secrete gastrin. These secretory funtions are frequently retained by metastatic tumors. For example, carcinomas of the beta cells of the pancreas metastasize, and both the primary and secondary tumors can secrete insulin. In fact, monitoring of blood glucose levels is a useful way to detect metastasis after surgical removal of the primary neoplasm.

Sometimes neoplasms secrete hormones or hormone-like substances not usually associated with the cell of origin. A good example of this phenomenon is provided by *humoral hypercalcemia of malignancy* (HHM). Most cases of HHM are the result of increased osteoclastic bone resorption mediated by humoral factors released by either tumor cells or

TABLE 6-8 Examples of Paraneoplastic Syndromes

TUMOR TYPE	CLINICAL SYNDROME	MECHANISM
Multiple myeloma	Nephrotoxicity	Secretion of immunoglobulin
Malignant lymphoma	Hypercalcemia	Osteoclast-activating factors
Canine carcinoma of the apocrine glands of the anal sac	Hypercalcemia	PTHrP
Sertoli cell tumor	Feminization	Secretion of estrogen
Mast cell tumor	Gastroduodenal ulcers	Secretion of histamine
Thyroid follicular epithelial cell tumor	Hyperthyroidism	Secretion of TSH
Thyroid C-cell tumor	Hypocalcemia	Secretion of calcitonin
Pancreatic β-cell tumor	Hypoglycemia	Secretion of insulin
Pituitary tumor	Cushing's disease	Secretion of ACTH
Adrenal cortical tumor	Cushing's syndrome	Secretion of cortisol
Pheochromocytoma	Hypertension	Secretion of catecholamines

normal host cells that act systemically and distant to the tumor. In addition, the presence of such systemic humoral factors may increase calcium reabsorption from the kidney or calcium absorption from the intestine, further contributing to hypercalcemia. Multiple humoral factors have been associated with the pathogenesis of HHM, including parathyroid hormone, and parathyroid hormone–like protein, cytokines, steroids, and prostaglandins. It is possible that different mediators participate in different kinds of tumors or that more than one mediator is involved in individual cases. For completeness, it should also be noted that cancer-associated hypercalcemia also occurs less frequently as a result of local humoral factors produced by tumors growing directly in bone.

HHM has been associated with many neoplasms in humans, including squamous carcinoma and carcinomas of kidney, breast, and ovary. Among domestic animals, dogs are most frequently affected with HHM, which occurs, for example, in approximately 25% of dogs with lymphoma. Another interesting example of HHM has been extensively studied in dogs with adenocarcinomas of the apocrine glands of the anal sacs. As compared to lymphoma, this is a less common tumor that usually occurs in older female dogs, the majority of which develop HHM. Also, as compared to dogs with lymphoma and HHM, dogs with adenocarcinomas of the anal sacs have greatly elevated circulating levels of *parathyroid hormone–related protein* (PTHrP). PTHrP was initially isolated from human tumors associated with HHM and has subsequently been shown to share 70% sequence homology with PTH at the amino terminuses of the proteins. Further similarities include the ability of PTHrP to compete with PTH for its receptors, to be inhibited by inhibitors of PTH, and to activate adenylate cyclase in bone cells

and cause resorption of bone *in vitro*. PTHrP is therefore believed to play an important role in the pathogenesis of HHM in dogs with adenocarcinomas of the anal sacs. As compared to PTH, which is produced only in the parathyroid gland, PTHrP is also produced in a variety of normal tissues, where its exact function is not known, but has been hypothesized to act as an autocrine or paracrine regulator. This implies that PTHrP and related molecules are not "aberrant hormones," as was once believed, but normal cellular products that have unforeseen actions when secreted, perhaps in quantity, by neoplastic cells.

Other distant effects of neoplasms are less easy to rationalize. For example, *hypertrophic osteoarthropathy* (also known as "pulmonary hypertrophic osteoarthropathy," or "Marie's disease") can occur in dogs with neoplasms in the lung or bladder. In this syndrome, the presence of the mass somehow causes the proliferation of osseous tissue in the bones of the distal limbs. The mechanisms involved are unknown, but removal of the mass may result in the resolution of the osseous lesions. The syndrome also may be associated with nonneoplastic intrathoracic masses, and such an association indicates that the lesions may not be the result of a specific function of the neoplastic cells.

CASE 6-2: PARANEOPLASTIC SYNDROME

Brandy, an 11-year-old, female golden retriever dog was presented with a history of depression, poor appetite, and obvious weight loss of about 1-week duration. Previous medical history was unremarkable. On being questioned, the owner reported that the dog had recently developed polydipsia (increased thirst) and polyuria (increased volume of urine). On physical examination the dog was lethargic and moderately weak, most noticeably in the rear limbs. A firm, nonpainful mass about 3 cm in diameter was palpated in the perineum adjacent to the rectum. A complete blood count (CBC) and blood chemistry panel was ordered. The CBC was unremarkable, but the chemistry panel showed mild elevations of serum enzymes (alanine aminotransferase, aspartate aminotransferase, and alkaline phosphatase) suggestive of liver damage. The serum calcium was elevated to 14.4 mg/dL (normal = 9.8 to 12.0 mg/dL). Abdominal radiographs seemed to show enlargement of the liver, but abdominal detail was poor as a result of ascites. The mass was resected surgically and noted at that time to be very vascular, firm, tan, and locally invasive. It extended along the wall of the rectum but was not closely adherent to it. The mass was fixed in neutral buffered formalin and submitted for histopathological evaluation. Two days after surgery, a second chemistry panel showed that the serum calcium had dropped to 10.3 mg/dL.

Histologically the mass was made up of cuboidal or polyhedral cells that were fairly regular in size (Fig. 6-31). They had uniform, round-to-oval nuclei and lightly stained, basophilic cytoplasm that was sometimes vacuolated. The cells were arranged into irregular-sized lobules that were separated by coarse, densely collagenous connective tissue septa. Occasional acinar structures were present, and their lumens often contained eosinophilic secretory product. Small invasive foci of neoplastic cells were present in the capsule surrounding the mass, and occasional emboli of neoplastic cells were found in lymphatics. Based on these characteristics, a diagnosis of adenocarcinoma of the apocrine glands of the anal sac was made. The pathologist commented that this type of tumor

was usually highly malignant and that metastasis to the internal iliac lymph nodes was common. Close clinical surveillance was therefore advised.

Two months after initial presentation, the dog was again examined because of recurrence of clinical signs. No mass could be palpated in the perineum, but the serum calcium was 16.2 mg/dL. Radiographs showed numerous dense masses in the lungs. Because of the poor prognosis, the owners decided on euthanasia. At postmortem examination a large, irregular, firm mass was found in the caudal abdominal cavity. The internal iliac lymph nodes were greatly enlarged and firm. Variably sized metastatic lesions were found in the lungs and in the liver. Histologically, all these closely resembled the original biopsy specimen.

Comments on Case 6-2

This neoplasm was diagnosed as an adenocarcinoma because it showed evidence of differentiation into acini and because of definitive evidence of malignancy, in the form of tissue and vascular invasion. The lobular arrangement with coarse fibrous septa and occasional acini is highly characteristic of tumors derived from the apocrine glands of the anal sacs. The pathologist was therefore confident in making this specific diagnosis. Also, these tumors behave in a very consistent way. Almost all cases metastasize to the internal inguinal lymph nodes early in the course of the disease and less commonly to other organs. This could be dependably predicted in this case and was

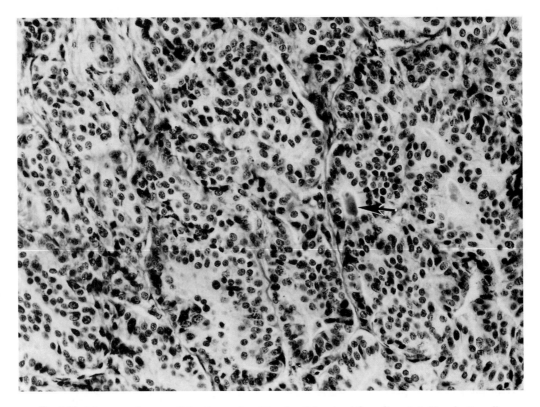

Fig. 6-31 Adenocarcinoma of the Aprocrine Glands of the Anal Sac. Case 6-2. Neoplastic cells form solid lobules separated by collagenous stroma. Occasionally the cells form acini containing eosinophilic secretory product, *arrow.*

confirmed at necropsy. Based on their knowledge of this neoplasm, the clinician and the pathologist had to offer a poor prognosis in this case.

This is also a good example of a paraneoplastic syndrome. Hypercalcemia is a frequent complication of this neoplasm and is believed to be associated with the secretion of PTHrP, a hormone with biologically activity similar to PTH. This finding is supported by the fact that resection of the primary mass was followed by normalization of the serum calcium levels. As in this case, the monitoring of serum calcium can be used as an indicator of recurrence or metastasis of the neoplasm when it is biologically active. This is true not only of neoplasms producing hypercalcemia, but also of all those secreting some measurable biologically active compound.

Lastly, this case of adenocarcinoma of the apocrine glands of the anal sac illustrates the likelihood of certain syndromes or lesions occurring in specific patient populations. This neoplasm occurs most commonly in old female dogs. Therefore, when such a dog shows signs of weakness, depression, polydypsia, and polyuria, this condition should be suspected. Of course, there are other diseases that can produce such signs, but it is in this way that lists of differential diagnoses are constructed. In this case, serum chemistry results revealed hypercalcemia, and physical examination revealed a perineal mass. With all this information the clinician can make a tentative diagnosis of adenocarcinoma of the apocrine glands of the anal sac with a high degree of confidence.

CACHEXIA

Very often the most important indirect result of malignant neoplastic disease is cachexia. Affected animals are often anorexic, have generalized wasting, and are weak. Inadequate food intake probably contributes to this process in many cases but is certainly not the sole explanation because many animals with neoplastic disease eat normally yet lose their body condition. It also has been postulated that tumor tissue competes with the host for nutrients. Although this may again contribute, it is difficult to explain cachexia associated with relatively small tumors on this basis.

There are profound changes in energy metabolism in animals with neoplasia. In general, neoplastic disease results in increased energy spending. Carbohydrate metabolism is altered, sometimes associated with changes in insulin sensitivity or secretion, as is lipid and protein metabolism. In addition there are alterations in the activity of many enzymes in animals with neoplasms, some being elevated and some decreased.

Many of the metabolic derangements associated with tumor cachexia have been attributed to *tumor necrosis factor-alpha* (TNF-α), also known as *cachectin*. This cytokine is produced by activated macrophages in a variety of chronic diseases, including neoplasia. TNF-α is capable of eliciting a variety of responses in the host. It has been implicated as a central mediator of wasting in chronic disease states. When administered to animals, it induces a cachectic state and is capable of suppressing the expression of many important metabolic enzymes. For example, it drastically reduces lipoprotein lipase activity in adipocytes as well as other enzymes contributing to lipogenesis, resulting in the depletion of body lipid stores. Beyond these effects, TNF-α (cachectin) also appears to be responsible for many of the changes in endotoxic shock.

IMMUNOSUPPRESSION

Most tumor-bearing patients are immunologically compromised one way or the other. This is especially true for tumors of the lymphoid system, those cells responsible for the immune response itself. This may involve defects in either the humoral, cell-mediated, or nonspecific host defense systems. It is probable that in most cases this results from rather than predisposes to the tumor. However, many carcinogens, such as irradiation, oncogenic viruses, and some chemicals are immunosuppressive, and it is still possible that this contributes to the establishment of tumors. The argument of what comes first, immunosuppression or neoplasia, is central to the concept of immune surveillance discussed later. The underlying mechanisms are poorly understood but likely include soluble factors, either secreted directly by tumor cells or by normal cells in response to the tumor. The importance of immunosuppression associated with tumors is best evidenced by the frequent necessity to protect tumor-bearing patients from intercurrent infectious disease.

Tumor Immunology

Observations made in naturally occurring cases of neoplasia sometimes reveal that the host can react against the presence of tumor cells. For example, canine mammary tumors, seminomas, some mast cell tumors, and, in particular, cutaneous histiocytomas often contain infiltrating lymphocytes (Fig. 6-32). In the case of canine mammary tumors, perivascular lymphocytic infiltrates have been associated with an improved prognosis and, in the case of canine cutaneous histiocytomas, the infiltrates have been associated with spontaneous regression of the tumors. Other neoplasms, such as the canine TVT, also frequently undergo spontaneous regression, indicating that the host can in some way defend itself against the neoplastic growth. The field of tumor immunology is, however, replete with contradictory results and controversy.

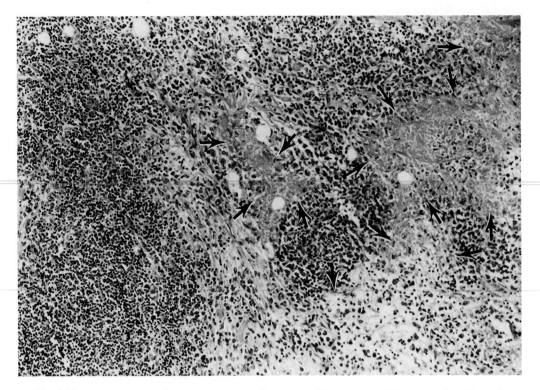

Fig. 6-32 Lymphocytic Infiltrate in a Canine Cutaneous Histiocytoma. This tumor is infiltrated by large numbers of small, densely staining lymphocytes. The lymphocytic infiltrate is associated with areas of necrosis within the tumor, *arrows.*

TUMOR ANTIGENS

There is no doubt that many tumors bear new antigens not found on normal host cells. These antigens are most common in experimentally induced tumors, whereas those demonstrated with spontaneous neoplasms are less frequently antigenic. The antigens borne on the surface of the neoplastic cells are known by a variety of names, including *tumor-specific antigens* (TSA), *tumor-specific transplantation antigens* (TSTA), or *tumor-associated transplantation antigens* (TATA). Transplantation antigens are detected by the elicitation of an immune response to transplanted tumor cells in syngeneic normal animals. Thus their detection depends on effective immunogenicity. This distinction is an important one because not all antigens expressed on tumor cells are effective immunogens. Some antigens therefore would not be able to induce immune-mediated destruction of tumor cells. Nor are all antigens expressed on tumor cells strictly abnormal. For example, many tumors in numerous animal species bear *embryonic antigens.* These are substances found normally on the surface of embryonic cells but not on normal adult cells. They do not usually function as transplantation antigens.

Neoplasms induced by oncogenic viruses bear antigens that are consistent and specific for the particular causative virus. These tumor-specific cell surface antigens are not part of the virion, though infected cells may, of course, contain antigenic viral material. The antigens are a consequence of cell transformation rather than infection and may represent the product of transformation-specific genes.

In contrast, neoplasms induced by chemical carcinogens bear antigens that are unique to each individual tumor. Different tumors induced by the same chemical bear different antigens even when several tumors occur on the same animal. There is, apparently, almost unlimited diversity in the antigens that may be expressed, and they vary widely in immunogenicity.

The first requirement for an immune-mediated attack on neoplastic cells, namely, antigenicity or more importantly immunogenicity, is therefore often satisfied. Nevertheless, since neoplasia is still clearly an important clinical disease, effective immunological rejection of tumors does not always occur. What must now be considered is the evidence that it can occur at all and, if it can, what allows some neoplasms to escape destruction.

THE CONCEPT OF IMMUNOLOGICAL SURVEILLANCE

Some years ago it was postulated that the immune system played an important role in preventing neoplastic disease. It was proposed that neoplasms arose frequently in all individuals and that the immune system of normal animals recognized the abnormal cells and destroyed them early in their development. Thus, clinically apparent neoplasms were believed to be attributable to a failure in the host's immune defenses. This theory, called *immunosurveillance,* was prompted partly by the fact that the only known function of T lymphocytes, at that time, was the rejection of foreign, grafted cells. The concept of immunological surveillance, at least in its original form, is currently much less attractive, and there is a large body of evidence that argues against it. Nonetheless, it is worthy of further discussion because it dominated and directed the field of tumor immunology for decades.

The concept of immunosurveillance was inherently attractive and provided a believable explanation for the role of T cells. Today it is known that T lymphocytes have a variety of additional functions, including regulation of the immune response and defense against viruses and other intracellular parasites. Additional evidence against the concept came from the study of immunodeficient animals and humans. It was reasoned that, if neoplasms arise commonly and are usually rejected, decreased immunocompetence should consistently be associated with an increased incidence of neoplasia. However, to the contrary, nude mice, which lack a thymus and thus have no T cells, do not develop an unusual number of tumors. They are, however, as susceptible as normal mice to chemical carcinogenesis and, as would be expected, are more susceptible to virus-induced tumors. Similarly, mice whose immune function is experimentally suppressed or immunodeficient humans develop no more tumors than usual. As a caution, it must be added that in all immunoincompetent animals, including humans, there is an increase in the incidence of neoplasms of lymphoid origin. This, however, is believed to be attributable to abnormal regulation of lymphoid precursor cells that results from the immunosuppressed state, rather than failure of a surveillance mechanism. Immunosuppressed people also have a somewhat increased incidence of tumors of the lip, skin, and cervix. All of these are suspected of being of viral origin, which might explain their increased occurrence in these individuals. Other evidence indicates that immunologically privileged sites, such as the cheek pouch of the hamster, are not subject to an unusual number of neoplasms and, contrary to what would be expected,

there is no increase in polyclonal neoplasms in immunosuppressed humans.

The original concept of immunological surveillance is thus probably incorrect, yet the rejection of the original hypothesis should not be taken as an indication that the immune system plays no role in combating neoplasia. For example, nude mice do possess other potent effector mechanisms that could destroy neoplastic cells. These include natural killer (NK) cells and macrophages. If neoplastic transformation occurs only rarely, there may not be a dramatic increase in the incidence of neoplasia in immunosuppressed individuals. It is well documented that, at least in some circumstances, neoplasms can elicit an immune response. The problem is to understand why this response is not always effective and how to manipulate it.

EVIDENCE FOR IMMUNITY AGAINST TUMORS

There is evidence in some experimental systems that the immune response can influence the fate of a neoplasm. These experiments usually are carried out in syngeneic strains of animals so as not to confuse responses to histocompatibility antigens with those to tumor antigens.

In the case of tumors induced by oncogenic viruses, there is clear evidence that the immune response can prevent the development of neoplasms. For example, polyomavirus injected into immunologically immature neonatal mice or immunosuppressed mice causes a variety of neoplasms. These neoplasms, when transplanted to normal, immunocompetent syngeneic hosts will survive and grow (Fig. 6-33). When the virus is injected into normal adult mice, it does not induce tumors. Furthermore, when polyoma-induced tumors are transplanted to syngeneic adult mice previously injected with the virus, the tumors fail to survive and grow. Similar results can be obtained when other viruses such as adenovirus or SV40 virus are used. As previously discussed, each of these viruses evokes antigens on the surface of transformed cells that are peculiar to the particular virus. Apparently an immune response against these can prevent the development of neoplasms. In the polyomavirus system, it appears that infection of the immunocompetent adult mouse induces surface antigens in some transformed cells that are recognized and destroyed. The resultant immunity prevents the subsequent establishment of transplanted tumors. This clearly demonstrates that effective antitumor immunity is possible but raises the question of why an effective response does not occur to the tumor transplanted to the previously unexposed host.

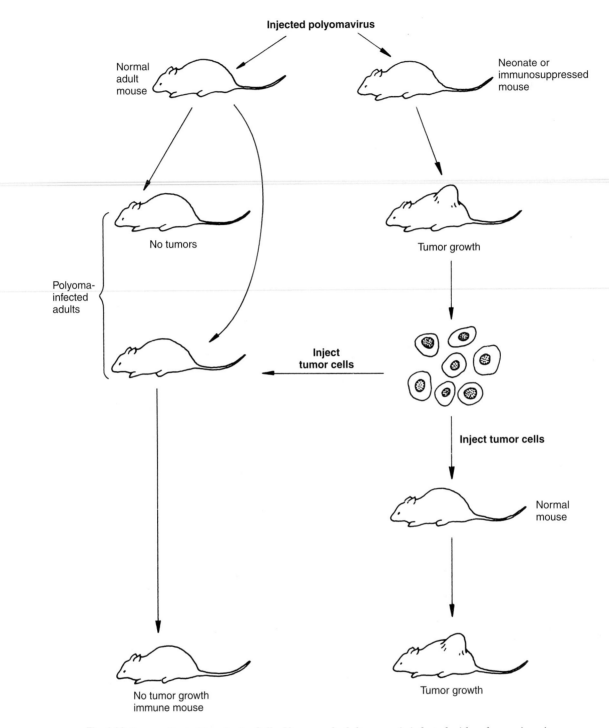

Fig. 6-33 Immunity to Neoplastic Cells. If a normal adult mouse is infected with polyomavirus, it does not develop tumors. If neonates or otherwise immunoincompetent mice are infected, they do develop tumors. The neoplastic cells may then be transferred to normal adult syngeneic mice, where they will grow and produce tumors. If cells are transferred to mice previously infected with polyomavirus, no tumors develop, a demonstration that these mice are immune to the development of the neoplasm. *(Modified from Olds LJ: Sci Am 236:62-79, 1977.)*

Effective immunity against naturally occurring virus-induced tumors is also well recognized. Two of the better understood examples include an oncogenic DNA virus–induced disease, Marek's disease of chickens, and an oncogenic RNA virus–induced disease, feline leukemia in cats. In both of these cases, antiviral as well as antitumor immunity are involved, and vaccines are available to provide protection against either infection or the development of tumors. The immune mechanisms involved in protection against these two important naturally occurring diseases are discussed in detail later in this chapter.

The situation in the case of chemically induced tumors is of course more complex because each tumor bears its own unique antigens. Immune-mediated rejection of such tumors can, however, be demonstrated under appropriate experimental conditions. If, for example, a tumor is induced in a mouse using a chemical carcinogen such as 3-methylcholanthrene, it can be transplanted to syngeneic animals where it will survive and grow. If the growing tumor is resected, the "cured" mouse that results is then resistant to further transplantation of the same neoplastic cells. This too indicates that immune rejection of tumor cells is possible, but, again, the primary tumor and the tumor transplanted to the nonimmunized host are not rejected. The reasons for failure of rejection of primary tumors are at present unknown, but some possibilities are discussed below. The whole problem of tumor immunity is additionally complicated by the fact that in many systems tumors are unaffected by the immune response. In some systems, in fact, tumor growth can be stimulated by an immune response. Many questions remain to be answered before we can understand and exploit the nature and effects of immunity to tumors. Nevertheless it is worthwhile to examine some of the effector mechanisms that are believed to be involved in tumor immunity and the ways in which the transformed cells may escape them.

EFFECTOR MECHANISMS IN TUMOR IMMUNITY

Potentially, tumor cells may be lysed or prevented from growing in many ways. Generally it is difficult to examine these mechanisms directly *in vivo*, and much of the available data has been obtained from *in vitro* assays, often correlated with *in vivo* behavior.

Cellular Cytotoxicity

The immune reaction cellular cytotoxicity, mediated by cytotoxic CD8 T lymphocytes, is believed to be one of the most important means by which the immune response can eliminate tumor cells. Sensitized T cells recognize antigens on the transformed cells and interact directly with them to induce "leakiness" in the cell membrane and eventually lysis (see Chapter 5 for a discussion of this process). This mechanism may be involved in canine TVT because peripheral blood lymphocytes (PBL) from dogs in which the neoplasm has regressed are cytotoxic for tumor cells *in vitro*; in contrast, PBL from dogs with progressive tumors are not. Similar evidence has been obtained in other systems. For example, the role of cytotoxic T cells has been studied in progressor and regressor UV-induced sarcomas. Regressor tumors contained three times the number of T cells compared to those of progressor tumors, whereas the numbers of other potential effector cells were comparable. T cells from the regressor tumors showed antigen-specific cytotoxicity against tumor cells *in vitro*, whereas those from the progressor tumors did not. These data support a role for cytotoxic T cells in immune reactions against neoplasms. Unfortunately, similar studies in other tumor systems often produce conflicting results, indicating that the outcome of such reactions depends on numerous events, which are not always predictable.

Antibody

The role of antibody in tumor immunology is somewhat controversial. Certainly cytolysis by antibody and complement has been shown to occur in some systems. Activation of complement is by the classic pathway, with the alternate pathway apparently being ineffective. This mechanism therefore requires that immunoglobulins bind to the surface of tumor cells to activate complement, after which the cell membrane is rendered "leaky," leading to lysis. Antibody also may play a role in tumor cell lysis by participating in *antibody-dependent cellular cytotoxicity* (ADCC). This mechanism has not been shown to occur *in vivo* but certainly is demonstrable *in vitro*. The reaction is mediated by a so-called *killer cell* that expresses Fc receptors that find Fc molecules on the surface of target cells causing target-cell lysis. Cells that might function as killer cells include monocytes, neutrophils, eosinophils, B cells, or natural killer (NK) cells.

Beside the potential for antibodies generated by the host against specific tumor antigens, there is also evidence that normal individuals carry natural antibodies. They may react with embryonic antigens or with cross-reactive antigens associated with infectious agents. In mice the antigens are often those of endogenous viruses. The potential of these antibodies to lyse tumor cells has been examined *in vitro,* where it has been found that several kinds of neoplastic cells could be lysed in the presence of complement. There is evidence that macrophage-dependent rejection of small tumor inocula may be dependent on natural antibodies. Immune reactions against tumors not dependent on specific cytotoxic T cells probably represent a mixture of mechanisms including natural antibodies, nonspecifically activated macrophages, and NK cells, depending on the type of tumor and the capacities of the host.

Natural Killer Cells

There is also evidence that certain tumor cells may be lysed by a form of natural immunity mediated by natural killer cells (NK cells). NK cells are a subset of lymphocytes distinct from T cells and B cells. They fall within the group of lymphoid cells known as *large granular lymphocytes.* Cytotoxicity mediated by NK cells also requires contact with the target cell. Tumor cells apparently are distinguished from normal cells by nonimmunological mechanisms. NK-cell activity is enhanced by exposure to tumor cells, viruses, and certain adjuvants and chemicals. This phenomenon is not immunologically specific, however, and is believed to be mediated by interferons and interleukin-2 (IL-2). Experimental evidence for a role for NK cells in the control of tumor growth and metastasis *in vivo* has been obtained by use of strains of mice deficient in NK activity. In these animals, injection of tumor cells selected *in vitro* for enhanced susceptibility to NK-mediated lysis led to increased growth rate, shorter induction times, and increased metastatic capability of the resultant neoplasms compared to those in control mice. On the other hand, induction of NK-cell activity reduced the rate of growth and metastatic capability of tumors. Additional evidence is that tumors rarely metastasize in nude mice, which have high NK-cell activity. Finally, adoptive transfer of NK cells to irradiated mice has been shown to increase the resistance of the recipients to NK-susceptible tumors. Most studies of the role of NK cells suggest that they are effective against small tumor loads but that they have little effect on established tumors. They may therefore play a significant role in surveillance against incipient tumors and in removing circulating tumor cells. There is a strong inverse correlation between levels of NK cells and the ability of tumors to metastasize in experimental animals. Enhanced resistance to metastasis has also been accomplished by transfer of NK cells.

Macrophages

Macrophages often form a major cellular component in neoplasms undergoing rejection, and they may be important effector cells in tumor immunity. Macrophages incubated with T lymphocytes sensitized to tumor cells become specifically cytotoxic for those cells. This activation of macrophages is mediated by a lymphokine, known as *specific macrophage-arming factor* (SMAF). The cytotoxic action of armed macrophages depends on direct contact with the target cells. The ability of activated macrophages to kill tumor cells *in vitro* has been correlated with reduced tumor growth *in vivo*. Additionally, transfer of specifically armed macrophages to experimental animals prevents the growth of tumor cells injected intravenously or intraperitoneally. Macrophages also may be toxic to tumor cells to which antibody is bound.

Macrophages may also be nonspecifically activated by a variety of substances such as endotoxin, aggregated IgG, and peptidoglycans from mycobacteria. Tumor cells may be lysed by such macrophages and are much more susceptible than normal cells. The mechanism by which such activated macrophages recognize tumor cells is not known but apparently is not dependent on immunologically specific processes or the presence of strong neoantigens. Presumably they are able to recognize some alterations on the surface of the neoplastic cells.

Escape Mechanisms

Given that a variety of mechanisms can mediate rejection of transformed cells, why do they fail to do so in naturally occurring neoplasms? Several reasons, outlined below, have been proposed.

Modulation of cell surface antigens occurs in some tumor cells exposed to high-titer antibody. Those antigens that undergo such modulation are known to be relatively mobile in the cell membrane leading to redistribution and in some cases to shedding. Under such circumstances, specific effector mechanisms cannot be activated. Antigenic modulation is apparently a specific response because transplantation of modulated tumor cells to seronegative syngeneic hosts leads to the reappearance of the antigens.

The rapid turnover and shedding of antigen may result in the presence of circulating antigen or immune complexes, which may act as blocking factors that interfere with immune effector mechanisms. Antibody molecules themselves also can act as blocking factors. For example, in the case of TVT, serum from dogs in which the tumor has regressed can inhibit the growth of tumor cells *in vitro,* and sera from dogs with progressive tumors can block this activity. In this example, both tumor inhibitory and blocking activity are in the IgG fraction. Immune complexes are apparently not involved. More to the point, the importance of the interplay of these phenomena is illustrated by the strong correlation between the relative reactivities of inhibitory and blocking activity and the clinical course of the neoplasm. In the case of the canine TVT, both cytotoxic T cells and antibody may be important as effector mechanisms, and antibody may act as a blocking factor.

It also has been proposed that tumor cells may produce substances that are toxic to effector cells, suppress the function of effector cells, or destroy antibody. For example, some tumor cells can suppress the activity of macrophages. This activity appears to be mediated by a low-molecular-weight substance that can inhibit mononuclear cell chemotaxis *in vivo* and *in vitro* and can, when administered to experimental animals, enhance the growth of transplanted tumors.

Another possible mechanism of escape is the emergence of cells resistant to immunological attack. Tumor heterogeneity would be suggestive that such cells exist in any malignant neoplasm. It is possible, using selection procedures similar to those described earlier in this chapter, to select cells that are less susceptible to immune-mediated lysis. Conceivably then, an immune-mediated attack on a tumor could destroy susceptible cells while allowing the emergence of a population resistant to the process.

Finally, it has been shown that the ability to mount an immune attack on circulating tumor cells can be influenced by the nature of the antigens of the major histocompatibility complex (MHC) displayed on the cancer cell. The class I MHC genes are involved in MHC restriction, regulating the ability of T cells to recognize antigens on cells. Experimental studies in mice comparing two clones of a carcinoma differing in metastatic capacity have shown that the highly metastatic clone displayed a high density of the class I MHC gene product H-2D but little H-2K, whereas the reverse was true for the low metastatic clone. This was found to correspond to immunogenicity; the highly metastatic clone generated a poor cytotoxic response, whereas the low metastatic clone generated a strong response. A series of gene-transfer experiments showed that the ratio of H-2K to H-2D determined the vigor of the immune response to the tumor cells and correspondingly the degree of metastasis. Expression of high levels of H-2D with low levels of H-2K appar-

ently suppressed the immune response. Similarly the loss of the appropriate MHC class I antigens resulted in reduced immunogenicity and enhanced tumorigenicity.

TUMOR-SPECIFIC SUPPRESSOR CELLS

It has been suggested that very small tumor cell loads escape detection by the immune system and that by the time the tumor cell load reaches the threshold required for an immune response the neoplasm is too well established to be rejected. Of course, in the case of naturally occurring tumors the initial tumor load is by definition small. This phenomenon has been referred to as "sneaking through." There is evidence to suggest that this is real and that it is not simply a passive event in which transformed cells are just not noticed. Rather, it appears to be attributable to the early generation of tumor-specific suppressor cells capable of inhibiting the immune-mediated attack on tumor cells, thus enhancing tumor growth. For example, if cells are taken from a tumor growing in one mouse and transplanted to a syngeneic mouse previously immunized with tumor cells, they will fail to grow because of immune-mediated rejection. If, however, the transplanted cells are given together with spleen cells from the tumor-bearing donor mouse, they will not be rejected but will survive and grow. Furthermore, if tumor-bearing mice are given antithymocyte antiserum, there is a significant enhancement of tumor regression. These phenomena have been shown to be attributable to a population of suppressor T cells, which are immunologically specific for antigens borne on the tumor cells. They apparently suppress the usual host effector mechanisms and allow enhanced growth of tumor cells.

Further evidence for the role of suppressor cells in carcinogenesis comes from studies of squamous cell carcinomas induced in mice by UV irradiation. These tumors are highly antigenic and, if transplanted to normal syngeneic mice, will be rejected. If, however, the recipient mouse is first subjected to a subcarcinogenic dose of UV radiation, a population of suppressor cells that enhances the growth of the transplanted neoplasm is induced. There is also evidence that suppressor cells may be produced as a response to very small doses of tumor cells, which can be regarded as a form of tolerance. In other words, the initial small number of tumor cells in a naturally occurring tumor could induce an effective suppressor cell population before any cytotoxic effector mechanisms were stimulated. The influence of suppressor cells on metastatic capacity also has been shown when this system is used. Some of the resultant tumors produce a higher rate of metastasis when transferred to mice treated with subcarcinogenic doses of UV irradiation than in control mice. This enhanced capacity for metastasis is again immunologically specific and can be transferred by the use of lymphocytes, presumably suppressor cells, from UV- irradiated animals.

There is evidence from studies in humans that suppressor cells may play an important role in influencing the outcome of naturally occurring neoplastic disease. It has been shown that patients with osteosarcoma may have circulating cells that are cytotoxic to tumor cells when tested *in vitro*. In some patients these cytotoxic cells can be demonstrated only when a suppressor cell population is first removed. The suppressor cells can inhibit the cytotoxicity reaction if returned to the incubation medium. The possible clinical importance of such observations is illustrated in a study in which 4 out of 4 patients with osteosarcoma who had such suppressor cell activity had pulmonary metastases. In contrast, only 1 out of 6 patients who did not have demonstrable suppressor cell activity had pulmonary metastases.

Finally, it should be added that suppressor activity also resides in cells other than T lymphocytes, including macrophages and possibly B cells. Suppressor activity also may be nonspecific in nature and could account for the immunosuppression found in tumor-bearing patients.

Etiology

In most naturally occurring cases of neoplasia, the specific cause is unknown. However, for some and in the case of most experimentally induced neoplasms, predisposing or direct causes have been identified. Certainly, many agents that can cause cancer have now been identified. Substances that cause neoplasia are referred to as *carcinogens,* or *oncogens.* More specifically, a carcinogen may be defined as any substance or agent that produces, in exposed individuals, an incidence of neoplasia greater than that observed in those who are unexposed (controls). Known carcinogens fall into three categories: physical agents, chemicals, and viruses. Voluminous literature is available on each of these, and each has developed into a discipline of its own.

PHYSICAL AGENTS

A naturally occurring example of the importance of physical agents in carcinogenesis is the development of osteosarcomas in dogs. These malignant tumors are much more frequent in large breed dogs, such as great Danes and Saint Bernards, and most often de-

velop at the ends of long bones especially in the forelimbs. It is believed that this is attributable to the greater proportion of body weight carried by the forelimbs and the constant trauma transferred to these sites associated with normal locomotion. Another example is the development of fibrosarcomas along the migratory path of the spiruroid nematode, *Spirocerca lupi,* in the esophagus of dogs. Although the specific mechanism of carcinogenesis is not known in this case, the intimate association of the nematode with neoplastic tissue is suggestive of a direct physical cause.

The *physical state* of a carcinogen can be important. This is best illustrated by certain plastic films that, when implanted into the tissues, produce sarcomas. When these same plastics are implanted in the form of a powder or as a perforated film, they are not carcinogenic. In this case, the physical state rather than the chemical nature of the material seems to be important.

Exposure to *radiation* is one of the best known physical causes of neoplasia. All ultraviolet (UV) rays and ionizing electromagnetic (x rays and gamma rays) and particulate (alpha and beta particles, protons, and neutrons) radiation can cause neoplasms. A striking example in animals is the occurrence of squamous cell carcinomas resulting from excessive exposure to UV rays of sunlight. White cats living in hot, sunny climates commonly develop tumors on the ears or nose, and Hereford cattle, which commonly have unpigmented eyelids, often develop ocular squamous cell carcinomas. In humans, epidemiological evidence indicates that excessive exposure to sunlight is associated with an increased prevalence of tumors such as squamous cell carcinoma, basal cell carcinoma, and malignant melanoma. The carcinogenicity of UV radiation is known to be attributable to mutations resulting from the formation of DNA pyrimidine dimers and subsequent errors in transcription. The development of tumors as a result of exposure to ionizing radiation is well documented in humans. Examples include leukemia in atomic bomb survivors from Hiroshima and Nagasaki, osteosarcomas in patients receiving radiographic therapy for spinal arthritis, and pulmonary carcinomas in miners of radioactive elements. The mechanisms underlying ionizing radiation–induced carcinogenesis are complex and involve direct as well as indirect somatic mutation of DNA.

CHEMICAL CARCINOGENESIS

A bewildering variety of chemicals has been shown to be carcinogenic. Some act locally at the site of application, and some act remotely. Some are synthetic experimental compounds, but many occur in the environment either naturally or as pollutants. Some chemicals are *complete carcinogens;* that is, they cause the development of neoplasms after a single dose and appear to be capable of both initiation and promotion. Other chemicals act as *incomplete carcinogens,* since they are capable only of initiation and require interaction with other compounds acting as promoters to express their carcinogenic potential.

Some chemicals are *direct acting;* that is, they do not require chemical transformation to be carcinogenic; however, most chemical carcinogens act *indirectly.* The latter are, in fact, *procarcinogens* and must undergo cellular metabolism to produce *proximate* or *ultimate carcinogens.* The P450-dependent monooxygenases located in the endoplasmic reticulum and particularly rich in the liver are the most important enzyme system involved in this metabolic conversion. For example, both polycyclic hydrocarbons and aflatoxins are metabolized to epoxides, which are the ultimate carcinogens. This phenomenon explains, in many cases, the species or organ specificity of certain carcinogens. Species specificity depends on the metabolic capability of the cells of particular species, whereas organ specificity depends on the site of metabolism. The liver therefore is a frequent target organ of carcinogens, with this frequency being consistent with its significant role in metabolizing toxins. The urinary bladder is also often affected by carcinogens whose metabolites are excreted through the urinary tract.

Simple *inorganic salts* also can act as carcinogens. For example, salts of nickel and beryllium have carcinogenic potential in humans. Proved cases with similar cause are rare in animals, but there is some evidence that similar mechanisms may be involved in some cases of osteosarcoma. In dogs in which metal fixation devices with multiple parts have been implanted for long periods, an unexpectedly high number of osteosarcomas occurs. Moreover, these are usually in the midshaft region of the bone rather than occurring at the usual predilection sites for this neoplasm. It is believed that electrolytic activity set up by slight differences in the composition of the components leads to relatively high local concentrations of metal ions, which in turn act as a carcinogen.

Chemical carcinogens, whether direct or indirect acting and whether complete or incomplete carcinogens, initiate carcinogenesis by a similar mechanism. The critical molecular lesion is the formation of adducts between electron-deficient chemicals and electron-rich sites in the cell, especially DNA, resulting in somatic mutation. The critical DNA tar-

gets remain to be identified, but protooncogenes and anti-oncogenes are likely targets. Subsequent development of a tumor requires cell proliferation to "fix" the lesion, and there are other promotional events as previously described. The final carcinogenic potential of the chemical is a result of a balance between metabolic activation (if required), detoxication and elimination of the chemical, and repair of the DNA defect.

VIRAL ONCOGENESIS

Both DNA and RNA viruses can cause neoplasia (Table 6-9). In many cases, analogous viruses that cause tumors in humans cause comparable tumors in animals. Several examples of specific oncogenic DNA and RNA viruses are discussed in more detail below.

Oncogenic DNA Viruses

DNA viruses, including hepadnaviruses, herpesviruses, papovaviruses, and poxviruses cause naturally occurring tumors. In addition, adenoviruses induce tumors in animals after experimental inoculation. Oncogenic papovaviruses include the papillomaviruses, which cause benign papillomas in many species and certain malignant neoplasms in humans. Poxviruses cause the Shope fibroma of rabbits and histiocytomas in rhesus monkeys. Herpesviruses are important oncogenic DNA viruses that cause malignant neoplasms in a variety of species, including humans. In chickens, Marek's disease virus and the resultant neoplastic disease is one of the most extensively studied DNA virus–induced neoplasms. Hepadnaviruses are the most recently recognized family of oncogenic DNA viruses and include hepatitis B virus in humans and the analogous woodchuck virus, both of which produce acute and chronic liver disease followed by the development of hepatocellular carcinoma.

One of two consequences may follow infection with potentially oncogenic DNA viruses. The infection may be *productive,* in which case the cells produce infectious virus and are lysed as a result. Alternatively, the cells may be transformed, in which case the infection is *nonproductive* and the cells are not killed. Such transformation does not require complete infectious virus; it can be produced by viral DNA or by portions of it. Therefore, transformation by DNA viruses appears to result from the introduction of specific gene sequences or gene products. Considerable advances have been made in understanding the nature and mechanism of action of these products.

TABLE 6-9 Representative Oncogenic Viruses

VIRUS	SPECIES	NEOPLASM
DNA VIRUSES		
Adenoviridae		
Various strains	Hamster	Experimental sarcomas
Hepadnaviridae		
Hepatitis B virus	Humans	Hepatocellular carcinoma
Woodchuck hepatitis virus	Woodchuck	Hepatocellular carcinoma
Herpesviridae		
Epstein-Barr virus (EBV)	Human	Burkitt's lymphoma, nasopharyngeal carcinoma
Marek's disease virus	Chicken	Lymphoma (Marek's disease)
H. saimiri, and *H. ateles*	Nonhuman primates	Lymphoma
Lucké virus	Frog	Renal adenocarcinoma
Papovaviridae		
Polyomaviruses	Mouse	Experimental carcinomas and sarcomas
Simian virus 40 (SV40)	Rodents	Experimental sarcomas
Papillomaviruses	Many species, including humans	Papillomas, carcinomas
Poxviruses		
Yaba virus	Rhesus monkey	Histiocytoma
Shope fibroma virus	Rabbit	Fibroma, myxomas
RNA VIRUSES		
Flaviviridae		
Hepatitis C virus	Human	Hepatocellular carcinoma
Retroviridae, subfamily Oncovirinae		
Type B		
Mammary tumor virus	Mouse	Mammary adenocarcinoma
Type C		
Murine leukemia and sarcoma viruses	Mouse	Leukemias, lymphomas, sarcomas
Feline leukemia and sarcoma viruses	Cat	Leukemias, lymphomas, sarcomas
Type D		
Mason-Pfizer monkey tumor–like virus	Sheep	Pulmonary carcinoma
Type E?		
Bovine leukemia virus (BLV)	Cattle	Lymphoma, leukemia
Human T-lymphotropic virus type 1 (HTLV-1)	Human	T-cell leukemia and lymphoma
Simian T-lymphotropic virus (STLV)	Nonhuman primates	T-cell leukemia and lymphoma

Oncogenic DNA viruses have been shown to contain oncogenes, that is, genes that can be responsible for neoplastic transformation, such as those that were originally described in oncogenic retroviruses. The origin of these DNA tumor virus oncogenes is not known. In contrast to the oncogenes of retroviruses, they are not related to proto-oncogenes. However, as shown in Table 6-10, the transforming capacity of several well-studied DNA tumor viruses is closely correlated with the interaction between the protein products encoded by the viral oncogenes and cellular proto-oncogenes.

Neoplastic transformation by oncogenic *adenoviruses* involves cooperation between two viral genes, *E1A* and *E1B*, each of which encode two proteins. The E1A proteins are involved in regulation of viral transcription, but both are required for neoplastic transformation. Different protein-binding domains are responsible for viral transcription versus transformation. The latter correlates with binding to the retinoblastoma gene product, Rb. The E1B gene products alone do not appear to be able to alter cellular phenotype, though both proteins contribute to the development of tumors. In this case, cellular

TABLE 6-10 Oncogene Products of DNA Tumor Viruses

VIRUS	VIRAL ONCOGENE PRODUCT	CELLULAR TARGET
Adenovirus	E1A (289aa)	Rb
	E1A (243aa)	Rb
	E1B (495aa)	p53
	E1B (175aa)	?
Polyomavirus	Large T-antigen	Rb
	Middle T-antigen	*src*
	Small T-antigen	?
SV40	Large T-antigen	Rb, p53
	Small T-antigen	?
Papillomaviruses		
BPV-1	E5	PDGF receptor
HPV-16	E6	p53
	E7	Rb

transformation correlates best with the interaction between the larger of the two E1B proteins and the tumor-suppressor p53 protein.

Both oncogenic *polyoma* and *SV40* viruses encode a multifunctional protein named *large T-antigen.* This antigen is involved in initiation of viral replication and cellular transformation, but these activities are mediated by different protein-binding interactions. Cellular transformation correlates with binding of large T-antigen of both viruses to Rb, as well as to p53 in the case of SV40. Both viruses also encode a *small T-antigen,* which binds cellular transcription factors. It also increases the efficiency of transformation in conjunction with the large T-antigen, but the mechanism of action is not known. Unlike SV40, polyomavirus encodes a middle T-antigen that contributes to other features of the transformed phenotype. The *middle T-antigen* becomes associated with the *src* proto-oncogene protein product on the inner aspect of the plasma membrane, greatly enhancing its tyrosine kinase activity.

Studies of oncogenic *papillomaviruses* have yielded additional important information on mechanisms of transformation by DNA tumor viruses. Early studies were performed with bovine papillomavirus-1 (BPV-1), frequently associated with benign cutaneous papillomas ("warts") in cattle. Cellular transformation by BPV-1 is closely correlated with binding of the *E5* oncogene product with the *beta receptor* of *platelet-derived growth factor* (PDGF), resulting in its tyrosine phosphorylation and activation. More recent studies have concentrated on "high-risk" human papillomaviruses (HPV) associated with the development of cervical carcinoma. Cellular transforma-

tion by HPV-16 correlates best with expression of the *E6* and *E7* genes. The HPV-16 E7 protein binds Rb protein through amino acid sequences similar to adenovirus E1A protein and SV40 large T-antigen. Although HPV-16 E7 is sufficient for transformation, E6 together with E7 increases the efficiency of transformation. Similar to SV40 large T-antigen and adenovirus E1B 495aa protein, HPV-16 E6 binds p53.

It is apparent that many DNA tumor viruses share common mechanisms of cellular transformation mediated by their oncogene protein products. A prominent shared mechanism is interaction with and functional inactivation of the tumor-suppressor gene products, Rb and p53. Other oncogenic DNA virus gene products interact with and overactivate critical signal transduction molecules. As discussed previously, interference with the function of these proteins has important implications for processes responsible for cellular homeostasis such as the cell cycle and apoptotic cell death.

Oncogenic RNA Viruses

Until recently, retroviruses were believed to be the only family of RNA viruses that caused tumors. There is now strong epidemiological evidence linking chronic infection with the flavivirus *hepatitis C virus* (formerly known as "non-A, non-B hepatitis virus"), with hepatocellular carcinoma in humans. No equivalent of hepatitis C virus has been identified in animals.

Most of what we know about *retroviruses* has been gained from the study of the Oncovirinae subfamily of this group of RNA viruses in animals. A wide variety of retroviruses cause naturally occurring neoplasms in many species of animals (Table 6-11). By comparison, only one retrovirus, human T-cell lymphotropic virus type 1 (HTLV-1), has been associated with tumors in humans. Retroviruses can be classified according to their ultrastructural appearance and designated by letters. Type B retroviruses cause mammary carcinomas in mice. Type C viruses cause leukemias, lymphomas, and other types of sarcomas in a variety of species. Besides the murine oncogenic retroviruses, feline leukemia virus (FeLV) is one of the most studied of the group. In addition to its neoplastic sequelae, FeLV also causes a variety of nonneoplastic conditions such as thymic atrophy, enteric disease, immunosuppression, anemia, and abortion. Bovine leukemia virus (BLV) and HTLVs have C-type morphology, but because of unique structural and functional characteristics, they have been assigned to a separate group, sometimes referred to as "type E retroviruses."

TABLE 6-11 Mechanisms of Cellular Transformation by Retroviruses

VIRUS CATEGORY	LATENCY PERIOD TO TUMOR FORMATION	EFFICIENCY OF TRANSFORMATION	ONCOGENIC MECHANISM
Acute transforming (sarcoma) retroviruses	Short (days)	High	Viral oncogene
Chronic transforming (leukemia) retroviruses			
cis-acting	Intermediate (weeks to months)	High to intermediate	Activation of cellular proto-oncogene by proximity of proviral integration
trans-acting	Long (months to years)	Low	Virus-encoded protein controlling transcription of cellular genes

Retroviruses are so named because they possess an enzyme, called *reverse transcriptase,* or, more correctly, RNA-dependent DNA polymerase, that is responsible for formation of a DNA copy of the RNA viral genome. This DNA intermediate becomes incorporated into the genome of the host, where it is known as a *provirus.* Replication-competent retroviruses contain three genes: *gag,* which codes for the precursor protein of virion core proteins; *pol,* coding for reverse transcriptase; and *env,* coding for virion envelope glycoproteins. In addition, the viral genome also contains regulatory sequences that, in the DNA provirus, are called *long terminal repeats,* or *LTRs,* with one being positioned at each end of the viral genome. The LTR contains the viral promoter and enhancer elements and, as discussed later, is likely important for the abnormal expression of proto-oncogenes in transformed cells.

All retroviruses associated with naturally occurring tumors are *exogenous* and transmitted horizontally as true infectious agents. These must be differentiated from vertically transmitted (through gametes) *endogenous* retroviruses, which are present in most vertebrate species and are generally nonpathogenic. Exogenous, oncogenic retroviruses can be divided into several categories based on the mechanism by which they cause cellular transformation (see Table 6-11). The *acute transforming retroviruses* can be isolated from tumor tissue but are relatively rare. They are sometimes called "sarcoma" viruses because they usually cause solid-tissue sarcomas. Examples of this group include feline sarcoma virus and Rous sarcoma virus. These viruses carry oncogenes that, when introduced into the cell, rapidly and efficiently induce tumors. As we have mentioned before, the viral oncogenes (v-*oncs*) are derived from cellular genes (proto-oncogenes) that have been transduced by the virus. Usually the proteins encoded by the v-*oncs* are abnormal, being fused to fragments of normal viral proteins, or otherwise mutated. In most cases (Rous sarcoma virus being the exception) the acutely transforming retroviruses are replication defective as a result of loss of part of the normal viral genome during the transduction process. Except for the Rous sarcoma virus, therefore, they require coinfection with a *helper virus* for productive infection to occur. As a result, most acute transforming retroviruses are (fortunately) not highly contagious.

From the point of view of naturally occurring neoplastic disease, the *chronic transforming retroviruses* are more important. These are sometimes referred to as "leukemia" viruses because of their frequent association with hematopoietic neoplasms. This group is further subdivided into *cis-acting* and *trans-acting* viruses. The *cis*-acting retroviruses include feline leukemia virus (FeLV), avian leukosis virus (ALV), and murine leukemia viruses (MuLV). These viruses do not contain oncogenes, and the mechanism or mechanisms of neoplastic transformation are different from those of the acute viruses. Several mechanisms have been proposed, with one of the most important being the insertion of the virus close to cellular oncogenes, resulting in their alteration or activation. The provirus of retroviruses can be integrated into multiple sites in the host genome, and the insertion process is believed to be essentially random. By chance, however, provirus may become inserted at a site critical to transformation that subsequently leads to neoplastic expansion and an infected cellular clone. This site often appears to be related to a proto-oncogene that, as a result of the proximity of the provirus, becomes overactivated or mutated. For example, in B-cell lymphomas caused by ALV, the provirus has been found to be inserted near the *myc* gene, and in erythroblastomas, caused by the same virus, the integration site is near the *erb* gene. These viruses are infectious agents and are readily transmitted horizontally from animal to animal. However, presumably because the infrequent integration of the provirus in the proximity of a proto-oncogene and the likely need for additional events, these viruses induce tumors after a longer latent period and with less efficiency than the acute transforming retroviruses do.

The *trans*-acting retroviruses have evolved the most complex mechanism for cellular transformation. This group includes bovine leukemia virus (BLV), human T-lymphotropic virus (HTLV), and simian T-lymphotropic virus (STLV). Two types of HTLV have been isolated from humans, HTLV-1 and HTLV-2. HTLV-1 is the first oncogenic retrovirus to be isolated from humans and is associated with both neoplastic (adult T-cell leukemia/lymphoma) and nonneoplastic (HTLV-associated myelopathy/tropical spastic paraparesis) disorders. The pathogenic potential of HTLV-2 remains uncertain. These agents are similar to the *cis*-acting retroviruses in that they do not contain a viral oncogene but are dissimilar in that they do not have a preferred integration site. In other words, although provirus is clonally integrated in all tumors from an individual patient, the site varies between tumors in different patients. These retroviruses are able to influence host cell gene expression in *trans*, that is, mechanisms acting at a distance. In addition to typical retroviral genes, these complex retroviruses also contain a unique set of genes located at the 3' end of the viral genome that was originally called the *X region*. The most well-characterized gene product encoded in this region is called *Tax*. Through interaction with host transcription factors, Tax *trans*-activates sequences in the viral LTR to help regulate viral replication. Important among the transcription factors with which Tax interacts is *nuclear factor-κB* (NF-κB). NF-κB plays a central role in immune activation of lymphoid cells, which are also the prime target cells of the BLV/HTLV group of retroviruses. Although incompletely understood, it is also believed that Tax acts as an oncoprotein by *trans*-regulating critical host growth-regulatory genes in addition to its own LTR. For example, Tax has been demonstrated to increase the expression of genes such as interleukin-2 and its receptor, interleukin-3, granulocyte-macrophage colony-stimulating factor, γ-interferon, transforming growth factor-β1, *myc*, *fos*, and lymphotoxin. Consistent with the general scheme that we have described for tumor progression, additional genetic or epigenetic alterations are required before tumors finally appear. Thus, neo-

plasms associated with *trans*-acting chronic transforming retroviruses have a long latency period and occur in only a small percentage of infected individuals.

Examples of Virus-Induced Neoplasms in Animals

To put some of the discussion of viral oncogenesis into the perspective of naturally occurring disease, three examples are discussed. These are Marek's disease of chickens, caused by a DNA virus; feline leukemia, caused by a conventional chronic transforming retrovirus; and bovine leukemia, caused by a *trans*-acting retrovirus.

Marek's Disease. Marek's disease is a form of lymphoma that occurs in chickens and is caused by a *herpesvirus* (Marek's disease virus, MDV). Characteristic lesions of Marek's disease include enlargement of peripheral nerves and lymphoid tumors of T-cell origin occurring in a variety of tissues (Fig. 6-34). Enlargement of nerves is attributable to neoplastic infiltration accompanied by demyelination, proliferation of Schwann cells, and a variable inflammatory infiltrate. Early in the course of infection, MDV causes degeneration of lymphoid tissue in the bursa of Fabricius, the thymus and the spleen, and the epithelium of the feather follicles. The degenerative lesions in the feather follicle epithelium are accompanied by the formation of intranuclear and intracytoplasmic inclusion bodies.

Chickens developing Marek's disease become infected at an early age. Infection is fully productive only in the epithelium of feather follicles, and virus is shed in dander, which serves as the source of infectious virus for susceptible chickens. In lymphoid cells, infection is essentially nonproductive, though limited production of viral DNA and antigens sometimes occurs. This nonproductive infection is accompanied by transformation. Tumor cells contain multiple copies of MDV DNA, with the number varying between different cases. The cellular location of viral DNA is not yet firmly established, though there is some evidence that viral DNA can be integrated into the host genome. Infection with MDV gives rise to numerous viral or virus-coded antigens in infected cells. One antigen, *Marek's associated tumor-specific antigen* (MATSA), was believed to be a virus-specific membrane antigen that could be used as a marker for neoplastic transformation in Marek's disease. However, it is now known that MATSA is expressed on nonneoplastic, activated T cells and that it is not specific for Marek's disease.

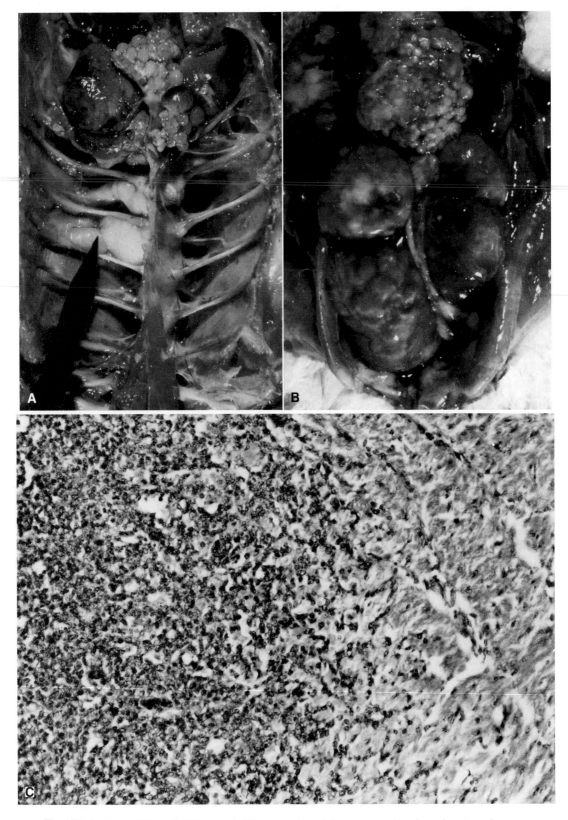

Fig. 6-34 Lesions of Marek's Disease. A, Nerves in this chicken are greatly enlarged, *pointer*, because of an infiltrate of neoplastic lymphocytes. These intercostal lesions are very suggestive of Marek's disease. **B,** Both the kidney and the ovary in this chicken are enlarged because of infiltration by neoplastic lymphocytes. **C,** In this photomicrograph, neoplastic lymphocytes, *left*, are invading the myocardium, *right*. (*Courtesy Department of Avian and Aquatic Animal Medicine, Cornell University.*)

Resistance to Marek's disease is influenced by host genetic factors, and high-susceptibility and low-susceptibility strains of chickens have been developed. Resistance is not against initial infection but against later amplification of infection and tumor development. Because thymectomy, but not bursectomy, reduces amplification of infection and tumor development, resistance seems to depend on intact T-cell function but not on antibody. However, antibody does develop to MDV antigens including, in some cases, MATSA. There is also some evidence that antibody may provide partial protection. For example, in chicks with maternal antibody the disease has a prolonged incubation period, and the extent of lesions may be reduced.

Chickens also may acquire active immunity to Marek's disease, and this disease provides the first example of successful vaccination against a neoplastic disease. Vaccination may be carried out either with an attenuated or nonpathogenic MDV or with *Herpesvirus* of turkeys. The latter is cross-reactive with MDV but is nonpathogenic for the chicken and may therefore be used as a vaccine. Vaccinated chickens remain susceptible to infection, though viremia and shedding of virus from the feather follicles is reduced. Once again, immunity against development of tumors is involved. Vaccination appears to prevent the proliferation of transformed cells as well as reducing the extent of virus replication. The mechanisms involved in this antitumor immunity are not clear but appear to be cell mediated. Cytotoxic T cells directed against both MATSA- and MDV-specific antigens are present in vaccinated chickens. The success of vaccination against Marek's disease is likely to be attributable to a combination of antiviral and antitumor immunity, involving several mechanisms.

Mechanisms by which MDV causes neoplasia are poorly understood. Although viral DNA exists in multiple copies in host cells and possibly is integrated into the host genome, no definitive oncogenes have been identified.

To recapitulate, Marek's disease illustrates several important features of neoplasia induced by DNA viruses. Transformed cells do not produce virus, but viral DNA is present in multiple copies in the cells, perhaps in an integrated form. Natural susceptibility is under genetic influence. Transformed cells contain viral and membrane-associated antigens, and immunity can be induced against the development of tumors. What makes Marek's disease unique is the fact that it is the first neoplastic disease to be successfully controlled by vaccination.

Feline Leukemia. Feline leukemia virus (FeLV), as indicated earlier in this chapter, can cause a variety of diseases in cats, with the one of interest to this discussion being lymphoma (lymphosarcoma). FeLV is one of the best studied of the oncogenic retroviruses. Its existence was first suggested by epidemiological studies of clusters of feline lymphoma, and its recognition was seminal to the realization that infectious viruses could cause naturally occurring cancers.

Infection by FeLV is common in random, outbred cat populations, particularly where groups of cats live in close association. The virus is excreted in saliva and is spread horizontally. Infection is usually followed initially by a mild, transient illness a few weeks after exposure. The majority of infected cats develop an immune response to the gp70 and p15E envelope proteins, clear the virus, and become immune. Those that do not become persistently infected, with some developing lymphoma months to years later and others dying of other FeLV-related diseases. The lesions in feline lymphoma consist of solid lymphoid tumors in a variety of organs (Fig. 6-35), or, less commonly, leukemia may occur. Neoplasms derived from T lymphocytes are most common, though B-cell tumors also occur. FeLV can also induce myeloid and erythroid leukemias. Tumors may be either virus positive or virus negative. In other words, transformed cells may or may not replicate virus. Lymphoma may also occur in cats in which FeLV cannot be detected though these animals often have a history of exposure to the virus. This lack of detection indicates that FeLV may also play an etiological role in such "FeLV-negative" lymphosarcomas.

FeLV-infected cells contain many virus-specific antigens. These include type-specific viral envelope antigens and group-specific internal virion antigens. Antibody to the envelope proteins, gp70 and p15E, is virus neutralizing and will protect against infection. An additional antigen, originally referred to as *feline oncornavirus cell membrane antigen*, or FOCMA, is expressed on FeLV-transformed cells. The exact nature of FOCMA is unclear. It is not expressed on normal lymphocytes or even those infected with FeLV. It may represent the expression of a recombinant gp70 envelope gene of a particular group of FeLV, FeLV-C, and endogenous cellular sequences. Interestingly, antibody to FOCMA does not protect against infection but, if present in significant titers, protects against the development of lymphoma in FeLV-infected cats and against sarcomas induced by feline sarcoma viruses (see below). FOCMA thus appears to be a tumor-specific antigen.

Cats in a natural population develop one of several outcomes after exposure to FeLV; they may fail to become infected and therefore not develop immunity; become infected, develop antiviral immunity,

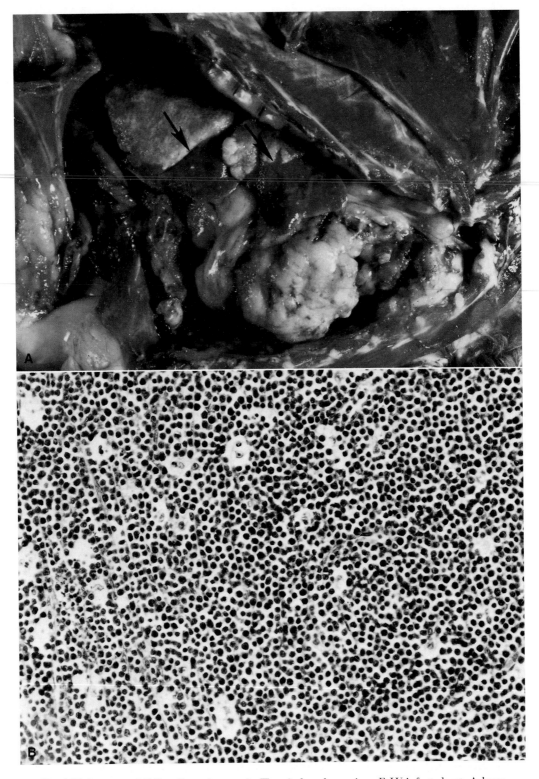

Fig. 6-35 Lesions of Feline Lymphoma. A, Thymic lymphoma in a FeLV-infected cat. A large mass of neoplastic tissue displaces the lungs dorsally. The lungs are partially atelectatic, *arrow.* This is one of the more common forms of feline lymphoma. **B,** Histologically, the mass consists of a sheet of relatively uniform neoplastic lymphocytes. The cells in the clear spaces are apoptotic cells or macrophages that have phagocytosed necrotic and apoptotic neoplastic lymphocytes.

and clear the virus; fail to develop immunity to the virus but develop anti-FOCMA antibodies, which protect against the development of tumors; or fail to develop either form of immunity and develop lymphoma or other forms of FeLV-related disease. Chronically infected carrier cats also can occur. The response of animals to infection depends, in part, on the dose of virus and the age at exposure. Young kittens often do not mount an adequate immune response and thus acquire active infection, which may lead to the development of neoplasia.

The mechanism of transformation by FeLV has not been fully elucidated. Presumably, mechanisms related to viral integration, similar to those of other chronic transforming retroviruses, are involved. Approximately 30% of naturally occurring FeLV-induced lymphomas contain rearrangements of the *myc* proto-oncogene, resulting from either transduction or proviral insertion.

FeLV also appears to be uniquely able to transduce proto-oncogenes to produce acutely transforming retroviruses, the *feline sarcoma viruses* (FeSV). Among the isolates of FeSV so far obtained from naturally occurring feline fibrosarcomas, seven different proto-oncogenes, namely, *fes, fms, sis, abl, fgr,* K-*ras,* and *kit,* have been shown to have been transduced. These FeSVs are associated with FeLV helper viruses. In each case so far examined, the gene product is a fusion of the product of the viral *gag* gene and the proto-oncogene. FeSV-induced fibrosarcomas do not occur in clusters, are not transmitted horizontally, but rather arise *de novo* in FeLV-infected cats.

The first commercially available antiretroviral vaccine was developed against FeLV. The first vaccine to be marketed consisted of inactivated viral antigens and FOCMA released from a FeLV-infected and transformed cell line maintained in tissue culture. A variety of other types of vaccines have been studied, including a more recently marketed FeLV gp70 *env* gene recombinant vaccine produced in a bacterial expression system. These vaccines have been reported to protect between 70% and 80% of cats exposed to FeLV under experimental or natural conditions.

Feline lymphoma or leukemia therefore also demonstrates several biological characteristics of virus-induced neoplasia, some of which it shares with Marek's disease. The infection is horizontally transmitted, may or may not be virus productive, and is associated with specific viral and cell membrane antigens. The association of productive infection with cell transformation is characteristic of oncogenic retroviruses viruses and contrasts with oncogenic DNA viruses. FeLV infection is also of interest because of the ability of antibody against a tumor-specific antigen, FOCMA, to protect against the development of neoplastic disease. Despite the controversy over the nature of FOCMA, the association between an effective anti-FOCMA antibody immune response and protection against neoplastic disease is one of the best-documented examples of tumor immunity.

Bovine Leukemia. Recognition of the occurrence of multiple cases of lymphoma or leukemia in herds of cattle, termed *enzootic bovine leukosis* (EBL), led to early suspicion that an infectious agent was involved. Additional evidence accumulated when EBL was linked to the introduction of a cow from a herd containing affected cattle to a naïve herd and the finding that it could be experimentally transmitted. The cause of the disease was discovered to be a retrovirus, *bovine leukemia virus* (BLV), when virus particles were recognized in cultures of lymphocytes of animals with *persistent lymphocytosis* (PL), a second syndrome associated with BLV infection. As already mentioned, because of structural and functional similarities, BLV is now classified with HTLV in a separate group of oncogenic retroviruses.

BLV is an exogenous, horizontally transmitted retrovirus that induces B-cell lymphoma or less commonly leukemia, as well as a nonneoplastic condition referred to as "PL." BLV remains highly cell associated and is therefore transmitted only under conditions where transfer of infected lymphocytes, especially whole blood, occurs. Iatrogenic infection through the use of common hypodermic needles is a frequent means of transmission. Hematophagous insects are suspected but not proved to be vectors of transmission. Despite the development of virus-neutralizing antibodies in BLV-infected cattle, the immune response cannot control the infection. Once infected, cattle are infected for life. Most BLV-infected cattle remain asymptomatic. Approximately one third develop PL, characterized by a nonneoplastic, polyclonal increase in circulating B lymphocytes. This is also an asymptomatic stage of the infection; however, it is a preneoplastic condition, since cattle with PL are approximately twice as likely to develop lymphoma as compared to BLV-infected cattle without PL. Less than 5% of BLV-infected cattle develop neoplastic disease and then only years after infection. Sheep can be infected experimentally and develop the same stages of infection but at an accelerated rate and with an increased incidence of tumors.

As discussed earlier, there are striking similarities between tumors induced by BLV and those induced by HTLV. Bovine tumors from a single animal have clonally integrated virus, but the site varies from animal to animal. Tumor cells contain one to four integrated copies of the provirus, but viral transcription and translation are extremely limited *in vivo*. BLV contains a unique region in the 3′ portion of the genome, *pX*, corresponding to the X region of HTLV. A product of this region, Tax, acts in *trans* to regulate viral transcription and is critical for initiation of infection and transformation but is not required for maintenance of the transformed phenotype. This is very similar to findings for HTLV and human T-cell neoplasms and again is suggestive that further genetic changes are required for development of the fully transformed cell.

Bovine leukemia and BLV therefore further illustrate the parallels that exist between neoplastic (and other) diseases in humans and other animals. Although a safe and efficacious vaccine is not yet available to protect against BLV infection, methods to control the horizontal spread of the virus and subsequent development of disease are clearly understood. The study of such animal models has been and will continue to be valuable to an understanding of mechanisms involved in human disease and, conversely, many principles established for human disease can be applied to those of animals.

Neoplasia in Perspective

In this chapter we have explored the nature and pathogenesis of neoplastic disease in some detail. From our discussion, it should be obvious that scientists have long been fascinated by the process whereby cell growth becomes uncontrolled in otherwise highly regulated and controlled biological systems. Our efforts to understand the factors underlying the initiation and subsequent development of neoplastic growth have led to an increased understanding of fundamental biological phenomena that control normal cell proliferation and differentiation. In retrospect, the convergence of these areas is not surprising. Neoplastic disease affects a phylogenetically diverse group of species. If the mechanisms responsible for neoplastic growth were that different from those involved in normal cell growth, it is likely that tumors would not have been maintained evolutionarily. Given the complexity of normal growth control mechanisms, neither is it surprising that neoplastic growth is a complex and multistep process. Our efforts to understand the basic biological phenomena that accompany neoplastic disease, or other diseases for that matter, are not simply a matter of academic curiosity. They will, in the long run, provide the tools by which we can provide better patient care.

RECOMMENDED READING

Albelda SM: Role of integrins and other cell adhesion molecules in tumor progression and metastasis, *Lab Invest* 68:4-17, 1993.

Cockerell GL, Reyes RA: Bovine leukemia virus–associated lymphoproliferative disorders. In Zinkle JG, Jain NC, editors: *Schalm's veterinary hematology*, ed 5, Baltimore, 2000, Williams & Wilkins.

Cordon-Cardo C: Mutation of cell cycle regulators, *Am J Pathol* 147:545-560, 1995.

Coussens LM, Werb Z: Matrix metalloproteinases and the development of cancer, *Chem Biol* 3:895-904, 1996.

Dorn CR, Priester WA: Epidemiology. In Theilen GH, Madewell BR, editors: *Veterinary cancer medicine*, ed 2, Philadelphia, 1987, Lea & Febiger.

Elangbam CS, Qualls CW Jr, Dahlgren RR: Cell adhesion molecules—update, *Vet Pathol* 34:61-73, 1997.

Folkman J: Tumor angiogenesis. In Mendelsohn J, Howley PM, Israel MA, Liotta LA, editors: *The molecular basis of cancer*, Philadelphia, 1995, Saunders.

Folkman J: Fighting cancer by attacking its blood supply, *Sci Am* 275:150-152, 1996.

Granville DJ, Carthy CM, Hunt DWC, McManus BM: Apoptosis: molecular aspects of cell death and disease, *Lab Invest* 78:893-913, 1998.

Hansen MF, Cavenee WK: Genetics of cancer predisposition, *Cancer Res* 47:5518-5527, 1987.

Hardy WD: Feline retroviruses. In Levy JA, editors: *The Retroviridae*, vol 2, New York, 1993, Plenum Press.

Harley CB, Kim NW, Prowse KR, Weinrich SL, Hirsch KS, West MD, Bacchetti S, Hirte HW, Counter CM, Greier CW, Piatyszek MA, Wright WE, Shay JW: Telomerase, cell immortality, and cancer, *Cold Spring Harbor Symp Quant Biol* 59:307-315, 1994.

Hoops TC, Traber PG: Molecular pathogenesis of colorectal cancer, *Hematol Oncol Clin North Am* 11:609-633, 1997.

Hunter T: Oncoprotein networks, *Cell* 88:333-346, 1997.

Kinzler KW, Vogelstein B: Lessons learned from hereditary colorectal cancer, *Cell* 87:159-170, 1996.

Levine AJ: Oncogenes of DNA tumor viruses, *Cancer Res* 48:493-495, 1988.

Levine AJ: p53, the cellular gatekeeper for growth and division, *Cell* 88:323-331, 1997.

Levine AJ: The tumor suppressor genes, *Annu Rev Biochem* 62:623-651, 1993.

Lugo M, de Klein A: Metaplasia: an overview, *Arch Pathol Lab Med* 108:185-189, 1984.

Marx JL: How cancer cells spread in the body, *Science* 244:147-148, 1989.

Misdorp W: Veterinary cancer epidemiology, *Vet Q* 18:32-36, 1996.

Nicolson GL: Organ specificity of tumor metastasis: role of preferential adhesion, invasion and growth of malignant cells at specific secondary sites, *Cancer Metastasis Rev* 7:143-188, 1988.

Nonoyama M, Tanaka A: Current developments in the molecular biology of Marek's disease. In Barbanti-Brodano G, Bendinelli M, Friedman H, editors: *DNA tumor viruses*, New York, 1995, Plenum Press.

Nowell PC: Cancer, chromosomes, and genes, *Lab Invest* 66:407-417, 1992.

Old LJ: Immunotherapy for cancer, *Sci Am* 275:136-143, 1996.

Onions D: Tumor immunology. In Theilen GH, Madewell BR, editors: *Veterinary cancer medicine,* ed 2, Philadelphia, 1987, Lea & Febiger.

Patnaik AK, Ehler WJ, MacEwen EG: Canine cutaneous mast cell tumor: morphologic grading and survival time in 83 dogs, *Vet Pathol* 21:469-474, 1984.

Pauli BU, Knudson W: Tumor invasion: a consequence of destructive and compositional matrix alterations, *Hum Pathol* 19:628-639, 1988.

Pauli BU, Lee C-L: Organ preference of metastasis: the role of organ-specifically modulated endothelial cells, *Lab Invest* 58:379-387, 1988.

Pitot HC, Dragon YP: Facts and theories concerning the mechanisms of carcinogenesis, *FASEB J* 5:2280-2286, 1991.

Powers BE, Hoopes PJ, Ehrhart EJ: Tumor diagnosis, grading, and staging, *Semin Vet Med Small Animals* 10:158-167, 1995.

Rojko JL, Kociba GJ: Pathogenesis of infection by the feline leukemia virus, *J Am Vet Med Assoc* 199:1305-1310, 1991.

Rosenblatt JD, Miles S, Gasson JC, Prager D: Transactivation of cellular genes by human retroviruses, *Curr Top Microbiol Immunol* 193:25-49, 1995.

Rosol TJ, Capen CC: Mechanisms of cancer-induced hypercalcemia, *Lab Invest* 67:680-702, 1992.

Schat KA: Marek's disease: a model for protection against herpesvirus-induced tumours, *Cancer Surv* 6:1-38, 1987.

Sell S, Pierce GB: Maturation arrest of stem cell differentiation is a common pathway for the cellular origin of teratocarcinomas and epithelial cancers, *Lab Invest* 70:6-22, 1994.

Shay JW: Telomerase in human development and cancer, *J Cell Physiol* 173:266-270, 1997.

Sherr CJ: Cancer cell cycles, *Science* 274:1672-1677, 1996.

Soini Y, Pääkkö P, Hehto V-P: Histopathological evaluation of apoptosis in cancer, *Am J Pathol* 153:1041-1053, 1998.

Stettler-Stevenson WG, Aznavoorian S, Liotta LA: Tumor cell interactions with the extracellular matrix during invasion and metastasis, *Annu Rev Cell Biol* 9:541-576, 1993.

Stoker M: Fundamentals of cancer cell biology, *Adv Cancer Res* 70:1-19, 1996.

Temin HM: Evolution of cancer genes as a mutation-driven process, *Cancer Res* 48:1697-1701, 1988.

Verma RS: Oncogenetics: a new emerging field of cancer, *Mol Gen Genet* 205:385-389, 1986.

Weidner N: Intratumor microvessel density as a prognostic factor in cancer, *Am J Pathol* 147:9-19, 1995.

Weinberg RA: Finding the anti-oncogene, *Sci Am* 259:44-51, 1988.

Weinberg RA: How cancer arises, *Sci Am* 275:62-70, 1996.

Woodhouse EC, Chuaqui RF, Liotta LA: General mechanisms of metastasis, *Cancer* 80:1529-1537, 1997.

Woodruff MFA: Tumor clonality and its biological significance, *Adv Cancer Res* 50:197-229, 1988.

CHAPTER 7

Nature and Causes of Disease

Interactions of Host, Pathogen, and Environment

Howard B. Gelberg
Barry J. Cooper

UNDERSTANDING DISEASE
Evolving Concepts of Disease

We live in a new age of discovery. Unlike the earlier intracontinental and intercontinental explorers, contemporary adventurers explore the mysterious unknowns of cells, tissues, and organs. Seminal discoveries made possible by the new tools of molecular biology and genetics have allowed probing of the uncharted waters of life. The more we know and the more we apply and adapt these new tools of discovery, the more we find that we, as complex organisms, have much in common with the simpler forms of life with which we share the planet. We also find that life is more complex than previously imagined.

Unraveling the genetic makeup of microbes and their hosts allows for a better understanding of the mechanisms of disease. Better understanding of the molecular and genetic basis of function and dysfunction allows for a more rational approach to preventive medicine and more focused targeting and development of treatment modalities. Unfortunately, with each new discovery come false hopes and expectations. Each report of a magic bullet for cancer or antiviral therapy for persistent infections is accompanied by heightened expectations of breakthrough cures such that none of us will die of disease. Such hopes are rarely realized. Concurrently, we read of new and reemerging pathogens, bacteria resistant to all known antibiotics as well as nosocomial and zoonotic infections with dire consequences.

Paradigms have shifted many times in our scientific lifetimes. For example, most gastric ulcers are now believed to be caused by a helical bacterium, at least in humans. (Such a link has not been proved in our domestic animal species, many of which, especially pet carnivores, harbor similar bacteria.) Proteins, void of nucleic acids, the blueprints for life, are capable of causing what used to be termed "slow viral diseases." What will be the next shift? How can we possibly foresee the future? How can we foretell when the next mad cow disease crosses from animal to man? How do we know that xenotransplantation will not introduce some new unrecognized scourge from swine to people?

Are we winning or losing the war against disease? How far can we push the longevity envelope? Will the machine (body) eventually wear out even if we eat properly, ingest antioxidants, insert genes into our cells to reverse hereditary diseases, get the proper amount of exercise, and understand and balance the increasingly complex and functionally redundant biochemical soup that maintains our bodies in homeostatic bliss?

Perhaps the answers to these questions lie in one definition of science: a self-correcting body of knowledge. Incremental advances in scientific understanding of function and dysfunction will likely lead to incremental advances in human and animal health. Scientists with open minds able to think outside the box will make those discoveries, thus correcting the body of knowledge. However, with each step forward there is likely to be a step backwards. Accompanying the development of each new miracle drug will be accelerated evolutionary pressure for the targeted organisms to survive by producing resistant mutations.

The margin between homeostasis and disease is razor thin. It is amazing how complex the regulatory processes within the body are and yet how simply elegant. Functional redundancy within the organism's machinery ensures that often several major changes must occur for disease to result. Pathogens must be extraordinarily clever, biologically, to overcome host defenses, exploit normal cell machinery for their functions, devise methods to survive in hostile intracellular environments, attach specifically to cell surface molecules to avoid washout, turn the host immune system into a weapon directed against the host, or incorporate into the host cell genome and survive under a variety of environmental extremes. Yet, at the same time it is a disadvantage for the pathogen to destroy the host until progeny pathogens are produced so that they can spread throughout the host population. Science is now directed at understanding how all this occurs. But the natural world is clever and adaptable. As we develop preventions and cures to many of the animal kingdom's ills, we will likely encounter new developments in the ways that pathogens survive. We may simply speed up the evolutionary process of the genetically plastic pathogens.

Koch's Postulates

The cause of disease is not always obvious and direct, and unfortunately, despite modern instrumentation and technology, establishing a cause is not always possible. To diagnosticians, this is frustrating. Fortunately, many illnesses and conditions without a specific known cause can be successfully treated symptomatologically. How then does one determine the cause of illness? Since 1882 this has been done by fulfillment of Koch's postulates. Koch's postulates require that one isolate an agent from a diseased individual, reproduce the disease experimentally using that agent, and reisolate the agent from the second diseased host.

Molecular Koch's Postulates

Until recently, fulfillment of Koch's postulates was the criterion standard for establishing causality of disease. However, there are many diseases not caused by infectious agents or caused by agents that cannot be isolated or cultivated *in vitro*. These require a new paradigm for establishing cause-and-effect relationships in disease production, hence the development of molecular Koch's postulates. To fulfill molecular Koch's postulates, at least for bacterial pathogens, one must demonstrate that the gene or gene product responsible for pathogenesis is present in virulent bacteria but not in avirulent strains of the same bacterium. Altering this gene should affect virulence. Removing the gene should render the organism avirulent, and adding the virulence gene should increase pathogenicity. The virulence gene should be expressed when in the host animal, and antibodies to the gene product should be protective.

The Tools of Molecular Biology

Our understanding of the mechanisms of disease is growing exponentially because of the widespread use of genetic and molecular tools. The human genome project is an example of a focused and detailed attempt to understand gene function by identifying all 3 billion human base pairs. Since there is extensive phylogenic conservation of gene structure and function among all life forms, such an endeavor, combined with similar studies in prokaryotes and eukaryotes of all types, will greatly add to our knowledge of function and dysfunction.

The polymerase chain reaction and *in situ* hybridization are techniques that have the ability to amplify and thus identify genes and eventually their products (proteins) present at low copy numbers in an infected host and help trace the pathogenic sequence of disease-producing events. They are also useful in identifying potential carriers of disease agents. These techniques employ single-stranded, chemically synthesized oligonucleotides called "primers," which delineate the sequence to be amplified. These techniques can amplify viral RNA or DNA as well as cellular RNA and chromosomal DNA.

Electronic fluorescent active cell sorting (FACS) can identify, separate, and collect an apparently homogeneous cell population into multiple subpopulations playing differing roles in homeostasis and injury. Isolation of individual cell populations allows for functional study. Knockout mice (missing functional genes) and transgenic animals (containing foreign or transplanted genes) are being used extensively for basic functional studies. These gene transfer techniques also have potential for applied or therapeutic procedures. Already cows are producing human clotting factors in milk, and genetically altered pigs are being developed as donors for human organ transplants (xenotransplantation). Recombinant DNA is being used for functional and diagnostic study. Genomic fingerprinting is routinely used in forensic medicine: witness the O.J. Simpson trial.

Emerging technologies such as "biochips" combining sensors made from a web of DNA and gold particles are being developed to detect precise nucleic acid sequences that change the electronic properties of the matrix, resulting in the absorption of specific wavelengths of light. The clinician recognizes the reaction and thus the presence of the pathogen, at bedside, by color changes. Such technology has potential application as an inexpensive, disposable, accurate, and rapid diagnostic tool. The applications of these new technologies are seemingly endless in understanding and diagnosing disease of all types.

These technological advances are largely based on recombinant DNA technology. The major reason that these techniques are possible is the availability of restriction endonucleases. A battery of well-characterized bacterial enzymes (endonucleases) cleaves nucleic acids at specific nucleotide sequences allowing DNA to be cut into relatively small specific fragments. It is possible to identify, clone, and amplify genes directly from DNA or to produce them from mRNA. The latter exploits reverse transcriptase from retroviruses to make a DNA copy of the mRNA molecule. Because it is a complementary copy, the product is referred to as "cDNA." In either case the cloned molecules can be used as probes to look for the presence of a gene and its mRNA and to assess their quantity. Furthermore, a variety of techniques allows the quality of the gene to be studied. Yet another remarkable dividend is the ability to quickly determine the sequence of a protein. It is much easier to sequence DNA than it is to do so for protein. Frequently, investigators who are interested in a particular polypeptide or protein will clone its gene, produce cDNAs, and sequence them. Because the genetic code is known, the sequence of the protein can very quickly be predicted. Throughout this book are many instances of knowledge that would not have been available without this technology.

During the discussion of the genetic basis of neoplasia, for example, passing reference was made to many such examples. The structure of the growth factors, for example, would be mostly unknown. The alterations in gene structure and the expression and amplification of oncogenes could not be measured. The nature of protein products encoded by the oncogenes would not be known. Finally, these techniques provide the ability to produce large quantities of purified protein products relatively easily and cheaply. The effect of this is enormous in all branches of the medical sciences.

NATURE OF THE PATHOGEN

Pathogens have been traditionally defined as disease-producing agents, usually those we can visualize such as viruses, bacteria, and protozoa. However, the definition of a pathogen perhaps needs some updating, since we now know that disease can be produced by a myriad of agents that do not fit into the traditional definition. Also, as we learn more about pathogenesis, we learn more about the mechanisms by which some of the traditional pathogens actually cause disease. We learn why some strains of *Escherichia coli*, for example, are more pathogenic than other strains. On a genetic and gene-product basis, we now know that mobile genetic elements transported through phages and plasmids can move from bacterium to bacterium taking with them the capacity to cause disease. We know that transposons encode virulence factors. These virulence factors include pili, adhesins, invasins, iron-binding siderophores, phagocytosis-resistant capsules, toxic proteins that kill the host cells or reduce the oxidative burst, changing surface antigens, proteases, and other factors. We also know that specific receptor molecules on certain host cells render them susceptible to infection. This knowledge opens wide doors to new approaches to prophylaxis and therapeutics.

The one constant thing about disease is its variability. The reasons for this become clearer when we recognize that there is an immense number of interdependent factors that influence the pathogenesis of a disease from inception to ultimate outcome. Some of these relate to the host and some to the various external causative factors such as bacteria and viruses. Many are also determined by alterations in the environment in which both the host and its pathogens dwell. We are now forced to recognize that, although certain organisms can cause disease, they do not always do so.

Prions

The nature of the pathogens keeps growing with our new knowledge. Prions (proteinaceous infectious particles, pronounced /pree-onz/), for example, are proteins that integrate into the host and affect protein folding and thus protein function. The prion theory, which earned Stanley Prusiner the Nobel Prize in medicine in 1997, is that prions are an entirely new class of infectious agents and may be responsible for a variety of neurodegenerative disorders besides the "slow virus diseases" such as scrapie, kuru, and bovine spongiform encephalopathy (mad cow disease). Also, prions can induce beta-pleated sheet conformations of proteins resembling but not identical to the plaque-like lesions in Alzheimer's disease. All known prion diseases are fatal and prions completely evade the host immune response. Traditional methods of inactivating pathogens in the food supply do not apply to prions, and such an incapacity makes them especially dangerous for cross-species transmission.

Viruses

Viruses may be thought of as delivery systems for nucleic acids (DNA or RNA). These nucleic acids may be single stranded or double stranded and, if composed of RNA, must be reverse transcribed to a DNA template for replication. Viruses are not capable of motility or replication outside of the host and therefore exploit numerous mechanisms for transport between hosts. These include aerosolization (coughing and sneezing), the fecal oral route, by insects (arboviruses) and other vectors, as well as vertically through the host genome (retroviruses). Viruses appropriate the host cell machinery to duplicate themselves, forming millions of self-copies. Some viruses leave cells by lysis, whereas others do not destroy the host cells. Many viruses have the ability to mutate frequently thus escaping host immune surveillance (as HIV can). Some viruses are associated with neoplasia. Of course, because viruses are intracellular pathogens, therapies aimed at control of virus-infected tissues must be directed at transmission of virus from infected to uninfected cells.

Pathologists often recognize viral diseases by their tissue tropism and pattern of necrosis, since many viruses do not produce crystalline arrays of viral particles (virus factories) in the host cell nucleus or cytoplasm. When they do occur, we recognize these viral factories at the light microscopic level as inclusion bodies (Fig. 7-1). Newer diagnostic techniques, such as *in situ* hybridization and the polymerase chain reaction, greatly increase the

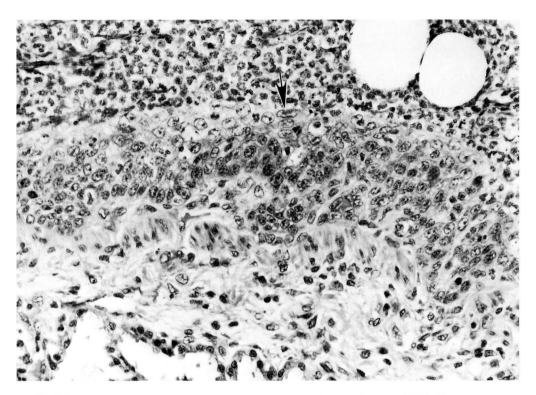

Fig. 7-1 Adenovirus Infection in Combined Immunodeficiency Disease (CID). There is suppurative bronchiolitis and dramatic hyperplasia of the bronchiolar epithelium in a foal with CID. One epithelial cell contains a viral inclusion body, *arrow*. The bronchiolar lumen is at top and is filled with necrotic debris and inflammatory cells.

number of viral infections that can be recognized at the light microscopic level or in the laboratory. Although "nested" PCR can be used to detect several pathogens from one nucleic acid extraction, specific reagents are generally required for each suspected pathogen, making these techniques generally unsuitable for use as pathogen "screens."

Bacteria

We know much about bacterial pathogens because they are visible on smears of exudates and with special stains in tissue sections (Gram's stain, acid-fast, and so on) (Figs. 7-2 and 7-3). Gram's stain, named after its Danish discoverer, separates most of the bacteria into two categories based on the constituents of their cell wall. In both gram-positive and gram-negative bacteria, protein molecules forming channels (porin channels) have evolved to allow the transport of hydrophilic compounds important in bacterial functioning.

Those bacteria that contain a high percentage of the sugar murein or peptidoglycan in their cell walls are gram positive (blue or purple). Since murein is unique to bacteria, it is a logical target for

antibiotic pharmaceuticals. Penicillin is an example of an antibiotic that inhibits murein synthesis. The cephalosporins are another. Gram-negative bacteria are generally more resistant to antibiotics. Gram-negative bacteria (red) have an outer membrane exterior to the peptidoglycan layers. This layer contains lipopolysaccharide (LPS), important in endotoxemia of bacterial infections. Lipopolysaccharides from gram-negative bacteria can cause septic shock by generating endogenous mediators of inflammation such as cytokines, nitrous oxide, superoxide anions, and lipid mediators.

The shape of bacteria are also used to classify them: either coccoid (round), bacilloid (rod-like), or helical (spiral). Currently, genera and species of bacterial pathogens are being reclassified and renamed based on genetic homology rather than Gram testing and other traditional approaches to bacterial taxonomy. 16S rRNA, found in all bacteria, is the current criterion standard for bacterial classification. Based on computerized databases, similarities among 16S rRNA sequences among bacteria help place a bacterium on a branch of the evolutionary tree. Sequencing techniques can be used in the classification of slow-growing or

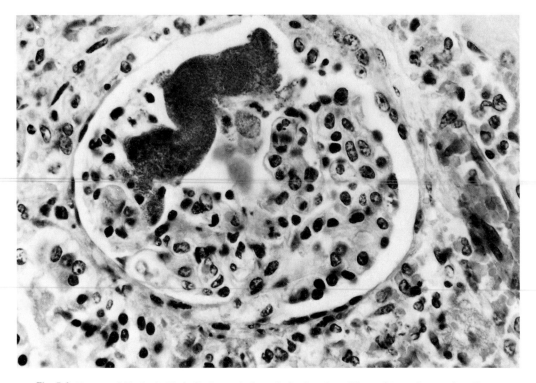

Fig. 7-2 Bacterial Emboli. Embolic bacteria have lodged and proliferated in a glomerulus. Eventually these would cause an inflammatory response. This lesion is from a case of actinobacillosis in a foal.

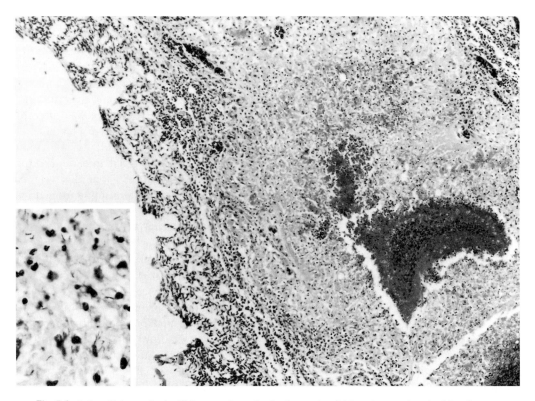

Fig. 7-3 Avian Tuberculosis. This granuloma in the lung of a chicken is associated with tuberculosis. A Ziehl-Neelsen stain for acid-fast bacteria clearly demonstrates the causative organisms in macrophages, *inset.*

difficult-to-culture bacterial species by means of PCR to amplify specific common sequences. These and other genotyping techniques will likely increase the numbers of bacterial species we can identify. (It is estimated that only 0.4% of bacterial species are currently known.) Although the resultant bacterial reclassification causes some consternation among students and practitioners, in the long run development of such a classification scheme should help to simplify an understanding of common pathways in bacterial pathogenesis.

Bacteria have no nucleus *per se* (prokaryotes) and have a single chromosome consisting of circular double-stranded DNA coiled in a nucleoid. Some antibiotics, such as the aminoglycosides, bind to bacterial ribosomes and inhibit transcription and translation of DNA.

Bacterial plasmids are bits of extrachromosomal DNA that replicate independently of nucleoid material. Although generally not necessary for bacterial survival, they are often important in antibiotic resistance and often encode virulence factors including those for toxin production.

Transferable genetic elements, particularly of bacteria, have also been shown to be virulence factors. As research progresses, bacteria have been found to have common (phylogenic?) similarities in these virulence factors. Genetic engineering techniques allow investigators to manipulate these factors in creating bacterial strains and vaccines containing molecules that may produce immunity without causing disease. Recombinant viral and bacterial vaccines are but one line of research that holds promise of providing immunity directed toward infectious agents.

Many bacterial agents have been established as the cause of disease by fulfillment of Koch's postulates. The mechanisms of disease production vary from bacteria to bacteria and are being elucidated with the new methods of molecular pathogenesis (molecular Koch's postulates). This new knowledge lends potential insight into the means of prophylaxis and control.

Nanobacteria

Recently, nanobacteria have been described. These are bacteria that are only slightly larger than viruses and have been implicated in kidney stone formation in humans. Apparently nanobacteria have the ability to utilize calcium and phosphorus in building protective shells that act as a nidus for stone formation. Nanobacteria are present in 80% of pooled bovine sera.

Chlamydiae, Rickettsiae, and Mycoplasmas

Chlamydia (causing avian psittacosis), *Rickettsia* (causing Potomac horse fever), and *Mycoplasma* (causing bovine contagious pleuropneumonia) are genera of organisms that have defied precise classification. They are considered to be bacteria (prokaryotes). The genome of *Chlamydia* is small compared to *Escherichia coli*. Chlamydiae are generally respiratory and genital intracellular pathogens. Chlamydiae enter nonprofessional phagocytes (epithelial cells) by a process called "parasite-directed endocytosis." They avoid digestion by inhibiting fusion of lysosomes with phagosomes.

Rickettsiae are parasites of eukaryotic cells and are also believed to be small bacteria. Many are zoonotic, with the most important being Rocky Mountain spotted fever. They cannot be stained by Gram's method, and all rickettsiae with a known mode of transmission implicate arthropods. They are thus transmitted into the body through the blood and are phagocytized by endothelial cells. They escape from the phagosome into the cytosol and spread to adjacent endothelial cells by cytoplasmic processes. Chlamydiae and rickettsiae are obligate intracellular pathogens.

Mycoplasmas are bacteria that lack a cell wall and are the smallest organisms that can grow in cell-free media. DNA hybridization studies indicate that mycoplasmas are only distantly related to the other bacteria. They are often commensal in the mucus membranes of the upper respiratory, genital, and digestive tracts and the bovine mammary gland. Some species become pathogens under appropriate conditions.

Fungi

Fungal pathogens are often dimorphic, appearing as either filamentous or yeastlike agents. They are eukaryotes; that is, they have a distinct nucleus with a nuclear membrane. They also contain a cell membrane, Golgi apparatus, mitochondria, and a cytoskeleton. Because they are eukaryotes, similar in many ways to host cells, they are difficult to kill without causing host cell damage. Many are free living in the environment and are opportunistic pathogens of animals secondary to debilitation, high glucose content, and antibiotic therapy (such as *Candida*). Fungi can be dermatotropic (ringworm) or systemic (such as *Aspergillus*, Fig. 7-4) and usually have both asexual and sexual stages in their life cycles. The systemic mycoses are generally geographically restricted diseases (as with *Blasto-*

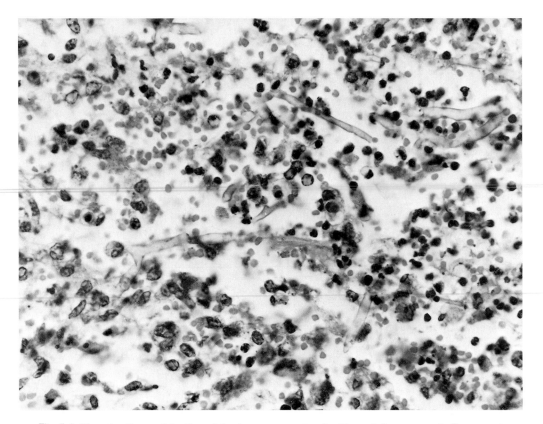

Fig. 7-4 Mycotic Abomasitis. Fungal hyphae are associated with an inflammatory infiltrate and hemorrhage.

myces, Fig. 7-5). They are believed to cause damage by direct injury to tissue together with the host's associated inflammatory response.

Algae

Colorless achlorophyllic algae of the genus *Prototheca* are believed to be opportunistic pathogens in animals and persons. They have been reported in cases of bovine mastitis and as local and systemic infections in pet carnivores.

Protozoa and Metazoa

Protozoal and metazoal parasites are eukaryotic pathogens that are biologically diverse, are intracellular to lumen dwelling in the host, and have evolved myriad methods for invading the host from simple ingestion to transmission by blood-sucking insects. Their life cycles (as with *Histomonas meleagridis* and *Strongylus vulgaris*) are often complex. Some parasites elicit a strong inflammatory response that interferes with function (*Spirocerca lupi*), whereas others (*Capillaria, Gonglyonema* spp.) do not. Many parasitic agents are zoonotic (*Toxoplasma, Cryptosporidium*) and may take a

lifetime (20 years plus) *(Echinococcocus)* to cause clinical disease in humans.

Besides attempting to poison the parasites without killing the host, successful treatment of parasitic diseases often hinges on understanding the life cycle of the parasite and intervening to break this cycle (such as pasture buildup of ova in ovine haemonchosis). Many parasites are limited geographically by climate and the presence of an intermediate or definitive host. Diagnosis of parasitic diseases is often by direct examination of feces, sputum, and other body fluids. Intracellular parasites are more difficult to identify, often requiring serological or biochemical testing.

Toxins

Toxins are important causes of disease, and although a specific toxin may not be identified in a particular case, often the type of tissue injury provides clues leading the clinician to suspect exposure to xenobiotics. Although some toxins are mucosal irritants (such as cantharidin from blister beetles), most enter the systemic circulation via the intestine. Fewer (such as paraquat) are inhaled. Since all materials absorbed from the gut travel to the liver, the

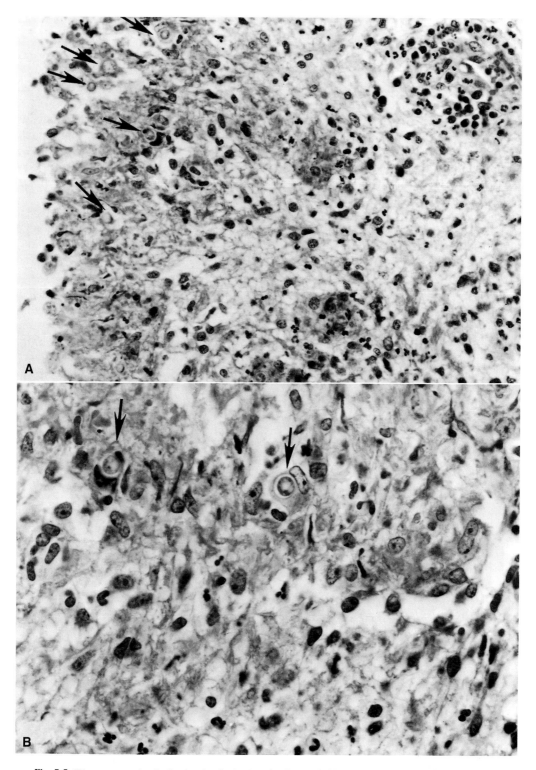

Fig. 7-5 Blastomycosis. A, Lesion in the brain of a dog with blastomycosis. *At left,* Fourth ventricle. There is necrosis of the ependyma and of the parenchyma of the brain and infiltration by macrophages and neutrophils. Several organisms are present, *arrows.* **B,** *Blastomyces dermatitidis* organisms are present in macrophages, *arrows.*

liver is often the first site of toxic injury. Although some toxins are direct acting and damage the first hepatocytes they contact in the periportal regions of hepatic lobules (as phosphorus does), most are biotransformed by the liver's microsomal oxidase system (cytochrome P-450) designed to convert fat-soluble compounds to water-soluble compounds, which can be excreted by the kidneys. The hepatocytes richest in these organelles and enzyme systems are located surrounding the central vein. Since the proximal convoluted tubules of the kidney are also high in microsomal oxidase enzymes, the biotransformed products of xenobiotic degradation may also damage this region. Although there are other mechanisms of toxicity such as glutathione reductase activity secondary to acetaminophen administration in cats, most toxins are recognized by the zone of tissue injury they induce in the liver or kidney. Likewise, the lung contains detoxifying enzymes that biotransform some inhaled toxicants. Oppositely, young animals without developed detoxifying systems may be relatively resistant to certain xenobiotics because they are unable to convert them to their toxic intermediaries. Under appropriate circumstances, toxins can contribute to cancer development (such as aflatoxins in trout).

Bacteria, viruses, and probably other infectious agents often have untoward effects on cells by virtue of the toxins they produce. These may be exotoxins, which are released from intact bacteria (Fig. 7-6) into the cellular milieu, or endotoxins released from the lipopolysaccharide within the cell wall of gram-negative and some gram-positive bacteria (Fig. 7-7). In either case, these toxins are not essential for bacterial growth but are useful for spread of the bacteria. They are generally encoded by DNA in plasmids, and their site of action may be local or far removed from the site of production. The role played by endotoxins in many disease states is not entirely clear, but it is certain that they exert a variety of profound biological effects, many of which have the potential to contribute to tissue injury. The general effects of endotoxins are well known and include the induction of fever, shocklike reductions in systemic blood pressure, and changes in peripheral blood counts and the blood coagulation system. Endotoxins induce the production, synthesis, or secretion of a variety of potent mediators and cytokines from other cell types. The diversity of such mediators that can be mobilized by endotoxin has made it difficult to define a unifying hypothesis for the mechanism or mechanisms of action of endotoxin. It has also confounded attempts to provide specific therapy for endotoxin-related diseases.

Many interactions of endotoxin with host systems have been described (Table 7-1). These include effects on the complement system, coagulation systems, platelets, neutrophils, monocytes and macrophages, and endothelial cells. Recent evidence indicates that critical interactions occur between endothelium and leukocytes mediated by β_2-integrin adhesion molecules as a result of LPS signals. Signal transduction by LPS occurs after binding to CD14 expressed on the surface of monocytes, macrophages, and neutrophils. The role of an identified acute-phase protein (LPS-binding protein) in plasma has not been determined. Current research efforts are directed at elucidating the mechanisms of endotoxin-mediated gene activation. How

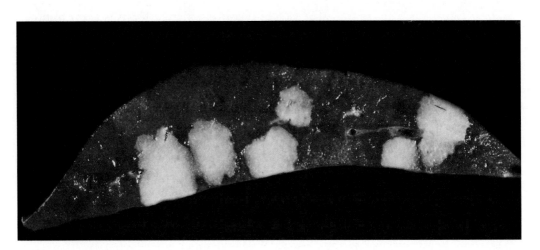

Fig. 7-6 Necrosis Caused by Bacterial Infection. There is multifocal hepatic necrosis in a case of necrobacillosis in a cow. This lesion is believed to be caused by toxins released by the causative organism *Fusobacterium necrophorum*.

all these events fit into the total puzzle of the effect of endotoxins on the whole animal is as yet not fully pieced together.

One property of endotoxin, which is probably of pathogenetic importance, is its ability to activate complement. Endotoxin can activate both the classical and alternate complement pathways *in vitro*, and in each case activation may be independent of antibody. In addition, if antibody to endotoxin is present, complement may be activated in the usual way by the interaction of antigen with antibody. The usual mechanism of classical and alternate pathway complement activation by endotoxin appears to be different, however, because the classical pathway is activated by the lipid A region of the endotoxin molecule through direct binding and activation of complement component C1 whereas alternative pathway activation depends on the polysaccharide portion of the endotoxin molecule. Complement activation leads to the generation of the potent anaphylatoxins C3a and C5a, but the role of these and other complement-derived mediators has been difficult to implicate in clinical endotoxic shock because of the complexity of overlapping *in vivo* events.

Clinical studies have established that selective inhibitors of arachidonic acid metabolism (nonsteroidal antiinflammatory drugs, NSAIDS) or inhibitors of the products of arachidonic acid metabolism can have a beneficial influence on the pathophysiological consequences of endotoxemia. Other studies, both *in vivo* and *in vitro*, have clearly established that endotoxins can elicit the production of both prostaglandins and leukotrienes. Macrophages and monocytes seem to be particularly sensitive targets for endotoxin-induced arachidonic acid metabolism, but neutrophils can respond similarly.

One of the key clinicopathological features of gram-negative sepsis with endotoxemia is the development of diffuse microvascular thrombosis. Some of this microvascular thrombosis is certainly related to the effects of endotoxin on endothelial cells, but endotoxin may also directly activate both the intrinsic and extrinsic coagulation pathways and leads to enhanced expression of tissue thromboplastin (factor III, tissue factor) on the surfaces of monocytes and macrophages. Tissue factor serves as a sort of receptor for factor VII that becomes activated to cleave factors X and IX by the extrinsic coagulation cascade. This highly procoagulant tissue factor activity remains largely cell associated with little released into the local microenvironment.

When two doses of endotoxin are administered to rabbits 24 hours apart, bilateral renal cortical necrosis results. This is known as the generalized Shwartzman reaction and has been shown to be attributable to intravascular blood coagulation. Thrombi form in the renal glomerular capillaries and, in this model, result in cortical necrosis of the kidneys. The generalized Shwartzman reaction therefore is a consequence of disseminated intravascular coagulation (DIC), which is discussed later in this chapter.

Platelets also are affected dramatically by endotoxin. Administration of endotoxin to some animal species causes thrombocytopenia with aggregation and trapping of platelets in vascular spaces. It causes secretion of platelet-derived mediators, which may in turn contribute to changes in blood pressure and to vascular permeability changes. Complement appears to be important in platelet aggregation, and endotoxin has relatively little effect on platelets in species in which these cells have no immune adherence receptors. The action of endotoxin on platelets may, however, be important in DIC and endotoxin-induced tissue injury.

Intravenous endotoxin administration or gram-negative bacterial sepsis is likely to produce a precipitous neutropenia followed by leukocytosis as a result of release of neutrophils (PMN) from the

TABLE 7-1	Summary of Effects of Endotoxin
TISSUE/SYSTEM	**EFFECT**
Whole animal	Fever, leukopenia followed by leukocytosis, microvascular injury, disseminated coagulation
Complement	Classical/alternate pathway activation; anaphylatoxin generation; many secondary effects
Neutrophils	"Primes" PMN for various enhanced functions; prostaglandin/leukotriene production; oxyradical generation; secretion; aggregation; enhanced adhesion *via* Leu-CAMs
Clotting system	Intrinsic/extrinsic activation; enhance TF expression on cell surfaces; DIC
Platelets	Aggregation; sequestration; secretion
Macrophages	Activation; "primes" for enhanced function; secretion of cytokines (GM-CSF, IL-1, TNF-α)
Endothelium	Direct damage (bovine); enhanced ELAM expression; mediator release

DIC, Disseminated intravascular coagulation; *ELAM,* endothelial cell adhesion molecules; *GM-CSF,* colony-stimulating factor; *IL-1,* interleukin-1; *Leu-CAMs,* leukocyte cell adhesion molecules; *PMN,* neutrophil; *TF,* tissue factor; *TNF-α,* tumor necrosis factor.

bone marrow. This initial shift of neutrophils from the circulating to the marginal pool is likely related to LPS-induced increased PMN adhesiveness to endothelium and clearly favors the interaction of PMN with vascular endothelium. LPS may interact with the PMN by simply binding to it. A specific receptor for LPS on PMN has been difficult to identify. It has been suggested that LPS may interact with part of the same CR3 receptor that recognizes C3bi and Mo-1. LPS may also indirectly activate PMN by liberation of the potent anaphylatoxin and PMN agonist C5a by complement activation.

Multiple PMN functions are known to be altered upon LPS exposure including increased adhesiveness to endothelium, PMN-PMN aggregation, lysosomal granule release, and enhanced respiratory burst activity. LPS seems to act as a PMN primer for some of these functions: enhanced release of toxic oxygen metabolites such as superoxide anion (O_2^-) and hydrogen peroxide (H_2O_2), and increased release of PMN lysosomal contents occurring after low-dose priming of PMN with endotoxin. The release of such PMN constituents as toxic oxygen radicals and lysosomal granule contents by adherent neutrophils may be an important feature of the pathogenesis of microvascular injury in endotoxemia. To complicate the picture, however, some studies suggest that animals depleted of neutrophils still react to endotoxin with the usual shocklike responses, and so under certain conditions PMN may not be essential to endotoxin-induced injury.

It has been established that monocytes and macrophages are very important in the pathogenesis of tissue injury produced by endotoxin. These cells are exquisitely sensitive to endotoxin and respond to it with changes in morphology, such as ruffling, increased phagocytic activity, and increased secretory activity. In short, endotoxin is capable of activating macrophages. Such activated cells secrete lysosomal enzymes such as collagenase, upregulate expression of surface tissue factor for activation of the extrinsic coagulation pathway, produce reactive oxygen species and nitrous oxide, and release potent cytokines like colony-stimulating factor (GM-CSF), tumor necrosis factor (TNF-α), and interleukins-1 (IL-1), -6, and -8. GM-CSF is in turn capable of stimulating the proliferation of granulocytes and mononuclear phagocytes, and IL-1 and TNF-α have a plethora of biological effects.

Endotoxin is one of the most potent known inducers of interleukin-1 (IL-1) and is biologically active at picogram quantities. Much of the released IL-1 is of mononuclear phagocyte origin, but other cell types may also contribute. The biological activities of IL-1 are as complex as is the activity of endotoxin and include a variety of effects on diverse cell types. Two classical IL-1 activities are the induction of fever (many of the activities of IL-1 were once attributed to a less-well-characterized "factor" known as "leukocyte endogenous pyrogen," now known to be IL-1), and the activation of lymphocytes. IL-1 also interacts with endothelial cells to enhance procoagulant (tissue factor) expression, enhances endothelial cell adhesiveness, and interfaces with the fibrinolytic system by inducing an inhibitor of tissue-type plasminogen activator (t-PA). Endotoxin-stimulated macrophages also produce tumor necrosis factor (TNF-α), a potent mediator that has many related and overlapping biological functions with IL-1.

It is well established that endothelial cell damage occurs *in vivo* in endotoxemia as evidenced by lesions as well as endothelial sloughing and the detection of circulating endothelial cells in the blood. The mechanisms of this injury, however, have been more difficult to define. Bovine endothelial cells seem to be particularly sensitive to endotoxin and can be directly injured by LPS *in vitro* in the absence of other factors. This may explain some of the sensitivity of cattle to diseases in which endotoxemia is involved. In most other species, however, endotoxin does not seem to play such a direct role, and several recent studies have implicated the neutrophil as a cellular intermediary. Under normal conditions, PMN marginated against the vascular endothelium or migrating through it toward tissue sites do not cause endothelial damage, but this picture may be quite different under the influence of endotoxin. In addition to causing enhanced adhesiveness of PMN to endothelium, endotoxin "primes" PMN for increased secretory and biochemical activity, possibly leading to endothelial cell damage by elaboration of toxic oxygen metabolites or lysosomal granule contents. Interestingly, direct contact and adhesion between the PMN and endothelium is apparently necessary for such injury to occur; when monoclonal antibodies are used to block upregulation of the leukocyte cell adhesion molecule (Leu-CAM) Mo-1 on activated PMN, greatly reduced injury occurs *in vitro*.

Not only do the PMN become stickier, but the endothelium itself also exhibits enhanced adhesiveness under the influence of endotoxin as a result of increased expression of endothelial cell adhesion molecules (ECAM). There has been a high level of interest in the role of the endothelial cell itself, apart from any other influences. One interesting observation is that the perfusion of one kidney by endotoxin, followed 24 hours later by systemic administration, produces a Shwartzman reaction limited to one kidney. This result indicates a role for local sensitization, which might be important in the pathogenesis of endothelial injury.

In conclusion, endotoxin produces a wide variety of effects on humoral and cellular mediation systems in the host. The contribution of each of these to the totality of effects of endotoxin in the intact animal are not entirely clear, but the remarkable sensitivity of monocytes and macrophages to endotoxin and the diversity of biological phenomena that they mediate makes these cells likely to be among the most important targets for endotoxin *in vivo*. It is also important to recognize that endotoxins are certainly not the only determinant of pathogenicity in gram-negative bacteria. Endotoxins may be present on bacteria that are not pathogenic, and, in some known pathogenic bacteria, factors other than endotoxin are clearly involved. In the case of human typhoid fever, for example, endotoxins derived from the causative organism *Salmonella typhi* can produce signs similar to those seen in the naturally occurring disease. However, the induction of tolerance to the endotoxin does not provide protection against the disease when individuals actually become infected.

Clostridium species generally cause tissue injury by means of exotoxin production. Tetanus, botulism, blackleg (Fig. 7-7), gas gangrene, and enterotoxemia of neonatal calves, foals, and piglets are examples of toxic clostridial diseases. Many of these toxins are among the most potent poisons known to man. Botulinum toxin, for example, if used in germ warfare, would be capable of killing 10 million people per gram of purified toxin. Botulinum toxin blocks presynaptic release of acetylcholine causing muscle paralysis and respiratory arrest. In waterfowl eating decayed vegetation containing *Clostridium botulinum* spores, production of toxin can lead to muscle relaxation resulting in a condition called "limberneck." It does not take much imagination to picture the consequences to waterfowl of not being able to keep their heads out of the water! Oppositely, tetanus toxin inhibits the release of inhibitory neurotransmitters from the synaptic junction resulting in extensor rigidity, especially after startle stimulation. Botulinum and tetanus toxin share a common A toxin but differ in the B toxin. One is inhibitory, and the other stimulatory.

In swine, both enterotoxic *E. coli* and enterotoxemic *E. coli* produce exotoxins in the gut. In enterotoxic colibacillosis, the target of the toxin is enterocytes. The toxin interferes with sodium and chloride equilibrium across the enterocyte host cells. This results in a "secretory diarrhea" subsequent to a fecal loss of sodium, chloride, and thus water. The volume of excess water exceeds the ability of the large intestine to resorb the excess fluid. In enterotoxemic colibacillosis, endothelial cells throughout the body are targeted by the toxin produced, resulting in edema.

As a final word on toxins, we should not leave the impression that only bacteria produce toxins that damage the host. Some enteric viruses have been shown to produce enterotoxins. Some bacteria and viruses can overstimulate T cells by producing toxins that activate the immune system by binding to class II MHC and T-cell receptors. These toxins are called "superantigens." Certain ectoparasites, in particular some ticks, cause a toxicosis in their hosts. Some ixodid ticks such as *Dermacentor andersoni* in North America and *Ixodes holocyclus* in Australia produce a potent neurotoxin that is capable of paralyzing and killing the host. In the case of *I. holocyclus*, the toxin apparently acts at the neuromuscular junction and inhibits the release of neurotransmitter. It is interesting to speculate on the various ways by which such parasites have developed these sophisticated mechanisms of interaction with the host.

Genetic Diseases

Genetic diseases are especially important in inbred animals. Many genetic disorders are incompatible with life. To mention just a few, conditions such as rod-cone dysplasia of dogs, globoid cell leukodystrophy of dogs and sheep, spider lamb syndrome (a hereditary limb deformity in some breeds of sheep), von Willebrand's disease, severe combined immunodeficiency of Arabian horses, and Duchenne muscular dystrophy have a suspected or identified genetic abnormality. The heritable nature of these diseases may be diagnosed by karyotyping or identification of abnormal genes or gene products. Although gene therapy is not widely available at present, identification of carrier animals is useful in eliminating these traits from the population through controlled breeding programs. Other genetic conditions are more subtle such as lactose intolerance, which involves deletion of a specific enzyme (lactase) on enterocytes. Most persons have a peculiar urinary odor after dining on asparagus. Theories abound as to whether this is attributable to a genetic difference in the gene coding for an enzyme that produces the odoriferous urinary metabolite of asparagus or more likely there is a genetic link to being able to olfactorally detect the peculiar odor. Either way, one would assume that the presence or absence of this gene or genes is not a factor in species survival.

Inborn errors of metabolism are those genetic diseases that arise because of the lack of a specific enzyme activity in a metabolic pathway. The net result

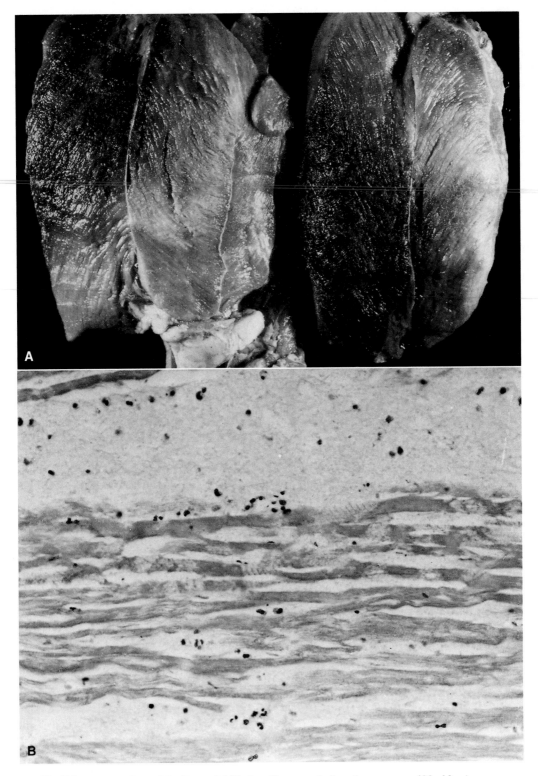

Fig. 7-7 Necrosis Caused by Bacterial Toxins. These are lesions from a case of blackleg in a cow. **A,** The necrotic muscle tissue is dark and hemorrhagic. **B,** The muscle fibers are necrotic and separated from one another by protein-rich edema fluid. There is minimal inflammation.

of this enzyme deficiency is the accumulation of the precursor substrate within the cell. Often these are called "lysosomal storage diseases." In some instances the storage product is glycogen, but in others, polysaccharides, mucopolysaccharides, glycoproteins, and the like. When these conditions are recognized in animals, they are thoroughly investigated as potential models for similar diseases in persons such as Tay-Sachs disease, Niemann-Pick disease, and many others. Still other diseases result in accumulation of amino acids with excretion in the urine (such as cystinuria of dachshunds). Dalmatian dogs have defective hepatocellular uptake of uric acid and cannot convert uric acid to allantoin. They are therefore prone to uric acid urinary bladder stones or calculi.

DNA can be damaged in a variety of ways. These include damage to individual bases: strand breaks (which can be single or double), altered base sequences, and abnormal cross-links between base pairs. The causes of such alterations are numerous and include radiation of various kinds as well as chemicals. In many cases, the nature of the damage caused by a particular agent is unknown. In other cases it is understood in detail. For example, ultraviolet (UV) irradiation is known to cause the formation of pyrimidine dimers in the DNA molecule.

Many mechanisms are available to the cell for the repair of damaged DNA molecules. In some cases single-strand breaks may be repaired by the enzyme polynucleotide ligase, which simply rejoins the broken ends of the strand. Excisional repair is a more complex and important mechanism for repair of DNA that involves several steps and the participation of many enzymes. It is used to repair DNA segments in which abnormal bases occur. It is likely that, despite the singular names used, the enzymes involved are part of complexes of cooperating enzymes and proteins that carry out the various steps. In the first step, an endonuclease causes a break in the DNA molecule adjacent to the defective base. An exonuclease then peels off, or excises, the segment in which the defect occurs, and DNA polymerase catalyzes the synthesis of a replacement strand using as a template the complementary bases on the opposite strand. The "patch" is then joined to the rest of the strand by the action of a ligase. This method of repair is capable of fixing defects in bases such as the dimers formed by UV irradiation. It is relatively error free. However, there is some evidence that, at least under some circumstances, it can exacerbate existing DNA damage. It apparently can generate double-strand breaks in DNA in which single-strand breaks already have been produced by some other agent. Double-strand breaks are more serious for the cell because they presumably are more difficult to repair, since no intact complementary strand is available as a template.

Postreplication repair is a second method of restoration of the damaged DNA molecule. This type of repair process takes place during the replication of DNA. The mechanisms involved are not clearly understood, but it is considered to be more error prone than excisional repair. The repair of double-strand breaks is also probably error prone.

The importance of discussing DNA damage at all is that faulty repair can occur and, when it does, it can result in mutation. When this occurs in a germ cell and is compatible with survival of the cell, it leads to an inherited mutation, which may be expressed as a defect in the progeny. In nongerm cells, faulty repair results in somatic mutation. A variety of phenotypic expressions may result from such mutations. When a structural gene is affected, there may be enzyme defects and the synthesis of abnormal proteins. When regulatory genes are involved, there may be changes in the rate or control of synthesis of gene products. Cells affected by somatic mutations may die or may remain viable.

Physical Agents

Physical agents such as trauma, heat, cold, and radiation, though not considered pathogens *per se*, are causes of disease and often death. An etiological diagnosis often depends largely on appropriate history taking and attention paid to environmental parameters. For example, actinic radiation can contribute to skin cancer in humans and other animals.

Metabolic Alterations

Alteration in lipid metabolism caused by fasting (fatty liver syndrome in cats, hepatic lipidosis in cattle, sheep, Shetland ponies, and miniature horses), vitamin A deficiency in cats, and iron deficiency in piglets are examples of diseases resulting from nutritional imbalances. Protein energy malnutrition delays healing by a variety of mechanisms, among them the decreased production of antibodies, depression of the complement system, and depression of cell-mediated immunity.

Hormonal imbalances and paraneoplastic syndromes disturb homeostasis and may cause disease. Often these conditions are diagnosed by functional tests (such as ACTH) rather than by biopsy and tissue examination. One needs to remember that in general, functionality of cells and tissues is not determinable by histological examination.

Idiopathic Diseases

All disease conditions that do not have an established cause and have not been experimentally reproduced (Koch's postulates) are considered idiopathic. Even though a great deal may be known about the disease, including circumstances surrounding the disease's appearance and effective therapy, if the cause is unknown the condition is considered idiopathic. Unfortunately, there are a great many diseases and conditions that fall into this nebulous category. They include acute pancreatic necrosis or its sequela pancreatitis. We know that this disease occurs most frequently in middle-aged, overweight, female dogs. We also know that it is often associated with a meal high in fat content. What we don't know is the precise trigger that causes intra-tissue activation of pancreatic trypsin. Likewise, equine serum hepatitis was believed to be associated with a reaction to the use of biological compounds of equine origin. However, the disease, characterized by massive liver necrosis (dishrag liver) and associated encephalopathy and death, occurs frequently in horses with no history of exposure to biological medical preparations of any kind. Likewise chronic (active) progressive hepatitis in the dog, though analogous histologically to the same condition in man (virus induced) has no identified cause. The list goes on and on and includes most neoplasms. It is worth considering that by the time clinical illness or tissue injury is present, the inciting agent may be gone. Such is the case in viral diseases of the newborn such as rotavirus infection in piglets and parvovirus infection of carnivores. By the time lesions and disease are present, virus isolation attempts may be fruitless. Such diseases are not, however, idiopathic.

Iatrogenic Diseases

Iatrogenic diseases are those caused by the clinician. "First do no harm" is a pedagogy that is not always easy to adhere to. For example, some years ago a dietary inoculant containing "friendly" intestinal flora was administered to neonatal foals to give their digestive system a jump-start. A percentage of these foals were dying at several days of age with what histologically looked like chronic liver disease, complete with fibrosis. Although initial efforts to establish a cause focused on an *in utero* toxin such as that generated by *Aspergillus* species, the culprit turned out to be excess iron fumarate in the dietary inoculant. We learned from this episode that hepatic fibrosis in the neonate occurs much more rapidly than in the adult (healing occurs without scarring *in utero*).

In many cases of iatrogenic diseases, medical intervention is responsible for breaching protective epithelial barriers. For example, repeated (or even single) jugular venipuncture can introduce bacteria directly into the bloodstream. Likewise, indwelling catheters may produce valvular damage. This damage may allow bacterial growth to occur on heart valves (bacterial endocarditis, Fig. 7-8) with eventual septic emboli to the kidney (from the left side of the heart) resulting in septic thrombi with attendant renal abscesses and infarcts.

RESISTANCE TO INFECTION AND DISEASE
Physical Barriers

Physical barriers to pathogen invasion include the integument and other epithelium-lined surfaces such as the conjunctiva, airways, and reproductive, urinary, and digestive tracts. These surfaces slough cells and produce organic acids from sweat and sebaceous glands, bile, surfactant, and a variety of other substances, including those from normal flora, that provide a first line of defense against pathogenic agents. Coughing, vomiting, expectoration, diarrhea, urination, and other impolite behaviors also help to rid the body of potentially threatening agents. Lymph nodes and the liver, armed with phagocytic and immunologically active effector cells (hepatic Kupffer cells), are a secondary line of defense against organisms and toxins, including endotoxin, that are able to traverse either an intact or a disrupted epithelial barrier.

In the respiratory tract an elaborate physical mechanism has evolved for the clearance of inhaled particles, including microorganisms. In the bronchi and trachea, mucus secreted by goblet cells is continually moved toward the pharynx by the action of the cilia of respiratory epithelial cells. Debris is therefore carried to the pharynx by the action of the ciliated bronchial cells where it is swallowed. This mechanism very efficiently removes particles large enough to impinge on the walls of the airways. Smaller particles such as bacteria (less than 2 μm) may reach the alveoli and escape mucociliary clearance by lodging in the lung at a level distal to where ciliated cells are found. Such small particles must be dealt with by other mechanisms such as phagocytosis by alveolar macrophages. Once interiorized by phagocytosis the particles are carried from the distal area of the lung to this mucociliary escalator by the motile alveolar macrophages. It is now clear that various kinds of pulmonary injury, which damage this mucociliary clearance mechanism or injure

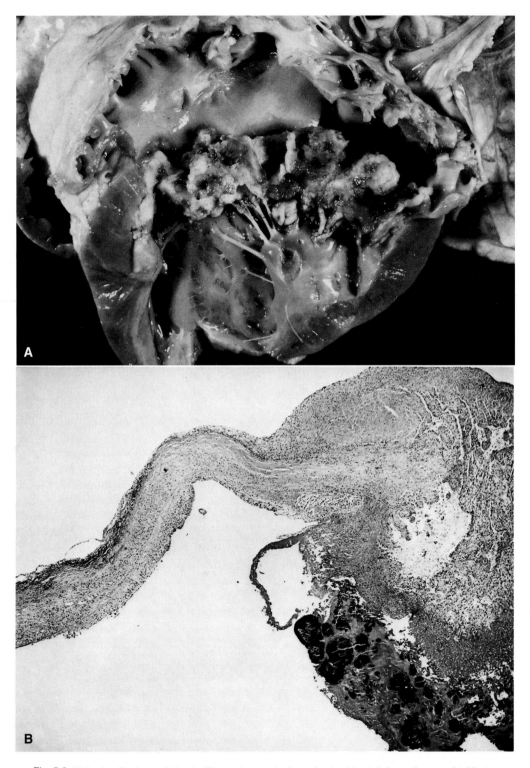

Fig. 7-8 Valvular Endocarditis. A, The atrioventricular valve in this pig's heart bears a friable inflamed mass caused by bacterial infection. **B,** The histological appearance of part of the mass is shown. The very dark material represents masses of bacteria embedded in necrotic inflammatory debris. Such masses often break off to form emboli, which can establish infection at other sites.

the alveolar macrophages, have an adverse effect on lung clearance and defense mechanisms.

Infection of the respiratory tract by certain viruses and *Mycoplasma* species can alter the function of ciliated cells, also interfering with the mucociliary elevator. This is important in interfering not only with clearance of the primary infectious agent but also with that of other inhaled particles or microorganisms, especially bacteria, and may result in secondary infections.

Alterations in the mucociliary elevator can also be brought about by excessively dry or cold air or, more importantly, by atmospheric pollutants. Ammonia, generated by bacterial breakdown of urea, can be an important pollutant in the environment of animals kept under intensive husbandry conditions. In pigs, ammonia contamination has been shown to impair bacterial clearance from the lungs, and in rats it has been shown to be an important predisposing agent to respiratory infections by *Mycoplasma* species. Similarly, a cold environment impairs pulmonary bacterial clearance in young pigs, and presumably a great variety of low-grade insults could predispose to pulmonary infection through similar mechanisms.

Genetic Resistance

Although living organisms are constantly bombarded with potential pathogens, most of us are not constantly ill, though students in the medical sciences often display symptoms of whatever disease is under study (hypochondria). The properly functioning body is quite adept at fending off disease-producing agents by a variety of mechanisms. Innate resistance includes chemotaxis, phagocytosis, natural cytotoxicity, and cytokines.

Important in this armamentarium is a genetic constitution that varies from individual to individual. Genetic polymorphism in populations, particularly at the major histocompatibility complex loci is particularly important in controlling infection through the immune system. Our genes, in combination with our healthful behaviors, largely determine our life span. Although it is true that one cannot outrun one's genes, proper care of the container in which we house our organs is critical in maximizing our genetic potential.

Examples of genetic predisposition to disease are numerous, and our knowledge of these factors is increasing exponentially and will continue to expand with genome mapping in humans and other species. Fortunately, through the study of knockout (gene-deleted or -inactivated) mice we have learned that many critical body systems are coded by more than one gene, making clinically significant gene deletion a relatively rare event. Functional genomics is the study of the effects of gene products on the organism as a whole.

In veterinary practice, important breed differences exist, especially in inbred strains of dogs. Basenji dogs are genetically prone to pyruvate kinase deficiency (an enzyme important in red blood cell formation), giant hypertrophic gastritis, and lymphoplasmacytic enteritis as well as an inability to vocalize. They also hunt lions! West Highland white terriers, cairn terriers, and Doberman pinchers may have inherited copper toxicosis caused by a lack of the appropriate enzyme to process copper. Abnormal porphyrin is formed in developing erythrocytes of some pigs, cattle, Siamese cats, and fox squirrels that have an inherited defect in uroporphyrinogen synthetase. Because the gene pool is relatively shallow in inbred animals, the chances of inadvertently breeding two animals carrying the same genetic defect are relatively high. Table 7-2 lists a small sample of known inherited disease in animals to illustrate their diversity.

Inherited diseases are attributable to mutations in particular genes and are passed on through the germ line. Many kinds of mutation can occur. These include point mutations, a change in a single base, deletions or duplications of variably sized segments of the genome, gene rearrangements, or a variety of chromosomal abnormalities. Mutations can be in coding portions of the gene or in regulatory elements. The result is the production of a defective protein or absence or reduction in the quantity of the protein product.

Many of the inherited diseases are inherited as simple mendelian traits. These include autosomal recessive, a very common mode of inheritance, autosomal dominant, or X-linked. They are usually the result of a mutation in a single gene, though syndromes occur where large deletions disrupt more than one adjacent gene. A clinician is often alerted to the possibility of an inherited disease by certain events. For example, inherited diseases occur most commonly in purebred strains. When a characteristic syndrome occurs in many animals of the same breed, an inherited problem might be suspected. Even more damning is the occurrence of more than one animal with the disease from the same litter or from the same breeding or from breedings of closely related animals. The nature of the disease can also be a clue to inheritance. For example, if a single case were shown by clinical or pathological examination to be a lysosomal storage

TABLE 7-2 **Some Genetic Diseases of Animals**

DISEASE	SPECIES	INHERITANCE
Myasthenia	Dog	AR
Globoid cell leukodystrophy	Dog, mouse	AR
G_{M1} gangliosidosis	Cat, dog, cow	AR
G_{M2} gangliosidosis	Dog, cat, pig	AR
Mannosidosis	Cow	AR
Muscular dystrophy	Dog, mouse, cat	XR
Collie eye anomaly	Dog	AR
Progressive retinal atrophy	Dog	AR
Hepatic copper storage	Dog	AR
Chondrodysplasia of malamutes	Dog	AR
Hip dysplasia	Dog	P
Patent ductus arteriosus	Dog	P
Subaortic stenosis	Dog	P
Persistent right aortic arch	Dog	P
Cyclic neutropenia	Dog	AR
Hemophilia A	Dog	XR
Hemophilia B	Dog	XR
Combined immunodeficiency	Horse	AR

AR, Autosomal recessive; *P*, polygenic; *XR*, X-linked recessive.

disease, it would be immediately suspected to be inherited. As a group, storage diseases are one of the most common of inherited diseases, and often affected animals show neurological signs. These kinds of occurrences, then, should raise a warning flag.

Sometimes genetic malfunctions in the host defense allow pathogens access to tissues from which they are normally excluded. Ciliary dyskinesia is sometimes a reproductive disorder (part of the reproductive tracts of both sexes is ciliated) but may also disrupt the pulmonary mucociliary elevator allowing respiratory pathogens access to the deeper reaches of the lung.

Genetic variation in organisms obviously can be very important. Microorganisms have an advantage in that their short generation period gives them a capacity for rapid change not enjoyed by the host. Nevertheless, the genetic characteristics of the host are just as important. Genetic characteristics of the host presumably are involved in determining the susceptibility of species to particular infectious agents. Most microorganisms can infect only a limited range of host species. The reasons for this are not clear. We do not know why, for example, canine distemper virus can infect dogs and mink but not cats, whereas feline panleukopenia virus infects cats and mink but not dogs. Why, in contrast, can rabies virus infect all warm-blooded animals including birds? Even within species, there are often dramatic differences between strains or breeds in the way in which they respond to various parasites or organisms. Zebu cattle, for example, are relatively resistant to ticks compared to European breeds. African swine fever virus causes devastating disease in domestic pigs but inapparent infection in the warthog. More than one mechanism is likely involved in these different processes.

Susceptibility to disease can be manipulated in the laboratory, and one can select strains of mice that are resistant to specific diseases such as mouse pox, salmonellosis, or mouse hepatitis. Very often such variations are determined by alterations in immune responsiveness, which is, in turn, controlled by immune response (Ir) genes. A vigorous immune response usually correlates with protection from disease, but this is not always the case. The "usefulness" of the immune response depends on how effectively and how quickly it eliminates the agent and how much tissue damage is incurred during the process. This can be exemplified when one considers that different strains of mice differ in their ability to respond to infectious agents. Studies of these mice demonstrate that resistance and susceptibility to infectious agents are determined by numerous genetic influences.

A large number of genes influence susceptibility to infectious agents. Our growing understanding of these genes and their functions will likely provide opportunities for novel means of prophylaxis and therapy.

Nutritional Balance

Although there is no scientific evidence that nutritional supplementation such as megadoses of vitamins, minerals, or other nutrients does anything other than cure deficiencies of the nutrient in question, evidence does exist indicating that disease states can arise from oversupplementation. That is not to say that trace minerals are not necessary for proper enzyme functioning because they are. It is also important to note that one cannot confidently extrapolate requirements for one species from another. For example, mineral blocks formulated for cattle will cause copper toxicity in sheep. Proper balanced nutrition is important for maintenance of homeostasis.

Immunological Resistance

The immunological system is also critical in resisting pathogens. Chapter 5 addresses this topic in detail. Accidents of nature and genetic manipulation of rodents have provided numerous models of the consequences of an imperfect immune system in disease susceptibility and pathogen clearance (Table 7-3). Human HIV infection and its analogs in domestic animals (FIV, SIV) are examples of infectious agents that deplete the immune system with the subsequent appearance of opportunistic and persistent infections such as microsporidiosis, cryptosporidiosis, and pneumocystosis (Fig. 7-9). Severe combined immunodeficiency disease (SCID) is a genetic defect of both arms of the immune system and occurs in mice, horses, particularly those of Arabian parentage (Fig. 7-10), beagles, and persons. Nude (hairless) mice are helper T-cell deficient and thus lack humoral, particularly IgA, activity. Since neither Nude nor SCID mice can reject xenografts, they are often used for immune reconstitution studies, tumor transplantation, and infectious disease research.

Heritable defects in defense mechanisms other than classical immune responses also occur. In particular, numerous defects in neutrophil function have been described. In the Chédiak-Higashi syndrome, abnormalities of lysosomes are prominent. This syndrome occurs in persons, mice, cats, cattle, and mink. It is associated with giant granules in all granule-containing cells, and although the cells are able to phagocytose normally, neutrophils exhibit defects in chemotactic migration and in lysosomal degranulation. Evidence has linked these abnormalities to defects in microtubular function, which in turn appear to be attributable to abnormalities in the regulation of the intracellular cyclic nucleotides cGMP and cAMP. Agents that elevate cGMP levels can correct the functional defects in this disease, and one of them, ascorbic acid (vitamin C), has been used successfully to treat human patients with Chédiak-Higashi syndrome. Hence, Chédiak-Higashi syndrome appears to involve a defect in control of the cytoskeleton. Whether this is attributable to abnormal cyclic nucleotide metabolism or to defects at the cell surface or to other abnormalities is unknown. Chédiak-Higashi syndrome provides an example of information obtained in the laboratory by researchers interested in the biology of the disease that can be applied in the field to help affected patients. This is no less true of diseases of animals than it is of man. In some species, including man and cattle, individuals with Chédiak-Higashi syndrome are abnormally susceptible to infections. In others, such as the cat, the disease does not predispose to infection, apparently reflecting differences in functional impairment of neutrophils.

In man there are several other neutrophil granulocytopathies. These include chronic granulomatous disease, in which there is a failure to generate a respiratory burst after phagocytosis. This in turn is associated with a failure to generate microbicidal

TABLE 7-3 Examples of Immune Deficiency Diseases in Domestic Animals

SPECIES	DISEASE	NATURE OF DEFECT
Equine	Combined immunodeficiency	Lack of functional T cells and B cells
Equine	Agammaglobulinemia	Lack of functional B cells
Equine	Selective IgM deficiency	Inability to synthesize or secrete IgM
Equine	Transient hypogammaglobulinemia	Delay in onset of antibody synthesis
Bovine	Lethal trait A-46	Defective T cell function; abnormal zinc metabolism
Bovine	Selective IgG_2 deficiency	Reduced IgG_2 synthesis
Canine	Cyclic neutropenia	Cyclic abnormalities of hematopoiesis
Canine	Granulocytopathy syndrome	Abnormal bacterial killing by neutrophils
Feline, bovine	Chédiak-Higashi syndrome	Abnormal granule-containing cells; possible microtubular defect (by analogy to man)

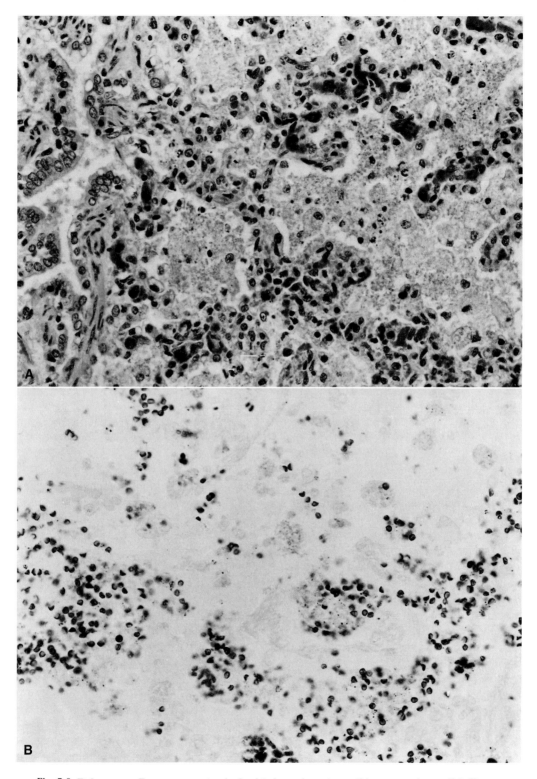

Fig. 7-9 Pulmonary Pneumocytosis. A, In this lung there is a mild mononuclear cell infiltrate, and the alveoli contain macrophages and exudate. This lesion is from an immunosuppressed horse. **B,** A silver stain reveals numerous *Pneumocystis carinii* organisms.

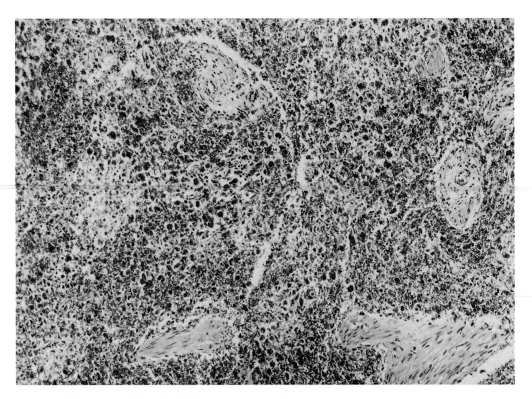

Fig. 7-10 Combined Immunodeficiency Disease (CID). In this spleen from an Arabian foal with CID there is no evidence of normal lymphoid follicle development (B-cell areas), and the periarteriolar sheaths (T cell–dependent regions) are sparsely cellular.

oxidizing agents. Defects in the myeloperoxidase system and other enzymes and lysosomal abnormalities also have been described. All these result in abnormal susceptibility to infection. In dogs a disease called "canine granulocytopathy syndrome," in which there is normal phagocytosis by neutrophils but defective intracellular killing of bacteria, has been described. Molecules such as CR3, a β_2-integrin, play a role in innate defense against microbiological agents by activating leukocytes, mediating phagocytosis, and promoting transmigration of leukocytes. Absence of this molecule may result in leukocyte adhesion deficiency. In cyclic neutropenia of collie dogs there is a periodic failure to produce neutrophils and other blood cells. In both of these canine diseases there is a greatly increased susceptibility to infections.

The ability to mount an immune response is of course affected by many nongenetic influences. The most important of these is simple failure to obtain passive immunity by means of colostrum. Because most domestic animals obtain their maternally derived antibodies from this source, deprivation of colostrum will result in immunodeficiency, and the animals are at increased risk for infections. Other causes of immunosuppression are too numerous to

deal with here but include neoplasia, treatment with drugs, especially with the commonly used corticosteroids, and infections. In dogs, for example, neoplasia, canine distemper, and generalized demodicosis have been associated with immunosuppression. In cats, infection with feline leukemia virus (FeLV) is associated with immunosuppression, and this and other feline viruses (FIV) are being intensely studied as models for human AIDS (acquired immunodeficiency syndrome). Some examples of immunosuppressive pathogens are listed in Table 7-4.

Many pathogens cause age-dependent disease usually affecting the very young and very old, likely the result of immunological deficiency. In this category are viral diseases such as rotaviruses and coronaviruses of infants of all species. The protozoan *Cryptosporidium parvum* falls into this category as well. However, other nonimmune factors are also players in this arena. For example, only piglets and calves, as opposed to adult animals, are susceptible to enterotoxigenic *Escherichia coli*. The development of gastric acidity is believed to protect older animals from *E. coli* infection. On the other hand, because of unknown factors, animals that have outgrown their susceptibility to *E. coli* are susceptible to *Salmonella* species infections. There is an age

SPECIES	AGENT	EFFECT
TABLE 7-4	Examples of Immunosuppression Caused by Infection in Animals	
Canine	Distemper virus	Lympholytic infection; depletion of B and T cells from lymphoid tissues; thymic atrophy; reduced PHA responsiveness
Canine	Parvovirus	Lympholytic infection; thymic atrophy; lymphopenia; functional deficiency unproved
Canine	*Demodex canis*	Serum factor suppressing PHA responsiveness of lymphocytes
Feline	Feline leukemia virus	Thymic atrophy; lymphoid depletion; depressed T-cell function
Feline	Panleukopenia virus	Lympholytic infection; thymic atrophy, lymphoid depletion; suppressed T-cell function in infected neonates
Bovine	Bovine virus diarrhea virus	B and T cell suppression
Equine	*Herpesvirus* type I	Lympholytic infection in neonates; thymic atrophy, lymphoid depletion

PHA, Phytohemagglutinin.

association in the susceptibility of pigs to swine dysentery *(Brachyspira hyodysenteriae)*, likely the result of the commensal growth of anaerobic bacteria, such as *Fusobacter* and *Bacteriodes* species, that are not present in young animals who have not yet developed climax flora.

Canine herpesvirus infection causes disease only in very young puppies even though previously unexposed older dogs also are susceptible to infection. The reasons for this are poorly understood though one possible explanation is that this virus prefers to grow at slightly lower temperatures than most. The relatively low body temperatures of young puppies, compared to that of adults, may enhance virus replication resulting in more extensive tissue damage. Another possible explanation might be that the immune response in such young animals is poorly developed.

PATHOGEN ESCAPE MECHANISMS AND TISSUE TROPISM

Disease-producing agents sometimes gain entry to the body upon contact, oblivious to host defense mechanisms. Many toxins act in this manner just as certain microbes such as *Bacillus anthracis* and *Leptospira* species do. For many pathogenic organisms however, mechanisms have evolved to allow the agent to escape, bypass, or otherwise exploit chinks in the armor of host defense and colonize the host. After all, it is a matter of survival for the pathogenic agent to outwit host defenses.

There is an almost infinite variety of ways in which pathogens circumvent host defenses to ensure their own survival. Many pathogens have specific cell types or targets to which they attach (tropisms). The enteropathogenic *E. coli* attach to host enterocytes by means of flagellar or pilial (fimbria) antigens that keep them from being washed out of the gut by peristalsis. Other bacteria such as *Vibrio* species are motile and can move through the surface intestinal mucus. They also produce a mucinase that helps in this process. *Salmonella* species enter the dendritic cells over Peyer's patches, which are designed to sample antigens. *Mycobacterium* species (causing tuberculosis [see Fig. 7-3], leprosy, Johne's disease) are able to survive and multiply in macrophages by virtue of their indigestible waxy coating consisting of mycolic acid, which they share with the *Corynebacterium* species. Some organisms produce zinc metalloproteases, which can digest ground substance causing necrotizing or hemorrhagic lesions. This may lead to edema and release of inflammatory mediators. Many of the anaerobic bacteria such as *Clostridium* species are able to reside within Kupffer cells until tissue injury and the resultant lowering of oxygen tension allow them to sporulate and multiply. *Helicobacter* species are able to survive in the harsh gastric environment by producing the enzyme urease, forming ammonia and neutralizing acid.

Frustrating Phagocytosis

Cell entry mechanisms vary by pathogen. Some microorganisms enter cells by specialized mechanisms involving ligand-receptor interactions, whereas others take advantage of host cell eating habits (phagocytosis). Because phagocytosis is such an important first line of defense against invading organisms, it is of great significance that many organisms have evolved methods of counteracting it. The ability to avoid phagocytosis is an important determinant of virulence in many bacterial species.

One mechanism involved in many bacterial infections is the ability of the organism to kill the phagocyte. Some strains of streptococci can produce substances called "streptolysins," which cause the degranulation of lysosomes inside intact cells. This kills the phagocyte. *Listeria monocytogenes* and some staphylococci utilize similar mechanisms. In cattle, certain strains of *Mannheimia (Pasteurella) haemolytica* are also toxic to alveolar macrophages and kill the phagocytes that ingest them. The importance of such phenomena can hardly be overemphasized. *M. haemolytica*, for example, is a major cause of pneumonia in cattle, and bovine pneumonia is one of the greatest causes of economic loss in the cattle industry today. *Corynebacterium ovis*, an important pathogen of sheep, possesses a toxic surface lipid that enables it to destroy phagocytes.

A second mechanism that may be used to interfere with the function of phagocytes is inhibition of chemotactic migration. Streptolysins, besides their ability to kill phagocytes, can interfere with chemotaxis. Relatively low concentrations are required to do this, and the production of streptolysins obviously confers some advantage on the bacteria.

Probably the single most important mechanism in preventing phagocytosis, however, is inhibition of the actual engulfment process. Many bacteria and some yeasts are able to do this. The ability to resist phagocytosis is commonly related to the possession of a capsule. Encapsulated (or smooth) strains of certain bacteria are pathogenic, whereas unencapsulated (or rough) strains often are not. *Streptococcus equi, E. coli, Pasteurella multocida,* and the yeast *Cryptococcus neoformans* are examples of organisms in which capsules are considered to enhance pathogenicity (Fig. 7-11). In some cases the thickness of the capsule correlates with the degree of virulence. Surface components other than capsules also can confer resistance to phagocytosis. For example, some strains of streptococci bear a surface protein called "M protein," which also is able to confer resistance to phagocytosis.

Although phagocytosis is an important mechanism of controlling infection, some organisms prefer to reside in phagocytes, since it protects them from host responses. Sometimes pathogen survival is ensured by a parasite-induced failure of phagosome-lysosome fusion and in other cases by neutralization of reactive oxygen derivatives or by failure of the parasite to generate an oxidative burst. Once inside the host cell, by whatever means of entry, the mecha-

nism by which the pathogen is able to maintain its own metabolic needs is, in general, poorly understood. Interference with host cell signaling mechanisms is a likely avenue by which obligate intracellular parasites inhibit host cell defense.

Obligate intracellular parasites such as *Toxoplasma gondii*, the microsporidia, and many others present a special problem to the host, since host defense mechanisms are useless inside cells. The most practical approach for the host is to be able to destroy the parasite as it leaves its host cell on the way to invading another cell. Eventually, or with exogenous immune stimulation, the host is able to clear the infection. In cases of immune dysfunction, as in HIV-infected patients, the very young, and the very old, these infections become chronic and sometimes life threatening.

Confusing Complement

Since the complement system is one of the most important means of host defense against infection, it is not surprising that pathogens have developed many different strategies for complement evasion. Evasion may occur on the surface of the organism itself because the complement cascade is not activated, because of complement inhibitors or inactivators released by the microorganisms, or because the membrane attack complex (MAC) either fails to form or does not lyse the organism. The binding of C1q may also actually facilitate entry into host cells of some organisms such as *Trypanosoma cruzi* and mycobacteria, whereas certain of the membrane proteins of *Campylobacter fetus* interfere with the deposition of C3 on the bacterial surface. The high concentrations of ammonia produced by *Pseudomonas aeruginosa* may also inactivate C3, whereas the same organism is known to produce elastase-like enzymes that can cleave many complement proteins. Lastly, certain microorganisms have developed sophisticated strategies for complement evasion based on such clever maneuvers as the generation of an inactivator of the C5a chemotaxin (group A streptococci), the proteolytic cleavage of bound C3 (*Leishmania donovani*), or the formation of a nonlytic C5b-9 complex (certain strains of *Salmonella* species and *E. coli*). In this latter escape mechanism, long-chain surface endotoxin (LPS) molecules apparently impart a steric barrier prohibiting access of the C5b-9 MAC to the hydrophobic domains of the membrane. Such studies of the means by which certain microorganisms evade the complement system have been very instructive in improving our understanding of the complicated interface between the host and its parasites.

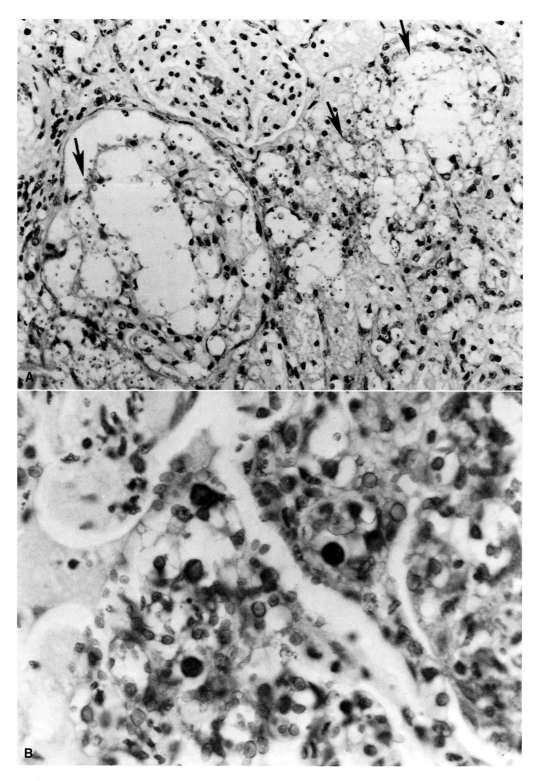

Fig. 7-11 Cryptococcosis. A, This micrograph shows a lesion in the kidney from a case of disseminated cryptococcosis in a dog. Cystic spaces contain many organisms, *arrows,* but there is minimal inflammation. **B,** A mucicarmine stain for acid mucopolysaccharides clearly shows the dark capsule surrounding the organisms. This capsule is believed to confer resistance to phagocytosis.

Intercurrent Infections

Some pathogens attack in concert with each other to allow colonization or multiplication. For example, in the shipping fever complex of cattle, diffuse viral injury (IBR, PI3, BVD, RSV) to the lung, associated with environmental stressers, causes relatively minor and repairable interstitial pneumonia. The damaged lung can then be colonized by a variety of opportunistic aerosolized bacteria including *Pasteurella multocida* and *Haemophilus somnus* (Fig. 7-12). Other experiments have shown that there is reduced phagocytic capacity in virus-infected animals as well as an impairment of killing of the bacteria that are phagocytosed (Fig. 7-13). The latter defect apparently is attributable to impairment of fusion of phagocytic vacuoles with lysosomes. Similarly, PI3 (parainfluenza type 3) virus has been shown to impair the clearance of *Mannheimia (Pasteurella) haemolytica* from the lungs of calves (Fig. 7-14). This virus is known to infect alveolar macrophages and, as a consequence, to reduce their phagocytic capacity.

In most of these experiments, aerosols containing very small particles are used, and therefore most of

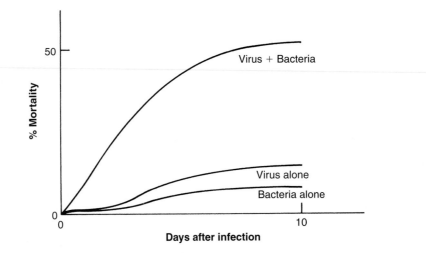

Fig. 7-12 Interaction of Viral and Bacterial Pathogens in Respiratory Disease. The percentage mortality is much higher in animals infected with both pathogenic viruses and pathogenic bacteria than in those infected with either viruses or bacteria alone. These experiments used combined infection in mice with parainfluenza virus and *Haemophilus influenzae*.

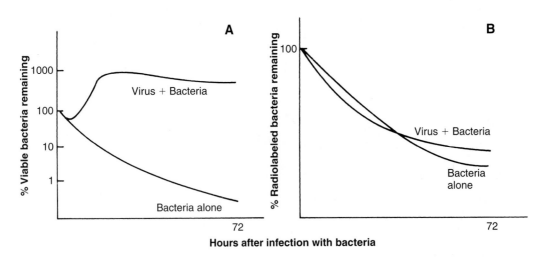

Fig. 7-13 Effect of Viral Infection on Clearance of Bacteria from the Lung. In dual infections with virus and bacteria, **A,** the population of bacteria in the lung progressively increases, rather than decreases as it does with infection by bacteria alone. **B,** When the bacteria used are radiolabeled, it can be shown that the introduced bacteria are removed from the lung as effectively in dual infections as in infections with bacteria alone. This type of data indicates that at least one effect of virus infections is to impair killing of bacteria by alveolar phagocytes.

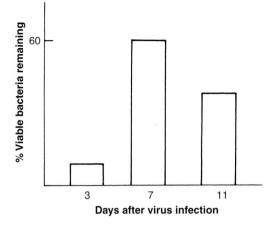

Fig. 7-14 Effect of Bovine Parainfluenza 3 Virus Infection on Bacteria. The time between viral injury and bacterial clearance is important. If *Mannheimia (Pasteurella) hemolytica* are administered 3, 7, or 11 days after virus infection, bacterial clearance is basically normal 3 days after virus infection but becomes severely impaired 7 days later, and the deficiency is still present 11 days after virus infection. *(Modified from data of Lopez A, Thomson RG, Savan M: Can J Comp Med 40:385-391, 1976.)*

the organisms are deposited in the deep lung where alveolar macrophages are most important for clearance. However, many viruses that infect the respiratory epithelium also are known to alter the function of the mucociliary apparatus. In PI3 virus infections, for example, infected cells soon develop morphological changes in the cilia and their basal bodies. Also, as a consequence of the hyperplasia of bronchiolar epithelium induced by this infection, immature cells line the bronchioles (Fig. 7-15). These cells lack the specialized functions of their mature counterparts, and this change must be accompanied by changes in mucociliary clearance mechanisms. A suppurative cranioventral bronchopneumonia, which may be fatal, often results.

In some instances, pathogens with the same age and tissue tropism gang up on the host to cause serious and perhaps fatal disease when the host is capable of controlling single uncomplicated infections. An example of this is concurrent infection with rotavirus, *Cryptosporidium*, Coccidia subclass organisms, and *E. coli*, all of which infect villous enterocytes of young animals. Swine dysentery requires an anaerobic flora in association with a pathogenic spirochete.

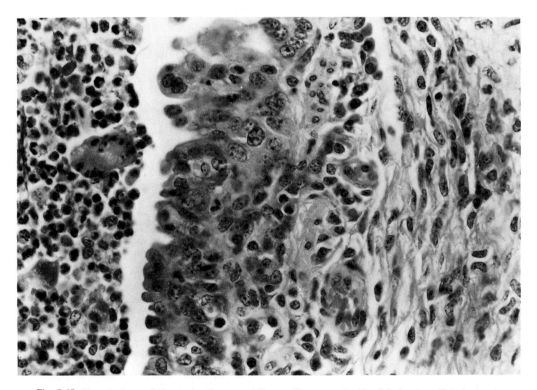

Fig. 7-15 Morphological Basis for Impaired Lung Clearance in Viral Infection. This lesion is from a case of bovine parainfluenza 3 virus infection. There is significant hyperplasia of bronchiolar epithelium. Notice that the surface epithelium is immature and lacks cilia. Such a lesion would result in defective mucociliary clearance.

Role of the Cell Cycle

Canine and feline (and other) parvoviruses require host cells in the S phase of mitosis to replicate and produce lesions similar to those caused by irradiation and radiomimetic toxins (mycotoxins). Viral destruction of intestinal crypt epithelium leads, in large part, to rapid enterocyte turnover, complete villous collapse, and eventual death. Susceptible carnivores, raised in a gnotobiotic environment, do not succumb to infection because their epithelial turnover rate is slow. In the same vein, since these parvoviruses are radiomimetic and replicate in rapidly dividing cells, one would suspect that in neonatal animals when most organs and tissues are rapidly dividing damage from viral infection would be widespread. In more mature individuals, the most rapidly dividing cells are intestinal crypt epithelium, lymphoid tissue, and bone marrow. Predictably, these sites turn out to be the age-dependent target tissues of parvovirus infection.

Microenvironmental Changes and Site-specific Nutrients

Microenvironmental changes can allow ubiquitous organisms a chance to displace normal microbiota and produce disease. For example, antibiotic treatment can displace normal flora and allow proliferation of pathogens (such as *Clostridium difficile*) as in lincomycin (an antibiotic) enteritis of rabbits and horses.

Lactic acidosis in cattle is brought about by a change in diet that results in a change in ruminal flora. A sudden change to feeds high in concentrates and low in cellulose promotes the rapid growth of acid-producing bacteria such as *Lactobacillus* species. The lowered rumen pH kills the cellulolytic bacteria. Lactic acid, in combination with the volatile fatty acids produced by rumen fermentation, cause chemical burning of the rumen epithelium (Fig. 7-16) allowing *Fusobacterium* and *Corynebacterium* species access to the hepatic circulation, where they form abscesses. Similarly, antibiotic therapy can kill off normal rumen flora resulting in the same end point as lactic acidosis causes.

Loss of normal flora secondary to antibiotic treatment can also result in colonization of oral, lingual, and esophageal mucosa by *Candida* species, a condition called "thrush." Although thrush is not a serious condition in itself, it does indicate a general debilitation secondary to antibiotic therapy, steroid administration (effect on the immune system), or increased glucose availability to epithelium, usually secondary to intravenous glucose administration.

Probiotics are viable microorganisms that are beneficial in the prevention and treatment of many en-

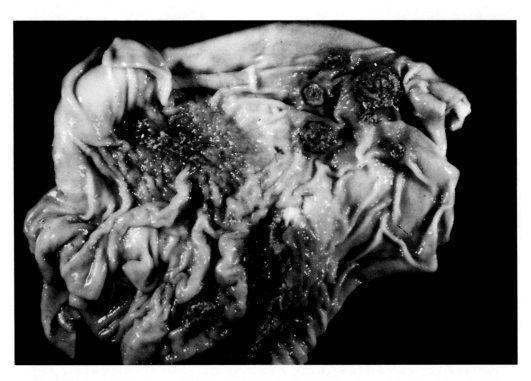

Fig. 7-16 Mycotic Abomasitis. This cow had multifocal ulcerative abomasitis caused by a fungal infection associated with a sudden change of feed.

teric diseases. After ingestion, their mechanisms of action are diverse and include immune stimulation, competition with pathogens for nutrients, inhibition of pathogen adherence to enterocytes, and production of antimicrobial chemicals. Many probiotics contain mixtures of bacterial species and strains.

In some cases the tissue involved contains unique nutrients required by the organisms. In ungulates, *Brucella abortus* shows a particular affinity for the placenta, fetal fluids, and chorion tissue. The tissue affinity of *B. abortus* is explained by the fact that the fetal fluids and placental tissues of susceptible ungulates contain significant amounts of erythritol, a nutrient for which the organism has a special requirement. In those animals in which *B. abortus* does not cause abortion, the placenta does not contain erythritol. Similarly, particular metabolic capabilities of the organism also may influence the site at which infections become established. *Corynebacterium renale* possesses the enzyme urease that allows it to metabolize urea, giving this organism a special affinity for the urinary tract. This organism is a common cause of pyelonephritis in cattle. Evidence for the importance of this metabolic capability in the pathogenesis of the disease is the observation that mutants lacking urease still colonize the renal medulla but fail to flourish and therefore produce little damage (molecular Koch's postulates).

Molecular Mimicry

True molecular mimicry, pathogen antigens similar or identical to host cell antigens, is an unproved theory. However, pathogens sometimes contain surface molecules that are structurally similar to naturally occurring ligands important in cell function and signaling. This allows these infectious agents to attach to host cells without the host recognizing them as foreign. Some of the newer approaches to disease prevention seek to occupy sites of pathogen attachment by exposure of the animal to nonpathogenic organisms. This approach has been successful in controlling pathogenic *Salmonella* infections of chickens by misting young birds with nonpathogenic bacteria.

Target Cell Oligosaccharides

An increasing number of pathogens such as group A rotaviruses are having the biology of the initial host-pathogen interaction elucidated. In the case of group A porcine rotavirus infection, the viral spike proteins attach to an enterocyte surface ganglioside (sialylated glycolipid). This initial interaction between sialic acid on the ganglioside and the spike protein of the viral capsid allows the virus to assume the correct spatial orientation to the host cell to allow viral entry, uncoating, and replication. New knowledge of this kind may lead to receptor therapy for diarrheal diseases, since adding exogenous receptor has the potential of binding virus before the virus can bind to enterocytes. This complex of virus and exogenously added receptor then passes harmlessly in the feces.

Other research has shown that *Vibrio cholerae* produces a sialidase that travels systemically and specifically removes α2-6–linked sialic acid from the podocytes. This anion loss results in collapse of podocyte cytoarchitecture and protein-losing glomerulopathy, a seemingly common event in glomerular injury.

Cellular oligosaccharides in general have been shown to be important cellular targets of microbes and toxins. The mechanisms by which pathogens have adapted to colonize and damage the animal host are diverse and are still being unraveled. Greater understanding of the mechanisms by which disease is produced will be instrumental in formulating novel and effective therapies.

Immune Evasion

Most mammals receive maternal antibody transfer either transplacentally or through colostrum. In those animals requiring colostrum for maternally derived passive immunity, failure to nurse in the critical first hours and days of life can be devastating. In veterinary practice, a field test to ensure that passive transfer of immunoglobulin has occurred is instrumental in predicting neonatal survival. In the absence of passive transfer, serum transfusions from the dam are often employed to provide some degree of protection against environmental pathogens. Similarly, a constant supply of antibodies bathing the gut lumen is necessary to protect offspring from the entry and establishment of enteropathogens. This necessitates frequent nursing.

A possible mechanism for avoiding the immune response of the host is the redistribution and possibly shedding of surface antigens. This is similar to the phenomenon of antigenic shedding that can occur in tumor cells. In this process, surface antigens usually distributed diffusely on the pathogen's surface become concentrated at one end, a process known as "capping." After this, the antigens may be shed. This mechanism has been demonstrated to occur *in vitro,* but its role *in vivo* is unclear. Other organisms may mask their inherent antigens by producing a capsule. Some organisms, such as *Streptococcus equi,* have capsules composed predominantly of hyaluronic acid, which is nonantigenic. It is possible that this protects against an immune response to deeper antigens. In many cases, though, capsular components themselves are antigenic and may elicit an effective immune response.

One tactic that does seem to be of considerable importance, being used by many organisms, is antigenic variation. It has been documented in African trypanosomiasis, for example, where there are fluctuations in the degree of parasitemia, which correspond to changes in the antigens carried by the parasite. After each antigenic change in the organism, the host generates antibody specific for the new variant. Antigenic variation appears to occur as a consequence of an immune response and to involve changes, presumably the synthesis of new antigens, in individual organisms. It is believed that these parasites have genes coding for a finite number of surface antigens, which can be varied in a regular sequence as a result of exposure to the host immune response. Antibody probably has both an inductive role, bringing about the change, and a selective one, destroying organisms with "old" antigens, against which antibody is directed. Antigenic variation also occurs in babesiosis in cattle and, at the other end of the biological spectrum, in the virus diseases, visna and equine infectious anemia (Fig. 7-17). The net result of antigenic variation is persistent infection. There are other diseases, such as Aleutian mink disease and African swine fever, in which persistent infection occurs despite the presence of large amounts of antibody. In such cases, although the antibody is directed against the virus, it is ineffective in ridding the host of infection. The mechanisms enabling the virus to persist in the face of specific antibody are essentially unknown.

Downregulation of MHC proteins is a mechanism by which some viruses avoid T-cell recognition. Downregulation of other surface molecules that permits adhesion of targets to T cells also occurs. This is countered by IFN-α, -β, and -γ upregulation. Some pathogens replicate in immunologically privileged sites or at least sites not exposed to immune surveillance such as the surface of the skin (papillomaviruses) or the luminal surface of secretory glands and kidneys (renal leptospirosis, mammary brucellosis). Some infectious agents evade the immune system by exploiting cellular apoptosis.

Vectors and Life Cycles

In many cases, especially when one is considering tropical diseases, the presence or absence of appropriate vectors, usually insects, limits the geographic spread of pathogenic agents. In more temperate regions, disease spread is possible only during the warmer months of the year when the appropriate vector is present. Examples of vector-borne diseases are legion and include malaria, Lyme disease, anaplasmosis, Rocky Mountain spotted fever, equine infectious anemia, West Nile virus, canine heartworms, and Potomac horse fever. In the last case, trematodes in freshwater snails, mayflies, and caddis flies have recently been implicated in disease transmission. *Spirocerca lupi,* a nematode parasite of canids, occurs in tropical regions where the dung beetle can serve as an intermediate host. It is an interesting parasite in that it induces fibrosarcomas of the esophagus after lodging in this location after migrating through the aorta.

Many pathogens, especially but not limited to parasites, have evolved complex multihost life cycles to gain entry to the tissues of animals of veterinary importance and to humans. A classic example is that of

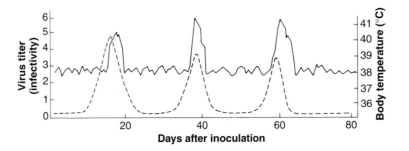

Fig. 7-17 Antigenic Variation in Equine Infectious Anemia (EIA) Virus. The clinical course of EIA is characterized by periodic exacerbations of anemia and fever, *solid line,* that are accompanied by surges of viremia, *dashed line.* Each increase in viremia is associated with the emergence of a new antigenic type of virus. *(This is a hypothetical case adapted from data of Kono Y: Recurrence of equine infectious anemia: approaches to an understanding of the mechanisms,* Proc Third Int Conf Equine Infectious Diseases, *pp 175-186, 1972, Paris, 1973.)*

Histomonas meleagridis, which causes multifocal necrotizing hepatitis and typhlitis (blackhead) in gallinaceous birds. The protozoon parasitizes earthworms that are then eaten by the bird. Therefore this is a disease of free-range chickens rather than commercial poultry that are raised indoors and not outside on dirt. San Miguel sea lion virus infection and vesicular exanthema of swine are epithelial blistering diseases of their respective species caused by serological variants of marine caliciviruses. Circumstantial evidence has accumulated to indicate that the virus may be harbored in the lungworm of seals, which is transported by the opal eye perch, a favorite food of seals and sea lions. Pigs get infected from eating marine waste, either fish or seals.

Persistent Infections

Some pathogens are content to live in harmony with their host by persistent infections. In some cases, as with many of the herpesviruses (such as pseudorabies virus of swine, cold sores and shingles of humans), the virus lies dormant in ganglia and is activated by stressers resulting in recrudescence of disease. Lesions then appear in tissue innervated by infected neurons. A herpesvirus of cattle, infectious bovine rhinotracheitis virus, can show similar behavior. The virus can cause lesions in the genitalia that resolve but leave the animals with a latent infection. When stress is mimicked by treatment of such animals with corticosteroids, genital lesions reappear. In such herpesvirus infections, free virus cannot be detected in infected ganglia during the latent stages though viral DNA is present. It is likely therefore that viral DNA is incorporated into the cell in some way though its exact form is not yet known.

Parasites such as trichinae *(Trichinella)* and *Cysticercus* species may encyst in muscle or visceral organs (lung, liver, respectively) of intermediate hosts waiting for an opportunity to be transmitted, usually through ingestion. Persistently infected animals often can act as sources of infection and thus are of considerable epidemiological importance.

The mechanisms by which infections persist are in general poorly understood. Certainly the avoidance of the immune response, as already discussed, plays some role, but it is equally certain that it is not the only factor involved. In both visna and equine infectious anemia, the virus undergoes periodic antigenic changes that allows a burst of replication and infection of new cells, which probably is important in the progression of the disease. Infection persists, however, in the quiescent stages when circulating antibody is able to neutralize free virus. In the case of these retroviruses, integration of the viral genome into the DNA of the host is probably of great importance in maintaining infection.

Environmental Factors

Human encroachment on isolated animal habitat or intimate human-to-animal or animal-to-animal contact that does not occur in nature may cause pathogen spread between species. Such is likely the case with HIV infection, which is believed to have originated from nonhuman primates in Africa, and simian herpesvirus B, which causes cold sores in monkeys but is fatal in persons. Hendra virus is a morbillivirus that caused an outbreak of respiratory disease in Queensland, Australia, and proved fatal to some persons. Morbilliviruses similar to that of canine distemper caused deadly epizootics among African lions and North Sea harbor seals. What outbreaks lie on the horizon?

DAMAGE TO THE HOST

The precise cellular and inflammatory events involved in protection and damage control of the host are discussed in detail in preceding chapters of this book. The major way we as clinicians are aware of this damage is that our patients exhibit signs or behaviors that vary from the expected norm of nearly perfect homeostasis. Taking careful inventory of signs, together with a detailed clinical history and physical examination, helps narrow possible organ system involvement. Biochemical measurement of body fluids and blood parameters, sometimes augmented with cytological and biochemical examinations of exudates and solid tissues, biopsy or fiberoptic examination of body compartments, together with modern imaging modalities including computerized tomography (CT) scans, magnetic resonance imaging (MRI), ultrasonography, and radiography further narrow possible causes. The result is that we recognize disease patterns by the causative agent's ability to damage the host in a specific location and in a specific manner and by the body's ability to respond to these injuries in a predictable fashion. More often than not, culture or direct examination of tissues and fluids does not identify an etiological agent. Still, the experienced and astute clinician is able to offer a reasonable differential diagnosis and with further testing is highly likely to identify the cause of the condition or at least apply a moniker to the condition that communicates what is known about idiopathic diseases.

In general, microorganisms can damage their host in one of four ways. They can kill their host outright. This is not the most efficient way for the pathogen to deal with the host, since if the host dies the pathogen dies also. The pathogen may cause disruption of cell machinery resulting in a wide variety of consequences for the host, ranging from cell death to cell proliferation. The microbe may cause a nonspecific inflammatory response as outlined in Chapter 4 or a specific immune response as outlined in Chapter 5.

Direct Injury

Physical and environmental agents such as heat, cold, and caustic materials often cause tissue coagulation. Such damage can be devastating as anyone who has experienced thermal burns or frostbite will attest. Often it is secondary bacterial infection of devitalized tissue that gives these injuries the potential of becoming systemic and life threatening.

Direct damage to the host by disease-producing agents is perhaps the most commonly recognized mechanism of damage to the host. This is true of many viruses. After infecting the cell, they shut down normal cellular metabolism and divert the activity of the cell to the production of virus. This results in alteration of membranes, dysfunction in homeostatic mechanisms, and eventually degeneration and cell death. There are many examples of virus-induced necrosis (Fig. 7-18). When viruses are grown *in vitro*, their cytotoxic effect often can be appreciated and is referred to as "cytopathic effect" (CPE).

Indirect Injury

Indirect injury implies a series of events that leads to loss of function or structure that, although etiologically linked, are not obvious. Renal failure for example, results in a cascading series of biochemical events that dramatically disrupt homeostasis. Failure to maintain acid-base balance and buildup of nitrogenous wastes in the blood result in hyperkalemia with cardiac dysfunction, hyponatremia with dehydration, anemia, and vascular damage. The parathyroid glands respond to calcium and phosphorus imbalance by becoming hyperplastic resulting in bone resorption (osteoporosis). Ammonia is split from urea by endothelial cells and at mucus membranes, resulting in vascular damage and a uremic or ammoniacal odor to the breath. Widespread vascular damage results in mineralization of many body tissues and basement membranes.

Likewise, liver failure results in a plethora of clinical signs, since the liver performs many essential body functions. These include integration of carbohydrate and fat metabolism and storage; protein and ammonia metabolism; and production of clotting factors V, VII, VIII, IX, X, fibrinogen, and al-

bumin. The liver additionally metabolizes vitamins and bile is required for fat-soluble vitamin absorption. The liver also degrades endogenous steroids and is important in activating, inactivating, and biotransforming drugs, toxins, and other xenobiotics by oxidation, reduction, and hydrolytic and conjugation reactions. Among the secondary effects of hepatic failure is hepatic encephalopathy, which is a central nervous system derangement resulting from ammonia and its split products in the brain (glutamic acid) resulting in morphological changes (status spongiosus) in the neuropil. As might be expected, other possible effects of hepatic failure include icterus, edema and ascites, diarrhea, photosensitization, and bleeding abnormalities.

Immune System

Immunosuppressive and immunostimulatory effects of pathogenic agents often cause the main signs recognized by clinicians. Kaposi's sarcoma, persistent cryptosporidiosis, and microsporidiosis as well as *Pneumocystis* pneumonia in humans are exceedingly rare conditions unless associated with immune suppression. The suppression is most often caused by infection with the HIV. Feline leukemia virus and bovine leukemia virus are examples of infectious agents that may result in neoplastic proliferation of lymphoid tissue. The coronavirus causing feline infectious peritonitis by itself causes little damage, but it induces deposition of immune complexes in blood vessels, resulting in pyogranulomatous vasculitis and clinical disease.

Toxic and Metabolic Injury

Toxic tissue injury has already been discussed regarding the nature of the pathogen (p. 386). Xenobiotics in general cause cell and tissue death by virtue of biotransformation pathways producing toxic intermediaries. Lesions therefore are common in the liver and kidney, but other tissues such as the lungs may also be affected, depending on the route of toxin entry and the host tissue's cytological levels of biotransformation enzymes. Idiosyncratic hypersensitivity reactions to xenobiotics such as penicillin occur in occasional individuals.

Many bacteria specifically produce toxic substances that are apparently involved in the production of disease. Some are responsible for the major signs of the disease. In most cases, however, the production of bacterial disease is multifactorial, and the role of toxins is poorly elucidated. For example, *Pseudomonas aeruginosa* produces some substances that may be of pathogenic significance. These in-

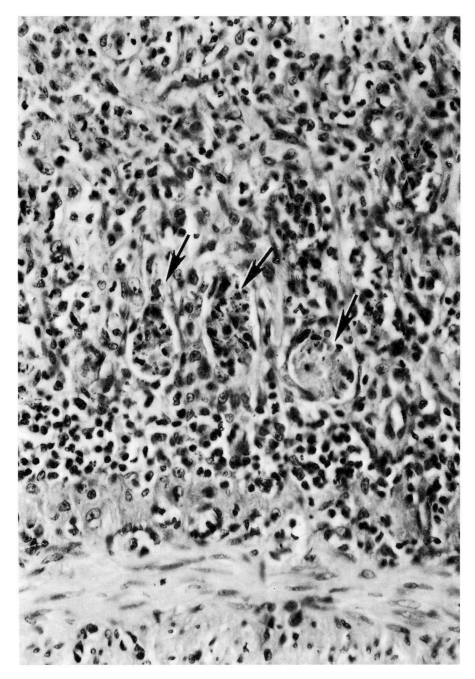

Fig. 7-18 Necrosis Caused by Viral Infection. This lesion is from a case of parvovirus infection in a dog. There is a loss of intestinal glands (crypts), and three remaining glands contain necrotic cellular debris, *arrows*. The necrosis of epithelial cells is considered to be a direct effect of the virus.

clude pigments, exotoxin A, phospholipase, proteolytic enzymes, so-called slime, and endotoxin. The relative role of each of these products in causing disease is still unclear.

Vitamin and mineral deficiency, calcium ionophores, and other pharmaceuticals can target a variety of tissues and interfere with normal metabolic processes.

Tissue and Species-specific Idiosyncrasies

Sometimes the tissue injury is relatively mild, but certain individuals overreact or underreact during the healing process resulting in large lesions, sometimes with loss of function. The resultant scar tissue has a habit of interfering with function, since maturation and cross-linking of collagen results in contraction and disruption of normal tissue architecture. "Proud flesh" in the horse is exuberant granulation tissue and a characteristic of equine organization of cutaneous scars.

Because of the lack of an adventitia, which provides suture-holding strength in all other parts of the tubular gut, esophageal injuries do not heal well. Therefore, even relatively minor damage to the epithelium can result in persistent vomiting and death caused by aspiration pneumonia. The brain-heart syndrome (neurogenic cardiomyopathy) is postulated to be attributable to catecholamine release from damaged neural tissue. It results in foci of necrosis within the myocardium. This sometimes results in sudden death, as the result of myocardial scarring and interference with electrical conductivity, often after recovery from the neural injury appears to have occurred. Thus a thorough knowledge of normal anatomy, histology, and physiology is critical to the competent clinician.

Neoplastic Injury

There is a variety of mechanisms by which neoplastic injury to the host occurs. Known causes vary from oncoviruses to lack of function of tumor-suppressor genes. These are discussed in Chapter 6. Many of us think of metastasis as the ultimate neoplastic injury. Although it is true that many metastatic cancers result in death, there are other ways in which even benign (nonmetastatic tumors) cause severe injury. One is by location. Brain tumors generally do not metastasize. They are capable of causing severe damage and often death, because they are inaccessible to surgery or to chemotherapeutic agents as a function of the blood-brain barrier, and are not particularly radiation sensitive, because of a low mitotic rate. They grow and displace normal parenchyma. Signs can vary from headaches to seizures. Eventually they may encroach on vital centers resulting in death.

Tumors of endocrine tissue often do not metastasize or reach sufficient size to result in massive tissue necrosis and death. However, if they are functional tumors producing and releasing hormones, they can interfere with homeostasis sufficiently to cause death. Examples are tumors of the islets of Langerhans, the pituitary, and adrenal glands. Beta-cell tumors of the islets result in hypoglycemia caused by excess insulin production. These tumors may be quite small, but the functional consequences of hypoglycemia (seizures) are quite severe. Although pituitary tumors can cause significant signs by occupying a nonexpansile space (sella turcica), they can also produce ACTH, resulting in a cushingoid syndrome. Pheochromocytomas may cause clinical disease by paroxysmal release of catecholamines and the associated symptoms. Hormone-like substances such as PTHrP (parathroid hormone–related protein) are produced by apocrine tumors of the anal sacs of dogs and by lymphoid neoplasms in a variety of species. The resultant signs are referred to as a "paraneoplastic syndrome" and is another example of a biochemical effect of a primary tissue injury at a distant site.

The war on cancer has not been won. Early detection and aggressive therapy have been largely responsible for increased survival rates, not new therapies or preventions. We know that the occurrence of many cancers can be reduced by elimination of destructive behaviors such as smoking and taking anabolic steroids. Still, hope springs eternal, and a molecular genetic understanding of neoplasia promises putative novel therapies in the future.

THE HOST'S RESPONSE

Although the specifics of injury and repair at the cellular and molecular level are rich with detail and becoming more so, observation and diagnosis of injury at the clinical, gross, and histopathological levels have not changed much over the years. What has changed however, are the tools by which we are able to diagnose the causes of disease and our understanding of the mechanisms of disease production. With this more detailed understanding comes a greater appreciation of the checks and balances that keep body processes in synchrony and the ability of the intact organism to maintain homeostasis. This knowledge allows for more rational and effective prevention and therapy.

Host killing mechanisms are diverse and include phagocytosis, sequestration of iron necessary for microbial growth, production of free radicals, oxygen-dependent mechanisms, production of cellular exports such as interferon-γ, immunological mechanisms, or the simple walling off of infected areas with granulation tissue. The body has remarkable powers of healing and great functional redundancy of cells, tissues, organs, and genes. It is exquisitely sensitive to its internal and external environment and constantly makes myriad adjustments to keep all systems in balance.

Fever

One of the most characteristic systemic reactions associated with infectious diseases is fever. Fever is an alteration or adaptation of normal thermoregulation. It is therefore distinguished from hyperthermia in which there is an uncontrolled elevation in body temperature. In fever, body temperature is still under control, but the so-called set point (or setting on the biological thermostat) is altered upwards.

In mammals, when body temperature needs to be changed, heat is generated or lost as required by both physiological and behavioral means. The former includes shivering and vasoconstriction to elevate body temperature and vasodilatation, sweating, and panting to lower it. Behavioral means consist in seeking a warm or a cool environment. In poikilotherms, only behavioral means are used to regulate body temperature.

Fever is caused by a variety of stimuli known collectively as exogenous pyrogens. These include bacteria, both gram-positive and gram-negative, viruses, fungi, antigen-antibody interactions, some drugs, and of course endotoxin. However, all fevers, of any cause except direct brain damage, are now believed to be mediated by the cytokine originally described as leukocyte endogenous pyrogen, now known to be interleukin-1. Other cytokines and lymphokines also appear to contribute to the pathogenesis of fever, including tumor necrosis factor (TNF-α), interleukins-1α, -1β, and -6, interferon-γ and -β, prostaglandin E_2, NO, and perhaps PAF.

The control center for body temperature appears to be in the hypothalamus, where both cold-sensitive and heat-sensitive neurons reside. Although circulating pyrogens should be size-excluded from the brain by the blood-brain barrier, circumventricular organs, specialized areas that have no blood-brain barrier, do recognize pyrogens. In these areas, at the edges of the ventricular system of the brain, the capillaries are fenestrated, and neurons contact substances directly from the bloodstream.

Of particular interest in this discussion is the role of fever in the host. Fever occurs in all mammals, in birds, and through behavioral adaptations in poikilotherms such as lizards, snakes, and fish. In response to infection, for example, a number of lizards and other poikilotherms have been shown to acquire a fever by seeking a warmer than usual environment. This indicates that fever has some beneficial effect because such an adaptation would not be expected to be so well preserved during evolution if it did not. In mammals, it is difficult to study the role of fever in host defense because any drugs or other means used to modify it might directly affect host defenses. On the other hand, fever can be prevented in poikilotherms simply by denying them access to a warmer environment. The use of this technique has shown that fever is probably a beneficial response. When lizards infected with *Aeromonas hydrophila* (a gram-negative pathogenic bacterium) were held at two temperatures, 35° C and 42° C, those at the

higher temperature generally survived, whereas most of those at the lower temperature died. Furthermore, it has been shown that lizards with fever have a more efficient inflammatory response than those held at normal temperatures. Similarly, mammalian leukocytes exhibit maximum phagocytic activity at temperatures equivalent to moderate fevers. Another advantage of fever might involve the utilization of iron by bacteria. Pathogenic bacteria ensure a supply of iron by synthesizing iron-binding siderophores. Bacteria can synthesize siderophores much less efficiently at relatively high temperatures, and fever may therefore interfere with bacterial growth by limiting the availability of iron. There is little direct evidence documenting a beneficial role for fever in mammals, but studies in rabbits correlating fever and survival have shown that modest fevers may be beneficial whereas high fevers apparently are not.

Some persons believe that the body should be largely able to regulate itself without much exogenous interference. For example, fever as a response to an infection may be nature's way to exterminate bacteria, since bacterial growth is often temperature dependent. Pain is seen as nature's way of forcing rest of injured body parts. On the other hand, common sense dictates that seizuring will result in permanent brain injury unless exogenous chemical intervention is applied. Similarly, large vessels will not cease bleeding even if the coagulation systems are intact and functioning. Therefore the clinician must be armed with sound knowledge of the body's ability to respond to different types of injury.

The Role of Iron

Iron is probably the single most important trace element required for bacterial growth. If it is lacking, bacteriostasis results. Suboptimal levels of iron interfere with the production of most bacterial products, including toxins. Host animals also have a requirement for iron, and both animals and bacteria have evolved specific mechanisms for acquiring it. Bacteria produce iron-binding substances, called "siderophores," that allow them to compete for the small amounts of free iron in the plasma and tissues. These products are synthesized and secreted, bind iron, and then are reabsorbed as iron chelates. Animals synthesize several iron-binding glycoproteins, the most important of which are transferrin and lactoferrin.

In animals, iron-binding proteins are found not only in the plasma but also in fluids at sites prone to infection such as milk, bronchial and intestinal secretions, and other body fluids. Transferrin is the major iron-binding protein in the plasma, and lactoferrin is important in secretions, especially in milk. It also is released from the specific granules of neutrophils and thus may be secreted locally at sites of infection. Animals can modulate the synthesis of these compounds in response to infection. For example, mice with experimental infections increase their rate of synthesis of transferrin, and infectious mastitis results in increased synthesis of lactoferrin in the bovine mam-

TABLE 7-5	Underlying Disease Entities Often Associated with Disseminated Intravascular Coagulation (DIC)

Septicemia, endotoxemia
Malignant neoplasia, including leukemia
Obstetrical complications
Some forms of hepatic disease
Severe trauma/tissue injury, including burns
Intravascular immune reactions (anaphylaxis)
Systemic vascular disorders
Certain venoms and toxins

mary gland. Within 90 hours of the onset of experimental *E. coli* mastitis there is a thirtyfold increase in the concentration of lactoferrin in the gland. Lactoferrin also is increased in amount in the involuting gland. Natural resistance–associated macrophage protein-1 (Nramp1) is an iron pump present in the membrane of the phagolysosome. It functions to further reduce the availability of iron to microorganisms.

In inflammatory disease, iron is sequestered in storage pools, and serum iron concentrations fall dramatically. This is a nonspecific effect that occurs in inflammatory disease of both noninfectious and infectious origin. It is tempting to speculate, however, that its purpose is to limit the availability of iron to bacteria that might infect the host.

Disseminated Intravascular Coagulation

Disseminated intravascular coagulation (DIC) is a potentially catastrophic systemic reaction in which there is generalized activation of the blood coagula-

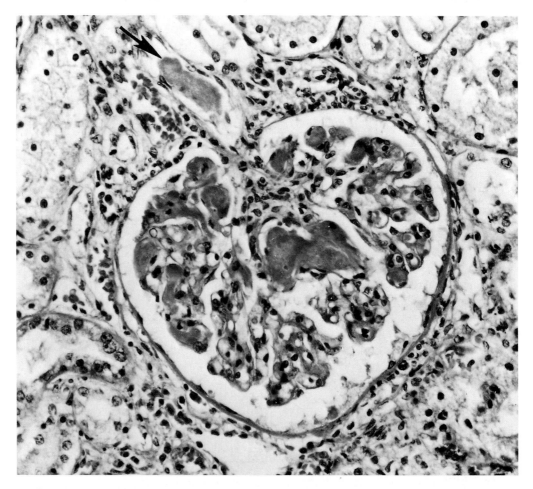

Fig. 7-19 Disseminated Intravascular Coagulation. Several fibrin thrombi are present in the capillaries of this glomerulus. A thrombus also is present in the afferent arteriole, *arrow.* Similar thrombi were present in many tissues from this dog.

tion system. DIC has many possible causes including extensive tissue injury, neoplasia, systemic immunological reactions (including anaphylaxis), and acute infections, especially those in which septicemia occurs (Table 7-5). In the latter case, coagulation is possibly activated by endotoxin or by widespread damage to the endothelium of vessels. A healthy endothelium balances antithrombotic and anticoagulant activity. The implication that endotoxin is involved either by direct activation of the coagulation system or through microvascular damage has become axiomatic. Coagulation may be initiated by either the intrinsic or the extrinsic pathways or, under some circumstances, by direct conversion of prothrombin to thrombin. DIC may prove to be an important pathogenetic factor in many infectious diseases. For example, it has been suggested that it may be involved in the pathogenesis of feline infectious peritonitis and of infectious canine hepatitis, a disease in which the causative virus can cause endothelial damage.

The immediate result of diffuse activation of the blood coagulation system is the deposition of microthrombi in small vessels of many tissues, including the renal glomeruli (Fig. 7-19). Tissue ischemia and infarction can result. The thrombi are rapidly removed by the fibrinolytic system. As a consequence breakdown products of fibrin and fibrinogen (fibrin degradation products, FDPs) can be detected in the circulation. Such massive activation of the coagulation system results in the consumption of platelets and numerous coagulation factors, the result of which may be a defect in coagulation. Because this is attributable to the utilization of clotting factors to the extent that normal coagulation cannot occur, it is referred to as a "consumptive coagulopathy." Some FDPs can further inhibit blood coagulation and exacerbate the tendency to bleed. Patients with DIC may therefore develop a hemorrhagic diathesis manifested by petechiae and ecchymoses in many tissues. Thus, regardless of its specific etiological background, DIC develops through a sequence of events in which the development of widespread microvascular thrombosis may paradoxically lead to bleeding tendencies and the emergence of a hemorrhagic diathesis (Fig. 7-20). Microthrombi may also cause bilateral hemorrhagic adrenal cortical necrosis, especially secondary to *Salmonella* species endotoxemia. This is termed the "Waterhouse-Friderichsen syndrome" and is a useful marker for making a postmortem diagnosis of endotoxemia.

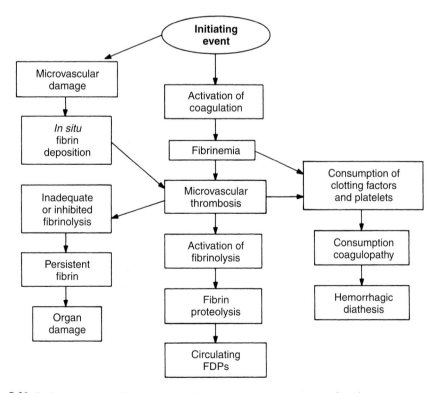

Fig. 7-20 Pathogenesis of Disseminated Intravascular Coagulation (DIC). The sequence of events in DIC includes initiation of coagulation followed by fibrin microthrombosis, consumption coagulopathy, and eventual hemorrhagic diathesis. The tissue outcome can be influenced by how effectively the fibrinolytic system operates. *FDPs*, Fibrin degradation products.

Inflammation

Neutrophils, which abound in acute, suppurative inflammatory reactions, release a variety of substances, including enzymes, that can damage host tissues. Inflammation is orchestrated by a changing series of mediators, the expression of adhesion molecules on leukocytes and underlying endothelium, cytokines, metalloproteases, and reactive oxygen species. The importance of inflammation to the host clearly is dependent on both the site and the persistence of the inciting cause. Obviously an abscess in the brain is of far greater consequence to the host than the same lesion in the subcutis or even in the lung or liver. Chronic inflammatory lesions, especially granulomatous lesions such as those caused by mycobacteria or pathogenic fungi, also can injure the host by acting as space-occupying lesions. Again, the significance of such a lesion varies with its site. Essentially all inflammatory lesions cause some damage, but the ideal outcome for the host is the rapid elimination of the inciting organism and minimal tissue damage. Fortunately for all of us this is usually the case.

MAKING A DIAGNOSIS

Examination of tissues and body fluids, fiberoptic probing into natural and man-made ostia, combined with histological examination and interpretation of lesions, are basic tools of both clinicians and pathologists. Special studies for antibodies, abnormal genes, proteins, carbohydrates, lipids, and other compounds in cells, fluids, secretions, and excretions often require targeted methodologies, use of special histological stains, and, in the case of tumors, histochemical and immunohistochemical labeling of intermediate filaments or cytodifferentiation markers.

We would be remiss if we didn't again pay homage to evolving methods in molecular pathology, especially as they relate to the diagnosis of disease and understanding of pathogenesis. These techniques are based on identification of specific sequences of nucleic acids, either DNA or RNA. With RNA-containing samples, reverse transcriptase provides for the base pairing to occur.

Molecular diagnostic tests may be manipulated to provide varying degrees of sensitivity. The probes used may be exquisitely sensitive and to be useful must not hybridize with the host's nucleic acids. These probes may be used to identify pathogens present in minute quantities without the necessity of culturing or isolation of infectious agents. Some techniques, such as *in situ* hybridization, may even be run on archived paraffin-embedded materials or formalin-fixed tissue samples. Other tests may be run on extracts of body fluids, feces, or tissue. All these tests work by complementary base pairing after denaturation, melting, or separation of extracted double-stranded nucleic acids. They are annealed, or joined back together, after specific synthetic oligonucleotide sequences (generally less than 30 nucleotides long) are used to promote matching of the single strand of DNA or RNA. In some cases a signal, either isotopic (radioactive) or nonisotopic (chemiluminescence, avidin-biotin, digoxigenin), is incorporated into the matching nucleotide sequences (hybridization), whereas in others the double-stranded product is separated and rematched through a process of amplification (thermocycling) until a signal can be detected on a gel. Only exact or near-exact base pairing provides a match allowing for annealing to occur. The conditions or stringency employed in this process determines the specificity of the reaction sequence.

The conclusion is that for an effective clinician to make a diagnosis much more than recognition of disease is required. It requires an understanding of the mechanisms by which the tissue's appearance or function becomes recognizably altered. Understanding the mechanisms of injury and the body's response to injury, which includes the time frame in which the injury and attempted repair occurred, is instrumental is providing the best care to our patients. It is not an academic intellectual exercise. Functional knowledge of the mechanisms of disease provides solid data on which to narrow the list of possible differential diagnoses, order additional more definitive tests, and formulate a plan to return the body to homeostasis.

RECOMMENDED READING

Afford S, Randhawa S: Apoptosis, *Mol Pathol* 53:55-63, 2000.

Bailar JC, Gornik HL: Cancer undefeated, *N Engl J Med* 36:1569-1574, 1997.

Bloom BR: Games parasites play: how parasites evade immune surveillance, *Nature* 279:21-26, 1979.

Burne RA, Chen YY: Bacterial ureases in infectious diseases, *Microbes Infect* 2:533-542, 2000.

Butel JS: Viral carcinogenesis: revelation of molecular mechanisms and etiology of human disease, *Carcinogenesis* 21:405-425, 2000.

Carson DA: An infectious origin for extraskeletal calcification, *Proc Natl Acad Sci* 95:7846-7847, 1998.

Carter GR, Chengappa MM, Roberts AW: *Essentials of veterinary microbiology*, ed 5, Baltimore, 1995, Williams & Wilkins.

Cotran RS, Kumar V, Collins T: *Pathologic basis of disease*, 6 ed, Philadelphia, 1999, Saunders.

Dinarello CA: Proinflammatory cytokines, *Chest* 118:503-508, 2000.

Donelson JE, Turner MV: How the trypanosome changes its coat, *Sci Amer* 252:44-51, 1985.

Ehlers MR: CR3: a general purpose adhesion-recognition receptor essential for innate immunity, *Microbes Infect* 2:289-294, 2000.

Esmon CT, Fukodome K, Mather T, Bode W, Regan LM, Stearns-Kurosawa DJ, Kurosawa S: Inflammation, sepsis, and coagulation, *Haematologica* 84:254-259, 1999.

Estes MK, Morris AP: A viral enterotoxin: a new mechanism of virus-induced pathogenesis, *Adv Exp Med Biol* 473:73-82, 1999.

Feldman S, Weisbroth S.: Diagnostic molecular microbiology; detection of pathogenic microorganisms in laboratory animals, *Lab Anim* 26:29-35, 1997.

Fraser J, Arcus V, Kong P, Baker E, Proft T: Superantigens: powerful modifiers of the immune system, *Mol Med Today* 6:125-132, 2000.

Gallin JI, Goldstein IM, Snyderman R: *Inflammation: basic principles and clinical correlates,* New York, 1988, Raven Press.

Gelberg HB, Healy L, Whiteley H, Miller L, Vimr E: Enzymatic removal of α 2-6 linked sialic acid from the glomerular filtration barrier results in podocyte charge alteration and glomerular injury, *Lab Invest* 74:907-921, 1996.

Ginaldi W, De Martinis M, D'Ostilio Q, Marini L, Loreto MF, Quaglino D: The immune system in the elderly: III. Innate immunity, *Immunol Res* 20:117-126, 1999.

Goebel W, Kuhn M: Bacterial replication in the host cell cytosol, *Curr Opin Microbiol* 3:49-53, 2000.

Hill AV: Genetics and genomics of infectious disease susceptibility, *Br Med Bull* 55:401-413, 1999.

Kajander EO, Çiftçioğlu N: Nanobacteria: an alternative mechanism for pathogenic intra- and extracellular calcification and stone formation, *Proc Natl Acad Sci* 95:8274-8279, 1998.

Kanter M, Mott J, Ohashi N, Fried B, Reed S, Lin YC, Rikihisa Y: Analysis of 16S rRNA and 51-kilodalton antigen gene and transmission in mice of *Ehrlichia risticii* in virgulate trematodes from *Elimia livescens* snails in Ohio, *J Clin Microbiol* 38:3349-3358, 2000.

Le J, Vilcek J: Tumor necrosis factor and interleukin 1: cytokines with multiple overlapping biological activities, *Lab Invest* 56:234-248, 1987.

Luheshi GN: Cytokines and fever: mechanisms and site of action, *Ann NY Acad Sci* 856:83-89, 1998.

Mauel J: Intracellular survival of protozoan parasites with special reference to *Leishmania* spp., *Toxoplasma gondii* and *Trypanosoma cruzi, Adv Parasitol* 38:1-51, 1996.

Mims CA, Dimmock N, Nash A, Stephen J: *The pathogenesis of infectious disease,* ed 4, London, 1995, Academic Press.

Miyoshi S, Shinoda S: Microbial metalloproteases and pathogenesis, *Microbes Infect* 2:91-98, 2000.

Mold C: Role of complement in host defense against bacterial infection, *Microbes Infect* 1:633-638, 1999.

Moulia C, LeBrun N, Renaud F: Mouse-parasite interactions: from gene to population, *Adv Parasitol* 38:119-167, 1996.

Mukaida N, Ishikawa Y, Fujioka N, Watanabe S, Kuno K, Matsushima K: Novel insight into molecular mechanisms of endotoxic shock: biochemical analysis of LPS receptor signaling in a cell-free system targeting NF-kappa β and regulation of cytokine production/action through beta 2 integrin *in vivo, J Leukoc Biol* 59:145-151, 1996.

Murphy FA: The public health risk of animal organ and tissue transplantation into humans, *Science* 273:746, 1996.

Naber S: Molecular pathology—diagnosis of infectious disease, *N Engl J Med* 331:1212-1215, 1994.

Nandan D, Knutson KL, Lo R, Reiner NE: Exploitation of host cell signaling machinery: activation of macrophage phosphotyrosine phosphatases as a novel mechanism of molecular microbial pathogenesis, *J Leukoc Biol* 67:464-470, 2000.

Ochman H, Lawrence JG, Groisman EA: Lateral gene transfer and the nature of bacterial innovation, *Nature* 405:209-304, 2000.

Pearson JD: Normal endothelial function, *Lupus* 9:183-188, 2000.

Prusiner SB: The prion diseases, *Sci Am* 272:45-87, 1995.

Rautemaa R, Meri S: Complement-resistance mechanisms of bacteria, *Microbes Infect* 1:785-794, 1999.

Relman DA: Detection and identification of previously unrecognized microbial pathogens, *Emerg Infect Dis* 4:382-389, 1998.

Rietschel E, Kirikae T, Schade FU, Mamat U, Schmidt G, Loppnow H, Ulmer A, Zahringer U, Seydel U, Di Padova F, Schreier M, Brade H: Bacterial endotoxin: molecular relationships of structure to function, *FASEB J* 8:217-224, 1994.

Rolfe RD: The role of probiotic cultures in the control of gastrointestinal health, *J Nutr* 130:396S-402S, 2000.

Rolsma MD, Kuhlenschmidt TK, Gelberg HB, Kuhlenschmidt MS: Structure and function of a ganglioside receptor for porcine group A rotavirus, *J Virol* 72:9079-9091, 1998.

Rostand K, Esko J: Microbial adherence to and invasion through proteoglycans, *Infect Immun* 65:1-8, 1997.

Rottman JB: Key role of chemokines and chemokine receptors in inflammation, immunity, neoplasia, and infectious disease, *Vet Pathol* 36:357-367, 1999.

Salyers AA, Whitt DD: *Bacterial pathogenesis: a molecular approach,* Washington, D.C., 1994, ASM Press.

Saper CB, Breder CD: The neurologic basis of fever, *N Engl J Med* 330:1880-1886, 1994.

Sauer FG, Mulvey MA, Schilling JD, Martínez JJ, Hultgren SJ: Bacterial pili: molecular mechanisms of pathogenesis, *Curr Opin Microbiol* 3:65-72, 2000.

Schaechter M, Medoff G, Eisenstein BI: *Mechanisms of microbial disease,* 2 ed, Baltimore, 1993, Williams & Wilkins.

Service RF: DNA ventures into the world of designer materials, *Science* 277:1036-1037, 1997.

Sriskandan S, Cohen J: Gram-positive sepsis: mechanisms and differences from gram-negative sepsis, *Infect Dis Clin North Am* 13:397-412, 1999.

Strauss EJ, Falkow S: Microbial pathogenesis: genomics and beyond, *Science* 276:707-711, 1997.

Sullivan GW, Sarembock IJ, Linden J: The role of inflammation in vascular diseases, *J Leukoc Biol* 67:591-602, 2000.

Sunder-Plassmann G, Patruta SI, Horl WH: Pathobiology of the role of iron in infection, *Am J Kidney Dis* 34:S25-S29, 1999.

Tang C, Holden D: Pathogen virulence genes—implications for vaccines and drug therapy, *Br Med Bull* 55:387-400, 1999.

Van der Ploeg LHT: Control of variant surface antigen switching in trypanosomes, *Cell* 51:159-161, 1987.

Varki A: Biological roles of oligosaccharides: all the theories are correct, *Glycobiology* 3:97-130, 1993.

Wagner JG, Roth RA: Neutrophil migration during endotoxemia, *J Leukoc Biol* 66:10-24, 1999.

Weinrauch Y, Zychlinsky A: The induction of apoptosis by bacterial pathogens, *Ann Rev Microbiol* 53:155-187, 1999.

Zetterström M, Sundgren-Andersson AK, Ostlund P, Bartfai T: Delineation of the proinflammatory cascade in fever induction, *Ann NY Acad Sci* 856:48-52, 1998.

Zijlstra RT, Donovan SM, Odle J, Gelberg HB, Petschow BW, Gaskins HR: Protein energy malnutrition delays small intestinal recovery in neonatal pigs infected with rotavirus, *J Nutr* 127:1118-1127, 1997.

Index

Page numbers followed by f indicate figures; t, tables; b, boxes.